In Vitro Diagnostic Industry in China

Haibo Song · Lizhong Dai
Editors

In Vitro Diagnostic Industry in China

Second Edition

Springer

图书在版编目（CIP）数据

中国体外诊断产业发展蓝皮书 = In Vitro Diagnostic Industry in China(Second Edition) : 英文 / 宋海波，戴立忠主编. -- 2版. -- 上海 : 上海科学技术出版社，2024.5
ISBN 978-7-5478-6584-2

Ⅰ. ①中… Ⅱ. ①宋… ②戴… Ⅲ. ①诊断剂－制药工业－产业发展－研究报告－中国－英文 Ⅳ. ①F426.77

中国国家版本馆CIP数据核字(2024)第066048号

Jointly published by Shanghai Scientific & Technical Publishers and Springer Nature Singapore Pte. Ltd.

In Vitro Diagnostic Industry in China (Second Edition)
Haibo Song • Lizhong Dai *Editors*

上海世纪出版（集团）有限公司
上海科学技术出版社 出版、发行
(上海市闵行区号景路159弄A座9F-10F)
邮政编码 201101 www.sstp.cn

字数：1150千字
2022年1月第1版
2024年5月第2版 2024年5月第1次印刷
ISBN 978-7-5478-6584-2/F·49
定价：498.00元

Preface

In recent years, China's in vitro diagnostic (IVD) industry has developed rapidly and has grown into a considerable industrial cluster. At present, China's IVD industry has a complete range of categories, numerous R&D and production enterprises, a comprehensive distribution of distribution enterprises, an increasingly perfect upstream, middle and downstream industrial chain, and constantly improved product quality, making it the fastest growing medical device segment.

At present, in vitro diagnostic products and technologies in China are developing towards integration, informatization, high-throughput, speediness, portability, and intelligence. The continuous emergence, updating, and iteration of some new technologies and new products such as mass spectrometry detection technology and gene editing technology make the development prospect of in vitro diagnostic industry very broad.

This book is the second edition of *In Vitro Diagnostic Industry in China*. The book is divided into 12 parts and 38 chapters, which comprehensively and systematically introduce the achievements and the latest development trends of the innovation and development of China's IVD industry in recent years. The contents include the 2021 China IVD industry report, the academic, technological development, market situation and research and development of related products in various subdivisions such as immunodiagnosis, clinical chemical diagnosis, molecular diagnosis, blood and humoral diagnosis, microbial diagnosis, instant detection, mass spectrometry analysis, pathological diagnosis, etc., the development report of China's IVD reagent raw materials, the development, investment and financing, acquisition and merger of China's IVD listed enterprises, etc. The updated contents of this book are China's IVD industry report, immunodiagnosis, clinical chemical diagnosis, molecular diagnosis, blood and humoral diagnosis, microbial diagnosis, real-time detection, China's IVD listed enterprise development, investment and financing, mergers and acquisitions, etc. New contents added include the development and application of molecular diagnostic products of COVID-19, flight mass spectrometry, tandem mass spectrometry, tumor markers, ELISA immune reagents, autoimmune diagnosis, concomitant diagnosis, fecal and intestinal microecology detection, pathological diagnosis, in vitro diagnostic reagent raw materials, in vitro diagnostic reagent reference materials and quality control materials, which make the book more innovative and richer. This book is characterized by a more comprehensive and systematic reflection of the new trends and new progress in the development of China's IVD industry, highlighting the hot technologies and innovative products in the industry, such as the novel coronavirus molecular diagnostic technology, instruments and reagents, COVID-19 nucleic acid emergency detection laboratory (gas membrane laboratory, shelter laboratory, mobile detection vehicle), and mass spectrometry detection technology.

This book was jointly written by well-known entrepreneurs, experts, professors, and elites in China's IVD industry, organized by the Medical Laboratory Science Industry Branch of the National Health Industry Enterprise Management Association, the Experimental Medicine Branch of the National Health Industry Enterprise Management Association, the IVD Branch of the China Medical Device Industry Association, and the Blue Book Editorial Department of China's IVD Industry Development. The editing and publishing of the second edition of China's IVD Industry will enable the world to have a more comprehensive and in-depth understanding of China's IVD products and technologies, promote international exchanges in the IVD industry, grasp new developments in the industry, constantly improve the level of prevention, diagnosis, and treatment of clinical diseases, and serve the health of all mankind.

Shanghai, China — Haibo Song
Hunan, China — Lizhong Dai
November 22, 2022

Declaration Lizhong Dai is an employee of Sansure Biotech Inc.

Contents

About the Editors

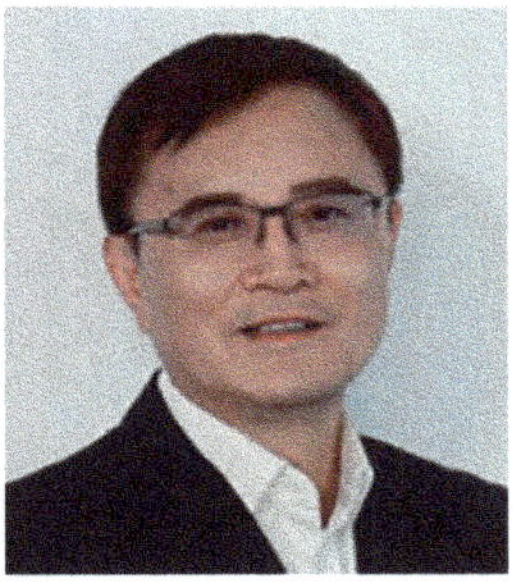

Haibo Song successively served as the Deputy Director of Anhui Provincial Center for Clinical Laboratories and as a senior technician. He is now Vice Chairman of National Association of Health Industry and Enterprises Management, Chairman of China Association of In Vitro Diagnostics, Vice Chairman of the Labeling Immunoassay Professional Committee of China Association for Instrumental Analysis, Vice Chairman and Secretary General of Professional Committee of Experimental Medicine, Standing committee member of the National Medical Clinical Laboratory and the Standardization Technical Committee of the In Vitro Diagnostic System, Associate Dean of Shanghai Academy of Experimental Medicine, and founder of CACLP.

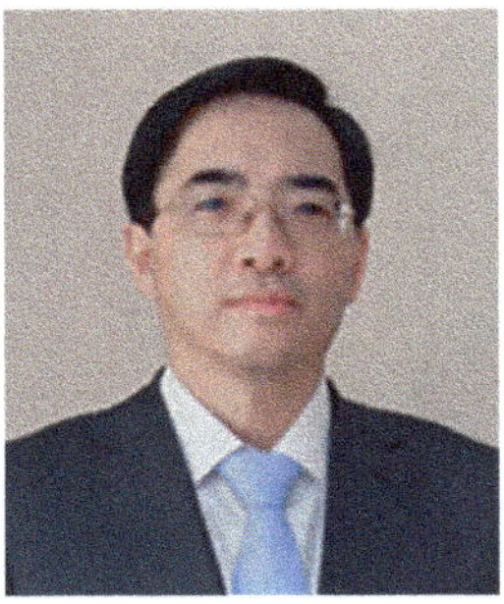

Lizhong Dai is a renowned molecular biologist, who obtained a PhD from Princeton University after graduated from Peking University and served as a postdoctoral fellow at the Massachusetts Institute of Technology. He is a famous leader of in vitro diagnostics in China and recipient of the State Council government special allowance for experts. He is Executive Director of China Medical Equipment Association, Vice President of Medical Laboratory Industry Branch of National Health Industry Enterprise Management Association, Vice Chairman of Hunan Federation of Industry and Commerce, Vice President of Hunan Preventive Medicine Association, Vice President of Hunan Pharmaceutical Industry Association, Vice President of Hunan Medical Device Association, and Chairman of Shengxiang Biotechnology Co., Ltd.

Part I

2021 China In Vitro Diagnostics Industry Development Report

Status and Progress

1

Haibo Song, Yaoyi Zhu, Linda Zhang, Qi Chen,
and Wenting Xiao

In 2021, China's in vitro diagnostics (IVD) industry had significant progress and development in all aspects. China Association of In Vitro Diagnostics and In Vitro Diagnostics Society of China Association for Medical Devices Industry jointly prepared the 2021 China In Vitro Diagnostics Industry Development Report.

1.1 IVD Market in China

1.1.1 Market Size of Domestic Enterprises and the Statistics of Listed Companies and Enterprises Listed on the National Equities Exchange and Quotations (NEEQ)

By summarizing domestic and foreign information about China's IVD market, based on the ex-factory price of manufacturers and the first-hand wholesale price of foreign-funded enterprises, and excluding the data of nonindustrial scope, it is

H. Song
China Association of In Vitro Diagnostics, Shanghai, China
e-mail: songhaibo@caivd.org

Y. Zhu
IVD Branch of China Association of Medical Devices Industry, Beijing, China

L. Zhang (✉) · Q. Chen · W. Xiao
Fosun Diagnostics (Shanghai) Co., Ltd., Shanghai, China
e-mail: zhanglinda@fosunpharma.com; chenqi@fosunpharma.com; xiaowt@fosunpharma.com

H. Song, L. Dai (eds.), *In Vitro Diagnostic Industry in China*,
https://doi.org/10.1007/978-981-99-3110-1_1

estimated that the size of China's IVD market will exceed RMB 130 billion in 2021 with a growth rate of about 15%. The proportion of imported products is higher than 50%.

Moreover, the data of 87 listed diagnostics companies and companies listed on the NEEQ in the first half of 2021 and the data of 94 listed diagnostics companies and companies listed on the NEEQ in the whole year of 2021 are summarized as follows:

In the first half of 2021, the total revenue of 87 listed companies was 74.65 billion CNY with a year-on-year growth of 54.79%; the attributable net profit was 17.92 billion CNY with a year-on-year growth of 82.06%.

In 2021, the total revenue of 94 listed companies was 163.486 billion CNY with a year-on-year growth of 33.72%; the attributable net profit was 35.52 billion CNY with a year-on-year growth of 39.42%.

See Tables 1.1, 1.2, 1.3, and 1.4 for data.

Tables 1.5, 1.6, 1.7, and 1.8 show the market value changes of A-share listed companies in recent 3 years, the list of newly listed companies, IPO queuing companies and delisted companies in 2021.

Table 1.1 Rankings of critical data of listed diagnostics companies in the first half of 2021 (10 thousand CNY)

Rankings	Operating revenue				Attributable net profit				Market value (2021.12.31)			
	Amount		Growth rate %		Amount		Growth rate %		Amount (100 million CNY)		Growth rate %	
1	Orient Gene	638,198	Hotgen	3904.13%	Orient Gene	339,425	Hotgen	74261.79%	Mindray Bio-Medical	4629.35	Gongdong Medical	249.25%
2	Dian Diagnostics	579,121	Orient Gene	670.63%	DA AN GENE	159,788	Tellgen	968.67%	Wantai BioPharm	1344.59	GenScript	230.21%
3	KingMed Diagnostics	545,545	Easy Diagnosis Biomedicine	216.55%	Hotgen	145,262	Orient Gene	547.82%	GenScript	724.96	Hotgen	197.90%
4	Runda Medical	433,331	Strong Biotechnologies	204.49%	Mindray Bio-Medical	134,690	Strong Biotechnologies	547.62%	KingMed Diagnostics	518.52	Huakang Biotech	131.78%
5	Mindray Biomedical	396,165	Tellgen	157.93%	Sansure Biotech	112,089	Leadman	327.68%	BGI Genomics	363.42	Easy Diagnosis Biomedicine	78.41%
6	BGI Genomics	364,621	HybriBio	156.88%	BGI Genomics	108,602	Bioeasy Biotechnology	316.45%	Snibe	346.52	Leadman	77.02%
7	Hotgen	359,972	Bioeasy Biotechnology	151.16%	Kingmed	105,923	Novogene	208.32%	Autobio	322.80	IVD Medical	54.60%
8	DA AN GENE	348,272	Wantai BioPharm	132.78%	Dian Diagnostics	72,709	HybriBio	203.15%	NanoMicro Technology	319.40	Wantai BioPharm	53.87%
9	KeHua Biology	239,997	NanoMicro Technology	111.64%	Wantai BioPharm	72,151	Wantai BioPharm	195.92%	DA AN GENE	281.53	Medicalsystem Biotechnology	30.23%
10	Yes!Star	232,270	Bioperfectus	97.46%	Easy Diagnosis Biomedicine	57,956	Easy Diagnosis Biomedicine	189.53%	Orient Gene	276.60	Runda Medical	19.95%
11	Sansure Biotech	202,832	HOB	87.11%	Wondfo Biotech	55,567	NanoMicro Technology	172.79%	Sansure Biotech	236.00	Orient Gene	13.55%
12	Wantai BioPharm	196,397	Gongdong Medical	70.76%	Maccura Biotechnology	53,168	KeHua Biology	148.64%	Sino Biological	235.08	Lifotronic Technology	9.53%
13	Maccura Biotechnology	196,037	Huakang Biotech	68.87%	Bioperfectus	50,203	HOB	136.32%	Dian Diagnostics	208.29	Tellgen	–0.20%

(continued)

Table 1.1 (continued)

Rankings	Operating revenue				Attributable net profit				Market value (2021.12.31)			
	Amount		Growth rate %		Amount		Growth rate %		Amount (100 million CNY)		Growth rate %	
14	Wondfo Biotech	185,622	KeHua Biology	64.35%	KeHua Biology	47,905	Chemclin Diagnostics	124.65%	Wondfo Biotech	175.22	HybriBio	−1.96%
15	Autobio	167,758	DA AN GENE	63.31%	Sino Biological	44,265	Yes!Star	117.48%	Sinocare	168.92	Dian Diagnostics	−2.07%
16	GenScript	160,698	Getein Biotech	58.02%	Snibe	42,861	Biosino	114.92%	Amoy Diagnostics	167.42	Amoy Diagnostics	−3.54%
17	HybriBio	129,863	KingMed Diagnostics	57.01%	Autobio	41,268	IVD Medical	106.07%	Novogene	165.28	KeHua Biology	−3.77%
18	Snibe	122,571	Chemclin Diagnostics	56.51%	HybriBio	39,102	DA AN GENE	105.25%	Maccura Biotechnology	162.43	Yes!Star	−5.17%
19	Thalys	119,779	Thalys Medical	55.23%	Liferiver Biotech	38,679	Gongdong Medical	97.74%	Gongdong Medical	161.36	DA AN GENE	−6.42%
20	IVD Medical	118,679	Runda Medical	47.25%	Alltest Biotech	32,610	KingMed Diagnostics	90.55%	YHLO Biotech	139.93	Mindray Biomedical	−10.61%
21	Easy Diagnosis Biomedicine	114,134	LBP	46.65%	Strong biotechnologies	22,118	Runda medical	86.10%	Strong biotechnologies	116.74	KingMed diagnostics	−11.92%
22	Sinocare	113,085	Yes!Star	44.96%	Runda Medical	20,699	Righton Gene	81.64%	Bioeasy Biotechnology	115.69	Thalys Medical	−12.64%
23	Bioperfectus	113,056	Amoy Diagnostics	40.96%	Gongdong Medical	17,706	Getein Biotech	78.08%	Liferiver Biotech	100.55	Improve Medical	−13.30%
24	Medicalsystem Biotechnology	112,135	Leadman	39.39%	Getein Biotech	17,086	Maccura Biotechnology	71.36%	Lifotronic Technology	97.11	Sinocare	−16.53%
25	Liferiver Biotech	90,690	Autobio	39.13%	Bioeasy Biotechnology	16,331	Succeeder	66.59%	HybriBio	86.73	Bohui Innovation	−17.14%
26	Strong Biotechnologies	80,781	GenScript	37.97%	Medicalsystem Biotechnology	13,305	Huakang Biotech	66.45%	Medicalsystem Biotechnology	81.62	LBP	−17.61%
27	Novogene	80,173	Lifotronic Technology	37.31%	Sinocare	11,901	AVE Science & Technology	63.29%	Bohui Innovation	80.95	Getein Biotech	−18.10%
28	Berry Genomics	73,361	Novogene	37.02%	Yes!Star	11,191	Bioperfectus	63.19%	Bioperfectus	80.60	Succeeder	−20.25%
29	Alltest Biotech	63,557	Maccura Biotechnology	34.97%	Amoy Diagnostics	11,132	LBP	56.09%	Runda Medical	77.72	Strong Biotechnologies	−20.79%

30	Sino Biological	63,470	Biosino	32.94%	Dirui	10991.92	Autobio	50.63%	Easy Diagnosis Biomedicine	77.61	Dirui	−23.55%
31	Getein Biotech	60,029	AVE Science & Technology	31.85%	Improve Medical	8980.38	Dian Diagnostics	45.02%	KeHua Biology	76.32	Bioperfectus	−28.51%
32	Gongdong Medical	57,604	Mindray Biomedical Mindray Biomedical	30.76%	YHLO Biotech	8856.16	Amoy Diagnostics	37.77%	Getein Biotech	72.98	BGI Genomics	−29.35%
33	YHLO Biotech	54,801	Alltest Biotech	30.48%	Lifotronic Technology	8242.52	Mindray Biomedical	35.99%	Hotgen	72.24	Snibe	−36.37%
34	Kindstar Globalgene	43,820	Dian Diagnostics	29.46%	Novogene	8158	Sino Biological	32.26%	Chemclin Diagnostics	71.86	Maccura Biotechnology	−37.43%
35	Dirui	41,762	Bohui Innovation	28.77%	IVD Medical	7889	Wondfo Biotech	23.76%	Berry Genomics	68.79	Wondfo Biotech	−42.68%
36	Improve Medical	41,624	Sino Biological	28.18%	Tellgen	7481	GenScript	19.43%	Alltest Biotech	66.31	Sansure Biotech	−48.22%
37	Amoy Diagnostics	39,895	YHLO Biotech	27.84%	Chemclin Diagnostics	7002	Lifotronic Technology	18.47%	Tellgen	51.97	Berry Genomics	−49.03%
38	Lifotronic Technology	35,608	Snibe	26.35%	NanoMicro Technology	6506	Alltest Biotech	3.57%	Kindstar Globalgene	51.70	Autobio	−50.70%
39	Bohui Innovation	34,869	IVD Medical	20.95%	LBP	5088	Dirui	1.65%	Dirui	49.44	NanoMicro Technology	–
40	Bioeasy Biotechnology	33,049	Sinocare	16.30%	HOB	4508	Bohui Innovation	−1.10%	Leadman	43.90	Sino Biological	–
41	Tellgen	30,329	Wondfo Biotech	15.53%	Succeeder	4172	Sansure Biotech	−9.00%	IVD Medical	43.57	Novogene	–
42	Leadman	24,552	Succeeder	11.59%	Berry Genomics	3123	Liferiver Biotech	−9.59%	Righton Gene	40.42	YHLO Biotech	–
43	Chemclin Diagnostics	23,693	Liferiver Biotech	10.79%	Righton Gene	2493	Snibe	−9.90%	HOB	39.73	Bioeasy Biotechnology	–
44	LBP	21,238	Improve Medical	3.59%	Leadman	1356	YHLO Biotech	−12.05%	Succeeder	36.44	Liferiver Biotech	–
45	Biosino	17,467	Kindstar Globalgene	2.02%	AVE science & technology	1262	Improve Medical	−14.74%	Improve Medical	32.93	Chemclin Diagnostics	–

(continued)

Table 1.1 (continued)

Rankings	Operating revenue				Attributable net profit				Market value (2021.12.31)			
	Amount		Growth rate %		Amount		Growth rate %		Amount (100 million CNY)		Growth rate %	
46	NanoMicro Technology	16,562	Berry Genomics	1.82%	Thalys Medical	326	Sinocare	−24.89%	Thalys Medical	29.50	Alltest Biotech	–
47	HOB	14,754	Medicalsystem Biotechnology	0.21%	Biosino	184	BGI Genomics	−34.24%	LBP	28.44	Kindstar Globalgene	–
48	Righton Gene	13,602	Righton Gene	0.03%	Huakang Biotech	−205	Medicalsystem Biotechnology	−41.12%	Yes!Star	26.81	Righton Gene	–
49	Succeeder	11,069	Sansure Biotech	−3.41%	Bohui Innovation	−1613	Thalys Medical	−57.66%	AVE Science & Technology	18.91	HOB	–
50	AVE Science & Technology	9731	Dirui	−9.82%	GenScript	−63,785	Berry Genomics	−73.41%	Biosino	2.46	AVE Science & Technology	–
51	Huakang Biotech	1217	BGI Genomics	−11.24%	Kindstar Globalgene	−150,170	Kindstar Globalgene	−1528.62%	Huakang Biotech	0.99	Biosino	–
Summary	**7,269,445**		**55.60%**		**1,776,536**		**81.61%**					

Note 1: The following table includes listed companies related to IVD on the main board, SME board, GEM and Hong Kong stocks
Note 2: Mindray's revenue adopts the revenue of the "in vitro diagnostics" product line in its financial statement, and the profit is calculated by multiplying the proportion of IVD product line in total revenue by the total profit, the same below

Table 1.2 Rankings of critical data of NEEQ companies in the first half of 2021 (10 thousand CNY)

Rankings	Operating revenue				Attributable net profit			
	Amount		Growth rate %		Amount		Growth rate %	
1	Huizhikang	25,142	Venture Bio-tech	1187.09%	Venture Bio-tech	2911	Surexam Bio-Tech	4607.17%
2	Darui Biotechnology	17,428	Wiz Biotech	608.66%	Wiz Biotech	2726	Venture Bio-tech	1085.38%
3	J.H. Bio-Tech	14,043	Zhongsheng Jinyu	243.02%	Huizhikang	2345	Wiz Biotech	812.52%
4	Venture Bio-tech	11,623	Promed	201.65%	J.H. Bio-Tech	1746	Darui Biotechnology	252.50%
5	Iprocom	10,478	Tianqi Medical	131.11%	Libo Medicine	1402	MultiSciences Biotech	222.72%
6	Xinle Medical	10,065	KeyGen BioTech	104.36%	Darui Biotechnology	1090	Huizhikang	196.24%
7	Wiz Biotech	10,027	MultiSciences Biotech	96.28%	Xincheng Biological	1020	Zhongsheng Jinyu	194.95%
8	Jiacheng Biotechnology	8066	GenePharma	74.65%	Jiacheng Biotechnology	1019	GenePharma	132.83%
9	Xincheng Biological	7618	Iprocom	56.74%	Iprocom	730	Yonghe-Sun Biotechnology	105.83%
10	Kangmei Biotech	7082	Sunshine Medical	55.83%	Keyu Biological	703	Kangmei Biotech	104.77%
11	Libo Medicine	7078	Baio Technology	50.79%	King Diagnostic	568	Libo Medicine	95.00%
12	Sunshine Medical	5646	Yonghe-Sun Biotechnology	50.70%	Babio Biotechnology	534	Promed	68.93%
13	Tzone Biotechnology	5523	Dahui Biotechnology	36.70%	Surexam Bio-Tech	521	King Diagnostic	66.80%
14	Surexam Bio-Tech	5508	Surexam Bio-Tech	36.65%	Oticon	494	Baio Technology	60.69%
15	Baio Technology	5029	Clinisciences	35.73%	Zhongsheng Jinyu	405	Tzone Biotechnology	51.89%
16	GenePharma	4773	Huizhikang	30.37%	Tzone Biotechnology	354	Dahui Biotechnology	38.89%
17	King Diagnostic	4519	Libo Medicine	30.13%	MultiSciences Biotech	238	Iprocom	24.65%
18	Newscen Bio-Pharmaceutical	4463	Xinle Medical	29.94%	GenePharma	206	Jiacheng Biotechnology	22.38%

(continued)

Table 1.2 (continued)

Rankings	Operating revenue				Attributable net profit			
	Amount		Growth rate %		Amount		Growth rate %	
19	Keyu Biological	4432	Keyu biological	27.34%	Dahui Biotechnology	107	J.H. Bio-Tech	18.62%
20	Babio Biotechnology	3404	Jiacheng Biotechnology	21.28%	Sunshine Medical	73	Haiyuan Medical	15.50%
21	Huamei Bio	3004	Kangmei Biotech	21.24%	Xinle Medical	67	Yasen Industrial	14.98%
22	Yonghe-Sun Biotechnology	2648	Haiyuan Medical	18.40%	Kangmei Biotech	44	Oticon	7.13%
23	KeyGen BioTech	2534	Oticon	14.48%	Yonghe-Sun Biotechnology	21	Keyu Biological	−5.57%
24	Zhongsheng Jinyu	2159	Darui Biotechnology	14.34%	Marr Bio	11	Marr Bio	−14.36%
25	Mokobio Life Science	1986	Huamei Bio	10.81%	Haiyuan Medical	−14	Zhongzhi Biotechnologies	−21.23%
26	MultiSciences Biotech	1911	Zhongzhi Biotechnologies	6.40%	Clinisciences	−47	Mokobio Life Science	−22.56%
27	Haiyuan Medical	1846	King Diagnostic	5.46%	Nymphavn Biotechnology	−57	Sunshine Medical	−28.16%
28	Oticon	1633	Tzone Biotechnology	5.35%	Yasen Industrial	−111	Xincheng Biological	−39.50%
29	Zhongzhi Biotechnologies	1538	Xincheng Biological	4.74%	Promed	−120	Babio Biotechnology	−76.57%
30	Dahui Biotechnology	1530	J.H. Bio-Tech	2.18%	Mokobio Life Science	−262	KeyGen BioTech	−81.90%
31	Promed	1279	Mokobio Life Science	1.35%	Zhongzhi Biotechnologies	−306	Xinle Medical	−85.70%

32	Tianqi Medical	667	Nymphavn Biotechnology	0.00%	Tianqi Medical	−392	Nymphavn Biotechnology	−112.23%
33	Clinisciences	574	Newscen Bio-Pharmaceutical	−11.94%	Baio Technology	−572	Clinisciences	−151.18%
34	Marr Bio	490	Marr Bio	−38.77%	Newscen Bio-Pharmaceutical	−631	Newscen Bio-Pharmaceutical	−241.09%
35	Yasen Industrial	196	Babio Biotechnology	−44.18%	Huamei Bio	−640	Huamei Bio	−259.76%
36	Nymphavn Biotechnology	0	Yasen Industrial	−53.64%	KeyGen BioTech	−910	Tianqi Medical	−3260.10%
Summary	**195,941**		**34.85%**		**15,271**		**157.16%**	

Table 1.3 Rankings of critical data of listed diagnostics companies in 2021 (10 thousand CNY)

Rankings	Operating revenue				Attributable net profit				Market value (2021.12.31)			
	Amount		Growth rate %		Amount		Growth rate %		Amount (100 million CNY)		Growth rate %	
1	Dian Diagnostics	1,308,261	Hotgen	945.54%	Orient Gene	492,019	Hotgen	1850.41%	Mindray Biomedical	4629.35	Gongdong Medical	249.25%
2	KingMed Diagnostics	1,194,322	Orient Gene	211.43%	DA AN GENE	361,819	Novogene	515.74%	Wantai BioPharm	1344.59	GenScript	230.21%
3	Orient Gene	1,016,917	Easy Diagnosis Biomedicine	195.05%	Mindray Biomedical	267,492	Bioeasy Biotechnology	261.38%	GenScript	724.96	Hotgen	197.90%
4	Runda Medical	886,011	Wantai BioPharm	144.25%	Sansure Biotech	224,270	Strong Biotechnologies	261.29%	KingMed Diagnostics	518.52	Huakang Biotech	131.78%
5	Mindray Biomedical	844,863	Bioeasy Biotechnology	131.20%	KingMed Diagnostics	221,964	Easy Diagnosis Biomedicine	201.37%	Vazyme	424.01	Easy Diagnosis Biomedicine	78.41%
6	DA AN GENE	766,426	NanoMicro Technology	117.74%	Hotgen	218,576	Wantai BioPharm	198.59%	BGI Genomics	363.42	Leadman	77.02%
7	BGI Genomics	676,614	Biotest Biotech	110.09%	Wantai BioPharm	202,147	Orient Gene	193.33%	Snibe	346.52	IVD Medical	54.60%
8	Wantai BioPharm	575,033	HybriBio	97.34%	BGI Genomics	146,154	NanoMicro Technology	158.75%	Autobio	322.8	Wantai BioPharm	53.87%
9	Hotgen	536,920	Strong Biotechnologies	88.58%	Easy Diagnosis Biomedicine	141,322	Leadman	143.97%	NanoMicro Technology	319.4	Medicalsystem Biotechnology	30.23%
10	Yes!Star	493,069	Alltest Biotech	64.98%	Bioperfectus	119,321	HybriBio	134.97%	DA AN GENE	281.53	Runda Medical	19.95%
11	Sansure Biotech	451,454	Bioperfectus	63.19%	Dian Diagnostics	116,288	Yes!Star	100.56%	Orient Gene	276.6	Orient Gene	13.55%
12	KeHua Biology	426,801	Acrobiosystems	56.30%	Snibe	97,370	Biotest Biotech	91.57%	Sansure Biotech	236	Lifotronic Technology	9.53%
13	Maccura Biotechnology	398,065	Hexin Instrument	48.66%	Autobio	97,366	Labway Clinical Laboratory	84.68%	Sino Biological	235.08	Tellgen	−0.20%
14	Autobio	376,592	KingMed Diagnostics	44.88%	Maccura Biotechnology	95,660	Huakang Biotech	63.71%	Dian Diagnostics	208.29	HybriBio	−1.96%

15	Wondfo Biotech	336,104	Gongdong Medical	43.95%	HybriBio	85,216	HOB	52.24%	Wondfo Biotech	175.22	Dian Diagnostics	−2.07%
16	GenScript	327,081	Labway Clinical Laboratory	43.62%	Biotest Biotech	83,359	Acrobiosystems	50.34%	Sinocare	168.92	Amoy Diagnostics	−3.54%
17	Bioperfectus	283,904	DA AN GENE	43.49%	Alltest Biotech	76,569	DA AN GENE	47.74%	Acrobiosystems	168.90	KeHua Biology	−3.77%
18	Easy Diagnosis Biomedicine	282,983	HOB	43.20%	Liferiver Biotech	75,852	KingMed Diagnostics	47.03%	Amoy Diagnostics	167.42	Yes!Star	−5.17%
19	IVD Medical	273,067	Lifotronic Technology	40.50%	Assure Tech	73,853	Bioperfectus	45.59%	Novogene	165.28	DA AN GENE	−6.42%
20	HybriBio	267,302	Tellgen	33.70%	KeHua Biology	72,102	Dian Diagnostics	44.83%	Maccura Biotechnology	162.43	Mindray Biomedical	−10.61%
21	Thalys Medical	259,955	Assure Tech	32.47%	Sino Biological	72,001	Univ Bio	42.15%	Gongdong Medical	161.36	KingMed Diagnostics	−11.92%
22	Snibe	254,542	GenScript	30.76%	Vazyme	67,829	Succeeder	40.73%	YHLO Biotech	139.93	Thalys Medical	−12.64%
23	Sinocare	236,131	Univ Bio	30.69%	Wondfo Biotech	63,443	Gongdong Medical	37.68%	Labway Clinical laboratory	139.10	Improve Medical	−13.30%
24	Medicalsystem Biotechnology	225,153	Mindray Biomedical	27.12%	Strong Biotechnologies	40,565	Tellgen	33.62%	Strong Biotechnologies	116.74	Sinocare	−16.53%
25	Liferiver Biotech	201,883	Autobio	26.45%	Getein Biotech	39,899	Amoy Diagnostics	32.86%	Bioeasy Biotechnology	115.69	Bohui Innovation	−17.14%
26	Alltest Biotech	187,343	Amoy Diagnostics	25.90%	Runda Medical	38,023	Lifotronic Technology	32.23%	Assure Tech	109.50	LBP	−17.61%
27	Vazyme	186,863	Runda Medical	25.33%	Gongdong Medical	31,099	Getein Biotech	30.93%	Liferiver Biotech	100.55	Getein Biotech	−18.10%
28	Novogene	186,640	Novogene	25.26%	Amoy Diagnostics	23,957	Autobio	30.20%	Lifotronic Technology	97.11	Succeeder	−20.25%
29	Biotest Biotech	181,808	Getein Biotech	24.78%	Bioeasy Biotechnology	23,651	Mindray Biomedical	27.11%	Univ Bio	89.27	Strong Biotechnologies	−20.79%

(continued)

Table 1.3 (continued)

Rankings	Operating revenue				Attributable net profit				Market value (2021.12.31)			
	Amount		Growth rate %		Amount		Growth rate %		Amount (100 million CNY)		Growth rate %	
30	Labway Clinical Laboratory	177,833	Dian Diagnostics	22.85%	Novogene	22,499	Righton Gene	22.26%	HybriBio	86.73	Dirui	−23.55%
31	Strong Biotechnologies	159,938	Thalys Medical	22.30%	Dirui	20,995	Chemclin Diagnostics	21.99%	Medicalsystem Biotechnology	81.62	Bioperfectus	−28.51%
32	Assure Tech	158,928	Yes!Star	20.06%	YHLO Biotech	20,475	Maccura Biotechnology	20.49%	Bohui Innovation	80.95	BGI Genomics	−29.35%
33	Berry Genomics	142,218	Leadman	19.63%	Labway Clinical Laboratory	20,384	Runda Medical	15.23%	Bioperfectus	80.6	Snibe	−36.37%
34	Getein Biotech	140,170	Wondfo Biotech	19.57%	Lifotronic Technology	19,035	Assure Tech	13.80%	Runda Medical	77.72	Maccura Biotechnology	−37.43%
35	Gongdong Medical	119,425	Vazyme	19.44%	NanoMicro Technology	18,809	Hexin Instrument	13.13%	Easy Diagnosis Biomedicine	77.61	Wondfo Biotech	−42.68%
36	YHLO Biotech	117,790	Huakang Biotech	18.94%	Medicalsystem Biotechnology	17,949	Alltest Biotech	12.73%	KeHua Biology	76.32	Sansure Biotech	−48.22%
37	Univ Bio	110,967	YHLO Biotech	17.91%	IVD Medical	17,454	IVD Medical	9.97%	Biotest Biotech	74.56	Berry Genomics	−49.03%
38	Sino Biological	96,527	Sinocare	17.17%	Acrobiosystems	17,421	KeHua Biology	6.76%	Getein Biotech	72.98	Autobio	−50.70%
39	Kindstar Globalgene	93,067	LBP	16.93%	Tellgen	16,108	AVE Science & Technology	3.90%	Hotgen	72.24	NanoMicro Technology	–
40	Amoy Diagnostics	91,703	AVE Science & Technology	16.91%	Chemclin Diagnostics	14,276	Snibe	3.68%	Chemclin Diagnostics	71.86	Sino Biological	–
41	Dirui	90,580	Snibe	15.97%	Univ Bio	10,873	Wondfo Biotech	0.04%	Berry Genomics	68.79	Novogene	–
42	Improve Medical	79,983	Chemclin Diagnostics	12.57%	Sinocare	10,757	YHLO Biotech	−2.75%	Alltest Biotech	66.31	YHLO Biotech	–
43	Lifotronic Technology	77,811	IVD Medical	12.46%	Succeeder	9737	LBP	−5.86%	Tellgen	51.97	Bioeasy Biotechnology	–
44	Bohui Innovation	71,475	Succeeder	7.88%	HOB	8619	Sansure Biotech	−14.29%	Kindstar Globalgene	51.7	Liferiver Biotech	–
45	Tellgen	65,459	Maccura Biotechnology	7.47%	LBP	7978	Vazyme	−17.46%	Dirui	49.44	Chemclin Diagnostics	–

46	Bioeasy Biotechnology	59,754	Biosino	7.06%	Hexin Instrument	7857	Liferiver Biotech	−18.61%	Leadman	43.9	Alltest Biotech	–
47	Leadman	56,406	Kindstar Globalgene	4.41%	Righton Gene	4733	Dirui	−21.39%	IVD Medical	43.57	Kindstar Globalgene	–
48	Chemclin Diagnostics	47,077	KeHua Biology	2.71%	AVE Science & Technology	3128	BGI Genomics	−30.08%	Hexin Instrument	41.96	Righton Gene	–
49	Hexin Instrument	46,424	Righton Gene	2.11%	Leadman	2242	Sino Biological	−36.15%	Righton Gene	40.42	HOB	–
50	NanoMicro Technology	44,635	Liferiver Biotech	−1.62%	Improve Medical	1857	Medicalsystem Biotechnology	−40.07%	HOB	39.73	AVE Science & Technology	–
51	LBP	43,899	Medicalsystem Biotechnology	−2.19%	Yes!Star	333	Sinocare	−42.44%	Succeeder	36.44	Biosino	–
52	Acrobiosystems	38,499	Bohui Innovation	−3.24%	Biosino	−114	Kindstar Globalgene	−49.32%	Improve Medical	32.93	Biotest Biotech	–
53	Biosino	34,823	Dirui	−3.35%	Huakang Biotech	−422	GenScript	−69.74%	Thalys Medical	29.5	Hexin Instrument	–
54	HOB	31,771	Sansure Biotech	−5.22%	Thalys Medical	−4951	Improve Medical	−88.57%	LBP	28.44	Vazyme	–
55	Righton Gene	29,095	Berry Genomics	−7.67%	Berry Genomics	−11,082	Biosino	−141.94%	Yes!Star	26.81	Assure Tech	–
56	Succeeder	23,992	Improve Medical	−12.99%	Bohui Innovation	−32,218	Berry Genomics	−152.60%	AVE Science & Technology	18.91	LabwayClinical Laboratory	–
57	AVE Science & Technology	21,067	BGI Genomics	−19.42%	Kindstar Globalgene	−145,443	Thalys Medical	−186.00%	Biosino	2.46	Acrobiosystems	–
58	Huakang Biotech	2613	Sino Biological	−39.53%	GenScript	−222,634	Bohui Innovation	−4393.4%	Huakang Biotech	0.99	Univ Bio	–
Summary	**15,916,033**		**34.03%**		**3,525,841**		**40.41%**					

Table 1.4 Rankings of critical data of NEEQ companies in 2021 (10 thousand CNY)

Rankings	Operating revenue				Attributable net profit			
	Amount		Growth rate %		Amount		Growth rate %	
1	Huizhikang	55,646	Venture Bio-tech	560.68%	Wiz Biotech	6813	MultiSciences Biotech	33290.59%
2	Darui Biotechnology	37,181	Wiz Biotech	375.47%	Huizhikang	4801	Venture Bio-tech	7284.55%
3	J.H. Bio-Tech	31,216	KeyGen BioTech	90.56%	Venture Bio-tech	3950	Wiz Biotech	341.44%
4	Wiz Biotech	27,645	Zhongsheng Jinyu	84.75%	J.H. Bio-Tech	3453	GenePharma	269.19%
5	Iprocom	23,908	Zhongzhi Biotechnologies	48.05%	Libo Medicine	3119	Zhongsheng Jinyu	160.47%
6	Xinle Medical	23,419	Nymphavn Biotechnology	46.54%	Xincheng Biological	2779	Kangmei Biotech	102.84%
7	Venture Bio-tech	19,319	MultiSciences Biotech	38.40%	Iprocom	2762	Mokobio Life Science	76.91%
8	Jiacheng Biotechnology	18,340	GenePharma	36.02%	King Diagnostic	1814	Promed	68.61%
9	Xincheng Biological	16,208	Promed	35.53%	Surexam Bio-Tech	1779	Yonghe-Sun Biotechnology	50.06%
10	Kangmei Biotech	15,702	Baio Technology	35.35%	Babio Biotechnology	1402	Surexam Bio-Tech	46.24%
11	Libo Medicine	15,625	Iprocom	34.30%	Keyu Biological	1354	King Diagnostic	43.86%
12	Sunshine Medical	12,102	Jiacheng Biotechnology	34.25%	Xinle Medical	1155	Dahui Biotechnology	26.15%
13	Tzone Biotechnology	11,726	Xinle Medical	34.24%	Jiacheng Biotechnology	1140	Libo Medicine	22.63%
14	Surexam Bio-Tech	11,457	Yonghe-Sun Biotechnology	32.82%	Oticon	914	Zhongzhi Biotechnologies	7.21%
15	King Diagnostic	11,168	Sunshine Medical	30.68%	KeyGen BioTech	638	Iprocom	4.72%
16	Baio Technology	10,550	Dahui Biotechnology	24.20%	GenePharma	364	Xincheng Biological	3.69%
17	GenePharma	10,218	Haiyuan Medical	19.69%	Tzone Biotechnology	330	Yasen Industrial	3.61%
18	KeyGen BioTech	10,039	Libo Medicine	18.66%	Zhongsheng Jinyu	317	Xinle Medical	0.63%

19	Keyu Biological	9665	Huizhikang	16.41%	MultiSciences Biotech	214	Huizhikang	0.24%
20	Babio Biotechnology	7713	Keyu Biological	16.07%	Dahui Biotechnology	187	Keyu Biological	−17.15%
21	Yonghe-Sun Biotechnology	6521	Surexam Bio-Tech	11.81%	Marr Bio	38	Jiacheng Biotechnology	−20.81%
22	Huamei Bio	5988	Darui Biotechnology	10.33%	Kangmei Biotech	29	Ocon	−25.14%
23	Newscen Bio-Pharmaceutical	5694	King Diagnostic	10.24%	Mokobio Life Science	−43	Baio Technology	−42.50%
24	Zhongzhi Biotechnologies	5073	Xincheng Biological	8.08%	Nymphavn Biotechnology	−110	J.H. Bio-Tech	−42.54%
25	Mokobio Life Science	4876	Clinisciences	6.82%	Clinisciences	−137	Marr Bio	−46.07%
26	Haiyuan Medical	4565	Tzone Biotechnology	3.11%	Yonghe-Sun Biotechnology	−144	Tzone Biotechnology	−46.38%
27	MultiSciences Biotech	3866	Oticon	2.48%	Promed	−186	Babio Biotechnology	−63.77%
28	Zhongsheng Jinyu	3862	J.H. Bio-Tech	1.72%	Yasen Industrial	−201	KeyGen BioTech	−76.44%
29	Oticon	3155	Kangmei Biotech	−6.26%	Zhongzhi Biotechnologies	−221	Huamei Bio	−116.24%
30	Dahui Biotechnology	3127	Huamei Bio	−6.59%	Sunshine Medical	−247	Darui Biotechnology	−124.55%
31	Promed	2359	Mokobio Life Science	−7.92%	Tianqi Medical	−556	Haiyuan Medical	−190.79%
32	Marr Bio	1795	Tianqi Medical	−36.83%	Haiyuan Medical	−813	Sunshine Medical	−221.07%
33	Clinisciences	1254	Babio Biotechnology	−37.18%	Huamei Bio	−1096	Nymphavn Biotechnology	−230.02%
34	Tianqi Medical	1190	Yasen Industrial	−41.18%	Darui Biotechnology	−1516	Tianqi Medical	−234.49%
35	Yasen Industrial	392	Marr Bio	−44.51%	Baio Technology	−2896	Clinisciences	−323.88%
36	Nymphavn Biotechnology	1	Newscen Bio-Pharmaceutical	−46.73%	Newscen Bio-Pharmaceutical	−5089	Newscen Bio-Pharmaceutical	−2460.94%
Summary	**432,568**		**23.35%**		**26,096**		**−28.59%**	

Table 1.5 Market value changes of listed companies in recent 3 years

Code	Company name	Listing date	Securities category	FY2019				FY2020				FY2021			
				Q1	Q2	Q3	Q4	Q1	Q2	Q3	Q4	Q1	Q2	Q3	Q4
002022	KeHua Biology	2004/7/21	SME board	58.07	52.24	48.95	60.1	82.76	92.44	93.32	79.31	89.64	92.16	67.88	76.32
002030	DA AN GENE	2004/8/9	SME board	105.9	87.08	80.78	91.7	138.20	239.25	307.04	300.86	294.11	298.09	260.54	281.53
002932	Easy Diagnosis Biomedicine	2018/7/10	SME board	30.7	27.59	25.21	24.11	27.57	42.55	51.04	43.5	75.28	67.33	42.78	77.61
300030	Improve Medical	2009/12/25	GEM	19.02	17.63	16.89	22.02	34.79	29.88	43.69	37.98	34.28	36.62	30.00	32.93
300244	Dian Diagnostics	2011/7/19	GEM	127.5	107.59	153.87	137.31	145.51	218.86	245.95	212.69	241.98	237.64	183.33	208.29
300289	Leadman	2012/2/16	GEM	32.72	26.78	23.12	24.51	24.21	29.72	32.88	24.8	28.25	25.89	26.78	43.90
300298	Sinocare	2012/3/19	GEM	68.4	67.72	77.34	84.74	83.90	181.59	226.17	202.38	210.58	177.06	132.94	168.92
300318	Bohui Innovation	2012/5/23	GEM	40.23	33.92	33.08	33.41	38.81	51.55	129.09	97.7	66.66	65.92	66.67	80.95
300396	Dirui	2014/9/10	GEM	43.31	48.17	43.86	46.73	55.39	74.19	74.60	64.67	66.14	57.50	48.80	49.44
300406	Strong Biotechnologies	2014/10/30	GEM	75.42	76.47	81.34	81.59	85.84	115.46	115.92	147.37	120.10	116.21	96.54	116.74
300439	Medicalsystem Biotechnology	2015/4/22	GEM	54.28	50.43	49.05	46.93	49.13	62.34	64.62	62.67	83.19	73.92	68.17	81.62
300463	Maccura Biotechnology	2015/5/28	GEM	108.25	144.27	144	150.41	155.01	324.34	295.10	259.61	264.72	234.37	160.53	162.43
300482	Wondfo Biotech	2015/6/30	GEM	116.26	131.66	168.24	177.41	265.89	356.72	284.86	305.71	347.58	287.91	191.35	175.22
300639	HybriBio	2017/4/12	GEM	31.91	31.85	42.24	53.13	59.32	110.09	106.62	88.46	93.89	97.01	93.43	86.73
300642	Tellgen	2017/4/12	GEM	37.97	37.32	36.99	37.39	39.44	47.15	51.20	52.08	61.76	78.15	59.99	51.97
300676	BGI Genomics	2017/7/14	GEM	289.83	230.74	257.06	274.87	301.72	623.64	575.80	514.37	534.90	490.90	362.29	363.42
300685	Amoy Diagnostics	2017/8/2	GEM	77.31	77.58	96.29	98.36	99.23	170.85	169.85	173.56	189.42	230.77	178.04	167.42
300760	Mindray Biomedical '	2018/10/16	GEM	1590.61	1974.28	2246.6	2211.34	3182.27	3717.31	4231.68	5178.84	5669.38	5835.93	4686.71	4629.35
300832	Snibe	2020/5/12	GEM						709.42	687.01	544.55	545.00	482.61	384.37	346.52
300942	Bioeasy Biotechnology	2021/2/9	GEM									124.75	120.57	113.48	115.69
301047	Sino Biological	2021/8/16	GEM											260.43	235.08

301060	Labway Clinical Laboratory	2021/9/13	GEM											72.98	139.10
301080	Acrobiosystems	2021/10/18	GEM												168.90
301166	Univ Bio	2021/12/28	GEM												89.27
603108	Runda Medical	2015/6/30	Shanghai A-share	68.33	61.6	59.11	57.61	57.88	77.26	77.78	64.79	69.49	65.08	59.33	77.72
603658	Autobio	2016/9/1	Shanghai A-share	271.7	287.36	378.92	404.8	502.07	700.12	695.29	654.73	551.01	444.22	312.34	322.80
603716	Thalys Medical	2016/10/31	Shanghai A-share	49.79	35.28	39.35	34.65	31.43	29.85	31.32	33.77	28.64	29.77	23.27	29.50
603387	Getein Biotech	2017/7/17	Shanghai A-share	66.7	67.29	61.04	60.02	82.89	104.75	95.42	89.11	90.57	81.79	66.79	72.98
603882	KingMed Diagnostics	2017/9/8	Shanghai A-share	132.24	159.02	256.46	234.53	257.81	409.91	469.36	588.7	667.41	739.11	475.23	518.52
603392	Wantai BioPharm	2020/4/29	Shanghai A-share						716.10	453.96	873.83	1336.10	1573.33	1347.54	1344.59
605369	Gongdong Medical	2020/9/16	Shanghai A-share											113.88	161.36
000710	Berry Genomics	2017/7/5	Shenzhen A-share	147.8	125.53	110.03	129.79	130.04	212.08	193.30	134.96	105.21	106.52	76.15	68.79
688068	Hotgen	2019/9/30	Science and Technology Innovation Board			44.27	29.19	28.29	42.92	30.76	24.25	140.25	117.55	72.37	72.24
688389	Lifotronic Technology	2019/11/4	Science and Technology Innovation Board				69.33	77.86	138.42	116.43	88.66	108.93	129.45	82.16	97.11
688399	Bioperfectus	2019/12/5	Science and Technology Innovation Board				33.94	42.90	162.96	152.05	112.75	104.96	98.83	66.82	80.60
688298	Orient Gene	2020/2/5	Science and Technology Innovation Board					87.95	183.96	192.70	243.6	220.21	261.12	187.81	276.60
688338	Succeeder	2020/8/6	Science and Technology Innovation Board							60.71	45.69	42.59	45.38	36.19	36.44

(continued)

Table 1.5 (continued)

Code	Company name	Listing date	Securities category	FY2019				FY2020				FY2021			
				Q1	Q2	Q3	Q4	Q1	Q2	Q3	Q4	Q1	Q2	Q3	Q4
688393	LBP	2020/8/20	Science and Technology Innovation Board							39.96	34.52	35.37	36.66	27.61	28.44
688289	Sansure Biotech	2020/8/28	Science and Technology Innovation Board							443.16	455.8	397.44	397.80	223.12	236.00
688656	HOB	2021/1/13	Science and Technology Innovation Board									49.53	46.90	33.04	39.73
688371	Liferiver Biotech	2021/1/18	Science and Technology Innovation Board									143.75	126.46	92.14	100.55
688606	Alltest Biotech	2021/3/25	Science and Technology Innovation Board									109.07	80.32	55.84	66.31
688468	Chemclin Diagnostics	2021/4/9	Science and Technology Innovation Board									86.17	89.46	66.08	71.86
688315	Novogene	2021/4/13	Science and Technology Innovation Board									172.69	195.30	207.52	165.28
688217	Righton Gene	2021/5/17	Science and Technology Innovation Board										46.35	35.41	40.42
688575	YHLO Biotech	2021/5/17	Science and Technology Innovation Board										179.82	118.46	139.93

688067	AVE Science & Technology	2021/6/16	Science and Technology Innovation Board										21.35	18.88	18.91
688690	NanoMicro Technology	2021/6/23	Science and Technology Innovation Board											317.96	319.40
688767	Biotest Biotech	2021/9/8	Science and Technology Innovation Board											61.25	74.56
688622	Hexin Instrument	2021/9/13	Science and Technology Innovation Board											48.35	41.96
688105	Vazyme	2021/11/16	Science and Technology Innovation Board												424.01
688075	Assure Tech	2021/11/18	Science and Technology Innovation Board												109.50

Note:

1. By the end of 2019, the total market value of 27 listed companies in the IVD industry was 471 billion CNY; by the end of 2020, the total market value of 33 listed companies in the IVD industry was 1183.6 billion CNY; by the end of 2021, the total market value of 52 listed companies in the IVD industry was 1201.6 billion CNY
2. By the end of 2019, the average P/E ratio of 27 listed companies in the IVD industry was 44.01 times; by the end of 2020, the average P/E ratio of 33 listed companies in the IVD industry was 65.09 times; by the end of 2021, the average P/E ratio of 52 listed companies in the IVD industry was 45.51 times

Table 1.6 Newly listed enterprises in diagnostics industry in 2021

Sector name	Code	Company name	Listing date
GEM	300942	Bioeasy Biotechnology	2021/2/9
GEM	301047	Sino Biological	2021/8/16
GEM	301060	Labway Clinical Laboratory	2021/9/13
GEM	301080	Acrobiosystems	2021/10/18
GEM	301166	Univ Bio	2021/12/28
Science and Technology Innovation Board	688656	HOB	2021/1/13
Science and Technology Innovation Board	688371	Liferiver Biotech	2021/1/18
Science and Technology Innovation Board	688606	Alltest Biotech	2021/3/25
Science and Technology Innovation Board	688468	Chemclin Diagnostics	2021/4/9
Science and Technology Innovation Board	688315	Novogene	2021/4/13
Science and Technology Innovation Board	688217	Righton Gene	2021/5/17
Science and Technology Innovation Board	688575	YHLO Biotech	2021/5/17
Science and Technology Innovation Board	688067	AVE Science & Technology	2021/6/16
Science and Technology Innovation Board	688690	NanoMicro Technology	2021/6/23
Science and Technology Innovation Board	688767	Biotest Biotech	2021/9/8
Science and Technology Innovation Board	688622	Hexin Instrument	2021/9/13
Science and Technology Innovation Board	688105	Vazyme	2021/11/16
Science and Technology Innovation Board	688075	Assure Tech	2021/11/18

Table 1.7 IPO Queuing Companies in Diagnostics Industry in 2021

Filing enterprise	Sponsor	Audit status
Main board of Shanghai Stock Exchange		
Cowealth Medical	Haitong Securities	Approved
GEM		
Orienter	Sinolink Securities	Inquired
InTec	CITIC Securities	Inquired
Fapon Biotech	Huatai Securities	Inquired
VivaChek	CITIC Securities	Inquired
Zeesan Biotech	CITIC Securities	Accepted
Quaero Life	CITIC Securities	Accepted
Science and Technology Innovation Board		
MGI	CITIC Securities	Submit registration
Rendu Biotechnology	Sinolink Securities	Submit registration
Innovita	CITIC Securities	Inquired
Hong Kong Stock Exchange		
Adicon	Morgan Stanley	Submitted
Bioer Technology	CICC	Submitted

Table 1.8 Delisted enterprises in the IVD industry in 2021

835236	Icubio	2016/1/6	NEEQ	Compulsory withdrawal

1.1.2 Investment and Financing Events of Domestic IVD Enterprises in 2021 (Table 1.9)

Table 1.9 Summary of investment and financing events of domestic IVD enterprises in 2021

S/no.	Time	Invested company	Round	Financing amount	Business	Investor
1	January 8	Calibra	Round B	Hundreds of millions of CNY	It is a high-tech enterprise under Dian Diagnostics that focuses on the R&D, clinical transformation and application of the new generation of multi-omics biomarker mass spectrometry	GL Ventures led the investment, followed by GL Capital Group and Green Pine Capital Partners
2	January 9	TargetingOne	Round B	150 million CNY	Digital PCR system	Lilly Asia Ventures led the investment, followed by China Growth Capital, GL Ventures, as well as the old shareholders Qingdao Yufeng, Chongyuan Huichen
3	January 11	NuProbe	Round A	42 million USD	Genomics and molecular diagnostics of ultra-sensitive tumor sequencing Panel test and Infertility Genetic Detection	BioTrack Capital and Yonghua Capital
4	January 14	Holosensor Medical	Round Pre-A	Over 100 million CNY	With microfluidics as the core technology, it provides a new generation of products of liquid biopsy for tumors and rapid test for infectious pathogenic microorganisms	Baidu Venture led the investment, followed by Kunshan Kechuang Fund, SND Ventures, and Purple Cow Startups
5	January 18	Inscinstech	Round Pre-A	Tens of millions of CNY	High-end intelligent protein purifier	Dynamic Balance Investment Management
6	January 26	Adicon	Strategic investment	88 million USD	Medical diagnostic test service	OrbiMed Asia
7	February 8	Monad	Round A	200 million CNY	Overall solutions for molecular and protein research in life science and R&D of raw enzyme	Luxin Venture Capital and ABclonal jointly led the investment, followed by Wuxi Jintou
8	February 10	Accunome	Round A2	Nearly 100 million CNY	Automatic and universal molecular diagnosis platform with molecular diagnosis, infectious diseases and severe diseases as the core	Sinovation Ventures

9	February 22	PushKang Biotechnology	Round C	Hundreds of millions of CNY	By using centrifugal microfluidic technology, combined with the original micro whole blood separation function and reagent freeze-drying technology, it studies and develops coagulation (i.e. thrombosis and hemostasis), chemiluminescence immunoassay, biochemical and other diagnostic test reagent chips and new supporting POCT detection systems suitable for the national conditions, focusing on the coagulation market	GL Ventures and Fu Rong Capital jointly led the investment, followed by Couplet Health Industry Fund
10	February 23	RainSure	Round B1	Tens of millions of CNY	Digital PCR supporting IVD kit	Qingke Asset Management led the investment, followed by Kaitai Capital
11	February 24	Wuxi Diagnostics	Round B	150million USD	Medical diagnostic test service	Shiyu Capital, etc.
12	February 24	AnchorDx	Round C	40 million USD	NGS products of early screening and early diagnosis for cancers	OrbiMed Asia, Yaoming Huiying Investment Fund
13	February 24	Calibra	Round B	150 million CNY	It focuses on the R&D, clinical transformation and application of the new generation of multi-omics biomarker mass spectrometry	GL Ventures led the investment, followed by GL Capital Group and Green Pine Capital Partners
14	February 28	Celula	Round B+	Tens of millions of CNY	Small flow cytometry and digital PCR, noninvasive prenatal screening	Peikun Fund led the investment, followed by Xiamen Silicon Valley Torch Fund
15	March 29	Dawei Bio	Round Pre-A	Undisclosed	Automatic digital PCR	Qingkong Jinxin Capital, Maccura
16	March 29	Histomed	Round B	100 million CNY - level	Medical diagnosis and pathological test services	Feitu Venture Investment, etc.
17	April 2	Sanmed Biotech	Round B	300 million CNY	Platform of liquid biopsy for tumors for early screening of serious malignant tumors such as lung cancer, intestinal cancer, breast cancer and liver cancer	CMG SDIC Capital

(continued)

Table 1.9 (continued)

S/no.	Time	Invested company	Round	Financing amount	Business	Investor
18	April 7	HRTJ	Round A	Tens of millions of CNY	It focuses on the allergen-specificIgE antibody detection system based on microfluidics and protein coating	River Head Capital led the investment, followed by TigerYeah Capital
19	April 8	YingSheng Biology	Undisclosed	Undisclosed	Based on metabonomics and genomics, it has built a domestic leading gene test platform and mass spectrometry platform, covering birth defect screening, disease prevention, human health services and other fields	Alibaba Health
20	April 8	Giant Med Diagnostics	Round Pre-A	20 million CNY	Medical diagnostic test service	Northern Light Venture Capital
21	April 19	Demeter	Round A	Tens of millions of CNY	Clinical mass spectrometry and chromatography	Fortune Venture Capital
22	May 10	Reliable Med	Round A+	Tens of millions of CNY	Liquid chromatography tandem mass spectrometry products	3H Health led the investment
23	May 10	ET Healthcare	A new round	More than 100 million USD	The biosensor Test-On-A-Probe (TOP) includes different detection technologies on a single probe to make the analysis of proteins, antibodies, nucleic acids, small molecules and cells	Sequoia Capital China and GL Ventures led the investment
24	May 10	Willingmed	Round Pre-A	Hundreds of millions of CNY	Infectious precision medical products and services provider	E-town International Investment, Songrui Phase I, Royal Capital, Biolink Capital, Delta Capital
25	June 1	Genskey	Round C+	Hundreds of millions of CNY	Medical diagnostic test service	CPE Fund
26	June 3	Accunome	Round A3	Tens of millions of CNY	Automatic and universal molecular diagnosis platform with molecular diagnosis, infectious diseases and severe diseases as the core	China Merchants Health

27	June 7	Conlight Medical	Round Pre-B	Nearly 100 million CNY	Medical diagnostic test service	Ehong Impact Capital
28	June 8	Qitan Technology	Round B	400 million CNY	Independent R&D, manufacturing and application of nanopore gene sequencer and supporting reagent consumables	CDH VGC and GL Ventures jointly led the investment, followed by BioTrack Capital, Huagai Capital and River Head Capital
29	June 10	Health Biotech	Round B+	200 million CNY	Clinical chromatography and mass spectrometry	Qiming Venture Partners led the investment, followed by BioVenture, C&D Emerging Investment and the long-term shareholder Sino-Ocean Capital
30	June 11	Reigncom Biotech	Round A	Hundreds of millions of CNY	Clinical mass spectrometry	Matrix Partners China led the investment, followed by Sinovation Ventures
31	June 15	Tongshu Gene	Round C	500 million CNY	It has the dual capabilities of LDT+IVD, and provides gene test services with NGS micro library building as the core barrier, and a big data transformation research center based on tumor genomics specimen bank	GL Capital Group, GCS Capital and Oceanpine Capital jointly led the investment
32	June 18	Gaugene	Round A+	Tens of millions of CNY	Flow fluorescent platform and multi-index combined determination	Qiming Venture Partners
33	June 25	Aivd Biotech	Round A	Nearly 100 million CNY	It provides a one-stop ODM service solution from upstream raw materials to reagents	Shenzhen HTI led the investment, followed by Shenzhen Nanling Equity Investment Fund
34	June 29	Kindstar Globalgene	Pre-IPO	140 million USD	Medical diagnostic test service	Carmignac, etc.

(continued)

Table 1.9 (continued)

S/no.	Time	Invested company	Round	Financing amount	Business	Investor
35	July 16	Wellgrow Technology	Round B	Approx. 100 million USD	New high-throughput flow fluorescence detection platform with independent intellectual property rights of magnetic fluorescence-encoded microsphere technology and flow fluorescence detection platform	China Pioneer Foundation & Capitals led the investment, followed by Cowin Asset Management, BioVenture VC, Beijing Life Science Park Venture Capital and the long-term shareholder Vinno Capital
36	July 19	RealMind Biotech	Strategic investment	Nearly 100 million CNY	Small chemoluminescence, automatic chemiluminescence POCT, microdroplet-controlled POCT and other platforms focusing on cardiac biomarkers, inflammation monitoring, reproductive function, growth and development, stomach function, brain damage, etc.	Ocean State Investment led the investment, followed by the original shareholders BGI Co-win and Portfolio
37	July 20	Hugo Biotech	Strategic investment	200 million CNY	A team that focuses on cell-free mNGS transformation clinical study and has the ability to self-develop algorithms	LYFE Capital led the investment, followed by the long-term shareholder Sinovation Ventures
38	July 22	Gene+	Round C	750 million CNY	Products such as large Panel gene detection and early screening for tumors	CCB International led the investment, followed by Fortune Capital, Jinmao Capital and GGV Capital
39	July 29	Healthcare Bio	Round B+	Tens of millions of CNY	Analysis platform of fluorescence in situ hybridization (FISH)	Chuchang Investment and Luojia Capital led the investment, followed by Hubei Provincial High Technology Industry Investment
40	September 2	Berry Oncology	Round B1	Nearly 700 million CNY	Gene tests focusing on the whole course of cancer	China Merchants Capital led the investment

41	September 3	Bioeast Biotech	Round A	100 million CNY	It has two series of products, namely bioactive materials and chemical synthetic materials (mainly including immunomagnetic beads used for chemiluminescence)	China Growth Capital led the investment, followed by BioVenture, Cowin Venture Capital and Portfolio
42	September 3	Thistory Bio-Medical	Round B+	Undisclosed	IVD thrombus and hemostasis track	Shenzhen Capital Group Co., Ltd.
43	September 6	RH Genetech	Angel round	Tens of millions of CNY	The fourth-generation gene sequencing, nanopore virus detection and other equipment related to biomacromolecule detection	Leaguer
44	September 8	Oncocare Life	Round A+	120 million CNY	Cancer gene methylation detection products	Oriza Seed led the investment, followed by Addor Capital
45	September 8	Shuwen Bio-Technology	Round B	Nearly 100 million CNY	Innovative products of tumor screening and in the field of maternal, infant and reproductive health	Guolian Investment led the investment, followed by Stream V, Anyuan Investment Fund and Kaichuang Fund
46	September 15	GeneMind	Round B	410 million CNY	It focuses on the R&D and manufacturing of upstream molecular diagnostic tool platforms based on gene sequencers, and has continuously innovated and accumulated a lot of intellectual property rights in underlying technologies such as instrument hardware, biochemical reagents, sequencing chips, software algorithms, etc	Sansure Biotech, Cowin Asset Management, Sino European Allied Capital
47	September 18	Precision Scientific	Round B+	150 million CNY	Companion diagnostics provides full support based on multi-omics and data mining for the full cycle of new drug development	Kington Capital and GTJA Investment jointly led the investment, followed by Qichen Investment andGrand Mount Capital

(continued)

Table 1.9 (continued)

S/no.	Time	Invested company	Round	Financing amount	Business	Investor
48	September 22	Sophonix	Undisclosed	Over 100 million CNY	Chemiluminescence POCT supplier, focusing on brain damage, central nervous system diseases, cytokine storm and other detection fields	ETP funds, CITIC Fund, Huajin Capital
49	September 26	Matridx	Undisclosed	Hundreds of millions of CNY	Pathogen metagenome mNGS automatic detection products	Huatai Zijin and Alibaba led the investment, followed by Proxima Ventures and Qianhai FOF
50	September 26	Promed	Undisclosed	Nearly 100 million CNY	IVD maternal and child health and coagulation diagnosis, maternal and child POCT and integrated photochemical signal transduction and transmission system and microfluidic chips	Qingke Asset Management
51	September 27	Sniper	Round B	200 million CNY	Automatic digital PCR instrument	HM Capital led the investment, followed by Apricot Capital and Huangpu Biomedical Fund
52	October 8	ChosenMed	Round C1	Hundreds of millions of CNY	Detect methylation canyon markers through an independently developed unique algorithm, and apply ctDNA methylation detection technology to early cancer screening	Yijing Investment, High-tech Health Care and Jingming Capital led the investment
54	October 15	Creative Biosciences	Round D	560 million CNY	Noninvasive early screening for intestinal cancer	Alibaba led the investment, followed by the old shareholders IDG Capital and China Renaissance

55	October 18	ATG Biotechnology	Angel round	Development technology and large-scale conversion and production of high-end molecular raw enzyme	mRNA synthetic raw material enzyme	Dynamic Balance Investment Management
56	October 18	Willingmed	Round A+	100 million CNY	Macrogenome high-throughput sequencing (mNGS) technology for rapid detection of complex infections	Runda Medical and Gongshu SDIC jointly invested
57	October 21	Pinnacles Medical Technology	Round A	300 million CNY	It quickly builds an IVD platform company with the Build-Buy-Collaborate model, and will continue to focus on building an efficient smart laboratory, and provide core products for a broader smart laboratory ecosystem	Lilly Asia Ventures (LAV) led the investment, and the new investors included Qingsong Investment Management and Vertex Ventures
58	October 22	Qlife	Strategic investment	Hundreds of millions of CNY	Clinical mass spectrometry devices	Centurium Capital, Cowin Asset Management
59	October 25	BiOligo Biotech	Round A	300 million CNY	It mainly has various DNA primers and fluorescence-labeled probes required for in vitro diagnosis, connectors & sealers & amplicon primers & targeted capture probes used for NGS library building, various RNA synthesis products, large size DNA&RNA synthesis, etc.	Carlyle led the investment, followed by CICC and Bio Venture
60	October 25	CoHealth	Round A	Tens of millions of CNY	Mobile digital medical detection system and its supporting consumables, intelligently manufactured biochip	Puhua Capital and Chengdu Technology Transfer led the investment
61	October 28	Holosensor Medical	Undisclosed	Tens of millions of CNY	Microfluidic chips, focusing on rapid test of tumors, infections, chronic diseases and other fields	CDIB Capital Group led the investment

(continued)

Table 1.9 (continued)

S/no.	Time	Invested company	Round	Financing amount	Business	Investor
62	October 31	Axbio	Strategic investment	Tens of millions of USD	The fourth-generation gene sequencer	5Y Capital, Kaitai Capital, MSA Capital and Yuanhe Puhua jointly invested
63	November 2	Asbios	Angel round	Millions of CNY	Molecular detection technology based on macrogenomic pathogenic microorganism detection (mNGS)	Undisclosed
64	November 2	Dynamic Biosystems	Round A	130 million CNY	Full-chain single-cell multi-omics technology	GL Ventures and HM Capital jointly led the investment
65	November 3	Oebiotech	Round A+	Nearly 100 million CNY	Multi-omics detection services and molecular diagnostic products	Sinopharm Capital led the investment
66	November 8	Biocomma	Round A	Over 100 million CNY	Adsorption & separation materials and filter materials	Shenzhen Capital led the investment, followed by SBCVC, BioVenture and Shenzhen HTI
67	November 8	Gloriousmed	Round B	100 million CNY	Gene test of tumors of the urinary system	The government funds, industrial companies and old shareholders participated.
68	November 9	Weimi Bio-Tech	Round B	Over 100 million CNY	Two high-end platforms: neural autoimmunity and flow fluorescence. The products mainly focus on pathogenic microorganism detection, inflammation detection, etc.	CICC Qide Fund led the investment, followed by Med-Fine Capital, Chuangyu Investment and Jiahong Medical
69	November 10	Singleron Biotechnologies	Round B	Nearly 100 million USD	It focuses on high-throughput single-cell multi-omics platform products	Lake Bleu Capital led the investment, followed by Firstmed, MSA Capital, as well as the existing shareholders Sherpa Healthcare Partners, Lilly Asia Ventures, ARCH Venture Partners, CDG Capital, CDH Investments, SuperString Capital, 3w Global Investment, SBCVC, etc.

70	November 10	Landing Med	Round D	320 million CNY	AI tumor diagnosis cloud	Alibaba Health led the investment, followed by Ether Investment
71	November 11	Yuce Biological	Round C+	Nearly 100 million CNY	Overall solution platform for tumor immune diagnosis and treatment. Focusing on the two research platforms, namely tumor genome and tumor microenvironment, the company builds a platform for the development and sales of clinical detection products for tumors and CRO service for pharmaceutical enterprises	Shenzhen Suizi Finance Management invested exclusively
72	November 24	Evergauge	Undisclosed	Tens of millions of CNY	Capillary electrophoresis and CE-MS	Haining Changhong Medical Industry Investment Partnership
73	November 25	Vision Medicals	Round D	300 million CNY	Infectious precision medicine, aiming at clinical departments such as ICU, infection, respiration, paediatrics, and neurology to build an AI diagnosis system for infectious diseases based on genomics, radiomics, and EMR	Boyu Capital led the investment
74	November 25	NeoImmune	Round Pre-A	30 million CNY	Key technologies for high-throughput reading and writing of T and B lymphocyte receptor repertoire and their applications in clinical detection and therapy	Ruijiang Kangsheng Fund
75	November 27	Hzymes Biotech	Round C	800 million CNY	Special enzyme creation platform	GL Capital Group led the investment
76	November 29	Willingmed	Round A+	100 million CNY	It has mNGS whole process high-throughput automation solution, focusing on the field of infectious precision molecular diagnosis	Shanghai Alliance led the investment exclusively
77	November 30	Ustar	Round E+	Over 300 million CNY	Molecular POCT	CPE Fund led the investment

(continued)

Table 1.9 (continued)

S/no.	Time	Invested company	Round	Financing amount	Business	Investor
78	November 30	Bio Guoke	Round A+	Tens of millions of CNY	Based on population genome research and focusing on the field of birth defects	Maccura and Chengdu Huiling Changxi Fund
79	December 13	ABclonal	Round D	1.2 billion CNY	Antibody, molecular enzyme reagent, CRO antibody discovery	Sequoia China, Luxin Venture Capital and China Merchant Bank International Capital jointly led the investment
80	December 20	Lychix Bio	Round B	150 million CNY	Based on the core technology platform μ-MPF, the company has built a number of application platforms, including an ultra-sensitive biomolecular detection platform, a multiple magnetic fluorescence-encoded microsphere platform for multi-index combined determination, and a high-throughput single-cell parallel control platform for cell multi-omics.	Legend Capital, HighLight Capital and CMG SDIC Capital jointly invested
81	December 20	ChosenMed	Round C2	Hundreds of millions of CNY	It covers tumor detection products in the whole industry chain, focusing on the guidance of targeted drugs for solid tumors, the prediction of the efficacy of tumor immunotherapy, especially the products regarding specific detection of nonsmall cell lung cancer and blood system tumors, etc.	Yijing Investment led the investment
82	December 22	Vacure	Round A	Tens of millions of CNY	Microfluidic POCT	Henan Jinggang Advanced Manufacturing Equity Investment Fund led the investment

1.2 Industry Development Questionnaire

The Medical Laboratory Society of the National Association of Health Industry and Enterprise Management cooperates with the In Vitro Diagnostics Society of the China Association for Medical Devices Industry to conduct a questionnaire, and invited the IVD Special Committee of the Shanghai Medical Instrument Trade Association, as well as the In Vitro Diagnostics and Precision Medical Investment and Industry Alliance, to hand out a questionnaire to the members of the industry associations. More than 400 valid questionnaires were connected in this industry development survey. The survey results are summarized and analyzed as follows:

1.2.1 The Growth in 2021 According to the Feedback from the Enterprises Is as Follows (Fig. 1.1)

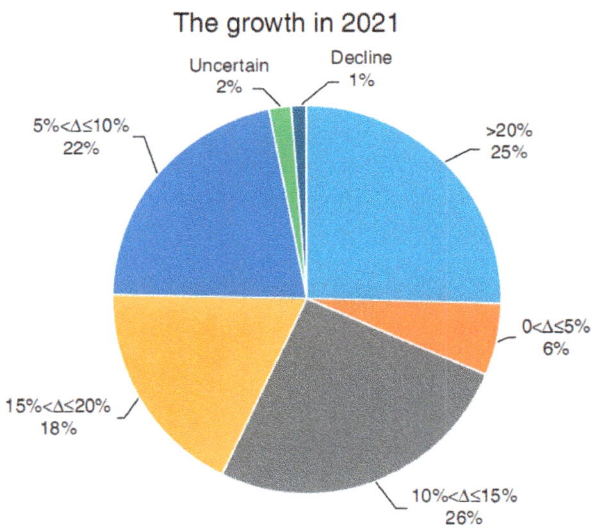

Fig. 1.1 Review of the growth in 2021 according to the feedback from the enterprises

1.2.2 The Estimated Growth in 2022 According to the Feedback from the Enterprises Is as Follows (Fig. 1.2)

To sum up:

(a) Based on the above enterprise feedback and relevant data summary, it is determined that the industry growth rate was more than 15% in 2021 and was expected to be more than 10% in 2022.

(b) **In terms of growth percentage:** The review shows that the industry growth rate in 2021 was concentrated at 10–20%, accounting for 44%; the growth rate was mostly concentrated at 10–15%, accounting for 26%. It is predicted that the industry growth rate in 2022 will also be concentrated at 10–20%, accounting for 51%; the growth rate will also be concentrated at 10–15%, accounting for 30%.

(c) **Compared with the survey data of the previous year:** In terms of growth percentage, it is believed that the industry growth rate in 2021 was concentrated at 10–20%, accounting for 44%. This result is about 7% less than the predicted value of 51% in the industry report of the previous year for the growth rate in 2021 being concentrated at 10–20%.

(d) The number of foreign investors participating in the questionnaire was slightly less than that in 2020 but higher than that in 2019: The results showed that, compared with the prediction in 2020, about 66% of the foreign-funded enterprises predicted that the industry growth rate would be concentrated at 10–20%, which was significantly higher than the predicted value of 44% in the general questionnaire for the concentrated industry growth rate. Compared with the previous survey data, the understanding and judgment of foreign investors on the Chinese market are getting closer to those of domestic companies.

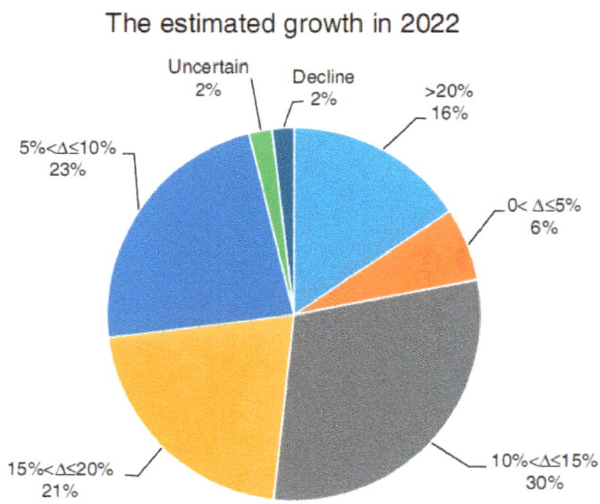

Fig. 1.2 Estimate of the growth in 2022 according to the feedback from the enterprises

(e) **It is noteworthy that:** In terms of growth percentage, the proportion of 44% of the considered industry growth rate being concentrated at 10–20% in 2021 was 1% less than that in 2020, which was the lowest in 6 years, but the proportion of growth rate > 20% reached 25%, which was the first time that the result in questionnaire was more than 20% in 7 years (the greatest value in previous years was 16% in 2015), indicating that the differentiation of enterprise development in the industry is increasing.

1.3 Review of Market Segment Development in 2021

According to the survey, in the range of 15–25% of the forecast of market segment development in 2021, the top three were Molecular Diagnostics, POCT and Immunoassay (this is consistent with the top three with the most development potential in the future, but the rankings were slightly different, in which POCT ranked before Immunoassay); followed by Microorganism, Blood and Pathology; Biochemistry also came last, which had been ranking last for three consecutive years (Fig. 1.3).

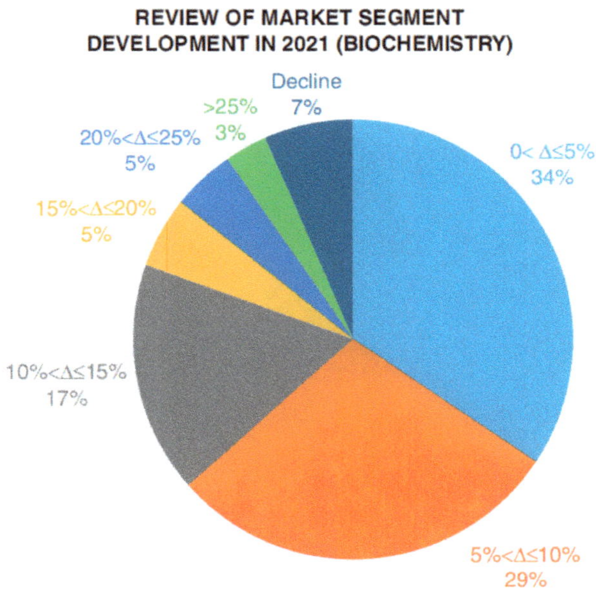

Fig. 1.3 Review of market segment development in 2021

Fig. 1.3 (continued)

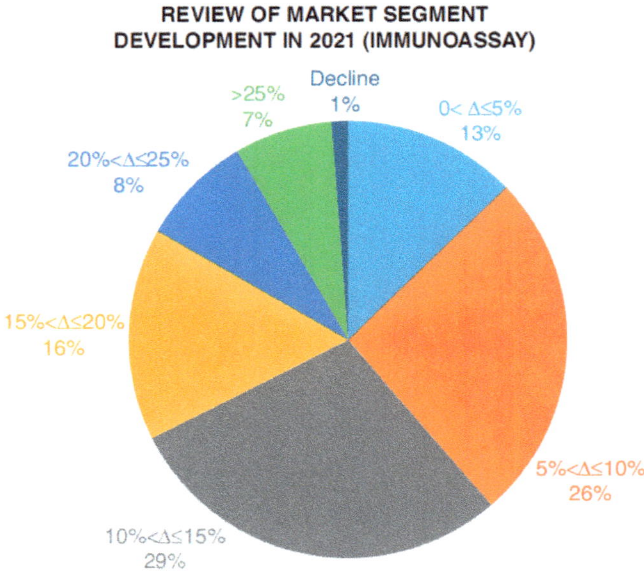

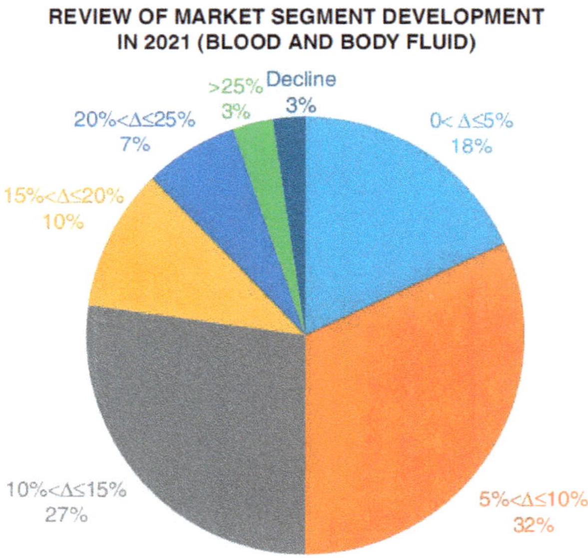

Fig. 1.3 (continued)

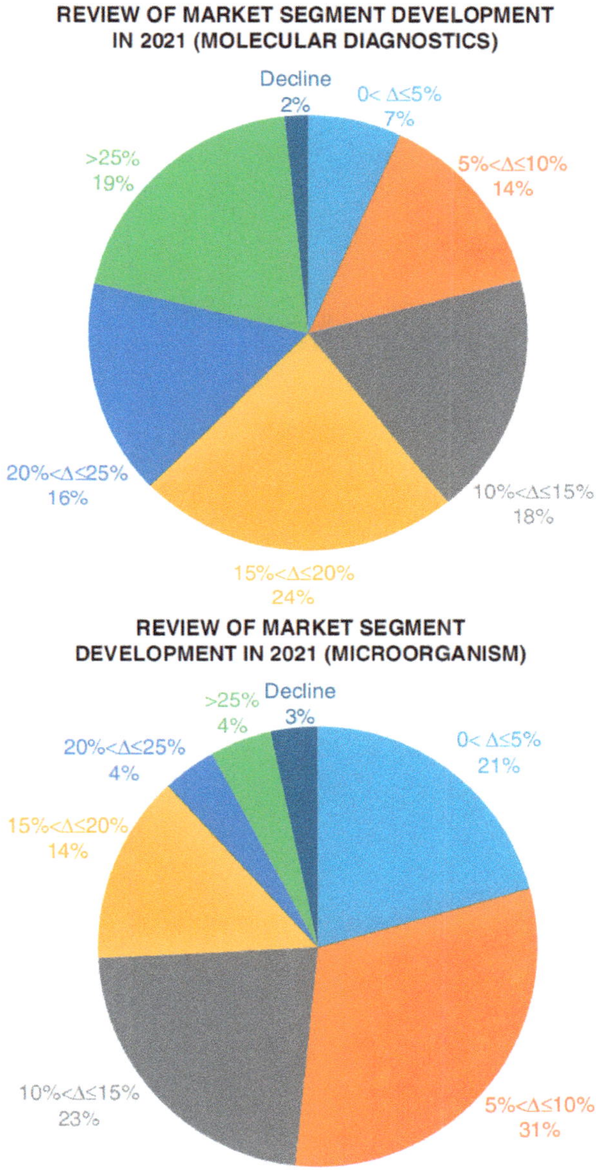

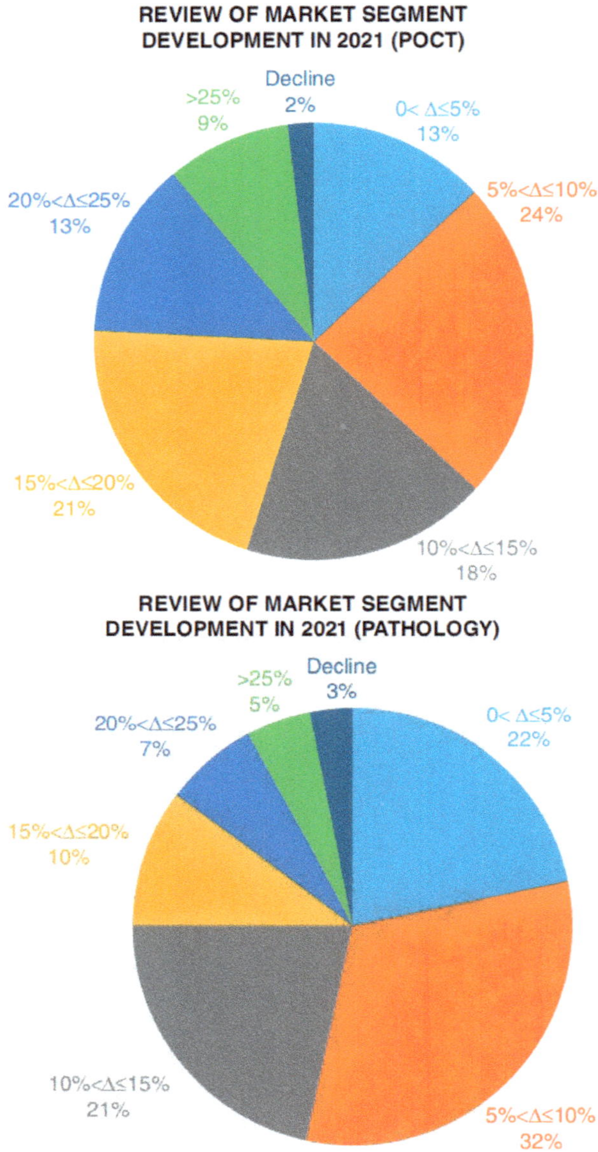

Fig. 1.3 (continued)

1.4 Forecast of Market Segment Development in 2022 (Fig. 1.4)

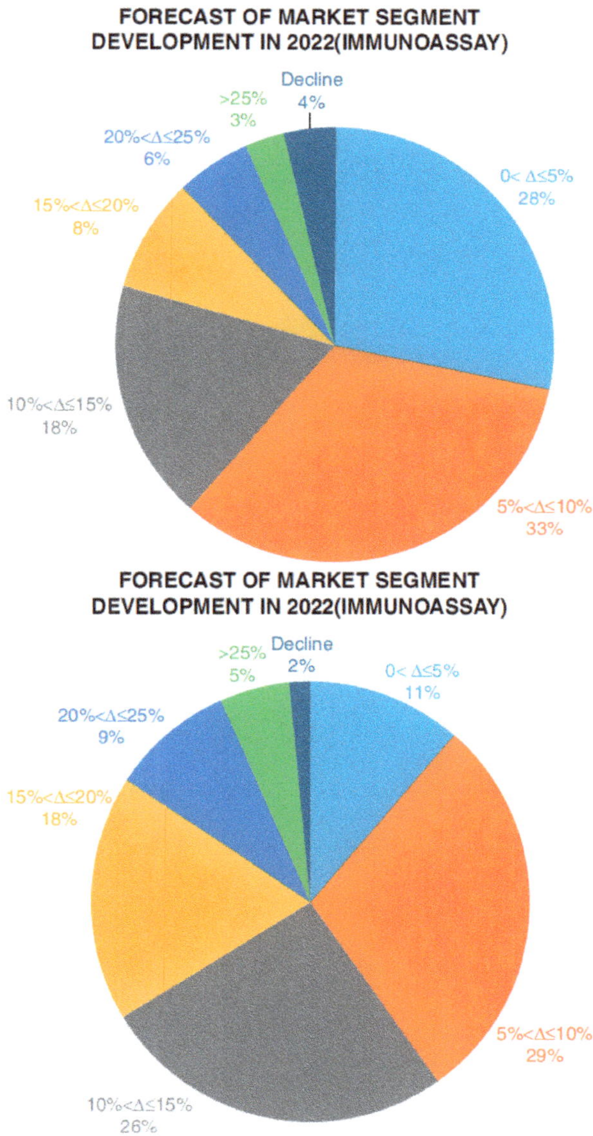

Fig. 1.4 Forecast of market segment development in 2022

Fig. 1.4 (continued)

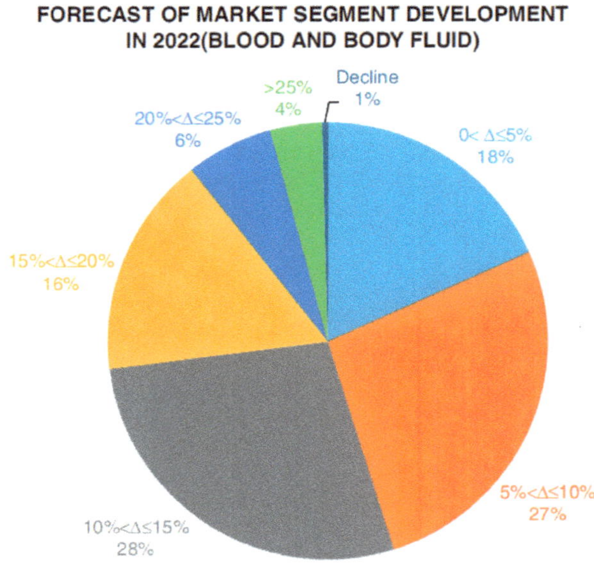

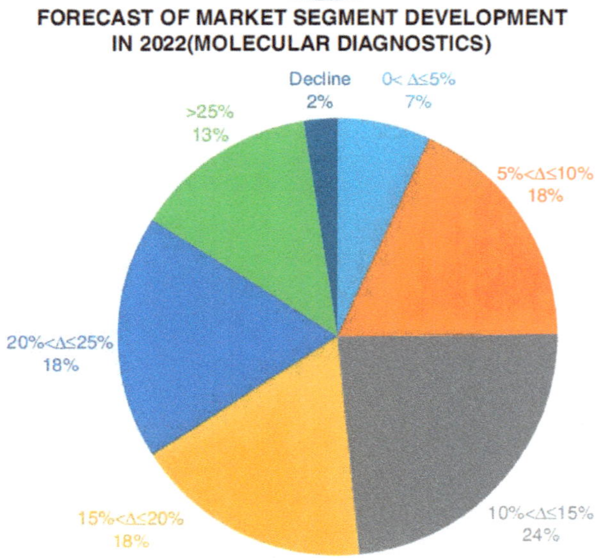

Fig. 1.4 (continued)

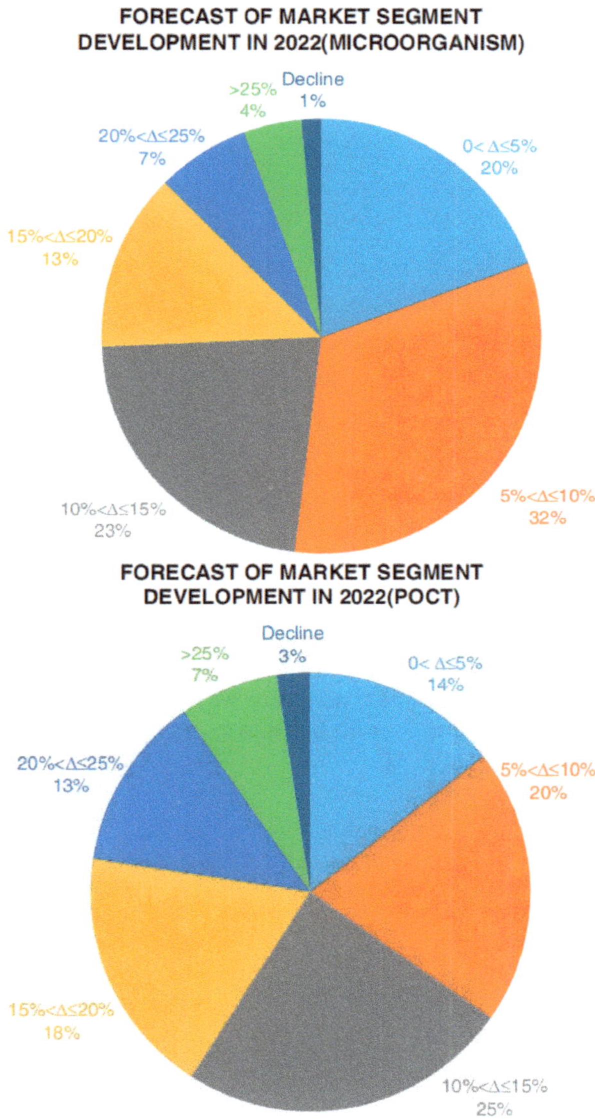

Fig. 1.4 (continued)

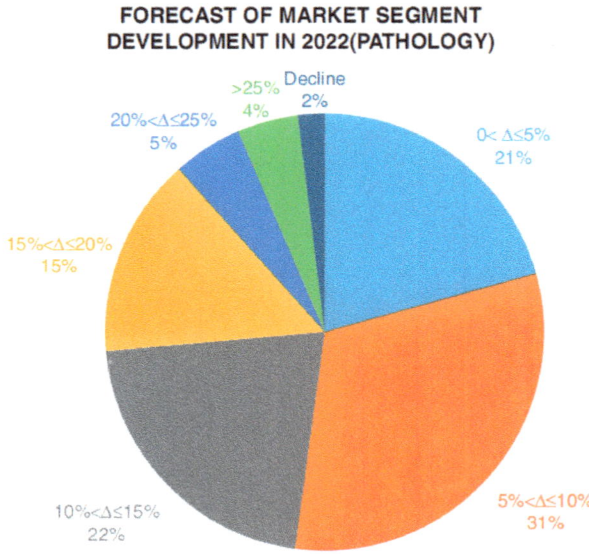

1.5 The Product Line with the Most Potential Development in the IVD Industry in the Next 3–5 Years According to the Feedback from the Enterprises Are as Follows (Fig. 1.5)

According to the comprehensive weighted order, the rankings were Molecular Diagnostics, Immunoassay, POCT, Blood and Body Fluid, Biochemistry, Microorganism, and Pathology, which were consistent with the survey results in 2020. The questionnaire also showed that the proportion of considering Molecular Diagnostics as the product line with the most development potential was 48%, which was less than 1% higher than the survey result in 2020, basically equal.

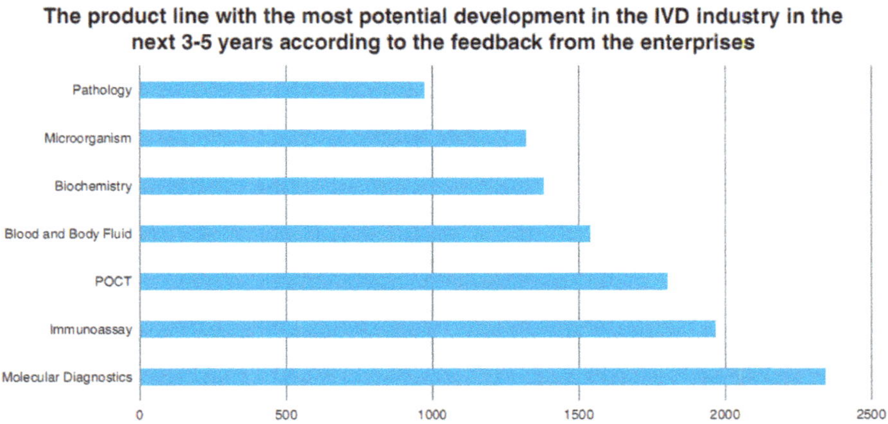

Fig. 1.5 The product line with the most potential development in the IVD industry in the next 3–5 years according to the feedback from the enterprises

1.6 The Factors Related to Industry Growth According to the Feedback from the Enterprises Are as Follows (Fig. 1.6)

According to the comprehensive weighted order, the rankings were "Overall Development of the Medical Industry, Clinical Needs, Technology and Product Innovation, Policy Support, and Promotion of Medical Reform". Compared with the survey results in 2020, the "Strengthening of Government Input" moved down to the seventh place, and the "Improvement of Living Standards" moved up to the sixth place. However, in the past 3 years, all factors had maintained the characteristics of rigid demand.

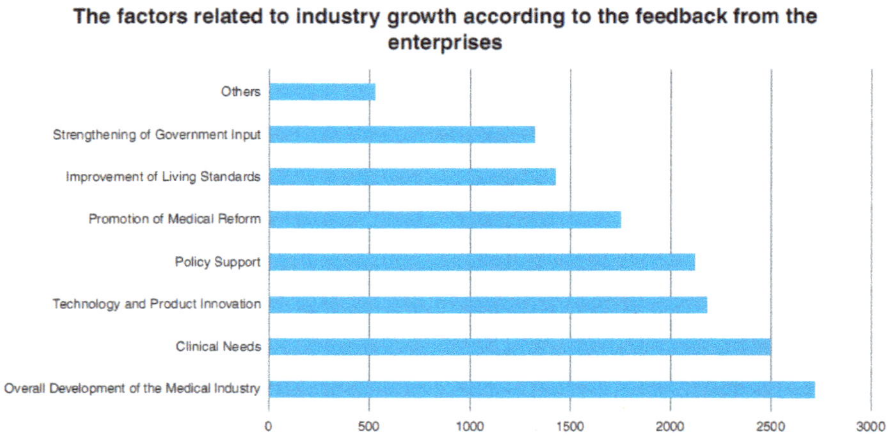

Fig. 1.6 The factors related to industry growth according to the feedback from the enterprises

1.7 Analysis of Difficulties Encountered in Industry Development (Fig. 1.7)

According to the comprehensive weighted order, the rankings were Product R&D, Product Registration, Medical Insurance Fees, Marketing, Talent Shortage, Capital and Financing. Compared with the 2020 survey results, "Marketing" and "Capital and Financing" swapped and the former ranked fourth, and it was the first time in the past 3 years that "Marketing" was second only to "Medical Insurance Fees".

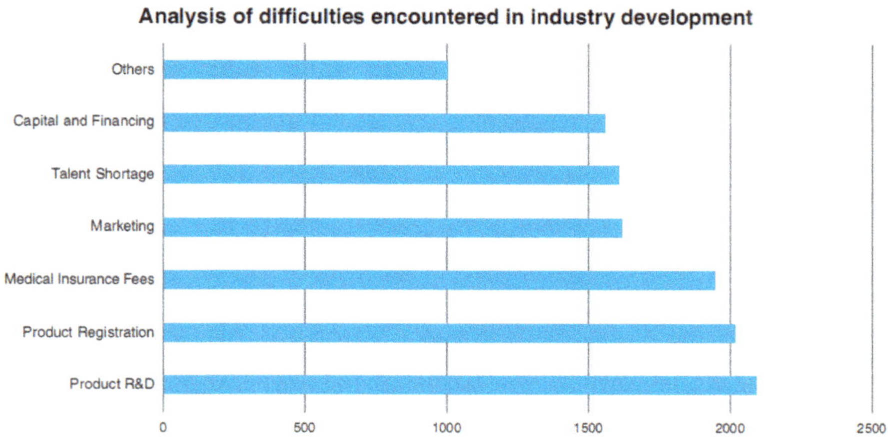

Fig. 1.7 Analysis of difficulties encountered in industry development

1.8 The Support That the Company Considers Most Urgently Needed (Fig. 1.8)

According to the comprehensive weighted order, the rankings were Medical Insurance Fees, Funds, Procurement Bidding, Optimization of Product Registration Process, Investment and Financing, Tax Policy, Government Project Funding, etc. Since this option was first added to the questionnaire in 2017, "Optimizing the Product Registration Process" has always been the first choice of support item, but it dropped to the fourth in this survey, "Medical Insurance Fees" moved up to the first, "Funds" moved up to the second from the fourth in 2020, and "Procurement Bidding" remained the third.

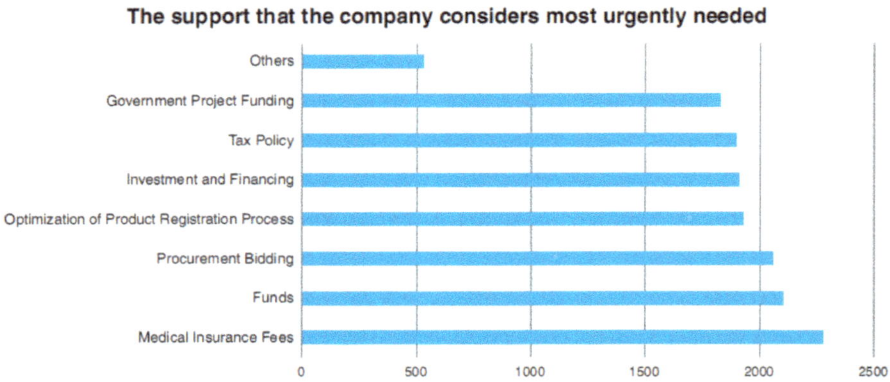

Fig. 1.8 The support that the company considers most urgently needed

1.9 Product Registration

According to the "Announcement on Approving the Registration of Medical Device Products" published by the NMPA (National Medical Products Administration) every month, the approval data are from the products registered for the first time, and the statistical data show that.

1.9.1 Registration of Domestic Products

By December 2021, the NMPA had approved 1710 medical device products (including IVD products) in 2021, an increase of 9% compared with 2020 [1]. Among them, there were 237 domestic Class III IVD products (including reagents and related testing instruments), accounting for about 14% of the total number of registered products. The distribution of registered products includes Beijing (34), Jiangsu (39), Guangdong (60), Shanghai (18), Zhejiang (15), Shandong (15), Jilin (3), Henan (10), Tianjin (9), Sichuan (10), Hubei (2), Chongqing (3), Fujian (14), Hunan (3), Anhui (1), Shaanxi (1).

1.9.2 Registration of Imported Products

By December 2021, the NMPA had approved the registration of 335 domestic Class III and imported IVD products, including 237 domestic Class III IVD products, accounting for 71% of IVD products; 98 imported IVD products, accounting for 29% of IVD products.

There is no exact data of the registration of domestic Class II and Filed Class I products approved by each provincial or municipal administration (Table 1.10).

Table 1.10 Data analysis of approved registration of medical device products (medical devices registered for the first time) issued by NMPA

Project content	2018	2019	2020	2021	Year on year
Medical device products approved by registration	1193	1726	1572	1710	9%
IVD products	307	524	448	335	−25%
Domestic Class III diagnostic products	172	352	326	237	−27%
Imported diagnostic products	135	172	122	98	−20%

(Unit: item)

It is noteworthy that:

1. The number of medical device products approved for registration in 2021 increased by 9% over 2020, which was close to the number approved for registration in 2019.
2. In 2021, the proportion of IVD products in all approved registration of medical device products decreased by 25% over 2020, indicating that in the second year of the COVID-19 outbreak, the registration of detecting products other than COVID-19-related products may still be affected.
3. In 2021, the NMPA approved 14 COVID-19-detecting reagents, including 9 nucleic acid-detecting reagents and 5 antibody-detecting reagents. At present, a total of 68 COVID-19-detecting reagents (including 34 nucleic acid testing reagents, 31 antibody-detecting reagents and 3 antigen-detecting reagents) have been approved in China.

1.10 Changes in Upstream, Midstream and Downstream of the Industry

Based on the summary of IVD-related industry analysis reports collected in 2021, we analyzed the upstream, midstream and downstream situations of the industry.

1.10.1 Upstream

The upstream scale of IVD was about 24 billion CNY with a growth rate of about 20%. The market share of imported brands was about 80%.

IVD raw materials include bioactive/nonbioactive materials used for preparing IVD reagents and key components required for developing IVD equipment. Among them, the quality of reaction enzyme, antigen, antibody and core component is the core factor of the performance of IVD product, which directly affects the accuracy, specificity and stability of the product and plays a key role in the IVD industrial chain. With the rapid development of the IVD industry in China, the market demand for IVD raw materials (enzymes, antigens, antibodies, etc.) as the upstream of the industrial chain is increasing rapidly. The market size was 8.2 billion CNY in 2019, and it is expected to grow to 20 billion CNY in 2024 at a CAGR of 19.4%. From the perspective of market structure, the key raw materials of IVD reagents in China mainly rely on imports: in 2019, imported products accounted for 88% of the market share of the raw materials for IVD reagents. The market size of domestic products was only one billion CNY, but it is growing rapidly with a CAGR of 30.6% in 2015–2019. As domestic enterprises gradually attach importance to the R&D of key technologies of raw materials and the localization of the supply chain of the biotechnology industry, it is expected that domestic products will gradually replace imported products. Domestic reagent manufacturers have reached a certain size by making great efforts to introduce, digest and absorb technology in recent years, and some manufacturers with reasonable size can meet part of the market demand. The quality of IVD products is largely determined by upstream IVD reagent raw materials. However, due to the fierce competition in the industry, some manufacturers have loosened quality control of raw materials in order to reduce production costs, which is an important factor for the uneven quality in the raw material production industry in China. In general, there is still a certain gap between the performance and stability of domestic products and foreign products, so the former cannot meet the needs of high-end projects. However, we can also see that some excellent domestic raw material suppliers, under the pressure of COVID-19, vigorously promote R&D, demand themselves with the highest international standard, and timely promote the replacement with domestic raw materials. The revenue of COVID-19-related antigens, antibodies, enzymes and other raw materials has increased dramatically, and many raw material manufacturers with revenue of more than 100 million have emerged. Among them, Fapon Biotech, Vazyme, Acrobiosystems, Sino Biological, Hzymes Biotech, Yeasen Biotechnology, Novoprotein, Cusabio and other companies have reached a certain market size. At present, Vazyme has been listed on the Science and Technology Innovation Board, and Acrobiosystems and Sino Biological have been listed on the GEM, with a total market value of more than 80 billion CNY. Fapon has also entered the waiting list for GEM IPO. In addition, many upstream raw material enterprises, such as Hzymes Biotech, Yeasen, Novoprotein, BiOligo, GeneMind, Bioeast, and Monad, have all achieved financing with a scale of more than 100 million CNY, and the accumulated financing amount is nearly two billion CNY.

1.10.2 Midstream

Biochemistry: Biochemical tests accounted for about 20% of the IVD market share with a growth rate of less than 5% and a localization rate of more than 60%.

Biochemical diagnosis is to obtain clinical judgment information based on biochemical indexes in the human body, such as enzymes, lipids, saccharides, proteins and inorganic elements, which is applied to routine testing items in medical institutions, CDC and third-party laboratories, including liver function, kidney function, blood glucose, blood fat, cardiovascular, and diabetes detection. Biochemical industry is one of the earliest and most mature diagnostic means of IVD in China. Its market growth is mainly driven by the sales of instruments and the pipeline of biochemical immunity, while reagents grow slowly. The substitution rate of domestic biochemical reagents is about 70%. At present, there are more than 200 domestic biochemical reagent manufacturers and more than 100 biochemical detection projects. The industry barrier is low, and the competition has entered the red ocean model. Domestic high-speed biochemical instruments are developing rapidly. Domestic biochemical analyzers with speeds below 800 account for 60–70% of the market share. More than 10 domestic enterprises can produce analyzers with speed of 1000 and 2000. In the biochemical field, the enterprise can maintain stable development by adhering to the route of R&D of high-quality products and reducing the cost of upstream raw materials. The cooperative development of pipelines, biochemical closed systems and biochemical instruments with other products (such as immunization) is an important direction for the development of biochemical enterprises in the future.

Immunization: Driven by the chemiluminescence market, immunodiagnosis is a segment with the largest scale and most new varieties in the IVD field in recent years. At present, it accounts for more than 30% of the IVD market share with a growth rate of about 15%. The localization rate is 25%–30%.

Immunodiagnosis is the largest sub-industry of IVD and is still developing rapidly. Immunodiagnosis can be classified into radioimmunoassay, ELISA, immunochromatography and chemiluminescence by methodological classification.

ELISA is still widely used because of its advantages such as fast detection and low cost. Domestic products account for more than 70% of the ELISA market share. Multinational enterprises and more and more domestic enterprises have ELISA product lines, and the market competition is similar to the biochemistry market. In recent years, most of the patent applications of Roche and other global leading enterprises adopt chemiluminescence technology, and the domestic immunization market also shows a trend of chemiluminescence replacing ELISA.

The market share of domestic products in the field of chemiluminescence is more than 20%. The domestic laboratory market is dominated by tertiary hospital customers, and the future growth momentum will come from the secondary and tertiary hospital market, which accounts for 65%. Under the background of medical insurance cost control, domestic luminescence enterprises are facing the pressure of price reduction. The fundamental competitiveness to become bigger and stronger lies in continuous R&D innovation and powerful sales channels. At present, some domestic reagent kits are fairly mature, but some core reagent kits with high-performance requirements are still mostly imported products. Analysis of patent applications for immunochemical raw materials shows that these segments are dominated by foreign biomedical giants. Therefore, for domestic enterprises to realize import substitution, firstly, they should improve the product performance, enhance the R&D of raw materials and the quality control of instruments, and ensure the stability and high quality of raw materials and instruments. Secondly, they should, according to the clinical needs, provide menus of test items that meet the requirements of domestic users and cannot be provided by foreign investors and increase the number of installed instruments in hospitals through substantial test menus and complete supporting reagents. Thirdly, domestic instruments and reagents should be more cost-effective than imported products.

Molecular diagnostics: As one of the fastest growing segments of IVD, driven by the demand for nucleic acid testing for COVID-19, molecular diagnostics has a market share of about 20% with a growth rate of 20%. The localization rate is more than 50%.

According to different technology platforms, molecular detection can be divided into polymerase chain nucleic acid amplification (PCR), gene sequencing (NGS), fluorescence in situ hybridization, gene chip and nucleic acid mass spectrometry. Molecular diagnostics is mainly used in infectious diseases, tumor diagnosis, genetic disease diagnosis, eugenics, personalized medication, etc. Multinational companies focus on high-end instruments, represented by ThermoFisher, Bio-rad, Roche Quantitative PCR and Illumina Sequencer. In the field of mid-range instruments, it is easy to make a breakthrough in technology, such as nucleic acid extractors, PCR amplifiers, nucleic acid hybridization ovens and gene chip instruments, localization has been achieved and domestic products have occupied the leading market, while the localization of gene sequencer is breaking through, mainly in three ways: (1) merge and acquire a foreign sequencer company, and launch its own-brand sequencers based on the core technologies of the acquired company, such as BGI; (2) develop independently with internal research capacity; (3) cooperate with a well-known foreign sequencer manufacturer, and transform its sequencer prototype to form the company's own-brand sequencers with special purposes, such as Berry and Daan. During the COVID-19 pandemic, the market size of China's molecular detection industry has surged, and the demand for nucleic acid testing has led to a doubling of the sales of domestic PCR amplifiers and nucleic acid extractors. According to the report of China Insights Consultancy, the market size of PCR amplifiers in China was 6.6 billion CNY in 2020, which is expected to reach 20.6 billion CNY by 2030, with a CAGR of 12.0% from 2020 to 2030 [2]. In the post-COVID-19 era, PCR technology will advance towards high precision, high throughput and automation by improving the performance of polymerase and the processing capacity of PCR equipment. The development of molecular diagnostics will largely depend on the process of substitution with domestic products of upstream equipment. With policy support and more excellent enterprises moving to the upstream instrument side, molecular diagnostic instruments are expected to be substituted with domestic products faster.

Looking forward to the future, the largest application market of molecular diagnostics will be in the tumor field, including tumor susceptibility gene screening, early diagnostics of tumors, companion diagnostics of tumors and drug guidance, and monitoring after tumor recovery, forming a whole course and life cycle management model. Among them, companion diagnostics is the fastest-growing sub-industry in the molecular segment. Micromolecule targeting drugs, macromolecular mAb drugs, immunological therapy and CART therapy all require gene screening for maximum efficacy. With the rise of precision medicine, based on AI, big data and Internet platforms, molecular diagnostics will be used more and more widely.

Blood and Body Fluid: The blood and body fluid test market mainly includes coagulation tests, blood cell analysis, urinalysis, urinary sediment analysis, etc. The overall market accounts for less than 10% of the IVD market with a growth rate of 10% and a localization rate of more than 50%.

Blood and body fluid test mainly involves blood cell, urine and blood coagulation test, including blood analyzer, coagulation analyzer, urine analyzer and other equipment, detection reagents and consumables. The basic principle is mainly to apply various physical and chemical methods, involving technologies such as flow cytometry, electrical impedance, and photoelectric colorimetry, as well as the detection of routine blood tests, thrombus and hemostasis, routine urine tests and other items.

Blood Coagulation At present, domestic enterprises have less than 20% of the share in the coagulation market, and foreign enterprises have absolute advantages, accounting for more than 80% of the market share. The three foreign giants of blood coagulation are IL (Werfen Group), Sysmex and Stago. With the deepening of hierarchical medical policy and the constant promotion of community hospitals and other related concepts in recent 2 years, the market for mid-range and low-end coagulation analyzers will increase significantly.

Blood Cell After decades of development in the field of blood cell tests, two blood cell giants have emerged, namely Sysmex and Mindray, accounting for 60% of the market share; at the same time, rising stars like Dymind have also emerged, and Maccura has also stepped up its layout in the high-end blood cell market in recent years. Blood cell analysis has also been upgraded from manual method to the current blood cell pipeline.

Urinalysis In the past market share of urine test analyzers, foreign brands have been occupying a high proportion. With the increasing maturity of the technology of domestic brands, domestic brands have gradually replaced imported products with a market share of more than 50%. Many domestic enterprises have started the ball rolling in the secondary and tertiary markets, such as Dirui and Urit. In the future, urinalysis will require higher speed, portability and accuracy to meet the needs of families, individuals and primary care; at the same time, in large hospitals and independent third-party laboratories, automatic pipelines for urinalysis will be more widely used.

With the continuous upgrading and improvement of automated instruments in the blood and body fluid market, another key competitive advantage in the future is the refinement and diversification of parameters. With the increasingly diversified demands for blood and body fluid test items in the Grade-A tertiary and Grade-A secondary hospitals, routine items obviously do not meet the clinical needs of the high-end market. Therefore, diversified parameters and reliable test results will be the key technologies for manufacturers to compete in the high-end market.

POCT: The current market size of POCT accounts for about 15% of the overall IVD market with a growth rate of about 15%. The localization rate is more than 50%.

From the perspective of the application field, POCT products can be used in clinical tests, chronic disease monitoring, emergency anti-terrorism, disaster medical rescue, infectious disease monitoring, inspection and quarantine, food safety, drug examination and other public health fields. From the perspective of application sites, POCT products can be used in a variety of occasions, including wards, outpatient departments, emergency departments, laboratories, operating rooms, and care units in large hospitals; primary hospitals, community clinics and private clinics; health service centers, disease prevention and control centers, medical rescue sites for disasters, food safety testing sites, environmental protection sites; customs quarantine control, fast screening of illegal drugs; forensic medicine sites; biological anti-terrorism sites, etc.

From the perspective of the growth rate of segments, POCT products for cardiac markers and infectious diseases are in a rapid growth period with rapid demand growth and large development space in the future. This is because saving cardiovascular patients requires much higher timeliness than treating other diseases, and POCT meets this demand with its high detection speed. Therefore, cardiovascular detection has become the fastest-growing application of POCT. POCT for infectious diseases is mainly a product for primary field screening and rapid detection of various common infectious diseases and major infectious diseases, including AIDS, syphilis, viral hepatitis, malaria, and influenza. Infectious diseases have attracted different degrees of attention worldwide because of their characteristics of infectivity, epidemicity, territoriality and seasonality. China has also gradually increased the prevention and monitoring of major infectious diseases. POCT products have become an important tool for the prevention and control of related infectious diseases. As in this pandemic, COVID-19-related POCT detection products are widely used in the domestic detection field abroad.

POCT is one of the fastest-growing fields in the IVD industry. Due to the increasing degree of aging and uneven distribution of medical resources, and thanks to the advancement of hierarchical medical policy and medicare reform policy, China's POCT industry will still maintain rapid growth in the next few years. With the development of precision medicine in recent years, there are higher requirements for the precision of medical detection instruments. Biochip, microfluidics, mass spectrometer, reverse transcription polymerase chain reaction, isothermal amplification, CRISPR gene editing and other technologies are combined with the POCT platform to promote the rapid development of POCT towards refinement. In addition, the combination of artificial intelligence, mobile intelligent devices, intelligent APP, wearable devices, biosensors and POCT detection technology can realize remote patient monitoring and home medical services, which is of great significance for chronic disease and health monitoring.

In the field of POCT, which is widely used and extensively demanded by the market, Chinese enterprises have made continuous progress in technology. They are not very far behind foreign enterprises and are more cost-effective. In the future, it is more and more likely to realize substitution with domestic products. "Miniaturization", "Integration", "Informatization" and "Intelligence" have become higher requirements for the technical development and integration of POCT. In the future, enterprises with the ability of upstream innovation and R&D and downstream channel promotion as well as the resources of industry–university–research collaboration will be more competitive.

Microorganism: China's microbiological diagnostics field started late with a share of no more than 5% and a growth rate of 10%. At present, the microorganism market is still dominated by imported products, and domestic products account for about 20%.

At present, the main microorganism detection platforms include conventional technologies, serum immunology, molecular diagnostics and mass spectrometry. Conventional methods and serum immunology are relatively mature. Immunoassay can only detect antibodies against known types of bacteria, which has high sensitivity, specificity and convenience, but the types of pathogenic bacteria that can be detected are not complete. Mass spectrometry and molecular diagnostics are new technologies. The core barrier of mass spectrometry is the traceability of bacteria banks. A cloud database of microbial protein fingerprints needs to be established. The representative domestic enterprises of mass spectrometry are Bioyong and Autobio, and the representative foreign enterprises are Bruker, Mérieux and BD; the core of gene test method lies in the establishment of bacterial gene databases and the selection of detection method. The cost of macro genome sequencing is high, and only known bacteria can be detected by PCR. The representative enterprises in molecular diagnostics are BGI, Jiangxi PrecisionGene, and Dynamiker Biotech, which focuses on the field of fungus detection. In the international market, Mérieux is a leading enterprise in the global microbiological diagnostics industry, covering all technical platforms in the field of microbiological diagnostics and accounting for 60% of the global market share of microbiological diagnostics.

Automation and intelligence are the future development direction of microorganism detection: due to emerging infectious diseases, nosocomial infection and increased antibiotic resistance, there will be an increasing demand for microbiology and virology in the next 5 years. Automated and intelligent microorganism detection equipment can improve the efficiency of testing microbial content of the sample, reduce the time required in routine testing, and detect the number and types of microorganisms in a short time; at the same time, the testing technology should guarantee the test results and improve the precision and scientific nature of the test.

Pathology: China's pathology market accounts for about 3% of the overall IVD market with a growth rate of 10%. The localization rate is about 20%.

Pathology usually includes histopathology, cytopathology and molecular pathology. Immunohistochemical technique is the most widely used in clinical practice, which can be used for the diagnosis and differential diagnosis of malignant tumors, the determination of the primary site of metastatic tumors, the further pathological typing of tumors, the determination of histological classification of soft tissue tumors, the discovery of micrometastases and the provision of a basis for clinical treatment.

At present, the commonly used molecular pathological examination techniques include chromosome karyotype analysis, fluorescence in situ hybridization, PCR, gene chip and first-generation sequencing. In the general trend of precision medicine, molecular pathology plays an important role in the detection of tumors, infectious diseases and genetic diseases. At present, molecular pathological examination equipment is dominated by international brands.

In China, cytopathology is mainly used for cervical cancer screening. TCT screening of cervical cancer accounts for 80% of the total cytopathology market, while there are too few examination items for other types of cancer.

The pain points of pathological diagnosis lie in the scarcity of pathologists and technicians and the seriously uneven distribution of resources. However, with the vigorous development of artificial intelligence, digital section scanning technology and the Internet, digital remote pathological consultation + AI-assisted diagnosis have taken root all over the country and become increasingly complete and mature, which could effectively give play to the technical advantages of the pathology department of superior hospitals, promote the subsidence of good pathologists and help promote hierarchical medicare.

The market size of immunohistochemical pathology in China is growing steadily. According to the data of Market & Market, the global immunohistochemistry market size was about 1.9 billion USD in 2020, and it is expected to grow to 2.7 billion USD in 2025 with a CAGR of 6.6% [3]. According to the data of Intelligence Research Group, the CAGR of China's immunohistochemistry market from 2012 to 2017 was 14.27%, which was significantly higher than the global average. With the promotion of national hierarchical medicare, the pathological diagnosis ability of primary care is bound to improve, which will bring a sustained and steady growth momentum to the development of the pathological diagnostics industry, and is conducive to the development of domestic brands.

1.10.3 Downstream

Most downstream users of IVD include medical institutions, independent medical laboratories, blood banks, physical examination centers and food testing markets. The downstream market was expected to grow by a two-digit percentage in 2021. On reason was that the routine business of medical institutions was expected to recover in 2021 from 2020. Another reason was the growing demand for nucleic acid testing of inpatients and the regular testing of COVID-19 prevention and control in various regions.

1.10.3.1 Medical Institutions

According to the statistics of the National Health Commission, as of the end of 2021, there were 1,030,935 medical and health institutions nationwide, an increase of 8013 over the previous year. Among them were 36,570 hospitals, 977,790 primary medical and health institutions and 13,276 professional public health institutions. Compared with the previous year, there were 1176 more hospitals and 7754 more primary medical and health institutions.

Person-times of diagnosis and treatment and person-times of hospitalization: In 2021, medical and health institutions nationwide had a total of 8.47 billion person-times of diagnosis and treatment, an increase of 730 million person-times over the previous year (an increase of 9.4%). In 2021, residents visited medical and health institutions 6.0 times on average. In the total amount of diagnosis and treatment in 2021, there were 3.88 billion person-times (45.8%) in hospitals, 4.25 billion person-times (50.2%) in primary medical and health institutions, and 340 million person-times (4.0%) in other medical and health institutions. Compared with the previous year, 560 million more person-times of diagnosis and treatment were in hospitals, and 130 million more person-times of diagnosis and treatment were in primary medical and health institutions. The total national health expenditure in 2021 was estimated to be 7559.36 billion CNY, including 2071.85 billion CNY on government health expenditure, accounting for 27.4%; 3392.03 billion CNY on social health expenditure, accounting for 44.9%; 2095.48 billion CNY on personal health expenditure, accounting for 27.7%. The per capita total health expenditure was 5348.1 CNY, and the proportion of total health expenditure in GDP was 6.5% [4].

1.10.3.2 Third-Party Medical Laboratory

In 2021, the third-party independent laboratory industry achieved rapid development with significant year-on-year growth. The third-party routine testing business developed well. At the same time, as the main force of nucleic acid testing, third-party laboratories play an important role in centralized screening in various regions and individual testing for individual customers. In the first three quarters of 2021, the performance of KingMed Diagnostics, Dean, BGI, Labway, Berry, Novogene, and other listed companies focusing on third-party business increased by 33%.

1.10.3.3 Physical Examination Center

With the gradual enhancement of the health awareness of urban residents, the health consumption demand of residents has increased significantly, and the per capita health care expenditure has increased significantly, which has strongly promoted the development of the physical examination industry. In 2020, the person-times of physical examination in China was about 464 million with a year-on-year growth of 4.5%; in 2020, the market size of physical examination in China was about 190.6 billion CNY with a year-on-year growth of 11% [5]. With the increasingly close integration of artificial intelligence, big data and people's physical examination, as well as the high-tech integration of people's physical examination-related data information, the past single service treatment model may be transformed into a modern information model of integrated "Prevention - Treatment – Maintenance". The revenue of Meinian Healthcare, a listed company engaged in physical examination, increased by 32% year on year in the first three quarters of 2021.

1.11 General Development Trends of Future Technology and Products

Integration, high throughput, immediacy, portability and precision medicine are the future development direction of products and technologies in the diagnostics industry. At the same time, the constant inburst and upgrade and iteration of new technologies and new products such as mass spectrometry and mobile detection system have brought broader application prospects to the IVD field.

1.11.1 Integration and High Throughput

In the process of China's health system reform, based on the establishment of the universal medical security system, a large number of medical needs have been released, and the number of patients and specimens has increased. The medical laboratory department urgently needs to obtain more reliable test data and information in the shortest time, so it is particularly important to provide faster and more comprehensive diagnosis and treatment basis for the clinic. Therefore, medical laboratories have a strong demand for high-throughput, high-efficiency and high-safety pipeline products. Secondly, with the promotion of hierarchical medicare, the workload of outpatient services has been transferred to lower-level hospitals, and the sample size of primary medical institutions has gradually increased. Secondary hospitals, including a large number of county-level hospitals, also have potential demand for pipelines. In addition, the localization of pipeline products is an important way to reduce the cost of clinical laboratories. China's pipeline market has great potential. In the next 10–20 years, there will be a large number of intelligent pipelines in the upstream product side of the IVD industry. A large number of whole laboratory pipelines, biochemical immunology pipelines, blood cell pipelines, molecular pipelines, urine pipelines, blood coagulation pipelines and pipelines for other segments will enter the end market. The nucleic acid testing pipeline is undoubtedly another direction of future industry innovation. It is feasible to focus on the pipeline development of infectious disease diagnosis.

1.11.2 Immediacy and Portability

POCT products are easy to operate, and can achieve spot sampling and timely results, which are very suitable for the application scenarios of primary medical institutions, emergency and critical wards and clinical departments. With the full implementation of the hierarchical medical policy, and the large-scale construction of five major emergency centers for pectoralgia, apoplexy, trauma, maternal near miss, and critical neonates with 4000 counties in China as the core units, POCT, as a representative of immediate and portable equipment, can release the needs of emergency and primary institutions and has a broad market. With the aging of the population and the prevalence of chronic diseases, especially in the prevention and control of public health, the conventional PCR nucleic acid testing technology cannot meet the needs of screening and detection due to its cumbersome process, complex operation, and the restrictions such as the need for centralized submission for testing. By contrast, by combining the characteristics of high sensitivity and specificity of molecular diagnosis and the advantages of the POCT platform, molecular POCT breaks through the restrictions of existing testing technologies on personnel and places, effectively shorting the testing time and improving convenience. Driven by the pandemic, molecular diagnostic POCT accelerated to the stage of clinical detection. In the future, the application of nucleic acid testing POCT will be able to detect a variety of pathogens and be applicable to multiple departments and a variety of application scenarios. At the same time, it can also detect human gene targets and promote precise and rational drug use.

1.11.3 Precision Medicine and Companion Diagnostics

According to 2020 statistics, the number of cancer cases in China is 4.57 million, and the number of cancer deaths is three million. China has a large base of cancer patients and many new cancer patients; the number of new cancer cases and cancer deaths ranks first in the world [6]. Both the number and the increment drive the patient's demand for companion diagnosis. At present, the top 10 sales of tumor drugs in China are tumor-targeting drugs, accounting for more than 50% of the global market share of anti-tumor prescription. More and more drugs used by pharmaceutical companies need diagnostic results as a reference, especially the introduction of many new drugs needs companion diagnostic testing. There is great potential for growth in companion diagnostics. In addition, with the deepening of the cooperation model of companion diagnostics and drug development, the R&D of diagnostic products will continue to accelerate.

1.11.4 Gene Sequencing Technology

Gene sequencing technology is the main technology of companion diagnosis, which is still in the development stage. With the research and development of sequencing technology, the development of the accompanying diagnostics market will change dramatically. The continuous investment of capital in recent years has provided "Logistics Support" for the field of companion diagnostics. To encourage the development of precision medicine in China, in 2015, the Ministry of Science and Technology determined to invest 60 billion CNY in developing the precision medicine strategy by 2030, providing strategic direction for the development of companion diagnostics.

1.11.5 Mass Spectrometry

At present, many domestic IVD enterprises have entered the mass spectrometry field, which started late and developed slowly. Developed countries in Europe and the United States have widely carried out mass spectrometry clinical chemical test projects, including neonatal screening, detection of hormones and their metabolites, therapeutic drug monitoring, vitamin D detection and trace element detection. From 2004 to 2020, dozens of innovative clinical mass spectrometry enterprises emerged in China. Due to the restrictions of factors such as access to fee list, access to reagent registration, standardization of methodology, laboratory conditions and lack of talents, the development of domestic enterprises is limited at present. With the constant improvement of such constraints, the mass spectrometry industry will enter the fast lane of development. Now more than 10 domestic mass spectrometers have obtained registration certificates. In addition, with the further development of LDT, many projects suitable for detection by mass spectrometers will continue to be launched, creating conditions for mass spectrometry to be extensively applied in clinical practice.

1.11.6 Mobile Testing System

Mobile sampling and mobile testing schemes have been widely used in public health prevention and control, played an important role and enhanced the emergency handling capacity of local authorities in public health emergencies. The mobile rapid nucleic acid testing vehicle is equipped with a low-throughput or medium-throughput nucleic acid tester and rapid virus inactivation equipment as well as mobile negative pressure disinfection chamber and 5G data real-time transmission function, which can be put into use in public places such as stations, squares, and airports. And it can provide timely and rapid testing services for remote areas and emergency scenes. This kind of testing system can meet urgent testing requirements under a variety of mobile scenarios. For example, onsite testing of multiple indicators can be realized in the ambulance in the future, and data can be transmitted to the first-aid consulting room in advance through the 5G network to improve treatment efficiency. At present, the development of various diagnostic technologies and products makes it possible to carry out all kinds of testing on a mobile vehicle, especially mobile nucleic acid testing systems designed for COVID-19, makes all kinds of mobile detection possible.

1.11.7 New Markers and New Inspection Items

There are many clinical needs for diagnosis and confirmation of the diagnosis of diseases. The country's annual investment in the field of basic science promotes the discovery and development of new markers by the research team, resulting in the continuous advancement of basic research.

Professor Yu Zujiang's team of The First Affiliated Hospital of Zhengzhou University and academician Li Lanjuan's team of Zhejiang University have jointly found that microbial markers could be used as an auxiliary tool for noninvasive diagnosis of COVID-19. ACE2 is a target of SARS-CoV-24, which is expressed in the lung, the liver, the kidney, the brain and small intestine epithelium. SARS-CoV-2 activates the intestinal ACE2 receptor and triggers inflammation, causing gastrointestinal symptoms and microbial dysbacteriosis. The treatise of the original research results has been published in "Gut", the official journal of the British Society of Gastroenterology.

The research team of the State Key Laboratory for Quality Research of Traditional Chinese Medicine of Macao University of Science and Technology has successfully designed the first TiO2-PGC chip in the world. Its extremely sensitive analytical technique can detect minor changes in the trace sugar chains of glycoproteins in complex sugar chains. The researchers analyzed the immunoglobulin in human serum and the serum of patients with rheumatoid arthritis (RA) with this innovative technology, and found that there were 21 diagnostic markers that could distinguish RA patients, among which, the specificity and sensitivity of the combination of two sulfonated N-glycan markers in diagnosing RA were about 85%, and it could differentiate RA from ankylosing spondylitis and osteoarthritis. This was an important breakthrough in the field of glycomics and rheumatoid arthritis diagnostics, which has provided a good technical platform for the in-depth study of glycomics.

A research team of Yokohama City University in Japan announced that it had jointly developed new diagnostic markers for ovarian clear cell carcinoma. Through analysis of protein components, it was found that ovarian clear cell carcinoma would characteristically produce TFPI2, in the hope of providing an effective reference for future diagnosis and treatment through the joint examination of "TFPI2" and existing ovarian cancer markers.

Innovative Technology: As IVD has a wide range of application scenarios and involves many techniques, and many detection needs have not been met, a variety of new technologies will continue to be developed, such as digital PCR systems, microfluidic chips, gene editing technology, noninvasive Blood Glucose Monitoring technology, intelligent wearables, third and fourth generation sequencing, etc.

In China, some manufacturers have obtained registration certificates for digital PCR instruments; however, no testing reagent has obtained registration certificate yet. Therefore, the market has not realized the advantages of digital PCR systems. There are various types of microfluidic chips, but until now, none of them has created a mainstream application scenario. All conditions above bring a lot of development potential to IVD enterprises. As a gene editing technology that has won the Nobel Prize, it is expected by everyone to generate specific products and application scenarios, bringing new surprises to the IVD industry. Although the Continuous Glucose Monitoring system is developing rapidly, the real noninvasive glucose monitoring system has not yet appeared. It is believed that with the continuous development of science and technology, the launch of noninvasive glucose monitoring will bring about a revolution in glucose monitoring.

The demand for intelligent wearables is increasing, and the relationship between manufacturers and end users has changed significantly. With the help of intelligent information, clinicians improve diagnosis, monitoring and prevention of diseases. At the same time, patients also avoid unnecessary visits. Both patients and consumers can obtain valuable advice on lifestyle and diet. In the context of increasing chronic diseases and aging, preventive and personalized care has become a new treatment. Those technologies that can support patients' behavior changes and bring positive changes in patients' lifestyles will be in high demand in the future.

The third-generation sequencer and the fourth-generation sequencer can complete single-molecule sequencing and direct RNA sequencing. After more than 10 years of development, the research on gene expression regulation based on single cell is gradually becoming mainstream. In third-generation sequencing, gene sequencing is studied in two dimensions of time (cell cycle) and space (organ distribution) with a single cell as a unit to record the mechanism details of gene expression regulation of cells in the original tissue. The fourth-generation sequencer can directly sequence RNA molecules at the single-cell level and single-molecule resolution and recognize the modified nucleotides not directly transcribed in the sequence. Therefore, the fourth-generation RNA direct detection technology must simultaneously utilize nanopore technology and on-chip Raman spectroscopy, which has the characteristics of fast sequencing and real-time monitoring of sequenced data.

Gene editing technology CRISPR: The gene editing technology CRISPR is on its way to commercialization. The latest progress in genetic engineering has started new changes in biological and translational applications. CRISPR-Cas9 and its variants can perform multiple operations on genome functions. This genome editing covers almost all industries involving biological systems, mainly including biotechnology, agricultural technology, therapeutics and diagnostics. A wide range of products in the biotechnology market, including CRISPR-Cas9, provide the required endonuclease and gene editing reagents. At present, CRISPR technology is still in the research stage in the diagnosis field. A lot of development work is still needed before the diagnostic test based on CRISPR technology can be used in practice. Today, only a few key institutions are committed to the diagnostic applications of CRISPR technology.

1.12 Industry Forums and Conferences

1.12.1 Major Chinese Forums in 2021

(a) 2021 The fourth Immuno-therapy & Companion Diagnostic Development Conference (Shanghai, December)
(b) 2021 China International Medical Innovation Forum (CMIF) (Suzhou, November)
(c) 2021 The 13th IVD China Summit (during CMEF) (Shenzhen, October)
(d) 2021 (The 5th) China Medical Laboratory Summit (Enmore) (Nanjing, September)
(e) 2021 The sixth World Precision Medicine (China) Summit (Guangzhou, August)
(f) The eighth China IVD Industry Investment CEO Conference (Taicang, July).
(g) 2021 The seventh Molecular Diagnostic Technology and Application Forum (Shanghai, May)
(h) 2021 (The 9th) Molecular Diagnostics Summit (Suzhou, March)
(During the Enmore EBC Bioindustry Conference)
(i) The eighth China IVD Industry Development Conference (Chongqing, March).

1.12.2 Major Chinese Expos

(a) The 85th China International Medical Equipment (Autumn) Fair CMEF (Shenzhen).
(b) The 12th National Conference of Clinical Laboratory Management and 2021 Clinical Examination Equipment and Products Exhibition CCLAB (Xi'an, postponed twice).
(c) The 17th National Conference & Expo of Laboratory Medicine of the Chinese Medical Association NCLM (Changsha, postponed twice to the beginning of 2022).
(d) The seventh National Conference of Clinical Laboratory Medicine Technology and Application, the 4th "Belt and Road" Laboratory Summit, and the seventh National Clinical Laboratory Equipment Exhibition CCLTA (Suzhou, offline + online).
(e) 2021 Annual Meeting of Laboratory Physicians of the Chinese Medical Doctor Association and the 16th National Laboratory and Clinical Conference (CDMA) (Zhuhai)
(f) The 84th China International Medical Equipment (Spring) Fair CMEF (Shanghai).
(g) The 18th China (International) Laboratory Medicine and Blood Transfusion Instrument and Reagent Expo (Chongqing, offline + online).
(h) "Voice of Innovation" The sixth China Experimental Medicine Conference CCEM (Chongqing, offline + online).

1.12.3 Major Overseas Expos

(a) 2021 MEDICA: This session of MEDICA was the first offline expo resumed after the pandemic in Germany with an exhibition area of 115,000 square meters, attracting excellent enterprises from nearly 70 countries. There were 3141 exhibitors in the MEDICA with a total number of 46,000 visitors. It also holds online expos and live broadcasts simultaneously so that the audience can learn about innovation in all medical fields.
(b) The 73rd AACC Annual Scientific Meeting & Clinical Lab Expo (AACC): The 73rd AACC was held in Atlanta, USA, from September 28 to 30, 2021. At the 73rd AACC, more than 400 exhibitors worldwide demonstrated the latest diagnostic technology, covering COVID-19 testing, artificial intelligence, mobile health, molecular diagnostics and automation equipment.
(c) The 2021 MEDLAB Middle East was held at Dubai International Exhibition Center, United Arab Emirates, from June 28 to July 1, and welcomed more than 600 exhibitors from nearly 40 countries and regions around the world. In the 4-day exhibition, 25,600 medical professionals from more than 120 countries were presented with the latest medical technology and the most forward-looking technology products.

1.13 Industry Associations (Table 1.11)

Table 1.11 Industry associations

National social groups related to IVD		
No.	Name	Subject
1	Chinese Society of Laboratory Medicine of the Chinese Medical Association	Academia
2	Laboratory Physician Society of the Chinese Medical Doctor Association	Academia
3	Laboratory Medicine Specialized Committee of the China Society of Integrated Traditional Chinese and Western Medicine	Academia
4	Chinese Hospital Association Clinical Laboratory Specialized Committee	Academia
5	Laboratory Medicine Specialized Committee of the Medical Science and Technology Commission, CPLA	Academia
6	Medical Laboratory Industry Society of the National Association of Health Industry and Enterprise Management	Industry
7	Experimental Medicine Society of the National Association of Health Industry and Enterprise Management	Academia
8	IVD Society of the China Association for Medical Devices Industry	Industry
9	China Society of Medical Laboratory Equipment	Academia & Industry
10	Branch of POCT Equipment and Technique for on-site Rapid Detection of the Chinese Association of Medical Equipment	Academia & Industry
11	Laboratory Medicine Society of the Chinese Geriatrics Society	Academia & Industry
12	Laboratory Medicine Specialized Committee of the Chinese Research Hospital Association	Academia
13	Molecular Diagnostic Medicine Specialized Committee of the China Research Hospital Association	Academia
14	Microbiology and Immunology Society of the Chinese Medical Association	Academia
15	Clinical Applied Biochemistry and Molecular Biology Society of The Chinese Society of Biochemistry and Molecular Biology	Academia
16	Laboratory Medicine Society of the China Association of Chinese Medicine	Academia
17	Chinese Society for Immunology	Academia
18	Labeling Immunoassay Committee (LIC) of the China Association for Instrumental Analysis	Academia
19	Medical Specialized Committee of the Laboratory Special Committee of the China National Accreditation Service for Conformity Assessment (CNAS)	Academia
20	Laboratory Society of the Chinese Association of Geriatric Research	Academia & Industry
21	Experimental Diagnosis and Social Services Specialized Committee of the China Health Culture Association	Academia & Industry

(continued)

Table 1.11 (continued)

National social groups related to IVD		
No.	Name	Subject
22	Medical Laboratory Engineering Society of the Chinese Society of Biomedical Engineering	Academia & Industry
23	Rheumatology and Molecular Immunology Society of the National Association of Health Industry and Enterprise Management	Academia & Industry
24	Laboratory Medicine Society of the Bethune Spirit Research Association	Academia & Industry
25	Clinical Diagnostics and Experimental Medicine Society of the Chinese Maternal and Child Health Association	Academia & Industry
26	Clinical Molecular Diagnostics Branch of the Biophysical Society of China	Academia & industry
27	Genetic Diagnosis of Genetic Society of China	Academia & industry
28	Clinical Laboratory Testing and Invitro Diagnostic Test Systems	Academia & Industry
29	Clinical Mass Spectrometry Committee of the Chinese Mass Spectrometry Association	Academia & Industry
30	Clinical Laboratory Medicine Society of the China International Exchange and Promotive Association for Medical and Health Care	Academia & Industry
31	Laboratory Medicine Specialized Committee of the China Medicine Education Association	Academia & Industry
32	Thrombosis and Hemostasis Specialized Committee of the Chinese Research Hospital Association	Academia
33	Intercollegiate Collaboration Council of Medical Laboratory Specialty of National Medical Colleges and universities	Academia
34	Hygienic Inspection Specialized Committee of the Chinese Preventive Medicine Association	Academia
35	Clinical Immunology Society of Chinese Society for immunology	Academia
36	Laboratory Medicine Specialized Committee of the China Medical Women's Association	Academia
37	Primary Laboratory Technique Standardization Society of the China International Exchange and Promotive Association for Medical and Health Care	Academia
38	Clinical Trial Society of the China Association for Medical Devices Industry	Academia
39	Clinical Laboratory Specialized Committee of the Chinese Antituberculosis Association	Academia
40	Biological Diagnostic Technology Society of the China Medicinal Biotechnology Association	Academia

Declaration Linda Zhang, Qi Chen and Wenting Xiao are employees of Fosun Pharm.

References

1. National Medical Products Administration 2021 Annual Report on the Registration of Medical Devices. https://www.cmde.org.cn/xwdt/zxyw/20220128091800763.html.
2. China PCR Assays and Instruments Market Analysis Report. https://www.cn-healthcare.com/articlewm/20210808/content-1250773.html.
3. Immunohistochemistry (IHC) Market by Product (Antibodies, Reagents, Equipment, Kits), Application (Diagnostics (Cancer, Infectious, Autoimmune Diseases), Research, Forensic), End user (Hospitals, Diagnostic labs, Academia)—Global Forecast to 2026. https://www.marketsandmarkets.com/Market-Reports/immunohistochemistry-market-121632939.html.
4. National Health Commission of the People's Republic of China. China's Statistical Bulletin on the Development of Health Services in 2021. http://www.gov.cn/xinwen/2022-07/12/content_5700670.htm.
5. Status and Development Trend Analysis of Health Examination Industry in China in 2020. https://www.chyxx.com/industry/202106/957920.html.
6. The World Health Organization's International Agency for Research on Cancer (IARC) released the latest global cancer data for 2020. https://www.sohu.com/a/443358070_120051436.

2 Opportunities and Challenges

Yaoyi Zhu, Linda Zhang, Qi Chen, and Wenting Xiao

With the coronavirus disease 2019 (COVID-19) outbreak in all countries worldwide and influenced by factors such as the global political environment, economy, technological innovation, and the Internet, in vitro diagnostics (IVD) enterprises are facing new opportunities and challenges.

2.1 Opportunities

2.1.1 Increased Medical Expenditure

According to the 2021 Statistical Communique of China's Health Development, the total national health expenditure in 2021 was preliminarily estimated to be 7559.36 billion CNY, the per capita total health expenditure was 5348.1 CNY, and the total health expenditure accounted for 6.5% of GDP. In 2021, the average outpatient cost of hospitals per time was 329.2 CNY, 1.5% higher than that of the previous year at the current price, and 0.6% higher at the comparable price; the average hospitalization cost per time was 11,002.9 CNY, 3.6% higher than that of the previous year at the current price, and 2.7% higher at the comparable price. The average daily hospitalization cost was 1191.7 CNY. The per capita financial subsidy standard for basic public health service projects increased from 74 CNY in 2020 to 79 CNY in 2021 [1]. It can be seen that China's overall health expenditure is constantly increasing, and the per capita health expenditure also shows a trend of synchronous growth.

Y. Zhu
IVD Branch of China Association of Medical Devices Industry, Beijing, China

L. Zhang (✉) · Q. Chen · W. Xiao
Fosun Diagnostics (Shanghai) Co., Ltd., Shanghai, China
e-mail: zhanglinda@fosunpharma.com; chenqi@fosunpharma.com; xiaowt@fosunpharma.com

H. Song, L. Dai (eds.), *In Vitro Diagnostic Industry in China*,
https://doi.org/10.1007/978-981-99-3110-1_2

2.1.2 Opportunities for Public Health Prevention and Control

IVD has significant advantages in the detection and prevention of infectious diseases and can play an important role in pathogen screening. There is great demand for the diagnosis and treatment of seasonal diseases and the examination of common respiratory and intestinal diseases, including a large number of outpatient and emergency examinations. Due to the needs for the prevention and control of COVID-19, many PCR testing products have emerged, which are basically operated based on gene amplification laboratories, but many primary prevention and control sites still lack effective nucleic acid testing means. If all provinces in the country delegate the authority of infectious disease testing to grassroots and communities, the primary prevention and control sites will gradually become the main battlefield. However, many epidemic areas do not have the nucleic acid testing capability, so samples need to be sent to qualified laboratories, which often take a long time. Therefore, in this case, mobile molecular rapid test is very suitable for the monitoring needs of infectious diseases at the grassroots level. At the same time, we predict that the state will pay more attention to nosocomial infection monitoring, and molecular rapid test products will be more favored.

2.1.3 Overseas Development

The export value of China's IVD products in 2021 should be more than ten billion USD, making China one of the major producers of IVD products in the world.

2021 was a more unpredictable year. At the beginning of the year, the market was still looking forward to the post-pandemic era of vaccination-based mass immunization, while the Omicron variant at the end of the year will probably lead to a record number of new infections per day. For the export market of COVID-19 testing, since antibody detection stepped down from the stage of history in the second half of 2020, antigen detection has cut a striking figure. After it was approved for the European OTC market for home testing in March 2021, it ushered in an unexpected outbreak. From March to May 2021, the export data of immunological products through customs were 1.07 billion USD, 2.06 billion USD, and 1.81 billion USD, respectively. By October 2021, the accumulative export value of immunological products in 2021 was more than 8 billion USD. In the fourth quarter of 2021, Acon and iHealth successively obtained the EUA of COVID-19 Antigen OTC Testing in the United States, opening up a COVID-19 testing market far larger than that of Europe to Chinese companies.

At present, China has one of the most complete product lines in the IVD field. There are Chinese enterprises engaged in R&D and production in all branches of the seven major product lines, and they are constantly expanding overseas exports. Some enterprises have set up production bases overseas, and invested in and held overseas enterprises. In the future, China's IVD industry will go global more and more significantly.

2.1.4 The Opening of Multi-Birth Policy Promotes the Test for Eugenics

According to the 2021 Statistical Communique of China's Health Development, in 2021, the antenatal examination rate of pregnant and lying-in women was 97.6%, and the postnatal visit rate was 96.0%. Compared with the previous year, the antenatal examination rate and the postnatal visit rate both increased. In 2021, the systematic management rate of children under the age of 3 was 92.8%, basically equal to that of the previous year, the systematic management rate of pregnant and lying-in women was 92.9%, slightly higher than the previous year. In 2021, free examination was provided to 8.23 million couples planning to get pregnant, covering an average of 93.5% of the target population. It is noteworthy that the proportion of second children in the births increased from about 30% in 2013 to about 43% in 2021 [1]. In the context of the full opening of the multi-birth policy, the risk of fetal chromosomal abnormalities will increase with the increase of the pregnant woman's age. This trend has led to the demand of the maternal and child market for prenatal screening, prenatal examination (such as monogenic inherited disease screening), assisted reproduction and genetic screening of newborns. In the next few years, the scale of relevant segments in China will expand rapidly.

2.1.5 The Policies of SFDA Drive Registration Fast and Convenient

This year is the year in which the State Food and Drug Administration issues most relevant laws and regulations on medical devices and IVD products, which will play a positive role in promoting the vigorous development of the IVD industry. Moreover, many regulations are new, such as the ones related to emergency registration procedure, LDT, registration and self-test, overseas clinical data use, and clinical exemption. It is believed that the promulgation of these laws and regulations will have a significant positive impact on the registration of IVD products.

2.1.6 Localization of Foreign Capital (Production, R&D, Decision-Making Process)

While foreign-funded enterprises set up production bases in China, more and more foreign-funded enterprises also set up R&D systems in China. The products developed and produced in China are not only supplied to the Chinese market but also re-exported to the world, from the original "in China, for China" to the current "in China, for the World". Moreover, the foreign-funded enterprises grant the Chinese team more decision-making authorities to actively and quickly respond to the development of the Chinese market. The localization of foreign capital makes foreign capital not only actively develop in China but also play a positive role in continuously stimulating and promoting the development of the Chinese market.

2.1.7 The Opening Up of the Capital Market Brings More Listing Opportunities

Since the opening of the Science and Technology Innovation Board in 2019, the number of IPOs in China's IVD industry has dramatically increased. The number of new listed companies in 2020 was 5 more than that in 2019. In 2020, a total of 9 companies were listed (including 4 in Science and Technology Innovation Board), 13 were approved (including 12 in Science and Technology Innovation Board), and 23 were accepted (including 18 in Science and Technology Innovation Boards), by the end of 2020, the market cap of listed companies was 1183.6 billion CNY, an increase of 151% over the end of 2019. In 2021, a total of 18 companies were listed (including 13 in Science and Technology Innovation Board), 3 were approved (including 2 in Science and Technology Innovation Board), and 9 were accepted, by the end of 2021, the market cap of listed companies was 1201.6 billion CNY, an increase of 1.5% over the end of 2020, and the CAGR of the market value of IVD-listed companies in 18–21 was 42.75%. From the perspective of the financing scale of the capital market, the net amount of funds raised by the four listed companies in 2019 totaled 1.35 billion CNYwith an average of 450 million CNY raised by each company, the 9 companies listed in 2020 (including Burning Rock and Genetron, the companies listed in NASDAQ) raised 9.53 billion CNY in total with an average of 1.19 billion CNY. In 2021, 18 listed companies raised 19.03 billion CNY with an average of 1.06 billion CNY. The incremental exit channels provided by GEM registration system and the establishment of the Beijing Stock Exchange will inevitably further expand the IPO in the medical and health sector in China in the future, which will also drive the investment in the primary market, stimulate capital to enter the IVD industry, and promote the rapid development of domestic IVD enterprises. According to incomplete statistics, as the industry that has benefited the most from COVID-19, IVD had 82 financing events in 2021 with a financing scale of more than ten billion CNY.

2.1.8 The State Increases Investment in the Construction of Medical Institutions and Facilities

In the middle of this year, the National Development and Reform Commission issued the Implementation Plan for the Construction of a High-quality and Efficient Medical and Health Service System during the 14th Five-year Plan Period (hereinafter referred to as the Plan) formulated by four departments. The state has made it clear that within 5 years, a high-quality and efficient integrated medical and health service system with complete system, reasonable layout, clear division of work, complementary functions, close cooperation, efficient operation, and resilience should be basically completed. With the policy support, a large number of medical device gaps emerged, and the medical device market ushered in a trillion-level allocation tide. The amount of investment subsidy within the central government budget for any single project of provincial, municipal, and county-level CDC shall not exceed 200 million CNY, 50 million CNY, and ten million CNY, respectively. The maximum amount of investment subsidies within the central government budget of regional medical centers, national serious infectious disease prevention and cure bases, and national major medical rescue bases shall not exceed 500 million CNY, 300 million CNY, and 300 million CNY, respectively. The Plan requires strengthening the construction of county-level medical communities, encouraging the construction of open and shared imaging, ECG, pathological diagnostics, medical examination and other centers based on county-level hospitals, strengthening the provision of telemedicine and information equipment, connecting with high-level provincial and municipal hospitals, and connecting with primary medical and health institutions [2]. With the policy support, products such as IVD and medical equipment, as an important link of the construction of medical institutions, will gain incremental market, and listed companies on related tracks are expected to benefit.

Recently, the National Health Commission and the Department of Finance jointly released the Notice on Issuing the 2022 Serious Infectious Disease Prevention and Control Budget in Advance. The Notice makes it clear that 15.57 billion CNY of financial funds will be issued in advance to expand the national immunization program, AIDS prevention and control, tuberculosis prevention and control, schistosomiasis and echinococcosis prevention and control, mental health and chronic non-communicable disease prevention and control, COVID-19 and other key infectious disease monitoring [3].

At the same time, the Ministry of Finance also issued the Notice on issuing the 2022 Basic Public Health Service Subsidy Budget in Advance. Compared with 2021, the basic public health subsidy in 2022 issued in advance this time has increased significantly, totaling 58.85 billion CNY [4]. The central and western regions received more subsidies, all exceeding 20 billion CNY. Sichuan, Henan, Shandong, Hunan, and other provinces received more funds. Nearly half of the subsidies will be invested into grassroots to improve basic public health services.

At the same time, aiming at the problem of insufficient cure capacity in public health emergencies, the National Health Commission pointed out that county-level hospitals were currently equipped with 9.7 ventilators on average (a minimum of 0 sets and a maximum of 24 sets), including 2.3, 1.9, and 5.5 on average for respiratory department, emergency department, and ICU, respectively. The number of ventilators in the eastern, central, and western regions shows a decreasing trend. The hospitals in poverty-stricken counties are equipped with 6.5 ventilators on average, and the respiratory department, emergency department, and ICU of hospitals in poverty-stricken counties are also equipped with less ventilators than the general level of county-level hospitals [5]. This also means that with the advanced issuance of subsidies, major primary medical institutions will further supplement the missing medical devices, so as to improve the comprehensive medical service capacity and complete the tasks indicators assigned by the state.

Undoubtedly, in the post-pandemic era, with the new requirements of the state for the construction of public health at the grassroots level, there will be more new opportunities for the industry. For example, the equipment configuration related to the testing of key infectious diseases such as COVID-19 will be the first problem to be solved.

2.1.9 The State Strengthens the Support of Medical Equipment Industrialization

IVD industry opportunities have always been highly related to the planning and deployment of the medical industry at the national policy level. The COVID-19 has reversed globalization and also made China's economic development environment face more profound and complex changes. "Innovation Driven" promotes economic development. In the "14th Five-year Plan", the investment in R&D of the whole society will increase by more than 7% annually, aiming to promote the transformation of clinical research achievements and speed up the solution of the "Bottlenecks" in a number of drugs, medical devices, vaccines, medical data, etc. Improve the facilities and equipment level of major medical research platforms such as key state laboratories; build high-level, international and open clinical research transformation platforms and innovative technology incubation bases for drugs, medical devices and equipment, vaccines, etc. Improve the infrastructure conditions for clinical diagnosis and treatment and appropriately allocate large medical equipment in advance. And deeply use 5G, artificial intelligence and other technologies to build global leading smart hospitals and serious disease data centers.

For national and regional medical centers included in the equipment plan, focus on building business houses, purchasing medical equipment, building IT and scientific research platforms, establishing telemedicine and education platforms, and accelerating the intelligent transformation and upgrading of medical equipment.

Select and build about 120 provincial-level regional medical centers. Improve the level of large-scale equipment, strengthen the construction of smart hospitals, and ensure the needs of telemedicine. Strengthen the construction of specialized centers for pectoralgia, apoplexy, trauma and respiration as well as comprehensive cancer treatment centers and chronic disease management centers. Strengthen the construction of county-level medical communities, encourage the construction of open and shared imaging, ECG, pathological diagnostics, medical examination and other centers based on county-level hospitals, strengthen the provision of telemedicine and information equipment, connect with high-level provincial and municipal hospitals, and connect with primary medical and health institutions. It is necessary to build county-level first-aid centers based on county-level hospitals, and establish and improve the county 120 emergency network based on qualified township health centers. Strengthen the construction of blood banks at all levels and improve the blood emergency linkage support capacity [2].

2.2 Challenges

2.2.1 Uncertainties Caused by COVID-19

The decline in routine works led by COVID-19 has affected the operation of routine testing items and the sales of corresponding IVD products. At the same time, problems in the supply chain of some products also affected the timely production and supply of products. There are also different effects on different enterprises. The differences between enterprises are enlarged, the performance of different products of the same enterprise varies, and the same product fluctuates greatly in different markets and regions.

2.2.2 Reform of Medical Service Price and Change of Medical Insurance Payment Mode

At present, there are great differences and discrepancies in medical service prices across the country, including charges for testing items. As the state prepares to advance the reform of medical service prices, it is worth paying close attention to whether a unified national charging standard for test items will be established. If this change occurs, corresponding response requirements and changes to IVD enterprises will definitely emerge. At the same time, with the in-depth and comprehensive operation of DRG and DIP in the country, the operation and arrangement of testing items by medical institutions will certainly have a great impact on the IVD industry, prompting enterprises to conduct in-depth research and actively explore the changes to adapt to this medical payment system.

2.2.3 Impact of Bidding

The one-size-fits-all bidding policy lacks the standard to judge the quality of reagents, and there is often a tendency for low price to win the bid, which often ignores the demand of medical institutions for services in the process of product application and ignores the fact that the clinical significance of products with different technical indicators is significantly different and the R&D and production costs of products are high. These may make some enterprises unable to attach importance to quality or performance, which is very disadvantageous for product users or end customers to expect more accurate diagnosis results and satisfactory services, and for promoting technological innovation in industries and enterprises.

2.2.4 Inadequate Innovation Ability

Relatively concentrated product categories, uneven product quality, and serious homogeneous competition in the industry have seriously hindered the healthy development of the IVD industry in China. Although the investment in R&D of enterprises in the industry has been increasing in recent years, the overall proportion is still low, generally below 10%, which is still far behind the international leading enterprises. Although various funds are active, there are few funds willing to invest in early projects and innovative projects. Most funds focus on mature and pre-IPO enterprises and projects. As a result, there are very few original and global leading projects every year.

2.2.5 Fiercer Market Competition

At present, domestic IVD enterprises face multiple challenges. On the one hand, foreign-funded enterprises have been expanding their presence in the Chinese market in succession. Danaher, Beckman, and Roche have constantly increased their investment in China during the pandemic period and built new production and R&D centers. The R&D centers and production bases of Perkin Elmer, Ortho, and other international enterprises in China have been increasingly put into use. The launch of Hitachi's first domestic 3500 biochemical analysis system in the Suzhou factory marks that the layout, acquisition, and strategic cooperation of international enterprises in China are accelerating. The pandemic is bound to further promote international brands to accelerate the pace of localized production, R&D, investment, M&A in the above ways. There is an objective gap between domestic enterprises and foreign enterprises in terms of global operation capability. In the international market, our domestic enterprises mainly focus on the markets of developing countries such as Asian, African and Latin American countries, and their market share in developed countries such as European countries and the United States is still small (except for COVID-19 reagents). Therefore, if a domestic IVD enterprise wants to become a company with global influence and obtain better development space, it must go abroad. The sooner the layout, the better. In the future, for excellent IVD enterprises, global operation is a must, which requires us to constantly accumulate experience and practice, strengthen the construction of our product lines and product quality, and build channels and systems for products to go abroad.

On the other hand, driven by COVID-19, a large number of IVD enterprises are vying to be listed. According to incomplete statistics, there are nearly 2000 IVD manufacturers in China, 52 A-share listed companies, 18 new listed companies in 2021, and 10–20 companies are expected to be listed in the next 2 years. This reflects the prosperity of the IVD industry and also means that competition among enterprises will be more intense in the future. Therefore, in the future, domestic IVD enterprises need to strengthen their quality control and the requirements for standardized and large-scale production. Only by improving their competitiveness can they stand out in the fierce competition and meet new development opportunities.

Declaration Linda Zhang, Qi Chen and Wenting Xiao are employees of Fosun Pharm.

References

1. National Health Commission of the People's Republic of China. China's Statistical Bulletin on the Development of Health Services in 2021. http://www.gov.cn/xinwen/2022-07/12/content_5700670.htm.
2. Notice on the issuance of the Implementation Plan for Building a High-quality and Efficient Medical and Health Service System during the 14th Five-Year Plan Period. https://www.ndrc.gov.cn/xxgk/zcfb/tz/202107/t20210701_1285212_ext.html.
3. Notice on the issuance of Budget for the Prevention and Control of Major Infectious Diseases in 2022 in advance. http://sbs.mof.gov.cn/zxzyzf/ggwsfwbzzj/202112/t20211203_3771887.htm.
4. Notice on the issuance of Budget for Subsidies for Basic Public Health Services in 2022 in advance. http://sbs.mof.gov.cn/zxzyzf/ggwsfwbzzj/202112/t20211203_3771890.htm.
5. Notification of the General Office of the NHC on the Service Capacity Evaluation of county-level Hospitals in 2019. http://www.nhc.gov.cn/yzygj/s3593g/202007/f124d3fe0ba64b408741f30a38e71dbf.shtml.

Part II

Immunoassay

Chemiluminescence Analyzers and Reagents

3

Shuang Li, Ting Peng, Ming Wang, and Yujie Cao

3.1 Introduction to Main Automated Chemiluminescence Immunoassay Analyzers

3.1.1 CL-8000i

Since 2013, Shenzhen Mindray Bio-Medical Electronics Co., Ltd., has released multiple automated chemiluminescence immunoassay analyzers including CL-2000i, CL-1000i, CL-900i, CL-6000i, and the latest CL-8000i. The detection system of CL-8000i uses alkaline phosphatase (ALP) as the marker and AMPPD as the substrate. CL-8000i performs up to 500 tests/hour on a single module and provides 36 refrigerated reagent positions and 300 sample positions. It is modularly scalable and compatible with the M6000 total laboratory automation system. CL-8000i helps to improve medical quality and operational efficiency in the following ways. First, the VU-Mix (vortex + ultrasound mixing) technology is used to remove non-specific conjugates and reduce fibrin interference; FS-Sampling (full-scene sampling) can automatically identify sample containers and intelligently identify and warn about abnormal liquid levels, which improves the accuracy of test results. Second, the calibrators and controls of CL-8000i carry their barcode and thus require no dispensing. This means they are ready for use in the test with a single press of a button. The system is equipped with an intelligent reagent management module that allows for the automatic mixing of magnetic beads and visualized loading, which simplifies the operational procedure. The high-throughput testing and emergency priority capabilities ensure a fast turnaround time (TAT) at all times.

S. Li (✉) · T. Peng
Shenzhen Mindray Bio-Medical Electronics Co., Ltd., Shenzhen, Guangdong, China
e-mail: lishuang_b@mindray.com

M. Wang · Y. Cao
Shenzhen YHLO Biotech Co., Ltd., Shenzhen, China

H. Song, L. Dai (eds.), *In Vitro Diagnostic Industry in China*,
https://doi.org/10.1007/978-981-99-3110-1_3

In addition, CL-8000i has won the iF Award for Product Design, User Experience, User Interface Design, and the Red Dot Award for User Experience and Interface Design. With an integrated intelligent alarm system and cross-media integration of information, CL-8000i can transmit information from far to near, so that the laboratory staff can accurately locate various unexpected risks and deal with them properly. Moreover, in line with Good Laboratory Practice, CL-8000i provides an end-to-end testing information traceability platform to support the analysis and investigation of results, making clinical testing safer and more reliable.

3.1.2 IFlash 3000-G

Shenzhen Yhlo Biotech Co., Ltd., has recently released iFlash 3000-G, which is powered by the magnetic microparticles-based acridinium ester direct chemiluminescence technology. With the ability to perform up to 600 tests/hour on a single module, it can report the first result in 12 min, greatly improving the work efficiency of the laboratory. IFlash 3000-G has 40 refrigerated reagent positions for the loading reagents with no downtime. It can accommodate either 140 sample positions or 480 sample loading units and support giving priority to emergency samples. It can be connected with other instruments in the same series and is compatible with a laboratory automation system. IFlash 3000-G is designed with independent sample and reagent needles, with no tips required. It is capable of liquid-level detection, clot detection, empty suction detection, and horizontal and vertical crash protection while reducing the carryover to less than 0.1 ppm. IFlash 3000-G can store 3000 cuvettes at one time. Its supports for pouring for loading at any time, in-line dilution of concentrated wash solution, and loading of all consumables with no downtime help to maintain the continuity of the sample testing process and ensure a fast TAT for the laboratory.

3.1.3 MAGLUMI X8

MAGLUMI X8 is the latest automated chemiluminescence immunoassay analyzer developed by Shenzhen New Industries Biomedical Engineering Co., Ltd. The analyzer is built upon direct chemiluminescence technology and uses ABEI as the luminescent maker. As the first ultra-high-speed automated chemiluminescence immunoassay analyzer with a throughput of 600 tests/hour, MAGLUMI X8 provides 42 reagent positions and 300 sample positions. It can be connected with instruments of the same model, biochemical instruments, and electrolyte analyzers, and be configured later to be compatible with Total Laboratory Automation (TLA) systems. It supports emergency priority and emergency position customization and features an auto-retest function. Its sampling process is achieved with disposable tips and a one-suction multi-injection method, which improves the utilization of tips. The analyzer can automatically detect liquid levels, clots, bubbles, and crashes. With the ability to load 576 tips at one time, it provides an intelligent loading mode that enables continuous loading and real-time display of quantity. Its reagent needle is made of titanium alloy and coated with TEFLON. A double-needle design realizes the simultaneous aspiration of different reagents. The product incorporates the 4-station cleaning technology in a high-speed single channel, the multi-magnetic separation technology, and the non-contact magnetic microbeads resuspension technology.

3.1.4 Smart 6500

Shanghai Tellgen Corporation uses acridinium ester as a luminescent marker for their chemiluminescence reagents, which are more suitable for the detection of thyroid function, hormones, and other small molecules. SMART 6500 automated chemiluminescence immunoassay analyzer provides a throughput of 360 tests/hour and a yield of 389 tests/hour/square meter. It can be connected with Immune Island, an innovative immunoassay solution of Tellgen, to incorporate flow fluorescence and chemiluminescence technologies for flexible combinations of multi-item testing and single-item testing. Users can determine how many of each instrument to use as per the testing needs of the laboratory and complete up to 3000 tests/hour. The Immune Island of Tellgen can also be connected with the Hitachi-Tellgen compatible automation line, the compact and unique immunoassay solution which provides a greater test throughput in a smaller area.

3.1.5 AutoLumo A6000

AutoLumo A6000 is the latest automated chemiluminescence immunoassay analyzer from Autobio Diagnostics Co., Ltd. The system adopts enzymatic chemiluminescence and uses HRP as the luminescent maker. The product is characterized by duplicate backup, ultra-fast detection, ease of use, scalability, and connectivity, and biosafety. The reagent tray, reagent needle, sample transfer channel, substrate solution, and wash solution are all designed with a backup, which minimizes downtime and ensures the uninterrupted running of the entire system. With a single-module testing speed of up to 600 tests/hour, up to four analyzers can be used online together to perform up to 2400 tests/hour. The reagents can be rapidly mixed within 5 min. The reagent chamber supports uninterrupted refrigeration even when the entire system is in sleep mode, which shortens the time it takes to prepare for an experiment. A dedicated emergency track is available for emergency samples to take precedence over on-test racks. The reagents, cuvettes, substrates, and wash solutions can be replaced with no downtime. A single analysis module has 50 reagent positions and supports RFID RF scanning to record reagent consumption in real-time. The concentrated wash solution is automatically prepared and supplied in real time, which facilitates storage, transportation, and replacement. With multiple systems working together, the analyzer can run offline for up to 6 h without interruption. The cuvettes can be discarded after solid-liquid separation. The sample loading/unloading and track modules are designed to be fully enclosed to minimize aerosol leakage. The pre-processing decapping module can realize rotary decapping, negative pressure-based filtration and discharge of aerosols, and UV disinfection of waste chambers.

3.1.6 i3000

i3000 is the latest automated chemiluminescence immunoassay analyzer from Maccura Biotechnology Co., Ltd. The analyzer is powered by the magnetic microparticles-based acridinium ester direct chemiluminescence technology. It offers benefits such as high speed, flexible scalability, excellent performance, ease of operation, and simple maintenance. Its multiple modules can work together to meet the needs of laboratories with different test volumes. Its single module runs up to 300 tests/hour. The time to the first result is 14 min. Up to 200 samples can be loaded at one time, with continuous loading allowed. An independent emergency channel is available for immediate loading. The Carry-over rate is less than 0.1 ppm. Up to 2000 cuvettes can be loaded at one time. A dedicated reagent loading channel allows reagents to be loaded at any time, while the analyzer is running. The consumables reservation function comes with an indicator light that tells when a replacement is needed. A reservation function is also available for the concentrated wash solution to allow automated preparation. The analyzer features a flexible set of washing methods, multiple magnetic separation techniques, and a patented magnetic field design. With the ability to perform daily maintenance automatically, without requiring any manual intervention, the analyzer can identify problems beforehand and support users in solving them.

3.1.7 Caris200

Caris200 is the latest automated chemiluminescence immunoassay analyzer from Beijing Wantai Biological Pharmacy Enterprise Co., Ltd. The analyzer is powered by the acridinium ester direct chemiluminescence technology. Impressive throughput: There are 50 reagent positions and an independent power supply, with no management required for 28 days after reagent loading; 50 items can be tested on one analyzer, offering a throughput of up to 200 tests/hour; 110 sample positions and 10 emergency priority positions ensure that various clinical testing needs can be met. Online continuous loading: Online continuous loading of samples and reagents; online continuous addition/replacement of buffers, pre-trigger solutions, trigger solutions, and other general reagents; online continuous addition of all consumables including disposable tips and cuvettes. Proper structure layout: The 3D robotic arm works flexibly and stably; the pressure-based liquid sensing technology is used to detect the liquid level; cost-saving disposable tips (non-carbon fibers) are used to prevent cross-contamination; the pre-heating cleaning function improves the efficiency in cleaning reagent loading needles; the anti-jamming design of cuvettes lowers the failure rate.

3.1.8 CM-320

CM-320 is the latest automated chemiluminescence immunoassay analyzer from Dirui Industrial Co., Ltd. The analyzer is powered by the acridinium ester-labeled direct chemiluminescence technology. It runs up to 320 tests/hour and comes with 620 sample positions and 36 reagent positions. It offers the ability to load reagents and cuvettes with no downtime and to automatically dilute concentrated wash solution in-line. This reduces the time spent on human-machine interaction and improves work efficiency. The three independent sample tracks, that is, Routine, Emergency, and Recycle, help to distribute samples efficiently. Up to 1500 cuvettes can be uploaded at one time. An optional auto decapping module is provided for decapping sample tubes automatically, which reduces the need for manual intervention. Real-time transmission of fault alarm data and communication with an online customer service team give users peace of mind. The waste cuvette recycling function is carefully designed to separate the liquid to prevent biological contamination in the laboratory. The analyzer can be integrated with any immune and biochemical modules. It can also be connected with Dirui LA-60 automated sample processing system to provide users with a centralized, intelligent and standardized laboratory automation solution.

3.2 Consideration in Reagent Development

3.2.1 Improving the Detection Sensitivity

Immunological detection is mainly for some analytes with very low content. Therefore, the detection sensitivity must be high enough to ensure satisfactory detection results. For example, by optimizing the conditions for immune response, newly emerging high-sensitivity troponins can enhance the detection sensitivity and the analytical precision of low concentrations, thereby greatly improving the ability to diagnose acute myocardial infarction at an early stage. In addition, high-sensitivity C-reactive protein and high-sensitivity procalcitonin are among the widely used items for testing in clinical practice. Studies have shown that these high-sensitivity tests are more clinically valuable than conventional detections.

3.2.2 Applicability for Multiple Sample Types

Serum and plasma samples are the types of samples commonly used in immunoassay. It is better to use the same sample type for the same test package; otherwise, two different tubes of samples will need to be collected, which affect detection efficiency. For example, pro-gastrin-releasing peptide (ProGRP) is the best marker for small cell lung cancer (SCLC) and the most reliable marker for lung cancer in clinical practice. However, ProGRP can be degraded by thrombin, which makes some companies' products not applicable for serum samples. ProGRP can be redesigned to make the coated antibody and labeled antibody avoid the thrombin cleavage site, thus ensuring good detection stability for both serum and plasma samples.

3.2.3 Improving the Anti-Interference Ability

Immunoassay works based upon the specific recognition of antigens by antibodies. How to prevent this specificity from interference is a permanent topic. Developing reagents requires thoroughly examining the structure and antibody characteristics of the markers for testing and designing appropriate reaction modes and blockers accordingly. It is also important to consider dozens of possible interferents, including drugs, analogues, serum endogenous substances, rheumatoid factors, and heterophilic antibodies. Therefore, a great deal of design and verification work is required to improve the anti-interference ability of reagents.

3.2.4 Controlling the Inter-Run Variation of Reagents

Inter-run variation is the key to ensure the stability and controllability of reagents, and can be controlled from three levels. From the raw material level, the physical and chemical properties and functions of different raw materials should be analyzed to eliminate problematic raw materials from the source. From the product design level, DOE should be used to identify the most inclusive formula and manufacturing process and minimize the risk of inter-run variation. From the production control level, it is critical to control indicators and implementation measures for each critical manufacturing step to circumvent the risk of inter-run variation that may possibly be introduced during the production stage.

3.2.5 Improving the System Stability

Immune response is affected by the intensity factors such as temperature and ionic strength. Immune products mostly use a closed system. It requires a good match and balance between the instrument and the reagent, so as to maintain good consistency in sample loading, incubation, cleaning, shaking, and other processes. Such consistency ensures that the instrument can deliver steady results across different temperatures and humidities, different days, and different places.

Declaration Shuang Li and Ting Peng are employees of Shenzhen Mindray Bio-Medical Electronics Co., Ltd.

Ming Wang and Yujie Cao are employees of Shenzhen YHLO Biotech Co., Ltd., Shenzhen, China.

Automatic Enzyme Immunoassay Instrument and Related Instruments

4

Yunqi Li, Rongbang Xia, Tao Zhao, Pengfei Lai, Nan Sun, Weijing Yi, and Wei Hu

4.1 Overview

Enzyme-linked immunosorbent assay (hereinafter referred to as ELISA) has been well received by numerous research institutes and enterprises due to high sensitivity, excellent specificity, easy operation, low cost, low requirements on instruments and equipment and other characteristics, and it has been extensively used in multiple detection fields like the HBVM, HIV, syphilis, prenatal and postnatal care, allergen screening and SARS-CoV-2 detection. ELISA is one of the most commonly used detection method at the moment [1–3]. The principle is to bond known antigen or antibody to surface of solid carrier to give it immunocompetence, which can be divided into antigen detection and antibody detection by different detection objects [4, 5]. Antigen detection mainly includes two-site sandwich enzyme immunoassay (Fig. 4.1) and sandwich competitive, while antibody detection mainly includes indirect method, double antigen sandwich method, sandwich competitive and capture ELISA.

At the beginning of ELISA, all steps were operated manually, and it relied on naked eyes for identification of chromogenic results. Accompanied with development of automation technology, various supporting instruments and standard consumables were introduced to the market. Over the past half century, ELISA-related reagents and instruments have been characterized by mutual promotion and development. Although chemiluminescence, PCR and other technologies have gone through constant iterations in recent years, ELISA is still irreplaceable and it's an essential detection technique in blood bank, hospital, family planning, disease

Y. Li · R. Xia · T. Zhao · P. Lai (✉) · N. Sun
Aikang MedTech Co., Ltd., Shenzhen, Guangdong, China
e-mail: laipengfei@aikang-medical.com

W. Yi · W. Hu
Zybio, Inc., Chongqing, China

H. Song, L. Dai (eds.), *In Vitro Diagnostic Industry in China*,
https://doi.org/10.1007/978-981-99-3110-1_4

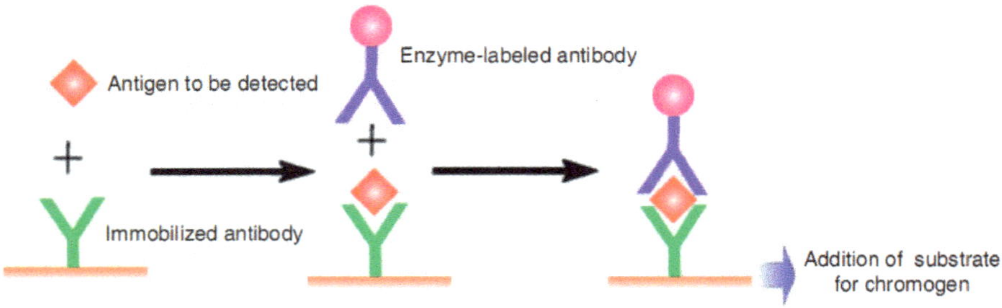

Fig. 4.1 Diagram for principles of two-site sandwich enzyme immunoassay

control, physical examination, biological product and other organizations. ELISA-based instruments and devices are still promising in the future. This paper analyzed past, present and future situations of enzyme immunoassay instrument from development stages of ELISA analyzer, development process of automatic enzyme immunoassay instrument in China, major domestic automatic enzyme immunoassay instrument manufacturers and their representative products, technical development direction of automatic enzyme immunoassay instrument, market profile of automatic enzyme immunoassay instrument and other major aspects.

4.2 Development Stages of Enzyme Immunoassay Instrument

The microplate reader first replaced human labor to identify the color of the reaction result. Then it developed into the automatic enzyme immunoassay instrument which can finish the process from original tube loading to automatic printing of result report sheet. According to its development degree of automation, enzyme immunoassay instrument can be divided into three stages, and it's moving toward the fourth stage at the moment.

4.2.1 The First Stage

Enzyme immunoassay instrument was a microplate reader that used to identifies concentration replace by naked eyes. The core idea is to analyze content of antigen or antibody to be detected through colorimetry with a dedicated spectrophotometer or photoelectrometer. To be specific, the instrument can adjust light wave emitted by light source to a single wavelength based on color of ELISA reaction result and get it into one end of the detected object, then use transducer to detect extent of loss of light intensity after passing the detected object, and thus calculate absorbance. According to the Lambert–Beer law, the absorbance is in direct proportion to sample concentration, and thus concentration of the detected object can be identified.

4.2.2 The Second Stage

ELISA analyzer developed devices of single functions and semi-automatic instruments that can replace most manual operations at the second stage, such as sampler, plate washer and integrated plate washing and plate reading. A certain proportion of complicated manual operations in detection process like sampling and microplate washing are replaced by instrument, but the whole ELISA process still needs manual intervention or operation. Those instruments often have disadvantages of small detection throughput and low speed, but they also have small size, great flexibility, low price and other characteristics, which make them still extensively used in some small medical institutions like township hospitals and health stations.

4.2.3 The Third Stage

At the third stage, the process from original tube loading to automatic printing of result report can all be finished by ELISA analyzer. Instruments of this stage have integrated semi-automatic instrument modules of the first and second stage, and built in automated liquid handling system with multiple pipetting channel, robot arm, rail and other modules. All ELISA steps are automatically finished inside the instrument, which significantly increased stability and consistence of detection results as well as detection throughput. Accompanied with increase in production capacity and reduction in production cost of different manufacturers, application of automatic enzyme immunoassay instrument has been extended from large medical institutions to small- and medium-sized medical institutions, which is gradually replacing semi-automatic instrument.

4.2.4 The Fourth Stage

Accompanied with further development of automation and intellectualization, to meet requirements of higher detection throughput and more detection items and realize interconnectivity between devices, expansion of automation from internal operations of a single device to total laboratory online automation of numerous different devices has become an inevitable trend. At present, total laboratory pipelining that combines and schedules multiple detection devices of the same type or different types of detection devices of laboratory has been gradually introduced to the market.

Accompanied with technological development, different instruments and modules of corresponding ELISA process have also gone through continuous iterations during change process of different stages. For instance, sampling accuracy has been continuously rising, while sampling channels have been constantly increasing from 1 channel to 8 channels and from one robotic arm to multiple robotic arms, microplate washing channels have increased from 8 channels to 96 channels, and washing solution can be detected and switched automatically, and the precision and linearity range of microplate reader have been continuously improving, which both improved precision of detection results and increased detection throughput.

4.3 Development Journey of Automatic Enzyme Immunoassay Instrument in China

Development and manufacturing of automatic enzyme immunoassay instrument started relatively late in China, but they have achieved continuous development under great efforts of developers. Some domestic automatic enzyme immunoassay instrument are almost as good as international first-class products at the moment, some of their performance indicators are even superior to international famous brands, and they suit Chinese users' use habit better in terms of operation and use. Development of automatic enzyme immunoassay instrument in China has experienced the following four stages.

4.3.1 Stage of Awareness (1978–1990)

Upon reform and opening up in 1978, domestic large hospitals started to import automatic detection devices from European countries and the US like semi-automatic microplate reader and semi-automatic plate washer, and laboratory operators of hospitals and blood banks used to finish ELISA laboratory detection through manual operation in conjunction with semi-automatic devices. Domestic enterprises couldn't produce the analyzer on their own during this device introduction stage.

4.3.2 Stage of Independent Production (1991–2000)

Accompanied with acceleration of China's reform and opening up, introduction of numerous overseas equipment manufacturing techniques had been accelerated. In 1991, the first set of semi-automatic micro-plate washer system introduced by DRAGON LABORATORY INSTRUMENTS LIMITED entered into the stage of mass production. In 1995, AusBio Bioengineering Co., Ltd., introduced the first set of HAMILTON automatic enzyme immunoassay instrument in China. Introduction of those devices greatly promoted improvement in independent R&D and production capacity of Chinese enterprises.

4.3.3 Stage of Rapid Development (2001–2015)

Domestic IVD device manufacturers started technological catching-up, who actively occupied the markets of blood bank, Grade III, Grade II and grassroots hospitals. A great number of excellent domestic automatic enzyme immunoassay instrument manufacturers emerged during this stage, such as Aikang MedTech Co., Ltd. (henceforth referred to as Aikang), Biobase Biodustry (Shandong) Co., Ltd. (henceforth referred to as Biobase) and Yantai Addcare Bio-Tech Limited Company (henceforth referred to as Yantai Addcare). Product configuration, performance, function and detection speed of automatic enzyme immunoassay instrument of those brands are superior to imported brands, particularly Aikang's URANUS AE

275 automatic enzyme immunoassay instrument. The product adopts multi-cartridge pipelined work mode, which enables circular sampling, pipelined operations, multi-work chamber's flexible deployment of tasks and rapid detection speed; it uses smart sensing system and boasts of high level of automation, which can avoid errors caused by manual interruption. Reagent and wash solution in laboratory process under intelligent management or reagent position uses Hall principle for intelligent identification to avoid placement of reagent added in wrong position during the laboratory process, drawer type stacked placement of wash solution bottles can realize real-time monitoring of wash solution volume, alarm will be sent automatically in case of insufficient liquid volume and standby wash solution can be switched to and used automatically without manual intervention; meanwhile, operating software's more human-oriented, and Chinese operating software and graphical wizard operation are customized for users, which are easy to understand and operate.

4.3.4 Stage of Comprehensive Replacement of Imported Products (2015 to Present)

At present, recognition of laboratory department of blood bank and hospital on domestic automatic enzyme immunoassay instrument has been increased. URANUS AE 288 High Throughput automatic enzyme immunoassay instrument and URANUS AE 368 fully automated ELISA post-processing system introduced by Aikang in laboratory of blood bank use partitioned management design, have reagent distribution module, oscillator, tower type incubator, automatic plate washer and microplate reader module, use flexible and smart robotic arms in combination with transfer track, transfer microplate between different modules, enable multi-task, multi-channel and parallel processing and thus realize fully automated completion of ELISA in a pipelined and efficient manner. Aforesaid products have been recognized by blood bank clients, which broke the long-term monopoly of imported automatic enzyme immunoassay instrument over laboratory of blood banks. Meanwhile, the country has introduced policies that give priority to purchase of domestic medical devices and encourage the medical industry's preference for domestic medical devices. In the future, domestic automatic enzyme immunoassay instrument are expected to replace imported brands to a greater extent.

4.4 Major Domestic Automatic Enzyme Immunoassay Instrument Manufacturers and Their Representative Products

4.4.1 Aikang MedTech Co., Ltd.

URANUS AE series automatic enzyme immunoassay instrument manufactured by Aikang can be mainly divided into four major categories, that is, High Throughput automatic enzyme immunoassay instrument, integrated automatic enzyme immunoassay instrument, combined automatic enzyme immunoassay instrument and automatic enzyme immunoassay instrument post-processing system. Whereas a new generation of high throughput automatic enzyme immunoassay instrument of Aikang, URANUS AE 288, has integrated multiple technologies and realized multi-task, multi-channel and parallel processing, which ensure optimal reaction process and high throughput processing capacity. Models of high throughput automatic enzyme immunoassay instrument also include URANUS AE 288 s, URANUS AE 188 s, URANUS AE 188 and URANUS AE 158. Integrated automatic enzyme immunoassay instrument manufactured by Aikang through independent R&D can provide different configurations based on different customers' actual requirements. Combined automatic enzyme immunoassay instrument created the design idea of combined analyzer with multiple cartridges and multiple robotic arms, reasonably assigned steps of ELISA to multiple cartridges for processing and pipelined operations and realized simultaneous detection of samples of multiple batches on the instruments, which enabled operation of different projects, different batches and different laboratory steps at the same time. Models of automatic enzyme immunoassay instrument Post-Processing System include URANUS AE 168, URANUS AE 268 and URANUS AE 368, which realized independent sampling and post-processing upon sampling of ELISA on different devices, and suitable for laboratories with large sample size and many items, which enabled batched and continuous insertion of micro-plates, broke imported brands' monopoly of automatic enzyme immunoassay instrument.

Aikang's automatic enzyme immunoassay instrument can realize sampling speed of no more than 85 s for continuous sample distribution of 96-well plate, and time for continuous reagent distribution of 96-well plate doesn't exceed 50 s, in terms of sampling accuracy, it can achieve sampling precision of 0.5% and below as well as interpretation repeatability of 0.5% and below under 1000 μL gradient, which enable laboratory process of high precision, high speed and high stability. Meanwhile, in plate washing procedure, immersion duration and cleaning times can be adjusted at will, which possesses high flexibility.

4.4.2 Yantai Addcare Bio-Tech Limited Company

Yantai Addcare is a domestic manufacturer engaged in R&D, production and distribution of automatic enzyme immunoassay instrument, which has automatic ELISA workstation of model ADC ELISA 1800, ADC ELISA 1100, ADC ELISA 600, ADC ELISA 400, ADC ELISA 300 and ADC ELISA 200.

4.4.3 Biobase Biodustry (Shandong) Co., Ltd.

Main models of fully automatic ELISA workstation of Biobase include BIOBASE1000, BIOBASE2000, BIOBASE2001, BIOBASE4000, BIOBASE4001 and BIOBASE8000.

4.4.4 JiaXing CRED Medical Instrument Co., Ltd.

Main models of automatic enzyme immunoassay instrument of JiaXing CRED Medical Instrument Co., Ltd. (henceforth referred to as JiaXing CRED), include HB-500E, HB-300E, HB-150E, HB-100E, HB-900E and HB-1000E.

4.4.5 Diasia Biomedical Technology Co., Ltd.

Main models of automatic enzyme immunoassay instrument of Diasia Biomedical Technology Co., Ltd. (henceforth referred to as Diasia), include AE1100, AE1100A, AE800, AE800A and AE600.

4.5 Technological Development Direction of Automatic Enzyme Immunoassay Instrument

Benefited from the country's vigorous expansion of medical device-related policies and improvement of supporting industry chain, domestic automatic enzyme immunoassay instrument manufacturers have actively improved core technological competence, made continuous product innovation and upgrade and broken several technical barriers of manufacturers of imported brands, which allowed the fully automated ELISA industry to experience rapid development. It can be learned from domestic patents search of automatic enzyme immunoassay instrument, China boasts of continuous active patent applications in such area, increase momentum of applications and gradual increase in enterprises' innovation awareness. According to incomplete statistics, the number of automatic enzyme immunoassay instrument-related patent applications was less than 10 in China before 2003, then, the number of patent applications increased to 12.5 per year on average between 2003 and 2010, domestic enterprises already started technical R&D and deployment in such field, and a few excellent enterprises received approval for marketing of fully automated ELISA analyzer, from 2011 to 2017, China moved on to the stage of rapid growth in patent application, and domestic enterprises continuously optimized their core technologies continuously, number of patent applications reached the peak in 2017, which was 62 for the whole year; number of patent applications reduced in 2018 and 2019, but it's still at the stage of active development with number remained above 40, number of applications reduced to 23 and 8 in 2020 and 2021, respectively, which indicated that related technologies have basically become mature (Fig. 4.2).

Aikang already started technical research on automatic enzyme immunoassay instrument in 2005, which allowed the company to become a relatively early entrant in the field. Aikang's URANUS AE series products received approval for marketing

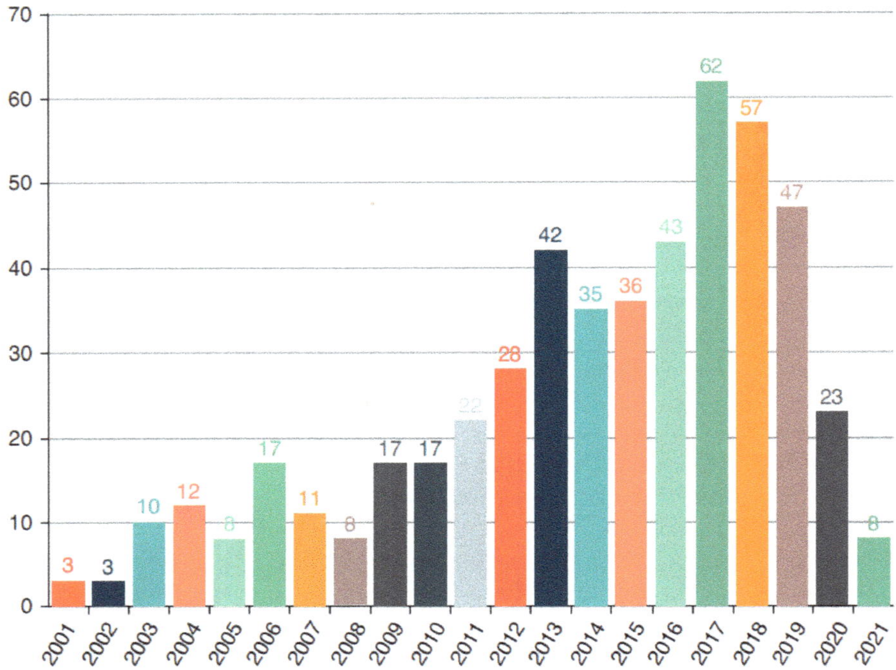

Fig. 4.2 Tendency diagram of number of automatic enzyme immunoassay instrument related patent applications in China

in 2006. Yantai Addcare started patent portfolios of ELISA workstation in 2007, and its pipelined fully automated ELISA workstation received approval for marketing in the same year. A bunch of excellent device manufacturers like Biobase, Diasia and JiaXing CRED also made deployment in the field and carried out technical studies, development and innovations in recent years, which further enriched automatic enzyme immunoassay instrument and offered users more choices.

It can be learned from analysis on automatic enzyme immunoassay instrument-related patent applications released in the 3 years from 2018 to 2021 that technical studies on it in recent years mainly focused on performance improvement of incubation temperature control technique, optical detection technique, sampling control technique, transfer control technique and other core modules, integration of fluorescence and chemiluminescence analysis function modules and other aspects. It can be seen that automatic enzyme immunoassay instrument will move toward directions of further improvement of performance, strengthening of degree of detection automation, extension of functional modules and automatic laboratory pipeline.

4.6 Market Situation of Automatic Enzyme Immunoassay Instrument

4.6.1 Market Size of Automatic Enzyme Immunoassay Instrument in China Between 2016 and 2027

According to network data, the market size of China's automatic enzyme immunoassay instrument was USD 30.69 million (approx. RMB 0.198 billion), it dropped a little bit to USD 29.02 million due to the outbreak of COVID-19. Market recovery is expected to be optimistic in 2022, which will reach USD 29.32 million. The hospital market is forecasted to pay more attention to automatic instruments, increase procurement and replace a certain proportion of microplate reader, and market size of China's automatic enzyme immunoassay instrument is expected to reach USD 30.97 million by 2026 (Fig. 4.3). According to network data of China's immunoassay devices in 2021, total amount of bid winning was around RMB 0.243 billion, which revealed the continued optimistic momentum of China's automatic enzyme immunoassay instrument market.

4.6.2 Market Shares of Segmented Application Scenario of Automatic Enzyme Immunoassay Instrument in China

Application scenario of China's automatic enzyme immunoassay instrument mainly includes hospitals, blood banks and other scientific research institutes. At present, in the field of hospitals, automatic enzyme immunoassay instrument can provide HBsAg, anti-HBs, HBeAg, anti-HBe, anti-HBc and anti-HBcIgM detection, HBsAg, anti-HCV, anti-HIV and TP detection, CMV, HSV, TOX, RV and TP detection as well as carcinoembryonic antigen and prenatal screening, and they can

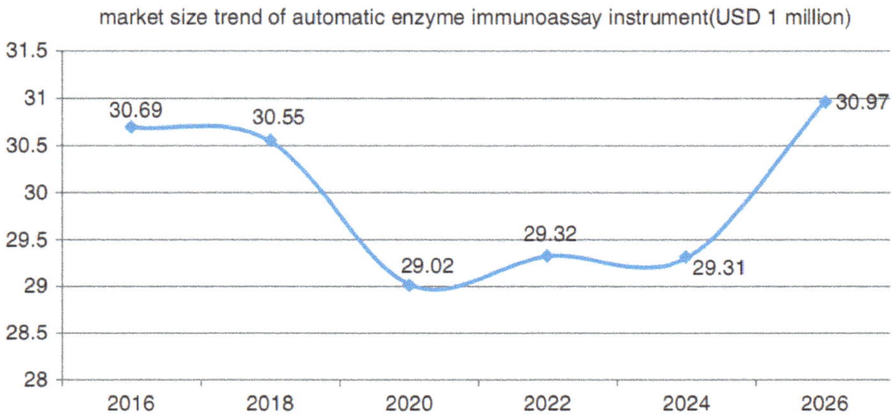

Fig. 4.3 Diagram of market size trend of automatic enzyme immunoassay instrument between 2016 and 2026 (data source: research on network data collation)

provide substantial detection items. Since grade-A tertiary hospitals normally have relatively large number of ELISA items and relatively large detection quantity, high throughput automatic enzyme immunoassay instrument that can handle multiple items at the same time are more suitable. Small hospitals boast of relatively large number of detection items and less detection quantity of each item, and detection of multiple items can often be conducted on the same microplate, based on this characteristic, highly integrated small automatic enzyme immunoassay instrument are comparatively more suitable. Blood banks use automatic enzyme immunoassay instrument for detection of blood collected, and the main detection items are infectious disease markers (HIV, HBV, HBsAg, HCV, TP, ALT, etc.), since blood banks have large sample size to be detected and relatively fixed detection items, high throughput automatic enzyme immunoassay instrument that can detect all items at the same time are more suitable.

According to a study conducted by network data, hospitals had the largest market share, about 78%, in China's automatic enzyme immunoassay instrument application scenario in 2020; followed by blood banks, which occupied the market share of about 15%. The market share of hospitals and blood bank is expected to remain relatively stable till 2027. Hence, it can be seen that the hospital market dominated the segmented application scenarios of automatic enzyme immunoassay instrument. Accompanied with hierarchical medical system's promotion of medical resources in lower tier cities, market demands of Grade II hospitals and township hospitals have become the new incremental of the automatic enzyme immunoassay instrument market. In case of domestic automatic enzyme immunoassay instrument manufacturers, they shall stay close to users' requirements in different application scenarios and create diversified products to provide comprehensive clinical detection solutions, which allow them to develop competitive advantages and create the greatest value for users.

4.6.3 Development Trend of Market of Automatic Enzyme Immunoassay Instrument Industry

Under the circumstance of continuous introduction of emerging detection techniques, ELISA will still be one of the mainstream detection techniques used in clinical laboratories of hospitals, blood banks, China Entry-Exit Inspection and Quarantine, Physical Examination Centers, Third Party Inspection Agencies and biological product companies, and domestic automatic enzyme immunoassay instrument still have relatively great development potentials.

At present, the recognition of laboratory departments of blood banks and hospitals has gradually been increasing due to relatively strong price advantage of domestic automatic enzyme immunoassay instrument in comparison with imported products as well as domestic manufacturers' continuous research and development. Taking High Throughput automatic enzyme immunoassay instrument and automatic enzyme immunoassay instrument post-processing system introduced by Aikang for laboratories of blood banks as examples, they have realized full automation of ELISA pipeline. Its products have been recognized by blood bank clients and broken the long-term monopoly of automatic enzyme immunoassay instrument of imported brands in laboratories of blood banks. Meanwhile, promulgation of hierarchical medical system policies and policies encourage hospitals' procurement of domestic medical devices will accelerate the replacement of imported instruments with domestic automatic enzyme immunoassay instrument.

Look into the future, accompanied with scientific and technological progress and particularly continuous development of biology, clinical medicine and materials science, interactive cooperation between different disciplines has become increasingly tight, users' requirements on performance of automatic enzyme immunoassay instrument have been constantly increasing as well, automatic enzyme immunoassay instrument have shown tendency toward fully automated detection in intellectualization and informatization of laboratories, and the field has extended outward to integrate sample processing system, sample transfer track and other laboratory devices through continuous technological innovation, functional expansion and performance improvement, which allow it to be total laboratory automation system.

Accompanied with development of national economy and improvement of people's livelihood, continuous deepening of urbanization and increasingly intensified population aging, reliance on fully automated instruments for medical diagnosis and treatment has been increasing, and the market size of IVD medical devices has been growing on a yearly basis. Despite the trend of CLIA's replacement of ELISA in the international market, China's immunologic diagnosis market is still characterized by co-existence of CLIA and ELISA. Besides, since ELISA boasts of more mature technology and relatively large cost advantage, market demand for ELISA is greater. In addition, accompanied with continuous deepening of China's healthcare reform, centralized procurement has been gradually implemented in the field of high value medical consumables, and concentration ratio of the industry will be gradually revealed. Domestic automatic enzyme immunoassay instrument manufactures shall seize the opportunity, give full play to their strengths in low cost and high acquaintance with domestic market, make plan and deployment in advance, stick to users' requirements, increase innovation inputs, facilitate new breakthroughs in quality and performance of automatic enzyme immunoassay instrument, promote greater diversity in product types and functions, meet constantly developing product requirements and offer more advanced products and better services for immunologic diagnosis.

Declaration Yunqi Li, Rongbang Xia, Tao Zhao and Pengfei Lai are employees of Aikang MedTech Co., Ltd.

Weijing Yi and Wei Hu are employees of Zybio Inc. (Nan Sun has resigned).

References

1. Hou J, Ren J, Song L, et al. Analytical performance of three diagnostic reagents for HBsAg on an automatic ELISA analyzer. J Clin Lab Anal. 2017;10(2):1002–8. https://doi.org/10.1002/jcla.22159.

2. Wang SH, Cao XH, Yuan LI, et al. Comparison of the test results between automatic enzyme-linked immunity analyzer and manual enzyme-linked immunoassay. J Kunming Med Univ. 2016;10:96–9. http://en.cnki.com.cn/Article_en/CJFDTOTAL-KMYX201610023.htm.
3. Créminon C, Taran F. Enzyme immunoassays as screening tools for catalysts and reaction discovery. Chem Commun. 2015;51(38):7996–8001. https://doi.org/10.1039/c5cc00599j.
4. UNIV CHUNG ANG IND ACAD COOP FOUND. Enzyme-linked immunosorbent assay system and method of using thereof: KR20190098504A. https://www.himmpat.com/browse?localId=142d0fce4f18dbbf7e87ca240d9e30a2. Accessed 22 Aug 2019.
5. Zhu Y, Alapati D, Costa J, et al. A comparison of enzyme-linked immunosorbent assay versus multiplex methodology using an in vitro model of pulmonary hypertension and inflammation. J Biomed Sci Eng. 2014;7(7):419–26. https://www.scirp.org/journal/PaperInformation.aspx?PaperID=46588.

5 Autoimmune Diagnostics

Haifeng Jin, Yanchun Guo, Tianshi Wang, Qiuping Yu,
Xuexin Deng, and Mu Wang

5.1 Overview of Autoimmune Diseases

5.1.1 The Concept of Autoimmunity

Autoimmunity refers to the destruction of the body's immune tolerance mechanism under the action of internal and external factors. On the one hand, the autoimmune B cells in the circulation increase in large quantities, and on the other hand, the self-reactive helper T lymphocytes promote the destruction of the self-tolerance of B lymphocytes. As a result, the immune system responds to its own components, producing antibodies against the self-components (auto-antibodies) and/or sensitized lymphocytes [1, 2].

5.1.2 Autoimmune Diseases

Autoimmune diseases (AIDs) generally refer to a large class of diseases when immune effector cells (cytotoxic T lymphocytes, natural killer cells, macrophages, etc.) or immune effector molecules (complement, antibodies, cytokines, etc.) produce pathological immune responses against self-tissue or cells, resulting in self-tissue damage. There are many AID classification methods, but they have not yet been unified. It can be divided into systemic autoimmune diseases and

H. Jin · Y. Guo · T. Wang · Q. Yu (✉)
Shenzhen YHLO Biotech Co., Ltd., Shenzhen, China
e-mail: yuqiuping@szyhlo.com

X. Deng
Tellgen Corporation, Shanghai, China

M. Wang
Shanghai Advanced Clinical Laboratory Science Co., Ltd. (ACLS), Shanghai, China

H. Song, L. Dai (eds.), *In Vitro Diagnostic Industry in China*,
https://doi.org/10.1007/978-981-99-3110-1_5

organ-specific autoimmune diseases according to the system involved. Systemic autoimmune diseases mainly include systemic lupus erythematosus, primary Sjogren syndrome, and systemic vasculitis. Organ-specific autoimmune diseases mainly include nervous system immune diseases, endocrine system diseases, digestive system diseases, and urinary system diseases disease.

5.1.2.1 Connective Tissue Disease

Connective tissue disease refers to a group of autoimmune diseases of pan-systemic rheumatic diseases, including systemic lupus erythematosus, primary Sjogren syndrome (pSS), systemic sclerosis (SSc), polymyositis/dermatomyositis, antiphospholipid syndrome, rheumatoid arthritis, ankylosing spondylitis, and vasculitis.

Systemic Lupus Erythematosus

Systemic lupus erythematosus (SLE) is a systemic autoimmune disease characterized by the involvement of multiple systems and organs, repeated relapses and remissions, and the presence of a large number of auto-antibodies in the body. The etiology of SLE is complex and is related to various factors such as genetics, sex hormones, and the environment (such as viral and bacterial infections). At present, the global prevalence of SLE is 0 to 241 per 100,000, and the prevalence of SLE is about 30 to 70 per 100,000 in China, with a male-female prevalence ratio of 1:10–12. With the continuous improvement of diagnosis and treatment, the survival rate of SLE patients has been greatly improved [3, 4].

Primary Sjogren Syndrome

Primary Sjogren syndrome (pSS) is a systemic autoimmune disease that causes dysfunction of the secretory glands, which results in dry surfaces of mucous membranes such as the mouth, eyes, nose, pharynx, larynx, and vagina. The etiology is unknown and may be related to genetic and environmental factors, affecting mainly middle-aged women, but can also affect children, men, and the elderly.

Systemic Sclerosis

Systemic sclerosis (SSc) is a rare autoimmune disease characterized by fibrosis of the skin and internal organs and microvascular lesions. SSc can be mainly divided into limited skin type (limited cutaneous SSc) and diffuse skin type (diffuse cutaneous SSc), in addition to scleroderma without skin sclerosis (sine scleroderma) and overlap syndrome (overlap syndrome). The prevalence of SSc is 1 per 10,000 in the world, and it is more common in women. At present, there is no relevant data on the incidence of this disease in China. Its clinical manifestations are complex and diverse, and the prognosis of patients with visceral involvement is biased. The etiology of SSc is complex, and it is currently believed that environmental, genetic susceptibility, and epigenetic factors are involved.

Rheumatoid Arthritis

Rheumatoid arthritis (RA) is a chronic, systemic inflammatory disease. The incidence rate of adults is 0.5 to 1% in the United States, and the incidence rate is 0.42%

in China [5]. It is more common in women and can occur at any age. The peak incidence is between 50 and 60 years old. Patients with the disease mainly present with symmetrical pain and swelling of the hands, wrists, feet, and knees (polyarthritis); other joints may also be affected, patients may also have monoarthritis or microarthritis, and some patients may show other organs symptom.

5.1.2.2 Nervous System Immune Diseases

Nervous system immune disease refers to a group of diseases that attack the nervous system by autoimmune cells and immune molecules, resulting in pathological changes such as damage to neurons or axons, demyelination, and destruction of nerve-muscle joints, and corresponding clinical symptoms. Nervous system immune diseases mainly include autoimmune encephalitis, neuromyelitis optica spectrum diseases, multiple sclerosis, paraneoplastic syndrome, myasthenia gravis, and Guillain-Barre syndrome (GBS).

Autoimmune Encephalitis

Autoimmune encephalitis (AE) generally refers to a type of encephalitis mediated by autoimmune mechanisms. In classic paraneoplastic limbic encephalitis, its target antigens are located in neuronal cells; while in the new AE represented by anti-NMDAR encephalitis, its pathogenic antibodies are mainly directed against neuronal cell surface proteins and receptors. At present, the incidence of encephalitis is 5–8 per 100,000, and the prevalence of AE accounts for 10–20% of encephalitis cases [6].

Neuromyelitis Optica Spectrum Disorders

Neuromyelitis optica spectrum disorders (NMOSD) is an immune-mediated inflammatory demyelinating disease of the central nervous system mainly involving the optic nerve and spinal cord. Clinically, it is characterized by severe optic neuritis and longitudinally extending long-segment transverse myelitis. It usually begins in young adults, and most of them are women. The recurrence rate and disability rate are high. The international incidence of NMOSD is 1–5 per 100,000 people. There is no accurate epidemiological data of NMOSD in China, but relevant reports indicate that non-white people are more susceptible.

Multiple Sclerosis

Multiple sclerosis (MS) is an autoimmune-mediated neurodegenerative disease characterized by inflammatory demyelination and axonal transection of the central nervous system. The global incidence of multiple sclerosis is 5–300 per 100,000, and it increases in high latitudes. Most of the patients with MS are young (the average age of onset is 20–30 years old), and there are more women than men with a ratio of nearly 3:1.

Paraneoplastic Neurological Syndrome

Paraneoplastic neurological syndrome (PNS) is a group of clinical symptoms caused by the nerve or/and muscular system affected by tumors or their products (including the production of ectopic hormones) leading to abnormal immune responses (including cross-immunity, autoimmunity, and immune complex deposition) or other unknown reasons, causing lesions in the endocrine, nerve, digestive, hematopoietic, bone and joint, skin, and other systems. Overt clinical symptoms of paraneoplastic syndromes can occur before, after, or at the same time as the onset of the tumor.

Myasthenia Gravis

Myasthenia gravis (MG) is an acquired autoimmune disease mediated by acetylcholine receptor (AchR-Ab) antibody, cellular immunity dependent, complement participated, postsynaptic membrane of neuromuscular junction involved, causing impaired junctional transmission, and characterized by weak skeletal muscle contractions. The annual incidence of the disease is 8–20 per 100,000 people. It can occur at any age. Before the age of 40, the incidence of women is higher than that of men, and the incidence of men and women between the ages of 40 and 50 is not much different. After the age of 50, the incidence of men is slightly higher than that of women.

Guillain-Barre Syndrome

Guillain-Barre syndrome (GBS) is an inflammatory disease involving the peripheral nervous system and is the most common cause of acute flaccid paralysis. The global incidence is about 1–2 per 100,000 person-years. All age groups can be affected, males are more common than females, and the incidence increases with age. The clinical symptoms of GBS disease vary widely, generally manifesting as weakness and sensory signs in the legs, progressing to the arms and cranial muscles.

5.1.2.3 Endocrine System Diseases

Autoimmune endocrine diseases refer to a class of diseases that cause multiple endocrine gland dysfunction due to loss of immune tolerance and manifest different clinical symptoms, mainly including Hashimoto's thyroiditis (HT) and type I diabetes.

Hashimoto's Thyroiditis

Hashimoto's thyroiditis (HT) is the most common thyroid autoimmune disease. The global annual incidence of Hashimoto's thyroiditis is estimated to be 0.3–1.5 per 1000 people. Decreased autoimmune tolerance of the thyroid is the main pathogenesis. After being stimulated, such as iodine intake, the immune cells that are originally tolerant to the thyroid are activated and lose their tolerance, causing leukocytes to infiltrate tissues and promote autoimmunity response development.

Type 1 Diabetes Mellitus

Type 1 diabetes mellitus (T1DM) is a chronic autoimmune disease with clinical manifestations of insulin deficiency and the resulting persistent hyperglycemia. Globally, the incidence of type 1 diabetes is increasing year by year, with an annual increase of about 2 to 3%. From 2001 to 2015, the annual incidence rate of people under the age of 65 was 22.9 per 100,000.

5.1.2.4 Digestive System Diseases

Immune-mediated digestive disorders involve all digestive organs from the mouth to the anus. The liver, gallbladder, and pancreas can all be affected. Common diseases include autoimmune gastritis, inflammatory bowel disease, coeliac disease, and autoimmune liver disease.

Autoimmune Gastritis

Autoimmune gastritis (AIG) is an immune-mediated organ-specific disease. The abnormal immune response leads to destruction of gastric parietal cells, loss of internal factors and decrease of gastric acid output, thus reducing the absorption of iron, vitamin B12 and other micronutrients. The incidence rate in Asia is lower than that in Europe and the United States.

Inflammatory Bowel Disease

Inflammatory bowel disease (IBD) is an idiopathic disease that is caused by genetic vulnerable sex and external environment, such as dietary changes and antibiotic use. Incidence rate can be affected in all regions of the world, with an upward trend. Other studies have shown that ulcerative colitis and Crohn's disease (CD) are two major types of IBDs, affecting approximately the world's 0.3% population.

Celiac Disease

Celiac disease is one of the most common food-related chronic diseases, with a global prevalence of 1.4%. Patients with coeliac disease may have gastrointestinal and other symptoms of varying severity, such as diarrhea, abdominal pain, anemia, and osteoporosis, but some may be asymptomatic. The pathogenesis of this disease is due to the ingestion of wheat, rye, and barley gluten proteins that cause villous atrophy, crypt hyperplasia, and intraepithelial lymphocytosis in the small intestine.

Autoimmune Liver Diseases

Autoimmune liver diseases (AILD) are a group of diseases with unknown etiology, liver tissue damage, and abnormal liver function caused by abnormal autoimmunity. Autoimmune liver diseases mainly include autoimmune hepatitis, primary biliary cholangitis, primary sclerosing cholangitis, and overlap syndrome. Autoimmune hepatitis (AIH) is a type of chronic hepatitis, which needs to be differentiated from chronic viral hepatitis, drug-induced and alcohol-induced hepatitis, and idiopathic chronic hepatitis. AIH can occur in all races worldwide, affecting children and adults of all ages, with a predominance of women. Primary biliary cholangitis (PBC) is the most common autoimmune liver disease, a lifelong disease, histologically manifested as chronic immune damage to small bile ducts. Primary sclerosing cholangitis is a rare chronic cholestatic liver disease characterized by strictures of the intrahepatic or extrahepatic bile ducts, or both, with bile duct fibrosis. Overlap syndrome is the most common combination of autoimmune hepatitis and primary biliary cholangitis. Patients having clinical manifestations of both diseases need to be differentiated clinically.

5.1.2.5 Hematological Diseases

Hematological diseases mainly include autoimmune hemolytic anemia, idiopathic thrombocytopenic purpura. Autoimmune hemolytic anemia (AIHA) is a relatively uncommon disease caused by anti-erythrocyte auto-antibodies. Immune thrombocytopenic purpura is an autoimmune disorder characterized by low platelet counts and mucocutaneous bleeding. The estimated incidence is 10 per 100,000 person-years, with about half of these occurring in children and about twice as high in women as in men.

5.1.2.6 Urinary System Diseases

The main causes of kidney damage in autoimmune diseases are auto-antibodies directed against intrinsic glomerular antigens (e.g., occur in membranous nephropathy and anti-glomerular basement membrane nephropathy) or nonspecific antibody deposition in the glomeruli (e.g., as neutrophil cytoplasmic antibody (ANCA) associated glomerulonephritis, C3 glomerulopathy and immunoglobulin A [IgA] nephropathy].

5.1.3 Antibody Markers for Autoimmune Diseases

As well-known effector molecules, the role of auto-antibodies in the pathogenesis of autoimmune diseases has become one of the main directions of research, although some auto-antibodies may not have pathogenic effects (such as natural auto-antibodies, tissue damage-producing auto-antibodies), or the pathogenesis is unclear. No matter auto-antibodies are pathogenic or not, it cannot be denied that auto-antibodies have important clinical significance, either as diagnostic tools, as indicators of disease activity monitoring, or both.

5.1.3.1 Auto-Antibodies Associated with Connective Tissue Diseases

There are many types of auto-antibodies in SLE, and the most widely used is anti-nuclear antibody (ANA). In SLE patients, the positive rate of ANA is as high as 90%. SLE-related antibodies mainly include anti-dsDNA antibodies, anti-Sm (Smith) antibodies, anti-U1-RNP (U1 ribonucleoprotein) antibodies, anti-nucleosome antibodies, anti-ribosomal P protein antibodies, anti-histone antibodies, anti-SSB/ La antibody, and anti-SSA/Ro antibody. Anti-dsDNA is a characteristic antibody of SLE, and its positive value is highly suggestive of the occurrence of systemic lupus erythematosus. Anti-U1-RNP (U1 ribonucleoprotein) antibody is generally a marker antibody for mixed connective tissue disease. Its positive rate is as high as 100%, and it is also a sign of clinical detection of SLE. Anti-nucleosome antibody is one of the early clinical detection indicators of SLE, earlier than anti-histone antibody and anti-dsDNA antibody. Anti-ribosomal P protein antibody is one of the clinical detection indicators of SLE. It is a highly specific index, which is closely related to the damage of SLE disease in the nervous system; anti-histone antibody is an important clinical detection index in SLE. The detection rate of anti-SSB/La antibody in SLE is about 10–15%. It has been confirmed by research that it is mainly related to hair loss, cheek erythema and serositis. It has high sensitivity in clinical detection, but low specificity. Anti-SSA/Ro antibody, mainly divided into anti-Ro52 and anti-Ro60, has a detection rate of about 40% in SLE. It mainly affects the formation of immune complexes of patients and has certain correlation with the inflammatory process of active lupus.

The biological markers of primary Sjogren syndrome (pSS) mainly include anti-SSA/SSB antibodies and anti-muscarinic receptor 3 (M3R) antibodies. The application of anti-SSA/SSB antibody in the clinical diagnosis and treatment monitoring of pSS is related to the occurrence and development of pSS and serious complications, and is included in the diagnosis and treatment guidelines of pSS, which has important clinical value. In recent years, it has been found that anti-M3R antibody plays a great role in the diagnosis and assessment of the severity of pSS and treatment. However, it has not been used in clinical practice.

Antinuclear antibodies in the blood of patients with systemic sclerosis (SSc) are above 95%. Among them, anti-topoisomerase I antibody (Scl-70) and anti-centromere antibody are classical antinuclear antibodies found in SSc. In recent years, more autoantigens have been discovered, including RNA polymerase III, fibrin, NOR90, Th/To, PM-Scl, Ku, and platelet-derived growth factor receptor (PDGFR). SSc-related auto-antibodies are associated with different disease subtypes, disease severity, including skin involvement, visceral manifestations, and prognosis.

In the myositis, auto-antibody spectrum, anti-Jo-l antibody, anti-PL-7 antibody, anti-PL-12 antibody, and anti-Mi-2 antibody are highly sensitive and specific. The combined detection of multiple myositis-specific auto-antibodies significantly increases the sensitivity and helps to improve the diagnostic rate of PM and dermatomyositis patients.

Antiphospholipid antibody (aPL) is a general term for a group of auto-antibodies targeting phospholipids and/or phospholipid-binding proteins. Among them, lupus anticoagulant (LA), anticardiolipin antibody (aCL) and anti-β2-glycoprotein I antibody (anti-β2GP1) are laboratory indicators in the classification criteria of antiphospholipid syndrome (APS). aPL plays a key pathogenic role in the development of APS. aPL positivity with systemic autoimmune disease is a risk factor for future thrombotic events.

The two most common auto-antibodies of patients with rheumatoid arthritis (RA) are rheumatoid factor (RF) and anti-cyclic citrulline polypeptide antibody (CCP). RF directly targets the Fc part of IgG. 70–80% RA patient's RF is positive. RF may also be positive in patients with SLE, pSS, or systemic infection, and in approximately 10% healthy people. The sensitivity of RF in RA is 80% and specificity is 85%. High concentration RF is associated with disease activity. The sensitivity of anti-CCP antibodies in RA is 67%, the specificity is 95%, and the anti-CCP antibodies are associated with radiographic progression.

The pathogenesis of vasculitis is a complex and multi-factor process. Antineutrophil cytoplasmic antibody (ANCA), B lymphocyte, T lymphocyte, monocyte, endothelial cell, and complement replacement pathway play an important role in this process. The two most common auto-antibodies of ANCA are anti-myeloperoxidase antibody (MPO-ANCA) and anti-protease 3 antibody (PR3-ANCA).

5.1.3.2 Nervous System Disease Auto-Antibodies

Autoimmune encephalitis antibodies are divided into two categories: anti-intracellular antigen antibodies and anti-cell surface antigen antibodies (Table 5.1) [7].

Table 5.1 Anti-neuronal antibodies associated with autoimmune encephalitis

Classification	Antigen	Antigen location	Encephalitic syndrome	Proportion of tumors	Main tumor type
Anti-intracellular antigen antibody	Hu	Neuron nucleus	Limbic encephalitis	>95%	Small cell lung cancer
	Ma2	Neuron nucleolus	Limbic encephalitis	>95%	Seminiferous cell carcinoma
	GAD	Neuronal cytoplasm	Limbic encephalitis	25%	Thymoma, small cell lung cancer
	Amphoteric protein	Neuronal cytoplasm	Limbic encephalitis	46–79%	Small cell lung cancer, breast cancer
	CV2	Oligodendrocyte membrane	Limbic encephalitis	86.5%	Small cell lung cancer, thymoma
Anti-cell surface antigen antibody	NMDA receptors	Neuron cell membrane	Anti-NMDA receptor encephalitis	Varies by gender and age	Ovarian teratoma
	AMPAR	Neuron cell membrane	Limbic encephalitis	65%	Thymoma, small cell lung cancer
	$GABA_BR$	Neuron cell membrane	Limbic encephalitis	50%	Small cell lung cancer
	LGI1	Neuron cell membrane	Limbic encephalitis	5–10%	Thymoma
	CASPR2	Neuron cell membrane	Morvan syndrome, limbic encephalitis	20–50%	Thymoma
	DPPX	Neuron cell membrane	Encephalitis, often with diarrhea	<10%	Lymphoma
	IgLON5	Neuron cell membrane	Encephalopathy with sleep disturbance	0%	–
	GlyR	Neuron cell membrane	progressive encephalomyelitis with rigidity and myoclonus (PERM)	<10%	Thymoma
	$GABA_AR$	Neuron cell membrane	Encephalitis	<5%	Thymoma
	mGluR5	Neuron cell membrane	Encephalitis	70%	Hodgkin lymphoma
	D2R	Neuron cell membrane	Basal ganglia encephalitis	0%	–
	Synapsin-3a	Neuron cell membrane	Encephalitis	–	–
	MOG	Oligodendrocyte membrane	acute disseminated encephalomyelitis (ADEM), etc.	0%	0%

The specific diagnostic biomarker for neuromyelitis optica spectrum disease (NMOSD) is aquaporin −4 antibody (AQP4-IgG). With the continuous progress of clinical and basic research, the oligodendrocyte glycoprotein antibody (MOG-IgG), aquaporin-1 antibody (AQP1-IgG), and glial fibrillary acidic protein antibody (GFAP-IgG) play an important role in the pathogenesis of NMOSD.

In myasthenia gravis (MG), antibodies against the muscle acetylcholine receptor (AChR) are detected in the majority of patients (85%), while antibodies against muscle-specific kinase (MuSK) are detected in 6% of patients. In 10% of MG patients, no auto-antibodies are found in the classic AChR and muskox antibody diagnosis (seronegative MG, SN-MG). Therefore, it is imperative to improve the known auto-antibody detection methods or discover new antigen targets.

5.1.3.3 Auto-Antibodies for Endocrine System Diseases

Autoimmune thyroid disease (AITD) is usually accompanied by anti-thyroid peroxidase (TPO), anti-thyroglobulin (TG), and anti-thyroid hormone receptor (TSHR) antibodies. Anti-TPO antibodies have been detected in 90–95% AITD patients, 80% Graves' disease(GD), and 10–15% non-AITD patients.

Anti-TPO antibodies may exert cytotoxic effects on thyroid cells in Hashimoto's thyroiditis (HT), but have not been determined in GDs. Anti-TPO antibodies can cross the placental barrier to some extent, but the effects on newborns are unknown. The positive rate of anti-TG antibody is 60–80% in HT patients and 50–60% in GD patients. Anti-TSHR antibodies are present in approximately 90% of patients with GD, 0–20% of patients with HT, and 10–75% of patients with atrophic thyroiditis.

The diagnosis and prediction of type 1 diabetes mellitus (T1DM) depend entirely on the determination of islet cell-related auto-antibodies. The titer of anti-glutamic acid decarboxylase antibody (GADA) usually reaches a peak at the age of 2 years, and then the positive rate and titer decrease along with the progress of the disease. However, it still exists for a long time in the adult, which can maintain good sensitivity (60–80%). GADA has become one of the diagnostic indicators for latent autoimmune diabetes in adults (LADA). Anti-insulin auto-antibodies (IAA) are the most important islet autoantigens in T1DM. IAA is usually the earliest antibody being detected with a peak titer at 2 years of age, and then the titer and positive rate decrease with age. The rate is very low, so it has limited diagnostic value for older T1DM. Anti-protein tyrosine phosphatase antibody (IA-2A) and its homolog IA-2βare both neuroendocrine molecules, members of the protein tyrosine phosphatase family, involved in the regulation of insulin secretion, and IA-2A drops before the diagnosis of T1DM. The degree of IA-2A increased gradually, and the positive rate of IA-2A in newly diagnosed T1DM patients is 60–80%. Zinc transporter-8 (ZnT8) is a specific Zn^{2+} transporter in islet D cells, which is only expressed in isletβcells. The positive rate of ZnT8 antibody increases with age at the age of >2 years, and the stability is high. The specificity of diagnosing TIDM in different age groups is basically similar, so ZnT8A is more valuable for diagnosing older T1DM patients.

5.1.3.4 Auto-Antibodies to Digestive System Diseases

Autoimmune gastritis (AIG) serological biomarkers include parietal cell antibody and intrinsic factor antibody. Gastric parietal cell antibody exists in 85–90% of patients with pernicious anemia. The serum positive rate of intrinsic factor antibody is lower than that of parietal cell antibody (about 60%), but the specificity of intrinsic factor antibody is higher. The level of parietal cell antibody and intrinsic factor antibody is significantly related to the atrophy degree of gastro-acid mucosa.

Inflammatory bowel disease (IBD) often includes ulcerative colitis (UC) and Crohn's disease (CD). The most commonly studied serological marker in IBD are anti-Saccharomyces cerevisiae antibody (ASCA) and anti-neutrophil cytoplasmic antibody (ANCA). ASCA occurs in 45–60% of CD patients and can reach 15% in UC. If ASCA and PAB are positive, and ANCA or GAB is negative, it indicates that CD is more likely to occur than UC.

Celiac disease-related antibodies mainly include human anti-tissue transglutaminase antibody (tTG) type IgA, endomysium antibody type IgA, and deaminated gliadin antibody types IgA and IgG. These serological antibody tests are becoming increasingly important in the diagnosis of coeliac disease. The sensitivity and specificity of endomysial antibodies reach 90%. Some studies have also found that the sensitivity and specificity of anti-tTG antibodies can reach 90%. About 50–75% of autoimmune hepatitis (AIH) patients in autoimmune liver disease (AILD) are positive for ANA antibody; anti-smooth muscle antibody (SMA) is not specific and can be used to identify and diagnose early AIH patients. The anti-liver and kidney microsomal (LKM) antibody helps to diagnose AIH2-type patients. It is not specific for AIH. The anti-soluble liver antigen/hepatopancreatic antigen (SLA/LP) antibody is specific for AIH. Ninety percent of patients with primary biliary cirrhosis (PBC) have positive anti-mitochondrial antibody. ANA and anti-sp100 antibodies may assist in the diagnosis of AMA-negative patients. Anti-sp100 antibodies can be detected in 20% patients with primary biliary cirrhosis, and anti-gp210 and/or anti-Lamin-B receptor antibodies can be detected in 30–50% AMA negative patients.

5.1.3.5 Auto-Antibodies for Urinary System Diseases

For decades, clinical studies have found that there are specific auto-antibodies in the serum of most patients with autoimmune nephropathy. Lupus nephritis is related to anti-C1q antibody, antinuclear antibody, and double-stranded DNA antibody. Primary necrotic crescentic glomerulus (NCGN) is associated with anti-myeloperoxidase antibodies. Nephritis induced by granulomatous vasculitis (GPA) is related to anti-protease 3 antibody. GBM is associated with pulmonary hemorrhage-nephritis syndrome. Membranous nephropathy is closely related to antiphospholipase A 2 receptor antibody (PLA2R). Specific auto-antibodies are an important part of the diagnostic criteria for autoimmune nephropathy.

5.1.4 Diagnosis of Autoimmune Diseases

The incidence of autoimmune diseases is increasing year by year, and it varies with regions and ethnic groups. It is more common in women. The disease course is longer and the disease is prolonged and repeated. The severity of the disease is parallel to the autoimmune response. It is easy to suffer from immunodeficiency diseases or malignant tumors. High-titer auto-antibodies and/or sensitized lymphocytes reacting with self-tissue components can be detected in blood. The pathological characteristics of tissues and organs are immune inflammation, and the damage scope corresponds to the distribution of antigens targeted by auto-antibodies or sensitized lymphocytes. Overlapping phenomenon: A patient can suffer from more than one autoimmune disease at the same time. The serological overlapping phenomenon is more common in some autoimmune diseases.

The development of diagnostic criteria for autoimmune diseases has undergone a long process and has been updated with the development of clinical and basic science. The general principles include clinical symptoms and signs, routine laboratory tests, functional tests of tissues and organs, and special immunological tests.

Taking SLE as an example, SLE is a systemic autoimmune disease. The main clinical features are as follows: systemic multi-system multi-organ involvement, repeated recurrence and remission, and a large number of auto-antibodies in the body. European League Against Rheumatism (EULAR), British Society of Rheumatology (BSR), Pan American League Against Rheumatism (PANLAR), and other influential academic organizations and institutions in the world have formulated their own SLE diagnosis and treatment guidelines. The Rheumatology Branch of the Chinese Medical Association published the Guidelines for Diagnosis and Treatment of SLE in 2010. In view of the continuous emergence of new diagnosis and treatment research results and new treatment drugs, the guideline formulation concept, methods, and technologies have also been developed and updated. The Rheumatology Branch of the Medical Association, the National Clinical Research Center for Skin and Immune Diseases, and CSTAR have formulated the "2020 China Systemic Lupus Erythematosus" based on the latest research evidence and the clinical practice in China. It is recommended to use the SLE classification criteria developed by the International Lupus Research Clinical Collaborative Group (SLICC) in 2012 or the EULAR/ACR in 2019 to diagnose suspected SLE. The sensitivity of the SLE classification standards of EULAR/ACR in 2019, SLICC in 2012, and 1997 is 96, 97, and 83%, respectively, and the specificity is 93, 84, and 93%, respectively. The sensitivity and specificity of the SLE classification criteria of EULAR/ACR in 2019 both are optimal.

5.2 Methods and Techniques for Auto-Antibody Detection

Determination of auto-antibodies plays an important role in the diagnosis and differential diagnosis of autoimmune diseases. At present, auto-antibody detection has been widely used in clinical practice in China. Factors such as the selection of detection methods, the professionalism of operators, and the selection of reagent quality are directly related to the quality of the test results, affecting the judgment and interpretation of the results by clinicians.

With the development of contemporary methods for quantitative detection of auto-antibodies, the identification of these antigen-antibody systems has been regarded as one of the milestones in clinical immunity in the past 60 years. As far as detection methods are concerned, microscopy and biochemical methods (often called morphological and immunological methods) play an important role in laboratory medicine. All derived immunological methods can be used for the diagnosis of autoimmune diseases. Based on methodological principles and application scenarios, methods for auto-antibody detection are divided into the following categories:

5.2.1 Indirect Immunofluorescence Assay

Indirect immunofluorescence is a method in which specific antibody components in serum or plasma form antigen-antibody complexes with antigens in tissues or cells. Fluorescein-labeled secondary antibody is used to recognize antigen-antibody complexes, and fluorescent microscope is used to observe bright fluorescence of fluorescein irradiated by external excitation light. The fluorescent pattern of the combined antigen-antibody complexes varies with different localizations.

5.2.2 Immunoblotting

The immunoblotting method is to transfer the natural or purified antigen to the nitrocellulose membrane, and then combine the antigen and antibody specifically to form an antigen-antibody complex with the antibody to be tested in the serum or plasma. The enzyme-labeled secondary antibody recognizes the complex and reacts with the chromogenic substrate to form a color band. According to the position of the band and the depth of the color, it is determined whether there is a corresponding auto-antibody.

5.2.3 Dot Immunobinding Assay

The dot immunology method uses the nitrocellulose membrane as a solid phase support to perform immunological detection of antigen and antibody reactions. After the antibody is being added, it can bind to the antigen on the membrane and then add the antibody labeled with a marker so that the marker is indirectly cross-linked to the cellulose membrane through the combination of the anti-antibody and the corresponding antibody. When the corresponding substrate is dispensed, the marker will react with the substrate to form insoluble products, which will be stained in dot shape to determine the results. According to the different markers being used, they can be divided into horseradish peroxidase dot immunological test (use horseradish peroxidase as the marker of anti-antibody), alkaline phosphatase dot immunological test (use alkaline phosphatase anti-alkaline phosphatase complex as the marker of enzyme), and gold-silver staining dot immunological test (use colloidal gold as the marker of anti-antibody). Among them, the most commonly used is the spot immunological test based on the horseradish peroxidase labeling system.

5.2.4 Enzyme-Linked Immunoassay

Enzyme-linked immunosorbent assay (ELISA) is a detection technology that combines the immune reaction of antigen and antibody with the high-efficiency catalytic action of enzyme. Auto-antibody detection usually adopts the indirect method. Enzyme-labeled antibody is used to detect the tested antibody that has been combined with the solid phase. The main steps are as follows: (1) The specific antigen is combined with the solid phase carrier to form the solid phase antigen. (2) Adding diluted serum: the specific antibody is combined with the antigen to form the solid phase antigen-antibody complex. (3) Adding enzyme-labeled anti-antibody: binding with the antibody in the solid phase complex so that the antibody is indirectly labeled with enzyme. (4) Color development by adding substrate: color depth represents the amount of tested antibody in the sample.

5.2.5 Chemiluminescence Immunoassay

Chemiluminescence immunoassay (CLIA) is a trace analysis method for determining the analyte content based on the linear and quantitative relationship between the analyte concentration and the chemiluminescence intensity of the system under certain conditions.

Mainstream reagent technologies being used internationally include: direct chemiluminescence [isoluminol (Snibe Diagnostic), acridine ester (Abbott, YHLO)], indirect (enzymatic) chemiluminescence (Danaher, Mindray, Autobio), and electrochemiluminescence (Roche). However, the major manufacturers involved in providing auto-antibody chemiluminescence immunoassay are YHLO, HOB, and Werfen.

5.2.6 Multiplex Immunofluorescence Assay

Multiplex detection is the simultaneous detection of multiple indicators (signals) of the same sample. Multiplex detection technology has superior methodological conditions in terms of detection speed. As the core, it is a multi-index parallel analysis technology platform integrating flow cytometry, laser analysis, high-speed digital signal processing, and other technologies, which can quantitatively detect a variety of different biomolecules at one time. Antibody molecules or gene probes for different analytes are bound to specific encoded microspheres in a covalently cross-linked manner, and each encoded microsphere corresponds to a specific detection item. First, the fluorescently encoded microspheres for different substances to be tested are mixed, and then the substances to be tested or amplified fragments to be tested are added, and the formed complex is then combined with the labeled fluorescein to react. Driven by the flowing sheath fluid, the microspheres pass through the detection unit in sequence in a single column, and through the analysis of the captured fluorescence code and the fluorescence intensity of the reporter molecule, the purpose of fast and accurate multiple detection is achieved.

5.2.7 Quality Control and Evaluation of Auto-Antibody Detection

There are various detection methods for auto-antibodies, including qualitative detection, quantitative detection, manual operation, and automatic detection. The traceability standards of each manufacturer are different, and the equipment level of each laboratory and the technical level of operators is different. The accuracy of laboratory test results may vary greatly, so the accuracy of auto-antibody test results is closely related to its quality control.

5.2.7.1 Improvement of Automation Level

The degree of automation of domestic auto-antibody detection is generally low, far behind European and American countries. With the continuous expansion of the overall demand for auto-antibody and the rapid growth of the market capacity and scale, more enterprises are attracted to develop automation devices and products. The automation degree and standardization degree of the overall auto-antibody detection have been improved. The improvement in the automation degree will reduce the problem of result difference caused by differences in personnel factors and technical capabilities.

5.2.7.2 Items Covered by Inter-Laboratory Quality Assessment

The auto-antibody items covered by the inter-laboratory quality assessment are limited, and the results are not satisfactory. The National Rheumatology Database Center (CRDC) has made some measures to improve this phenomenon: increasing the number of auto-antibody inter-laboratory quality assessment items and the types of diseases covered, provide data analysis for quantitative detection. CRDC aims to further improve the standardization of auto-antibody testing in each center, establish a laboratory quality management concept, and provide guarantee for individualized and precise treatment of clinical rheumatism. Existing coverage items are ANA, dsDNA, antiphospholipid antibodies, autoimmune liver disease auto-antibodies, autoimmune vasculitis, and rheumatoid arthritis-related auto-antibodies. It meets the basic inter-laboratory comparison needs for major items in each laboratory center.

5.2.7.3 Coverage of Quality Control Materials in Internal Quality Control

Due to the limitation of domestic auto-antibody detection methodologies such as western blotting, ELISA, and indirect immunofluorescence (IFA) method, all of which are mainly operated manually. There are often no quality controls for internal quality control, and only negative and positive quality controls are being monitored. Due to the increased level of automation, increased quality control requirements, increased clinical demand for accuracy of test results, the demand for internal quality control has also been increased. Some companies have begun to develop third-party quality control products for auto-antibodies to meet laboratory needs to further improve laboratory management capabilities. Items covered by auto-antibody quality control products include ANA-related auto-antibodies, antiphospholipid antibodies, autoimmune liver disease-related auto-antibodies, and rheumatoid arthritis-related auto-antibodies.

5.2.7.4 Limited Standardization

The lack of recognized official standard reference materials for auto-antibody testing is a major cause of discrepancies in auto-antibody testing results. Different methods of obtaining raw materials, genetic engineering of proteins and extraction of natural substances, inconsistent selection of binding sites, and inconsistent assignment systems can all lead to large differences between auto-antibody detection platforms, and poor inter-laboratory comparability.

5.3 Status of Domestic Autoimmune Diagnostic Products

5.3.1 Registered Products of Domestic Autoimmune Diagnostics

At present, the most commonly used autoantibody detection methodologies in China include indirect immunofluorescence, immunoblotting, enzyme-linked immunosorbent assay, chemiluminescence, and flow cytometry fluorescence/liquid-phase microarray chip. Although immunoblotting is slightly less automated, it is still the mainstream methodology for autoantibody detection because of its simplicity of operation, the ability to combine dozens of parameters, and high efficiency. In recent years, traditional autoimmune manufacturers, such as Shenzhen YHLO Biotech, Suzhou HOB Biotech, Guangzhou Kangrun Biotech, and emerging manufacturers, such as Sichuan C-Luminary Biotechnology and AVIC Saiwei Biological Science & Technology, have started to focus on promoting high-throughput, fully automated chemiluminescence equipment and supporting autoimmune reagents, and there is a trend to gradually replace immunoblotting and enzyme-linked immunosorbent assay. In addition, some domestic manufacturers (e.g., Shanghai Tellgen Diagnostic Technology, Zhuhai Livzon Diagnostics) have also applied the flow cytometry fluorescence/liquid-phase microarray chip platform for autoantibody detection, which has a unique advantage in screening multiple parameters of autoantibody profile with its parameter co-testing function.

In China, the most commonly used methodologies for autoantibody detection are immunoblotting (51%), followed by chemiluminescence (16%), enzyme-linked immunosorbent assay (16%), and indirect immunofluorescence (13%), with less use of multiplex assays (4%).

5.3.2 The Main Instrument Products of Domestic Autoimmune Diagnosis

5.3.2.1 Automated Indirect Immunofluorescence Equipment

There are very few domestic automated equipment for indirect immunofluorescence, and only Shenzhen YHLO Biotech has products that support indirect immunofluorescence experimental operation and (or) fluorescence karyotype analysis equipment in China. Because of the differences in the position and size of the cell wells coated on the fluorescent slides of different manufacturers, and the interpretation principles of different manufacturers are different, and the secondary antibody dyes are also different, so the fluorescent karyotype analysis equipment is a closed system and does not support the reading of fluorescence results of other brands. The pretreatment equipment for indirect immunofluorescence is basically open, and the position of the addition needle and the height of the wash plate can be adjusted according to the position of the slide hole and the thickness of the slide of the target manufacturer.

iSlide240 Indirect Immunofluorescence Pre-Treatment System

iSlide240 is an indirect immunofluorescence pre-treatment system developed and manufactured by Shenzhen YHLO Biotech. It can realize the pretreatment of fluorescence experiments, including serum dilution, sample addition, incubation, cleaning and reagent addition processes. Subsequent manual blocking and interpretation of results under a microscope or automatic interpretation of the fluorescence results using iReader600 is required. The iSlide240 has a sample position of 240, with 2 addition needles, and supports 24 fluorescent slices for simultaneous operation, supporting automated experiments with most of the indirect immunofluorescence carriers on the market.

iReader600 Indirect Immunofluorescence Karyotype Analysis System

iReader600 is an indirect immunofluorescence karyotype analysis system launched by Shenzhen YHLO Biotech and iSlide240 simultaneously, which can realize the automatic reading of ANA, dsDNA and ANCA fluorescence karyotype and the automatic photographing of ALD fluorescence results, and can issue graphic report sheets. The iReader600 supports 50 fluorescence slices on the machine at the same time, and supports three fluorescence channels: FITC, DAPI and Evans Blue. The average reading time is about 10 seconds per well, which is fast and efficient.

5.3.2.2 Fully Automated Immunoblotting Instrument

Shenzhen YHLO Tenfly Immunoblotter Series

There are three models: Tenfly Blot, Tenfly Auto and Tenfly Phoenix, of which Tenfly Blot supports simultaneous experiments on 44 membrane strips, and can automatically complete the steps of incubation, cleaning, and reagent addition, requiring manual serum addition and additional scanning to interpret the results. Tenfly Auto is an upgraded version of the immunoblotting analyzer that supports simultaneous experiments on 48 membrane strips. It can automatically complete the steps of incubation, washing, reagent addition, drying and automatic interpretation of results. Only manual serum addition is required. Tenfly Phoenix is a fully automatic immunoblotting analyzer that can support 60 membrane strips for simultaneous experiments. It can automatically complete the steps of adding serum samples, incubating, washing, adding reagents, drying and automatically interpreting the results. It also supports LIS two-way communication, which is the most automatic immunoblotting analyzer available at present.

Shenzhen Rayto Life and Analytical Sciences Immunoblotter Series

The commonly used equipment models are Biotray 866 and Biotray 933, and currently, HOB Biotech, Unicorn and other manufacturers are using Rayto's immunoblotter solution. Biotray 866 is a semi-automatic immunoblotting analyzer that supports simultaneous experiments on 40 membrane strips. It can automatically complete the steps of incubation, cleaning, and reagent addition, requiring manual sample addition and interpretation of results. Biotray 933 is a fully automatic immunoblotting analyzer that can support 50 membrane strips for simultaneous experiments. It can automatically complete the steps of serum sample addition, incubation, washing, reagent addition, drying, and interpretation of results, and supports LIS two-way communication.

Shanghai Xun-Da Medical Instrument XD Immunoblotter Series

XD series commonly used equipment models are XD236 and XD248. XD236 supports simultaneous experiments on 30/36 membrane strips, and XD248 supports simultaneous experiments on 48 membrane strips. Both are semi-automatic immunoblotting analyzers, which can automatically complete the steps of incubation, washing, and reagent addition, requiring manual sample addition and interpretation of results.

5.3.2.3 Chemiluminescence Immunoassay Analyzer

iFlash3000 Fully Automated Chemiluminescence Immunoassay Analyzer Series

iFlash3000 was launched in 2016 by Shenzhen YHLO Biotech, which adopts the direct chemiluminescence principle of acridinium ester. The iFlash3000C model is targeted for laboratories with large sample volume, with 140 sample positions (another 15 emergency positions), 30 reagent positions, supporting 2000 reaction cups, and a maximum test speed of 300 T/h. It also has a cascade function, supporting up to 4 devices in a cascade. The iFlash3000H is a desktop instrument with a small footprint, targeted at smaller laboratories, with 50 sample positions, 20 reagent stations, supporting 1000 reaction cups, and a maximum test speed of 180 T/h.

SMART6500 Fully Automated Chemiluminescence Immunoassay Analyzer
The manufacturer is Chongqing Keysmile Biological Technology, and the main cooperative manufacturer of SMART6500 equipment in the panels of autoimmunity is Suzhou HOB Biotech. HOB Biotech's SMART6500 adopts enzymatic chemiluminescence, has 96 sample positions, 24 reagent positions, supports 1000 reaction cups, the one-step test speed is 360 T/h, two-step test speed is 300 T/h, and the first result time is 47 min. In addition, the SMART6500 is available with a syringe TIP solution to reduce cross-contamination.

LEACL-600 Single Packaged Fully Automated Chemiluminescence Immunoassay Analyzer
In 2019, Zhuhai Livzon Diagnostics released a single packaged chemiluminescence immunoassay analyzer LEACL-600. In addition to detecting autoantibodies, it can also diagnose AMH, PCT, IL-6, tuberculosis infected T cells, bacterial vaginosis and other parameters/diseases. LEACL- 600 adopts enzymatic chemiluminescence method, with a total of 30 sample positions, 12 reagent positions, a test speed of 60 T/h and a first result time of 18 min.

Lumiray Chemiluminescence Immunoassay Analyzer Series
Lumiray series were produced by Shenzhen Rayto Life, and HOB Biotech has used Rayto's Lumiray1200 chemiluminescence immunoassay analyzer. Currently, Sichuan C-Luminary Biotechnology is developing a series of autoimmunity reagents based on the Lumiray platform. Lumiray1600 and Lumiray630 both use enzymatic chemiluminescence, the test speed is 120 T/h and 80 T/h respectively, and the first result time is 20 min and 15 min respectively.

AVIC Saiwei Biological Science & Technology (Beijing Beier Bioengineering) Fully Automated Chemiluminescence Immunoassay Analyzer
The analyzer was launched in 2016 by Beier Bioengineering Holdings Beijing AVIC Saiwei Biological Science & Technology. Its VI-200 adopts enzymatic chemiluminescence method, with a total of 100 sample positions, 30 reagent positions, supporting 1200 reaction cups, a test speed of 240 T/h, and a first result time of 19 min. The sample needle adopts a disposable Tip solution.

Kaeser Fully Automated Chemiluminescence Immunoassay Analyzer Series
It is a product of Chongqing Keysmile Biological Technology, Guangzhou Kangrun Biotech is developing autoantibodies, reproductive hormones and other reagents based on this instrument. Kaeser chemiluminescence immunoassay analyzer series

use acridinium ester-labeled direct chemiluminescence technology. The Kaeser 6600 has 96 specimen positions, 24 reagent positions, and supports 1000 reaction cups, with a test speed of 360 T/h and a first result time of 35 min . The Kaeser 1000 has 24 specimen positions, 15 reagent positions, and supports 130 reaction cups, with a test speed of 120 T/h and a first result time of 15 min.

5.3.2.4 Multiplex Detection Platform

Fully Automated Flow Cytometry Fluorescence Immunoassay Analyzer TESMI F4000

The first domestic flow cytometry fluorescence immunoassay analyzer was launched in 2018 by Shanghai Tellgen Diagnostic Technology. The platform is developed based on Luminex 200 flow cytometry fluorescence multiplex detection technology. It combines the advantages of Luminex 200 flow cytometry fluorescence technology, such as high throughput, capable of joint inspection, and quantification, and also has automatic sample processing function, which realizes high-speed, random to the performance of on-call testing and fully automatic processing. The platform has a total of 125 sample positions, the test speed is 120 samples/h, and the first result time is 38 min. For the 16 detection parameters of the antinuclear antibodies, a maximum of 1920 results can be generated per hour. The platform has 25 reagent positions. For example, if the number of reagent detection indicators in a single channel is 4, then a single machine can simultaneously detect 100 indicators online (the number of indicators depends on the actual number of indicators of each reagent), which can greatly reduce the number of instruments required and the need for multiple-instrument assignment of samples.

MCLIA-800 Fully Automated Multiplex Immunoassay Analyzer

It is a multiplexed assay platform launched by Zhuhai Livzon Diagnostics, which applies laser microengraving technology to carry out laser lithography on chips. It can encode up to 4096 chips in total, which can achieve the purpose of detecting multiple markers simultaneously in one reaction tube, with high throughput, full automation, fast speed and random injection and other characteristics. MCLIA- 800 has 128 sample positions, 5 reagent positions, with a first result time of 37 min, and can complete 60 samples testing per hour.

5.3.3 Main Reagent Products of Domestic Autoimmune Diagnosis

5.3.3.1 Indirect Immunofluorescence Reagents

Almost all imported brands of autoimmune reagents manufacturers have products using indirect immunofluorescence method, while there are fewer domestic brands of reagents using this method. At present, the domestic manufacturers who independently develop and produce indirect immunofluorescence products include Shenzhen YHLO Biotech, Beijing H&J NoVoMed and Suzhou HOB Biotech (Table 5.2).

Table 5.2 Detailed list of manufacturers of indirect immunofluorescence reagents

Diseases	Markers	YHLO	H&J	HOB
Connective tissue diseases	Anti-nuclear antibody (ANA)	√	√	√
Systemic lupus erythematosus	Anti-double-stranded DNA (dsDNA) IgG antibodies	√	√	√
ANCA-associated small vessel vasculitis	Anti-neutrophil cytoplasmic antibody (ANCA) IgG	√	√	√
Autoimmune hepatitis	Autoimmune hepatitis-related IgG antibodies	√	–	√
Rheumatoid arthritis	Anti-keratin antibody (AKA) IgG	–	√	√
Rheumatoid arthritis	Perinuclear factor	–	√	–

Table 5.3 Detailed list of immunoblotting reagent manufacturers

Markers	YHLO	SDR	Kangrun	HOB	Kexin	Huian	Uniten
Anti-nuclear antibodies	√	√	√	√	√	√	√
Vasculitis antibodies	√	√	√	√	√	–	–
Autoimmune hepatitis antibodies	√	√	√	√	√	–	–
Myositis antibodies	√	√	–	–	–	–	–
Autoimmune diabetes antibodies	√	√	–	–	–	–	–
Autoimmune gastrointestinal disease antibodies	√	–	√	–	–	–	–
Autoantibodies screening	√	–	–	–	–	–	–

5.3.3.2 Immunoblotting Reagents

There are more than ten manufacturers of immunoblotting reagents, and the only brands with a high market share and a complete disease spectrum are Shenzhen YHLO Biotech, Beijing SDR Diagnostics, Guangzhou Kangrun Biotech, Suzhou HOB Biotech, Shanghai Kexin Biotech, Shenzhen Huian Biosci Technology and Guangdong Uniten Biotechnology (Table 5.3).

5.3.3.3 Chemiluminescent Immunoassay Reagents

The growth momentum of chemiluminescent reagent manufacturers is obvious, and more and more manufacturers are joining the ranks of autoantibody reagent product development and production to provide more high-quality products (Table 5.4).

5.3.3.4 Multiplex Assay Reagents

At present, there are only two domestic multiplex assays, Shanghai Tellgen Diagnostic Technology and Zhuhai Livzon Diagnostics. The multiplex assay has the characteristics of high throughput and fast detection, and it is likely to replace the immunoblotting method in the future, especially for the panels that require multiple assays such as antinuclear antibodies detection.

The tests performed by Shanghai Tellgen Diagnostic Technology include ANA-16s and ANA-15s for antinuclear antibodies, AAV-3s for vasculitis, IgG and

Table 5.4 Detailed list of registered products of chemiluminescent reagent manufacturers

Diseases	Markers	YHLO	HOB	C-Luminary	AVIC Saiwei	Kangrun
Connective tissue diseases	ANA	√	√	√	–	–
	dsDNA IgG	√	√	√	√	√
	RNP IgG	√	√	√	√	√
	Sm IgG	√	√	√	√	√
	Nuc	√	√	√	√	√
	His	√	√	√	√	√
	P0	√	√	√	√	√
	PCNA	√	√	√	√	√
	SS-A IgG	√	√	√	√	√
	SS-B IgG	√	√	√	√	√
	Ro52 IgG	√	√	√	√	√
	Scl-70 IgG	√	√	√	√	√
	PM-scl	√	√	√	√	√
	CenpB	√	√	√	√	√
	Jo-1 IgG	√	√	√	√	√
Rheumatoid arthritis	RF IgA	–	√	√	–	√
	RF IgG	√	√	√	–	√
	RF IgM	√	√	√	–	√
	RF	√	√	–	√	–
	Anti-CCP	√	√	–	√	√
	MCV	–	–	√	–	–
	RA33 IgG	√	√	–	–	–
Autoimmune hepatitis	ASMA IgG	√	–	√	–	–
	AMA-M2	√	√	√	–	√
	LKM-1	–	√	√	√	√
	SLA/LP	–	√	√	√	√
	LC-1	–	√	√	√	√
	sp100	–	√	√	√	√
	gp210	–	√	√	–	–
ANCA-related small-vessel vasculitis	PR3 IgG	√	√	√	√	√
	MPO IgG	√	√	√	√	√
	GBM IgG	√	√	√	√	√
Antiphospholipid syndrome	Cardiolipin IgM	√	√	√	√	√
	Cardiolipin IgA	√	√	√	√	√
	Cardiolipin IgG	√	√	√	√	√
	Anti-Cardiolipin	√	√	√	√	–
	β2-glycoprotein I IgG	√	√	√	√	√
	β2-glycoprotein I IgA	√	√	√	√	√
	β2-glycoprotein I IgM	√	√	√	√	√
	Anti-β2-glycoprotein I	√	√	√	√	–

(continued)

Table 5.4 (continued)

Diseases	Markers	YHLO	HOB	C-Luminary	AVIC Saiwei	Kangrun
Autoimmune diabetes	GADA	√	√	–	–	–
	IAA	√	√	–	√	–
	IA-2A	√	√	√	–	–
	ICA	√	√	√	√	–
	ZnT8A	√	–	√	–	–
Autoimmune thyroiditis	TSHR	√	–	–	–	–
	TG	√	√	–	√	√
	TPO	√	√	–	√	√
Others	PLA2R	–	–	√	–	–
	M2-3E IgG	–	–	–	√	–
	KL-6	–	–	√	–	√
	MMP-3	–	–	√	–	√
	IgG1/IgG2/IgG3/IgG4	√	–	–	–	–

IgM antibodies of anti-cardiolipin (aCL) and anti-β2 glycoprotein I (aβ2GPI) for antiphospholipid syndrome, anti-CCP antibodies for rheumatoid arthritis, ALD-6s for autoimmune hepatitis, and M-type phospholipase A2 receptor (PLA2R) for membranous nephropathy. The tests available at Zhuhai Livzon Diagnostics include ANA-17s, ANA-15s, ANA-13s, ANA-9s for antinuclear antibodies, AAV-7s and AAV-3s for vasculitis, ALD-7s for autoimmune hepatitis, and 5s for myositis.

5.4 Introduction of Major Domestic Autoimmune Diagnostic Companies

5.4.1 Shenzhen YHLO Biotech Co., Ltd.

Shenzhen YHLO Biotech Co., Ltd is an innovative company committed to independent research and development, focusing on academic research. YHLO's autoimmune diagnostic products cover connective tissue disease, autoimmune vasculitis, autoimmune hepatitis, antiphospholipid syndrome, rheumatoid arthritis, autoimmune diabetes, autoimmune gastrointestinal disease, autoimmune thyroiditis and other disease areas.

The chemiluminescence platform mainly includes two models, iFlash3000H and iFlash3000C. The detection speed and throughput are different, and they are suitable for different customer usage scenarios. In addition, the iFlash3000C has cascade capability and can be accessed to a Total Laboratory Automation, allowing up to four devices to be connected and share the same sampling system to improve the detection speed and throughput.

The immunoblotting platform mainly includes three models of immunoblotting analyzers, Tenfly Blot, Tenfly Auto and Tenfly Phoenix. Among them, Tenfly Blot is a semi-automatic immunoblotting analyzer, and Tenfly Auto and Tenfly Phoenix are fully automatic immunoblotting analyzers, supporting the process of incubation, washing, reagent addition, drying, and interpretation. Tenfly Phoenix is the most automated immunoblotting analyzer on the market.

Also, YHLO has indirect immunofluorescence reagents and automated operation and interpretation equipment for parameters including anti-nuclear antibodies, anti-neutrophil antibodies, anti-dsDNA antibodies, and anti-tissue antibodies.

5.4.2 Jiangsu HOB Biotech Group Suzhou Co., Ltd.

HOBo's autoimmune antibodies detection methodologies are mainly chemiluminescence as well as immunoblotting methods.

The fully automated chemiluminescence immunoassay analyzer of HOB adopts Chongqing Keysmile Smart 6500 platform, based on which we have developed chemiluminescence reagents for diseases related to connective tissue disease, vasculitis, autoimmune hepatitis, antiphospholipid syndrome, rheumatoid arthritis, autoimmune diabetes, autoimmune thyroiditis, etc.

HOB immunoblotting reagents mainly have three panels: antinuclear antibodies, vasculitis, and autoimmune hepatitis. Its automated equipment models mainly come from Shenzhen Rayto, including Biotray-866 and Biotray-933.

5.4.3 Shanghai Kexin Biotech Co., Ltd.

Currently, Shanghai Kexin has a series of specialized experimental platforms ranging from gene cloning, protein expression and preparation, antibody preparation to cell culture, etc. In the research and development of diagnostic reagents, Shanghai Kexin has mature technology platforms such as enzyme-linked immunosorbent assay (ELISA), immunoblotting (Blot) and colloidal gold immunochromatographic assay (GICA). In terms of raw material preparation, Shanghai Kexin has E. coli expression system technology platform, yeast expression system technology, large-scale fermentation and renaturation purification technology, CHO cell expression system technology, large-scale transient gene expression technology, hybridoma technology, and large-scale animal cell culture technology.

Shanghai Kexin focuses on the research and development and production of autoimmune diagnostic reagents. In 2010, Shanghai Kexin independently developed and produced an anti-cyclic citrullinated antibody detection kit (enzyme-linked immunosorbent assay), and achieved a high market share. In addition, Shanghai Kexin also has a combination of testing parameters such as anti-nuclear antibodies, vasculitis, autoimmune hepatitis, and autoimmune diabetes.

5.4.4 Beijing H&J Novomed Co., Ltd.

Beijing H&J was established in May 2005 and is located in Beijing Yizhuang Economic and Technological Development Area, where high-technology is concentrated. Beijing H&J focuses on the development, production and sales of in vitro diagnostic reagents based on autoantibodies for rheumatic diseases. The product methodologies include indirect immunofluorescence method, enzyme-linked immunosorbent assay and immunoblotting method, and the detected disease panels includes antinuclear antibodies, vasculitis, autoimmune hepatitis, and rheumatoid arthritis. As an early domestic autoimmune brand, it has a certain popularity.

5.4.5 Shanghai Tellgen Life Science Co., Ltd.

Shanghai Tellgen Life Science Co., Ltd. (hereinafter referred to as "Tellgen Life") has been dedicated to the development, manufacturing and promotion of in vitro diagnostic products since its establishment in 2003. The products developed by Tellgen Life include more than 250 products in multiple technology platforms such as flow cytometer fluorescence, chemiluminescence, biochemistry, molecular diagnosis and Total Laboratory Automation. Flow cytometer fluorescence technology is a specialty of Tellgen Life, which is a high-throughput assay that can detect up to 100 parameters at a time. It can greatly improve detection efficiency and is particularly suitable for multiplex testing.

By the end of 2020, Tellgen Life has received approval from the China Food and Drug Administration (CFDA) for six products in the FlowAI® series of flow cytometer fluorescence autoantibodies immunoassay tests, including 16 parameters in the antinuclear antibodies, 4 in the antiphospholipid antibodies, 3 in the vasculitis antibodies, and 24 in the rheumatoid arthritis including anti-CCP antibody. Combined with the TESMI F4000 fully automated flow cytometer fluorescence immunoassay system, it is high throughput, fully automated, fully quantitative and on-call. In particular, the maximum speed of 1920 tests per hour can greatly improve the efficiency of the laboratory when testing a multi-marker combination such as the antinuclear antibodies.

5.4.6 Zhuhai Livzon Diagnostics Inc.

Founded in 1989, Zhuhai Livzon is the first high-tech subsidiary of the listed company Livzon Pharmaceutical Group (an A-share/H-share listed company), specializing in the R&D, production and marketing of in vitro diagnostic reagents and supporting equipment, and is one of the earliest in vitro diagnostic reagent manufacturers in China.

Livzon Reagent currently has enzyme-linked immunosorbent assay technology platform, colloidal gold rapid detection platform, microorganism detection platform, as well as newly established molecular nucleic acid detection technology platform, automatic digital liquid-phase chip multiplex detection platform and single-packaged chemiluminescence platform. The product lines of Livzon Reagent cover many fields such as infectious diseases, respiratory infections, tumor marker detection, drug concentration monitoring, autoimmunity, allergen detection and blood safety.

In the field of autoantibody detection, Livzon adopts the fully automated digital liquid-phase chip multiplex assay platform (MCLIA-800) and single-packaged chemiluminescence platform (LEACL-600). Available test panels include antinuclear antibodies, vasculitis antibodies, autoimmune hepatitis and myositis antibodies.

5.4.7 Guangzhou Kangrun Biotech Co., Ltd.

Founded in 2002, Kangrun has independently developed and produced dozens of products such as reproductive endocrine hormones, thyroid function, and EBV. In recent years, Kangrun has started to develop and produce reagents for reproductive hormones and autoimmunity fields on the chemiluminescence platform of Chongqing Keysmile, and has now launched some quantitative assays such as antiphospholipid antibody and vasculitis. It is worth mentioning that Kangrun has launched autoimmunity quality control products through its subsidiary Guangzhou Bochi Biotechnology, which has filled the vacancy of quality control in domestic autoimmunity laboratories.

5.4.8 Sichuan C-Luminary Biotechnology Co., Ltd.

Founded in 2018, Sichuan C-Luminary specializes in the development and production of core raw materials for in vitro diagnostic reagents, while the company also provides diagnostic products for clinical users for autoimmune diseases and allergic diseases. At present, more than 20 kinds of core raw materials of diagnostic reagents (mainly recombinant autoimmune antigens and component allergens) developed by the company have been widely used in the development of downstream kits.

In addition, the company has established a technology platform for chemiluminescence assay based on Rayto's Lumiray series chemiluminescent immunoassay analyzer, on which it has developed quantitative multiple autoantibody assay kits as well as allergen assay kits. It has launched tests for conventional autoimmune parameters such as antinuclear antibodies, autoimmune hepatitis, antiphospholipid antibodies, and rheumatoid arthritis. In addition, it has developed special autoantibody parameters such as membrane membranous nephropathy (e.g., anti-PLA2R antibodies), infertility (e.g., anti-sperm antibodies, anti-ovarian antibodies, anti-clear band antibodies) and interstitial lung disease-related antigen tests (e.g., KL-6).

5.4.9 Beijing Beier Bioengineering co Ltd. (Beijing AVIC Saiwei Biological Science & Technology Co., Ltd.)

Beijing Beier is located in Beijing Economic and Technological Development Area, a high-tech enterprise integrating R&D, production, sales and service of fully-automated chemiluminescent instruments and reagents. In 2016, Beier Bioengineering held Beijing AVIC Safeway Biotechnology Co., Ltd, which greatly expanded Beier's chemiluminescent product line, especially the fully-automated chemiluminescent immunoassay analyzer, and the current chemiluminescent reagents cover a wide range of panels including thyroid function, sex hormones, tumor markers, autoantibodies, liver fibrosis and many other parameters.

5.4.10 Other Enterprises

In addition to the above-mentioned enterprises, there are other small enterprises such as Shenzhen Anqun Biology Engineering Co., Ltd., Shenzhen Sciarray Biotechnology Co., Ltd., Weifang Kanghua Biotech Co., Ltd., Shenzhen Huian Bioscitech Co., Ltd., and Guangdong Uniten Biotechnology Co., Ltd. These enterprises mainly promote traditional methodologies such as ELISA and immunoblotting, and they have few detection assays, no obvious competitive advantages, and small user groups.

5.5 Market Analysis of Autoantibodies Products in China

After 20 years of development in China, autoantibody detection has gradually developed from an emerging project of immunodiagnosis to a segmented field that hospitals and IVD companies attach great importance to. Autoantibody detection has been used in clinical diagnosis and treatment for more than 50 years, providing comprehensive diagnosis and treatment information for 50 million rheumatology patients nationwide. In recent years, new methods such as chemiluminescence and multiplex detection technology have also been gradually applied in the field of autoimmune disease diagnosis, improving the level of autoantibody detection technology and providing more efficient clinical services. In the past 10 years, domestic manufacturers have entered the field of autoimmune diagnosis and occupied a place. The development of China's intelligent manufacturing has promoted the development of autoantibody detection and diagnosis and treatment technology. In the future, the development of China's autoimmune disease diagnosis market is bound to enter the fast lane.

5.5.1 Market Volume of Autoimmune Diagnostic Products

According to the literature, about 7.6% to 9.4% of the global population suffers from various types of autoimmune diseases, and more than 100 autoimmune diseases have been identified, commonly including rheumatoid arthritis, systemic lupus erythematosus, Sjögren syndrome, psoriasis, and ankylosing spondylitis. Among the top 100 global drug sales in 2019, 25 immune drugs entered the list, of which Adalimumab (Humira) is firmly at the top of the list. In terms of diseased groups, due to the large population base, according to the survey on the number of patients with major autoimmune diseases in China in 2019, it is expected that China will still have the largest number of patients with autoimmune diseases in the world by 2030, with a stable growth and autoimmune disease diagnosis market. The demand is huge. In addition, the national emphasis on autoimmune diseases has promoted the development of rheumatology and immunology clinical departments (Fig. 5.1).

5.5.1.1 The National Policy Supports the Construction of Rheumatology and Immunology Departments

In recent years, China has paid more and more attention to the diagnosis of autoimmune diseases, and on October 31, 2019, the National Health Commission issued the Guidelines for the Construction and Management of Rheumatology and Immunology Departments in General Hospitals (for Trial Implementation) (hereinafter referred to as "Guidelines"). The Guidelines state that tertiary general hospitals with conditions should, in principle, set up independent rheumatology and immunology departments, and encourage secondary general hospitals and other types of medical institutions with conditions to set up independent rheumatology and immunology departments, while hospitals should have independent testing departments to support the routine examination of rheumatology and immunology diseases. The continuous attention and vigorous construction of clinical departments of rheumatology and immunology by the state will be beneficial to the rapid development of the autoimmune disease diagnosis market.

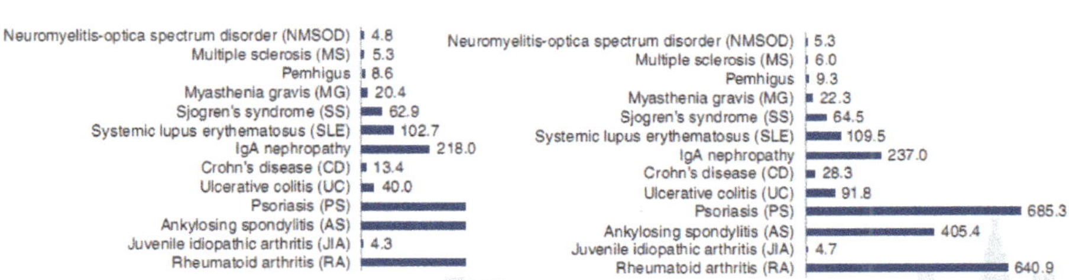

Note: 1) According to Everest Medicines prospectus, the number of patients with atopic dermatitis Wai in China is about 61.5 million in 2019 and will reach 65.9 million in 2030, and according to Lancet data, the number of Chinese asthma patients is about 45.7 million in 2019 and COPD patients about 100 million, which are not marked in the figure because of the huge scale of the number of patients.

(2) According to the Chinese journal of Dermatology, the incidence of psoriatic arthritis in Chinese patients with psoriasis is 6% to 13%.

Fig. 5.1 Population of major autoimmune diseases in China in 2019 and forecast in 2030

5.5.1.2 An Aging Population Leads to an Increase in the Prevalence of Autoimmune Diseases

Autoimmune diseases are caused by abnormalities in the immune system due to external stimuli, and as age increases, the prevalence of autoimmune diseases increases. An expanding aging population will inevitably lead to an increasing demand for autoimmune disease diagnosis.

5.5.1.3 The Growth of Autoimmune Diagnostic Market Is Driven by Policies Such as Graded Treatment

In 2014, the Ninth Committee of the Rheumatology Branch of the Chinese Medical Association proposed the plan of "one city, one department, one center," which has led to the popularization and sinking of autoantibody testing, and many county-level people's hospitals are now carrying out autoantibody testing. At the same time, to further strengthen the graded treatment of rheumatic immune diseases and enhance the medical service capacity of primary care institutions for rheumatic immune diseases, the Chinese Rheumatology Center Alliance (CRCA), initiated by Peking Union Medical College Hospital, was officially established in Beijing in November 2017, which will further promote the popularity of autoantibody testing in primary care institutions. The establishment of the CRCA will further promote the spread of autoantibody testing in primary care settings, and will also lead to the spread of testing groups, which will lead to a greater understanding of autoimmune diseases and increased compliance with testing, leading to new developments in autoantibody testing. According to MARKETS AND MARKETS data, the global autoantibody testing market was $3.365 billion in 2017 (Fig. 5.2).

The autoimmune disease diagnostics market in China continues to grow at a high rate, and based on laboratory data obtained from expert research and public data, the autoimmune disease diagnostics market is forecast to grow at a CAGR of nearly 30% per annum from 2018 to 2023. The autoimmune disease diagnostic market size is forecasted to reach RMB 3.37 billion in 2023. Due to the outbreak of the COVID-19 epidemic in 2020, the diagnosis and treatment of autoimmune diseases market has been impacted, mainly reflected in the reduction in the number of hospital visits, and the growth rate of the market size in 2020 will be reduced to 10% (Fig. 5.3).

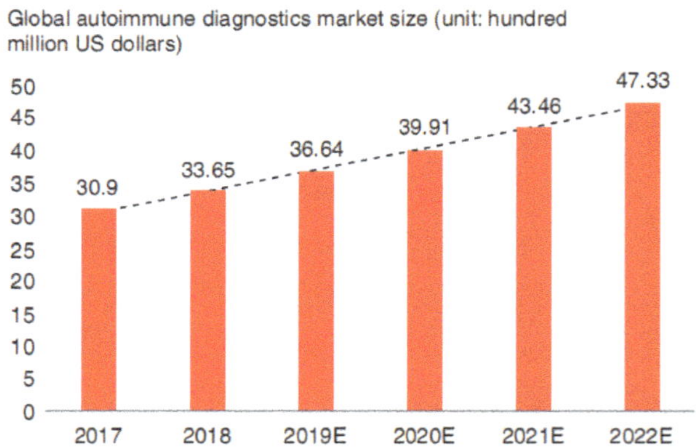

Fig. 5.2 Global autoimmune diagnostics market size (unit: hundred million US dollars). (Source: MARKETS AND MARKETS, Founder Securities Research Institute)

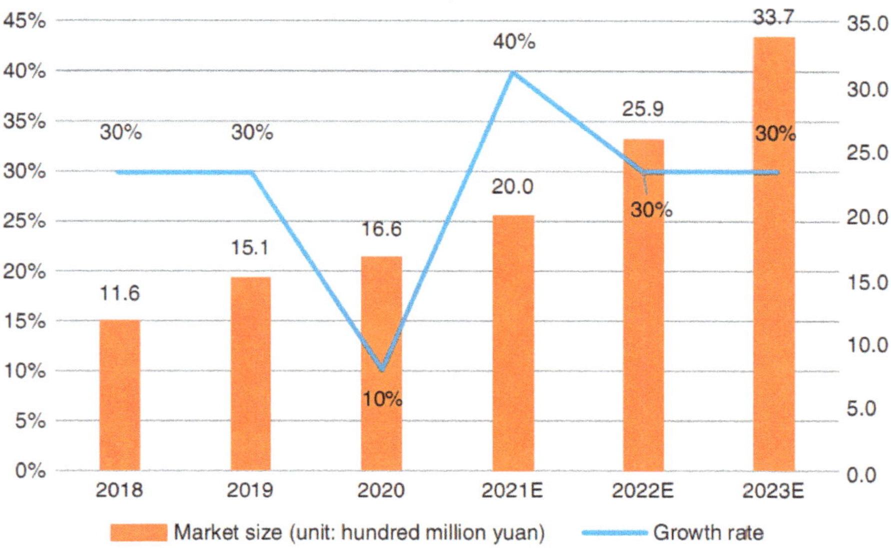

Fig. 5.3 Autoimmune disease diagnostics market size (unit: hundred million yuan), 2018 to 2023. (Data Source: Domestic and Foreign Medical Devices and In Vitro Diagnostics Industry Research Report)

5.5.2 Methodology Proportion of Autoimmune Diagnostic Products

Hundreds of autoantibodies have been identified so far, and the methodologies for detecting these autoantibodies are diverse, mainly including indirect immunofluorescence (IIF), latex agglutination test, double diffusion test, counter immunoelectrophoresis (CIEP), radioimmunoassay (RIA), linear immunoassay (LIA), enzyme linked immunosorbent assay (ELISA), chemiluminescence assay (CLIA), and multiplex assay.

There were 271, 408, and 642 laboratories participating in the external quality assessment of autoantibodies organized by the Chinese Rheumatism Data Center (CRDC) in 2018, 2019, and 2020, respectively. The data showed that the most commonly used methodology for autoantibody testing in China was immunoblotting (51%), followed by enzyme-linked immunosorbent assay (16%), chemiluminescence (16%), and indirect immunofluorescence (13%), with less use of multiplex testing (4%) (Figs. 5.4, 5.5 and 5.6).

5.5.3 Autoimmune Diagnostic Market Pattern

After years of development, the autoimmune disease diagnostic market has formed a situation in which multinational manufacturers are leading, followed by domestic manufacturers, and multiple manufacturers are "competing for a hundred flowers."

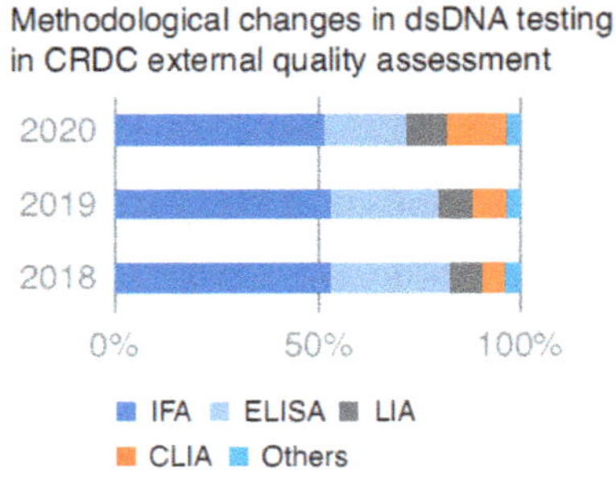

Fig. 5.4 Methodological changes in dsDNA testing in CRDC external quality assessment

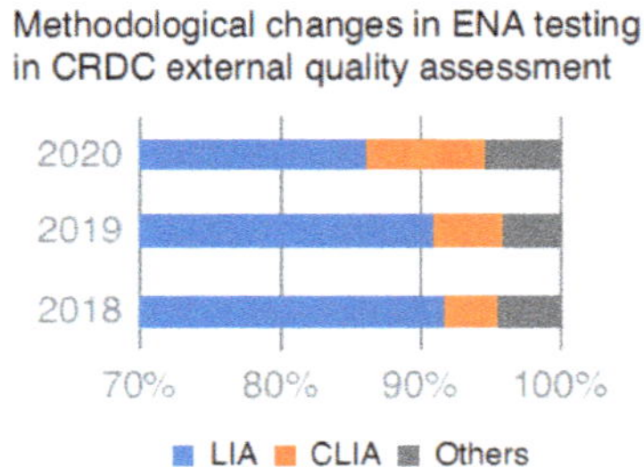

Fig. 5.5 Methodological changes in ENA testing in CRDC external quality assessment

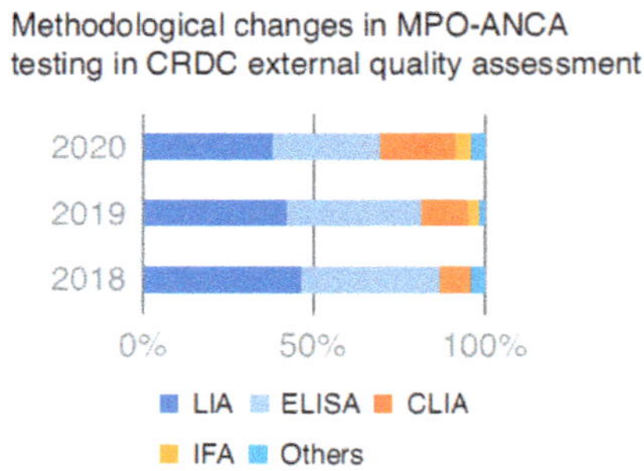

Fig. 5.6 Methodological changes in MPO-ANCA testing in CRDC external quality assessment

As foreign companies entered the domestic market earlier, they almost monopolized the entire autoantibody testing market through high quality products, unique brand advantages and continuous academic education. It was not until 2009, when YHLO Biotech launched its autoantibody diagnostic reagents by immunoblotting and 2010, when Kexin Biotech launched its anti-CCP antibody diagnostic reagents, that the situation where imported brands completely monopolize the market has been changed.

With the rise of domestic chemiluminescence companies, more and more chemiluminescence companies have differentiated themselves from routine projects through the development of autoimmune antibody diagnostic product lines and acted as a stepping stone to enter the hospitals, such as YHLO Biotech, HOB Biotech and AVIC Saiwei Biological Science & Technology. At the same time, these companies have actively deepened basic scientific research and improved their clinical transformation capabilities, and finally occupied an important position in the autoimmune diagnosis market.

In the application market of autoimmune diagnostic products in China, the share of each company varies, among which the highest share (48%) is accounted for by Oumeng Medical Diagnosis (China), the second ranked company is YHLO Biotech(18%), the companies with market share between 5% and 7% are HOB Biotech(7%), Kangrun Biotech (6%), Kexin Biotech (6%), HUMAN Diagnostics(5%), the companies with share below 5% are Wolfen (4%), H&J NoVoMed (2%), Anqun Biology Engineering(1%), Kanghua Biotech (1%), and the other companies with a total of about 2%.

5.6 Future Changes and Trends in the Development of Autoimmune Diagnostic Technologies and Products

5.6.1 Localization of Autoantibody Testing

Imported medical manufacturers in Europe and the United States started early, with mature and perfect products, and have occupied the Chinese market for a long time, while training a large number of technicians. In recent years, with the technological progress of China's medical device companies and the maturity of the supporting industry chain, as well as the promotion of national policies such as medical reform, graded treatment, and support for domestic equipment, localization of product testing is the main theme of future development; on the other hand, domestic brands use chemiluminescence and fully automated, high-throughput detection platforms such as flow cytometry fluorescence/liquid-phase chip, which have obvious advantages over the traditional methodologies of imported brands. This is also one of the reasons that drive customers to replace imported products.

5.6.2 Development of Intelligent and Automated Autoantibody Diagnostic Technology

The clinical application value of autoantibody testing mainly includes early warning of disease, diagnosis and differential diagnosis of disease, judgment of disease process and efficacy, and prognosis evaluation. At present, most hospitals still use qualitative immunoblotting method. Due to the limitation of detection technology, the qualitative results can only guide the diagnosis or differential diagnosis, and cannot meet the more in-depth clinical needs for disease progression judgment and efficacy monitoring. Compared with qualitative assays, quantitative assays can set the optimal laboratory threshold value, so the results are more accurate, while quantitative results can also be more effective in tracking the disease, predicting the occurrence and prognosis of the disease, and monitoring the effectiveness of treatment. The development of automated detection technologies such as chemiluminescence and flow cytometry fluorescence/liquid phase microarray provides a strong guarantee for quantitative, precise, microscopic and efficient testing, which is conducive to the development of rational clinical treatment strategies and protocols.

In addition, with the improvement in clinical treatment technology, the number of patients with autoimmune diseases increases year by year, and the clinical demand for autoantibody testing also increases year by year, and the existing testing equipment can no longer meet the needs of testers. Therefore, chemiluminescence, flow cytometry fluorescence and other fully automated, high-throughput detection technologies applied to autoantibody testing have received the attention of laboratory workers since their introduction.

5.6.3 Popularization and Sinking of Autoantibody Testing

Autoantibody testing is generally carried out in tertiary hospitals because of its strong professionalism, strong demand for interaction between clinical and testing, high clinical requirements for testing, and strong expertise of clinical prescribers; thus, it is a special testing program. In 2014, the ninth Committee of the Rheumatology Branch of the Chinese Medical Association, with Professor Zeng Xiaofeng of Peking Union Medical College as the chairman, proposed the plan of "one city, one department, one center," which has led to the popularization and sinking of autoantibody testing, and autoantibody testing is now carried out in many county-level people's hospitals.

To further strengthen the graded treatment of rheumatic and immune diseases and improve the medical service capacity of rheumatic and immune diseases in primary care institutions, in November 2017, the Chinese Rheumatology Center Alliance (CRCA), initiated by Professor Zeng Xiaofeng of Peking Union Medical College Hospital, was officially established in Beijing, which will also further popularize autoantibody testing in primary care institutions.

5.6.4 Laboratory Standardization of Autoantibody Assays and Standardization of Traceability

Autoantibody testing is an important tool in the diagnosis and treatment of autoimmune diseases. However, due to the lack of a standardized test method for autoantibody testing and the influence of working conditions, traditional treatment habits, interpretation of results and health insurance restrictions, there are inconsistencies and irregularities in the clinical application of autoantibody testing.

According to the results of domestic autoantibody quality control in the past decade and recent data from a national multicenter laboratory survey, the rate of conducting and correctness of some autoantibody tests is not satisfactory. At the same time, there are errors or misinterpretations in the interpretation of autoantibody results. Standardization and uniformity of autoantibody testing is the future trend, and the challenge is how to standardize and correctly interpret them. The standardization of autoantibody testing includes the whole process of reagent development and production, specimen testing and report review, which involves many aspects such as reagent and instrument manufacturers, suppliers, technical level of testing personnel, testing management system, and clinicians' awareness. At the manufacturer's end, the national administration, national standardization committee and industry association should unify the management, top-level design and unified deployment in terms of reagent access, instrument audit, system regulations, standard development and technical requirements, so as to solve the problem of standardization of autoantibody testing from the source, improve the accuracy of autoantibody testing results, and lay the foundation for high-quality autoantibody testing results. In terms of laboratories, there are still a large number of laboratory workers whose experimental procedures and inspection reports are not standardized. It is necessary to provide standardized training and education for laboratory workers, to obtain certificates, to standardize the testing process, report review and interpretation of results, so as to better serve the clinical.

Traceability standardization is a must for autoantibody testing to ensure traceability consistency, achieve true quantification of autoantibody testing, and serve the clinic more efficiently.

5.6.5 Autoantibody Diseases Testing Parameters and Expansion of Clinical Application Scenarios

Due to the specificity and sensitivity of autoantibody tests, autoimmune diseases cannot be diagnosed by the results of individual antibody tests. One reason is that multiple different autoantibodies can be present at the same time in a particular autoimmune disease (e.g., anti-dsDNA antibodies, anti-Sm antibodies, anti-ribosomal P (anti-Rib-P) antibody can be present at the same time in SLE patients), and the same autoantibody can be present in multiple different autoimmune diseases (e.g., both SLE patients and SS patients may have positive anti-SSA antibodies). Therefore, laboratories often need to combine multiple autoantibodies for simultaneous testing to improve the sensitivity and specificity of the test. For example, for connective tissue diseases such as SLE, laboratories often combine as many as a dozen autoantibodies (collectively referred to as the antinuclear antibodies or connective tissue disease antibodies). Another reason is that even when laboratories combine multiple programs for simultaneous testing, there are still cases of missed tests. In the case of antiphospholipid syndrome, for example, the laboratory tests included in the 2006 Sydney International Classification of Antiphospholipid syndrome include lupus anticoagulant (LA), anticardiolipin IgG/IgM, and anti-β2 glycoprotein 1 antibody IgG/IgM [8]. However, the combination of these three tests only detects about 70% of patients with APS, so there is a need to find new biomarkers to complement the existing anti-phospholipid antibodies. The more popular new parameters in recent years mainly include anti-PS/PT antibody, anti-β2 glycoprotein 1 structural domain 1 antibody, and anti-membrane linked protein A5 antibody, which, combined with traditional antiphospholipid antibody, can greatly improve the detection rate of antiphospholipid syndrome.

In addition, the field of application of autoantibodies has been expanding. Since the 1980s, a series of classical autoantibodies associated with paraneoplastic syndromes such as anti-Hu antibodies were discovered one after another, the relationship between tumors and abnormal immunity has attracted more and more attention. Autoantibody diagnostic kits for cancer diagnosis have already appeared on the market, for example, Oncimmune (UK) and Hangzhou CancerProbe Biotech have launched autoantibody kits related to lung cancer, and Provista Company (USA) has launched autoantibody kits for breast cancer diagnosis.

5.6.6 Autoantibody Discovery for Newly Discovered/Newly Categorized Autoimmune Diseases

Common skin diseases such as psoriasis and vitiligo are now considered to be autoimmune diseases, and autoantibodies such as ANA are often detected in patients with these diseases. At present, the detection of ANA mainly relies on the Hep2 cell-based indirect immunofluorescence method. In the course of clinical practice, a considerable number of laboratory workers and clinicians focus only on familiar known fluorescence patterns, and for special rare fluorescence patterns are in many cases subjectively considered as non-specific staining or impurities and ignored. In fact, detailed documentation of unknown fluorescence patterns encountered in clinical work should be made and analyzed in the context of the patient's disease or clinical symptoms, which may lead to the discovery of new fluorescence patterns in relation to the disease and also facilitate the discovery of novel autoantibodies with high specificity.

Secondly, the discovery of novel autoantibodies has helped clinical diagnosis and treatment, for example, neuromyelitis optica (NMO) was long thought to be a subtype of multiple sclerosis (MS) until 2004 when Professor Lennon reported the discovery of specific IgG-type autoantibodies, the target antigen of which is aquaporins 4 (AQP4), hence the name anti-aquaporin 4-immunoglobulin [9]. The discovery of this biomarker led to the recognition that neuromyelitis optica is a completely different disease from multiple sclerosis.

5.6.7 Genetic Testing and Individualized Medicine

Autoimmune diseases are currently considered to be genetic in nature. For example, ankylosing spondylitis is associated with the HLA-B27 gene, and celiac disease is associated with HLA-DQ2/DQ8. Genetic testing can help clinical assessment of patients' disease susceptibility and facilitate clinical detection of patients in the latent or pre-onset stage, and through early clinical intervention, can delay or even stop the progression of the disease, thus improving the quality of life of patients.

In addition, starting from the susceptibility genes of autoimmune disease patients, we can conduct more in-depth research on the pathogenesis of autoimmune diseases, so as to realize personalized treatment for patients. Taking autoimmune hepatitis (AIH) as an example, current studies have confirmed that HLA genes are closely associated with AIH occurrence, clinical manifestations and prognosis, especially the different alleles of HLA DRB1. In the US population, HLA DRB1*0301 was associated with younger age of onset and poor response to glucocorticoid therapy in patients with AIH-1. HLA DRB1*0401 is associated with older age of onset, higher female incidence, combined with other immune diseases, and lower treatment failure rates in AIH-1 patients. The tumor necrosis factor-α (TNF-α) allele, TNF-α*2, is associated with hormone therapy failure and poor prognosis in AIH-1 patients [10].

Precision medicine, a new medical model with precision and individualized diagnosis and treatment as its core, has become a direction and hot spot for medical research. Researchers have discovered genetic susceptibility loci in different autoimmune disease populations, explored the genetic molecular mechanisms of individual differences in drugs, and actively searched for biological markers for precise diagnosis and prognosis prediction. These studies have greatly deepened the understanding of autoimmune diseases among clinicians and are expected to improve the overall benefit of autoimmune disease diagnosis and treatment. Autoimmune diseases are characterized by complex etiology, diverse clinical manifestations, and the need for long-term maintenance of treatment. It is expected that the results in the field of genetics will provide clinicians with better ideas in terms of individualized and precise management.

Declaration Qiuping Yu, Haifeng Jin, Yanchun Guo and Tianshi Wang are employees of Shenzhen YHLO Biotech Co., Ltd., Shenzhen, China.

Xuexin Deng is an employee of Tellgen Corporation, Shanghai, China.

Mu Wang is an employee of Shanghai Advanced Clinical Laboratory Science Co., Ltd (ACLS), Shanghai, China.

References

1. Patakas A, Benson RA, Withers DR, Conigliaro P, McInnes IB, Brewer JM, et al.Th17 effector cells support B cell responses outside of germinal centres PloS One 2012;7:e49715.
2. Taylor JJ, Martinez RJ, Titcombe PJ, Barsness LO, Thomas SR, Zhang N,et al.Deletion and anergy of polyclonal B cells specific for ubiquitous membrane-bound self-antigen.J Exp Med 2012;209:2065–2077.
3. Li M, Zhang W, Leng X, et al. Chinese SLE Treatment and Research Group (CSTAR) registry: I. Major clinical characteristics of Chinese patients with systemic lupus erythematosus. Lupus. 2013;22(11):1192–9. https://doi.org/10.1177/0961203313499086.
4. Rees F, Doherty M, Grainge MJ, et al. The worldwide incidence and prevalence of systemic lupus erythematosus: a systematic review of epidemiological studies. Rheumatology. 2017;56(11):1945–61. https://doi.org/10.1093/rheumatology/kex260.

5. Jin S, Li M, Fang Y, et al. Chinese registry of rheumatoid arthritis (CREDIT): II. Prevalence and risk factors of major comorbidities in Chinese patients with rheumatoid arthritis. Arthritis Res Ther. 2017;19(1):251. https://doi.org/10.1186/s13075-017-1457-z.
6. Granerod J, Ambrose HE, Davies NW, et al. Causes of encephalitis and differences in their clinical presentations in England: a multicentre, population-based prospective study. Lancet Infect Dis. 2010;10(12):835–44. https://doi.org/10.1016/S1473-3099(10)70222-X.
7. Dutra LA, Abrantes F, Toso FF, et al. Autoimmune encephalitis: a review of diagnosis and treatment. Arq Neuropsiquiatr. 2018;76:41–9.
8. Miyakis S, Lockshin MD, Atsumi T, Branch DW, Brey RL, Cervera R, Derksen RH, De Groot PG, Koike T, Meroni PL, Reber G, Shoenfeld Y, Tincani A, Vlachoyiannopoulos PG, Krilis SA. International consensus statement on an update of the classification criteria for definite antiphospholipid syndrome (APS). J Thromb Haemost. 2006;4(2):295–306. https://doi.org/10.1111/j.1538-7836.2006.01753.x.
9. Pache F, Wildemann B, Paul F, Jarius S. Neuromyelitis optica [Neuromyelitis optica]. Fortschr Neurol Psychiatr. 2017;85(2):100–14. German. Epub 2017 Feb 24. https://doi.org/10.1055/s-0042-124186.
10. Oliveira LC, Porta G, Marin ML, Bittencourt PL, Kalil J, Goldberg AC. Autoimmune hepatitis, HLA and extended haplotypes. Autoimmun Rev. 2011;10(4):189–93. Epub 2010 Oct 7. https://doi.org/10.1016/j.autrev.2010.09.024.

Tumor Markers 6

Zhiyu Cai, Ye Sheng, Li Zhu, Jianer Yao, and Wei Deng

6.1 Overview

Tumor markers are substances that reflect the existence of tumors. They do not exist in normal adult tissues but only in embryonic tissues; their content in tumor tissues is much higher than in normal tissues. Their existence and quantitative change can indicate the nature of tumors, and help understand the histogenesis, cell differentiation, and cell function of tumors, thus aiding the diagnosis, classification, prognosis judgment, and treatment monitoring.

Traditionally, tumor markers are markers used to detect protein levels in serum. However, in a broad sense, all kinds of gene mutation, expression, methylation, and other indicators related to tumor screening, diagnosis, medication, and prognosis can be regarded as tumor markers. This part mainly involves the tumor markers of immunoassay, also called "tumor markers" in the traditional sense. Other tumor markers for molecular diagnostics, such as gene mutation and methylation, do not belong to the scope of this section.

Currently, there are more than 20 serum tumor markers commonly used in clinical practices. Few of these tumor markers are related to one type of tumor, while most may indicate multiple tumors. To be more specific, no "universal" tumor markers have been found yet, which means one marker cannot detect all tumors. Therefore, no tumor markers with superior sensitivity and specificity have been found. Therefore, one of the current principles for applying tumor markers is to select several relevant tumor markers for joint examination.

Z. Cai (✉) · Y. Sheng · L. Zhu · J. Yao
Tellgen Corporation, Shanghai, China
e-mail: caizhy@tellgen.com

W. Deng
Shenzhen Mindray Bio-Medical Electronics Co., Ltd., Shenzhen, Guangdong, China

H. Song, L. Dai (eds.), *In Vitro Diagnostic Industry in China*,
https://doi.org/10.1007/978-981-99-3110-1_6

6.2 Market Prices of Common Tumor Markers in Major Provinces and Regions

The charge of tumor marker detection varies wildly among provinces; some provinces may even have a 2–3 times difference.

Table 6.1 shows the charge of commonly used tumor markers collected nationwide in central provinces and cities as of December 2021. In terms of different regions, the cost in Guangdong Province is the highest, with an average charge of 94.5 CNY for each tumor test item, followed by an average charge of 93 CNY in Hunan Province. Zhejiang Province has the lowest cost of 47 CNY per test item.

Table 6.1 Charges for tumor markers in major provinces and regions (as of Dec. 2021)

Item abbreviation	Shanghai	Beijing	Zhejiang	Guangdong	Shandong	Jiangsu	Chongqing	Hunan	Hubei	Fujian
AFP	32	50	25	69	60	40	55	60	80	36
CEA	32	40	35	69	60	45	50	60	80	36
NSE	64	95	40	70	70	65	80	90	80	77
Cyfra21-1	100	95	40	90	70	65	80	90	80	103
SCCA	100	95	40	115	100	65	80	60	80	86
TPSA	64	80	40	90	70	65	60	120	80	68
FPSA	64	90	40	90	70	65	70	120	80	68
PGI	100	120[a]	80	76	160	90	44	100	80	70
PGII	100	120[a]	80	76	160	90	44	100	80	70
CA50	55	50	40	138	80	65	55	120	80	68
CA125	55	95	40	138	80	65	55	120	80	68
CA15-3	55	95	40	138	80	65	55	120	80	68
CA19-9	55	95	40	138	80	65	55	120	80	68
CA242	55	95	40	138	80	65	55	120	80	68
CA72-4	55	95	40	138	80	65	55	120	80	68
HE4	100	60	120	100	85	125	90	90	80	100
ProGRP	40	100	80	60	200	115	52	80	50	90
β2-MG	30	45	40	50	60	45	25	30	50	27
Ferritin	40	35	20	50	40	55	50	60	50	20
Free-β-HCG	50	50	40	57	100	95	70	60	50	45

[a]The charges for PG I and PG II tests in Beijing are determined independently by service providers and are about 120 CNY in general

6.3 Main Serum Tumor Markers Approved by the Domestic Drug Administration

As of December 2021, about 90 tumor marker manufacturers were found on the National Medical Products Administration (NMPA) websites, with nearly 1300 registration certificates. Table 6.2 shows the leading manufacturers of tumor markers.

In addition, the NMPA degraded the registration classification of most tumor markers from Class III to Class II by the end of 2020 and updated the intended use of these tumor markers. The intended use of auxiliary diagnosis has been deleted from all Class II serum tumor markers and unified into treatment monitoring, efficacy monitoring, recurrence monitoring, and metastasis monitoring. This change reflects the caution of the regulatory authorities on the definition and

Table 6.2 Leading manufacturers of tumor markers

Serial no	Corporate name	Number of registration certificates	Main methodology
1	Tellgen Corporation	39	Multiplexed flow fluorescence immunoassay, chemiluminescence immunoassay
2	Snibe Co., Ltd.	35	Magnetic particle chemiluminescence immunoassay
3	Autobio Diagnostics Co., Ltd.	32	Plate type luminescence assay, magnetic particle chemiluminescence immunoassay
4	Beijing Dacheng Biotechnology Co., Ltd.	29	Plate type luminescence immunoassay, magnetic particle chemiluminescence immunoassay
5	Beijing North Institute of Biotechnology Co., Ltd.	28	Enzyme-linked immunosorbent assay, chemiluminescence immunoassay, time-resolved fluorescence immunoassay
6	Bioscience (Tianjin) Diagnostic Technology Co., Ltd.	26	Chemiluminescence immunoassay
7	Suzhou Hybiome Biomedical Engineering Co., Ltd.	24	Direct luminescence of acridine ester immunoassay
8	Fosun Diagnostics Co., Ltd.	21	Chemiluminescence immunoassay
9	Weihai Wego Biotech Co., Ltd.	20	Plate type luminescence immunoassay, magnetic particle chemiluminescence immunoassay
10	Shenzhen Mindray Biomedical Electronics Co., Ltd.	20	Enzymatic reaction chemiluminescence immunoassay

Note: Statistics from the official website of the National Medical Products Administration application of tumor markers in tumor screening and auxiliary diagnosis. Because most tumor markers lack sufficient specificity and sensitivity in detecting early tumors to meet clinical satisfaction, the clinical application guidelines of many tumor markers abroad also do not support screening and auxiliary diagnosis. However, many Chinese experts have different opinions since much valuable information can still be obtained from detecting tumor markers in high-risk groups. After all, laboratory tests in China are very cheap compared with those in Europe and the United States. It is still prevalent to carry out the corresponding tumor marker detection for the high-risk groups in outpatient service to assist the diagnosis.

The point worth noting is that the guiding principles of various foreign medical treatments are formulated in reference to the results of health economics so that they will calculate whether it is cost-effective to invest in specific tests to decrease certain diseases' mortality and medical insurance expenditure.

The systems of charge in China, Europe, and the United States have massive differences. The differentiation of charges for general testing items in Europe and the United States is about 8 to 10 times as high as that in China. It is inappropriate to apply the guiding principles of Europe and the United States in China because diverse charges will lead to inconsistency of health economics calculation. Among nearly 20 serum tumor markers, alpha-fetoprotein (AFP) and prostate-specific antigen (PSA) belong to Class III. The value of these two indicators in tumor screening and early diagnosis is relatively clear, so the NMPA has preserved the two markers' Class III registration.

Table 6.3 shows the information about the adjustment of the subcategory of tumor markers by the NMPA.

Table 6.3 Summary of suggestions on proposed adjustment of 6840 in vitro diagnostic reagent classification subcategory

	Original contents				Adjusted contents	
Serial no	Directory No	III-7 Reagents related to tumor markers—Product classification name	Intended use	Manage categories	Manage categories	Intended use
1	171	Carcinoembryonic antigen (CEA) detection reagent	Used to detect CEA in human samples, and mainly used for efficacy observation, prognosis judgment, and recurrence monitoring of malignant tumors in clinical practice	Class III	Class II	Used for quantitative test of CEA, and efficacy observation, prognosis judgment, and recurrence monitoring of malignant tumors in clinical practice
2	175	Cytokeratin 19 fragment (CYFRA21-1) detection reagent	Used to detect CYFRA21-1 in human samples, and mainly used for efficacy observation and recurrence monitoring of non-small cell lung cancer in clinical practice	Class III	Class II	Used for quantitative test of CYFRA21-1, and efficacy observation and recurrence monitoring of non-small cell lung cancer in clinical practice
3	176	Squamous cell carcinoma antigen (SCC) detection reagent	Used to detect SCC in human samples, and mainly used for auxiliary diagnosis of cervical cancer and non-small cell cancer in clinical practice	Class III	Class II	Used for quantitative test of SCC, and treatment monitoring of cervical cancer and non-small cell cancer in clinical practice
4	177	Neuron specific enolase (NSE) detection reagent	Used to detect NSE in human samples, and mainly used for auxiliary diagnosis of small cell lung cancer (SCLC) and differential diagnosis of non-small cell lung cancer (NSCLC), and monitoring of the change, treatment response, and recurrence of SCLC and neuroblastoma in clinical practice	Class III	Class II	Used for quantitative test of NSE, and treatment and recurrence monitoring of lung cancer and neuroblastoma in clinical practice

5	178	Human epididymal protein 4 (HE4) detection reagent	Used to detect HE4 antigen in human samples, and mainly used for auxiliary diagnosis and efficacy monitoring of ovarian cancer in clinical practice	Class III	Class II	Used for quantitative test of HE4, and efficacy monitoring of ovarian cancer in clinical practice
6	179	Cancer antigen 125 (CA125) detection reagent	Used to detect CA125 in human samples, and mainly used for auxiliary diagnosis and treatment monitoring of ovarian cancer and other diseases in clinical practice	Class III	Class II	Used for quantitative test of CA125, and treatment monitoring of ovarian cancer and other diseases in clinical practice
7	180	Cancer antigen 15-3 (CA15-3) detection reagent	Used to detect CA15-3 in human samples, and mainly used for efficacy and prognosis observation of breast cancer in clinical practice	Class III	Class II	Used for quantitative test of CA15-3, and efficacy and prognosis observation of breast cancer in clinical practice
8	181	Carbohydrate antigen 19-9 (CA19-9) detection reagent	Used to detect CA19-9 in human samples, and mainly used for auxiliary diagnosis and efficacy monitoring of pancreatic and other gastrointestinal malignant tumors in clinical practice	Class III	Class II	Used for quantitative test of CA19-9, and efficacy monitoring of pancreatic and other gastrointestinal malignant tumors in clinical practice
9	182	Carbohydrate antigen 242 (CA242) detection reagent	Used to detect CA242 in human samples, and mainly used for auxiliary diagnosis and efficacy monitoring of pancreatic cancer, colorectal cancer, and other gastrointestinal malignant tumors in clinical practice	Class III	Class II	Used for quantitative test of CA242, and efficacy monitoring of pancreatic cancer, colorectal cancer, and other gastrointestinal malignant tumors in clinical practice

(continued)

Table 6.3 (continued)

	Original contents				Adjusted contents	
Serial no	Directory No	III-7 Reagents related to tumor markers—Product classification name	Intended use	Manage categories	Manage categories	Intended use
10	183	Carbohydrate antigen 50 (CA50) detection reagent	Used to detect CA50 in human samples, and mainly used for disease progression and efficacy monitoring of digestive system tumors (such as pancreatic cancer) in clinical practice	Class III	Class II	Used for quantitative test of CA50, and disease progression and efficacy monitoring of digestive system tumors (such as pancreatic cancer) in clinical practice
11	184	Cancer antigen 72-4 (CA72-4) detection reagent	Used to detect CA72-4 in human samples, and mainly used for auxiliary diagnosis and efficacy monitoring of gastrointestinal system and other malignant tumors in clinical practice	Class III	Class II	Used for quantitative test of CA72-4, and efficacy monitoring of gastrointestinal system and other malignant tumors in clinical practice
12	185	Tissue polypeptide specific antigen (TPS) detection reagent	Used to detect TPS in human samples, and mainly used for auxiliary diagnosis and efficacy monitoring of breast, ovary, digestive system, and other tumors in clinical practice	Class III	Class II	Used for quantitative test of TPS, and efficacy monitoring of breast, ovary, digestive system, and other tumors in clinical practice
13	186	β2 microglobulin(β2-MG) Test reagent	Used to detect β2 MG in human samples, which is mainly related to tumors and multiple myeloma	Class III	Class II	Used for quantitative test of β2 MG, and treatment monitoring of tumors and multiple myeloma in clinical practice
14	187	Ferritin test reagent	Used to detect ferritin in human samples, and mainly used for recurrence and metastasis monitoring of malignant tumors in clinical practice	Class III	Class II	Used for quantitative test of ferritin, and recurrence and metastasis monitoring of malignant tumors in clinical practice

15	188	S100 protein detection reagent	Used to detect S100 protein in human samples, and mainly used for treatment monitoring of central nervous system neoplasm in clinical practice	Class III	Class II	Used for quantitative test of S100 protein, and treatment monitoring of central nervous system neoplasm in clinical practice
16	191	Prostate alkaline phosphatase (PAP) detection reagent	Used to detect PAP in human samples, and mainly used for auxiliary diagnosis and efficacy/prognosis evaluation of prostate cancer, as well as differential diagnosis of metastatic bone tumors in clinical practice	Class III	Class II	Used for quantitative test of PAP, and efficacy and prognosis evaluation of prostate cancer, as well as treatment monitoring of metastatic bone tumors in clinical practice
17	192	Prostate acid phosphatase (PACP) detection reagent	Used to detect PACP in human samples, and mainly used for monitoring of bone metastasis of prostate cancer in clinical practice	Class III	Class II	Used for quantitative test of PACP, and monitoring of bone metastasis of prostate cancer in clinical practice
18	193	Thymidine kinase (TK) detection reagent	Used to detect TK in human samples, and mainly used for monitoring of tumor proliferation in clinical practice	Class III	Class II	Used for quantitative test of TK, and monitoring of tumor proliferation in clinical practice
19	194	Pro-gastrin releasing peptide (ProGRP) test reagent	Used to detect ProGRP in human samples, and mainly used for auxiliary diagnosis of SCLC in clinical practice	Class III	Class II	Used for quantitative test of ProGRP, and treatment monitoring of SCLC in clinical practice
20	195	Pepsinogen (PG) I test reagent	Used to detect PG I in human samples. The concentration level of PG I and the ratio of PG I/II can be used in auxiliary diagnosis of gastric cancer	Class III	Class II	Used for quantitative test of PG I, and monitoring of the concentration level of PG I and the ratio of PG I/II, which can be used to monitor the treatment of gastric cancer, in clinical practice

(continued)

Table 6.3 (continued)

	Original contents				Adjusted contents	
Serial no	Directory No	III-7 Reagents related to tumor markers—Product classification name	Intended use	Manage categories	Manage categories	Intended use
21	196	Pepsinogen (PG) II test reagent	Used to detect PG II in human samples. The concentration level of PG II and the ratio of PG I/II can be used in auxiliary diagnosis of gastric cancer	Class III	Class II	Used for quantitative test of PG II, and monitoring of the concentration level of PG II and the ratio of PG I/II, which can be used to monitor the treatment of gastric cancer, in clinical practice
22	199	κ Light chain detection reagent	Used to detect κ light chain in human samples (such as serum and urine), and mainly used for auxiliary diagnosis of multiple myeloma in clinical practice	Class III	Class II	Used for quantitative test of κ light chain, and treatment monitoring of multiple myeloma in clinical practice
23	200	λ Light chain detection reagent	Used to detect λ light chain in human samples (such as serum and urine), and mainly used for auxiliary diagnosis of multiple myeloma in clinical practice	Class III	Class II	Used for quantitative test of λ light chain, and treatment monitoring of multiple myeloma in clinical practice
24	203	Insulin-like growth factor-I detection reagent	Used to detect insulin-like growth factor-I in human samples, and mainly used for auxiliary diagnosis and treatment guidance of lung cancer in clinical practice	Class III	Class II	Used for quantitative test of insulin-like growth factor-I, and mainly used for treatment monitoring and guidance of lung cancer in clinical practice
25	204	α-L-fucosidase test reagent	Used to detect α-L-fucosidase in human samples, and mainly used for auxiliary diagnosis of liver cancer in clinical practice	Class III	Class II	Used for quantitative test of α-L-fucosidase, and treatment monitoring of liver cancer in clinical practice

26	205	Prolactin test reagent	Used to detect prolactin in human samples, and mainly used for auxiliary diagnosis of prolactinoma in clinical practice	Class III	Class II	Used for quantitative test of prolactin, and treatment monitoring of prolactinoma in clinical practice
27	206	Calcitonin (CT) test reagent	Used to detect CT in human samples, and mainly used for auxiliary diagnosis of medullary thyroid carcinoma and SCLC in clinical practice	Class III	Class II	Used for quantitative test of CT, and treatment monitoring of medullary thyroid carcinoma and SCLC in clinical practice
28	207	Arylsulfatase detection reagent	Used to detect arylsulfatase in human samples, and mainly used for auxiliary diagnosis of breast cancer and colorectal cancer in clinical practice	Class III	Class II	Used for quantitative test of arylsulfatase, and treatment monitoring of breast cancer and colorectal cancer in clinical practice
29	217	Hematopoietic cell removal reagent	Used to remove red blood cells, white blood cells, and other components in whole blood in vitro, so as to obtain the non-hematopoietic cells in blood for downstream analyses, such as circulating tumor cell test, immunocytochemistry analysis, construction of genomic map, etc.	Class III	Class II	Hematopoietic cell sample treatment reagent, which is used to remove the white blood cells from whole blood by immunoassay methods

Note: Source from the official website of the National Medical Products Administration

6.4 Market Situation of Tumor Marker Detection Reagents

Previously, radioimmunoassay, enzyme-linked immunosorbent assay, and solid chip method were used to detect tumor markers in China. Fewer and fewer customers used these methods. At present, most customers use fully automatic chemiluminescence instruments for single assay. A fully automated multiplexed bead flow fluorescence analyzer is used in the application scenario of joint assays. Therefore, in general, the market capacity of tumor marker detection reagents is usually calculated under the classification of luminescent immunoassay.

According to the *Annual Report on the Data of Medical Device Industry in China (2022)*, the chemiluminescence market in China was about 32.79 billion yuan in 2021 and is forecasted to be 40 billion yuan in 2022. At the same time, the domestically made luminescence immunoassay accounts for about 25%, and it is expected to accelerate the domestic substitution process through centralized procurement and other governmental policies. Among them, tumor markers account for about 35% of the chemiluminescence market, with a market volume of about 11.5 billion. It can be considered that Roche has been dominating the tumor marker detection market. However, until the recent decade, domestic tumor marker manufacturers led by Tellgen, Snibe, Mindray, and Autobio actively participated in the market. The quality and comprehensiveness are also catching up with and even surpassing oversea companies.

6.5 Leading Domestic Manufacturers of Tumor Marker Test Kits

6.5.1 Tellgen Corporation

Tellgen has been dedicated to tumor detection and developed products for early tumor screening, auxiliary diagnosis, personalized medication, and prognosis judgment. From the beginning, the company has been committed to the research, development, and promotion of the unique high-throughput flow fluorescence technology. In 2008, the company was the first to launch high-throughput joint immunoassays of tumor markers, based on multiplex bead flow fluorescence technology. It has industry-leading detection throughput and a comprehensive menu of tumor markers. Additionally, the company has established technical platforms covering immunoassay, molecular diagnostics, biochemical assay, and mass spectrometry. The application of Tellgen products covers cancer prognosis, cardiovascular disease, autoimmune disease, pathogen infection, and reproductive health, using multiplexed bead flow fluorescence, chemiluminescence, fluorescence PCR, and liquid chromatography with tandem mass spectrometry (LC-MS-MS). Moreover, Tellgen launched ground-breaking products, such as the first flow fluorescent tumor marker joint assay in China, the first NMPA-approved Y chromosome microdeletion detection kit, and the SHOX2 + RASSF1A dual gene methylation detection kit for malignancy characterization of small nodules in lungs. In 2018, Tellgen and Hitachi jointly launched the Hitachi-Tellgen compatible modular automation lines, which use Hitachi's high-throughput and stable sample pre-processing module, orbit, and biochemical analysis systems, connecting Tellgen Super Multiplex Immunoassay System (TESMI). They can be compatible with international mainstream immune analyzers, achieving a good balance between quality and price, opening a new era of domestic compatibility pipeline.

6.5.2 Shenzhen Mindray Bio-Medical Electronics Co., Ltd.

The serological tumor marker panel has always been the superior product of Mindray's chemiluminescence platform. It has a perfect quality control and traceability system. Relying on the AmpEr chemiluminescence test system, it adopts the innovative substrate luminescence enhancement technology and ALP enzyme labeling technology to achieve super sensitivity and ultra-high precision test. It has the advantages of good repeatability, small inter-batch variation, strong on-board stability, strong anti-interference ability, and high HOOK threshold. In combination with stable and high-speed chemiluminescence testing equipment, the panel can provide users with an accurate and efficient diagnostic solution. There are 20 tumor marker assays covering the complete testing panel of lung cancer (5 test items), gastrointestinal tumors, thyroid tumors, male reproductive tumors, gynecologic tumors, etc. These panels have been subjected to a comprehensive evaluation of application in treatment monitoring scenarios in large tertiary level cancer hospitals of China, fully meeting the clinical needs under different diagnostic and treatment scenarios. With the acquisition of HyTest, the world's leading supplier of raw materials for immunoassay, Mindray will further strengthen its ability in independent research of core materials, accelerate the enrichment of tumor marker projects, and provide more and better packages for first-line medical institutions, to promote clinical diagnosis and treatment.

6.5.3 Autobio Diagnostics Co., Ltd.

In vitro diagnostic (IVD) projects of serological tumor markers series have always been the popular products of Autobio chemiluminescence platform. The automatic chemiluminescence analyzer for tumor marker products has the advantages of high automation, good precision, and little cross-contamination. To fully meet the clinical needs under different diagnosis and treatment scenarios, there are 19 tumor markers, covering a complete assay menu of lung cancer, gastrointestinal tumors, thyroid tumors, male tumors, and gynecological tumors. The key raw materials are independently developed by Yimeinuo Bio, a subsidiary of Autobio. The self-sufficiency rate of raw materials for tumor marker reagents is more than 50% with stable supply and small inter-batch variation (which can be controlled within 5%), and the personalized HRP enzyme labeling technology ensures high sensitivity, high precision, and small difference between batches of reagent products. With the independently developed third-party tumor marker compound quality controls from Biaoyuan Company, Autobio strictly controls the inter-batch variation of reagents from R&D to production, and the quality controls are highly compounded to facilitate the use. Autobio has a perfect quality control and traceability system, raw materials, quality control products, reagents and instruments supporting, providing more abundant products for medical laboratories.

6.6 Certification of New Tumor Markers

There are few newly discovered serum tumor markers worldwide that have been developed into assay kits and approved by relevant national regulatory authorities in the past decade. The vast majority of domestically manufactured products are imitation of existing serum tumor marker detection products. However, a few new tumor markers or marker combinations have been approved in China. Examples are as follows:

6.6.1 Human Fibrinogen Degradation Products (DR-70)

First time of obtaining the certificate: In January 2019, Jiangsu Weizhen Biomedical Technology Co., Ltd.

The target of DR-70 detection is serum fibrin degradation products (FDP) in human blood. In the human body, FDP is generally derived from the decomposition of blood clots. When blood vessels are damaged and lead to bleeding, fibrinogen coagulates and forms fibrin clots for the wound, slowing and stopping the bleeding. After the vascular wound is healed, the fibrin clot will be decomposed to form a soluble fibrin degradation product—FDP. Under normal conditions, the FDP content in the blood is in a relatively stable range. When a malignant tumor occurs in the body, it may cause abnormal FDP content in the blood through three mechanisms: (1) tumor cells may secrete coagulant substances to activate blood coagulation; at this time, the corresponding physiological mechanism of the human body will promote the increase of serum FDP concentration; (2) The tumor caused necrosis of normal cells, and the death of cancer cells led to the release of a large number of procoagulant substances into the circulatory system; (3) In the process of recognizing tumor cells, immune cells may also release procoagulant substances to cause exogenous coagulation. Among them, the increase of procoagulants caused by the second and third mechanisms will intensify the progress of the first mechanism, thus increasing FDP in blood.

Intended use: It is used to detect the content of fibrinogen degradation product DR-70 in human serum, and the detection results can be used for auxiliary diagnosis and disease monitoring of gastric cancer.

6.6.2 Tissue Polypeptide Antigen (TPA)

First time obtaining the certificate: In August 2019, Suzhou Lihe Biomedical Engineering Co., Ltd.

The molecular weight of tissue polypeptide antigen is 17,000–43,000, composed of three subunits, B1, B2, and C. Its activity is mainly in B1. TPA primarily exists in the placenta and most tumor tissues. The detection rate of serum TPA in patients with various malignant tumors (ovarian cancer, colon cancer, rectal cancer, hepatocellular carcinoma, pancreatic cancer, lung cancer, breast cancer, endometrial cancer, and testicular tumor) can range from 20% to 90% (with a positive serum of >130 U/L). It is as high as 80–100%. Its existence does not correlate with the location and tissue type of the tumor.

6.6.3 Quantitative Fecal Occult Blood Test with Dual Indicators of Hemoglobin and Transferrin

First time obtaining the certificate: In March 2018, Tellgen Corporation.

The dual indicators of hemoglobin and transferrin are not tumor markers but a combination for the quantitative fecal occult blood test. However, the clinical practical intended use of fecal occult blood is for early colorectal cancer screening, thus, falling under the classification of tumor markers. The gold standard for clinical screening of colorectal cancer is endoscopy. However, endoscopy is a semi-invasive test, and the tested patients lack general compliance. Therefore, the quantitative fecal occult blood test is recommended to be the first choice by the national colorectal cancer screening guidelines. The innovation of this test is to detect dual indicators of fecal occult blood quantitatively. There was no quantitative fecal occult blood approved by NMPA before Tellgen, especially the dual indicator quantitative detection of fecal occult blood. This reagent can achieve a sensitivity of as high as 90% for lower gastrointestinal bleeding by combined testing of hemoglobin and transferrin in feces. Hemoglobin and transferrin dual-indicator quantitative fecal occult blood detection will become an economically effective and preferred method for colon cancer screening.

6.7 Future Outlook

As the most extensive application in the field of domestic chemiluminescence, tumor markers have received great attention from many companies. Most IVD companies with luminescence products have developed and registered tumor marker products. Since the enormous consumption of tumor markers takes place in large tertiary hospitals, and the primary market of domestic brands is still in hospitals below Grade II. Therefore, the domestic substitution of overseas brand tumor markers is still in early stages. However, at present, both instruments and test kits manufactured by domestic companies are rapidly catching up with oversea companies. In the next decade, manufacturers taking a significant share in the routine immunoassay projects of tertiary hospitals, especially tumor markers, will be the leading players of the immunoassay market in the future.

Innovative research in tumor detection is very active, not in serum tumor markers, but in genetic testing. Many new serum tumor markers are reported in the literature, but few of them have been approved for clinical use. Even the most famous multinational companies have not launched any new commercialized serum tumor marker in the past two decades. It can be seen how difficult it is to find a new marker that can pass clinical validation. On the contrary, there is countless innovative development in other testing methodologies, such as gene mutation, methylation, ctDNA, NGS, and ddPCR. It is expected that molecular detection will be the main channel for innovative research on tumor markers in the future.

Declaration Zhiyu Cai, Ye Sheng, Li Zhu and Jianer Yao are employees of Tellgen Corporation. Wei Deng is an employee of Shenzhen Mindray Bio-Medical Electronics Co., Ltd.

ELISA Immunological Reagents 7

Chao Chen, Yuming Ji, Jianfang Liu, Haifeng Shi,
and Wan he Ding

7.1 ELISA Immunological Reagents Overview

Enzyme-linked immunosorbent assay (ELISA) has experienced vigorous development for nearly 50 years since it was proposed in 1971. At present, the common detection methods of ELISA immunoreagents include double antibody sandwich method and double antigen sandwich method, competition method, indirect method, capture method, and biotin-avidin ELISA [1]. Because of its simplicity, stability, ease of automated operation, and variety of detection reagents (Table 7.1), ELISA detection is widely used in laboratory departments of large and medium-sized hospitals, and it is the main technical means of blood source screening at present. Common ELISA immunodetection items mainly cover: hepatitis series, respiratory series, venereal disease series, tumor marker series, TORCH (Toxoplasma, Rubella virus, Cytomegalovirus, Herpes simplex virus, and others) series, children's digestive tract series, etc.

C. Chen (✉) · Y. Ji · J. Liu · H. Shi
Shanghai Kehua Bio-Engineering Co., Ltd., Shanghai, China
e-mail: chao.chen@skhb.com

W. h. Ding
Jiangsu Yingke Xinchuang Medical Technology Co., Ltd., Nanjing, Jiangsu, China

H. Song, L. Dai (eds.), *In Vitro Diagnostic Industry in China*,
https://doi.org/10.1007/978-981-99-3110-1_7

Table 7.1 List of mainstream ELISA immunological reagents

Serial no.	Diagnostic category	Mainstream detection reagents	Clinical applications
1	Hepatitis series	Hepatitis A virus IgM antibody test kit	Infection detection and treatment monitoring for hepatitis A, B, C, D and E
		Hepatitis A virus IgG antibody test kit	
		Hepatitis B virus surface antigen diagnosis kit	
		Hepatitis B virus surface antibody test kit	
		Hepatitis B virus e antigen test kit	
		Hepatitis B virus e antibody test kit	
		Hepatitis B virus core antibody test kit	
		Hepatitis B virus core antibody (IgM) test kit	
		Hepatitis B virus pre-S1 antigen test kit	
		Hepatitis B virus nucleic acid associated antigen test kit	
		Hepatitis B virus surface antigen confirmation kit (neutralization test)	
		Hepatitis C virus antibody diagnosis kit	
		Hepatitis C virus core antigen test kit	
		Hepatitis D virus IgM antibody test kit	
		Hepatitis D virus IgG antibody test kit	
		Hepatitis E virus antigen test kit	
		Hepatitis E virus IgM antibody test kit	
		Hepatitis E virus IgG antibody test kit	
2	Respiratory series	Mycobacterium tuberculosis IgG antibody test kit	Auxiliary diagnosis of novel coronavirus infection, as well as screening, diagnosis and treatment monitoring of other respiratory diseases
		Tuberculosis infection T-cell test kit	
		Influenza A (H1N1) virus (2009) HA antigen test kit	
		Novel coronavirus(2019-nCoV) IgM/IgG antibody test kit	
		Novel coronavirus (2019-nCoV) IgM antibody test kit	
		Chlamydia pneumonia IgM antibody test kit	
		Chlamydia pneumonia IgG antibody test kit	
		EB virus VCA IgA antibody diagnosis kit	
3	Venereal disease series	Human immunodeficiency virus antibody diagnosis kit	Infection detection and treatment monitoring of sexually transmitted diseases
		Human immunodeficiency virus antigen antibody diagnosis kit	
		Treponema pallidum antibody diagnosis kit	

Table 7.1 (continued)

Serial no.	Diagnostic category	Mainstream detection reagents	Clinical applications
4	Tumor marker series	Alpha fetal protein test kit	Screening, diagnosis, and postoperative monitoring of common cancers
		Carcino-embryonic antigen test kit	
		Six tumor markers test kit	
		Total prostate-specific antigen test kit	
		Free prostate-specific antigen test kit	
5	TORCH series	Toxoplasma IgM antibody test kit	TORCH, pre-pregnancy, or early pregnancy examination, differential diagnosis of prenatal infection
		Toxoplasma IgG antibody test kit	
		Rubella virus IgM antibody test kit	
		Rubella virus IgG antibody test kit	
		Cytomegalovirus IgM antibody test kit	
		Cytomegalovirus IgG antibody test kit	
		Herpes simplex virus type I IgM antibody test kit	
		Herpes simplex virus type I IgG antibody test kit	
		Herpes simplex virus type II IgM antibody test kit	
		Herpes simplex virus type II IgG antibody test kit	
6	Children's digestive tract series	Coxsackie virus A16 IgM antibody test kit	Screening and diagnosis of hand-foot-mouth disease in children
		Enterovirus 71 IgM antibody test kit	
7	Others	Hantavirus IgM antibody test kit	
		Hantavirus IgG antibody test kit	
		Human rabies virus IgG antibody test kit	
		Leukocyte differentiation antigen CD8 test kit	
		Leukocyte differentiation antigen CD4 test kit	
		Talaromyces marneffei antigen test kit	
		Dengue fever virus NS1 antigen test kit	
		Dengue fever virus IgG antibody test kit	
		Nucleoprotein resistance Sp100 IgG antibody test kit	
		Varicella-zoster virus IgG antibody test kit	
		Neutrophil gelatinase-associated lipocalin test kit	
		Anti-m2 mitochondria IgG antibody test kit	
		Anti-cyclic citrullinated peptide antibody test kit	
		Anti-cyclic citrullinated peptide IgG antibody test kit	
		Encephalitis B virus IgM antibody test kit	
		Autoimmune disease ENA antibody test kit	

7.2 Introduction of ELISA Immunological Reagents from Different Manufacturers

According to the projection of the number of approvals reported by the Chinese Academy of Inspection and Quarantine, the ELISA immunological reagents are estimated to be about 1.5 billion servings in 2021, and the total number of blood screening (pharmaceuticals) is about 670 million servings, and the market capacity is estimated to be about 1.6 billion RMB. At present, the domestic market in China is basically dominated by domestic reagents, and the representative manufacturers of domestic reagents are Shanghai Kehua, Beijing WANTAI, InTec, etc. The details are as follows:

7.2.1 Shanghai Kehua Bio-Engineering Co., Ltd.

Shanghai Kehua Bio-Engineering Co., Ltd. was founded in 1981, and it was listed in the SME Board of Shenzhen Stock Exchange in 2004. The main business of the company covers enzyme-linked immunity, chemiluminescence, colloidal gold immunity, biochemistry, nucleic acid and supporting medical testing instruments, and it is the earliest company in China to launch test kits for two-half detection of hepatitis B. Kehua has rich products in hepatitis diagnosis, providing users with antigen and antibody test kits for hepatitis A, B, C, and E, and also providing test kits for HIV, syphilis, and tumor markers. The above products meet the needs of clinical and blood collection and supply systems.

7.2.2 Beijing WANTAI Biological Pharmacy Enterprise Co., Ltd.

Beijing WANTAI Biological Pharmacy Enterprise Co., Ltd. founded in 1991, is a high-tech enterprise engaged in the research, development and production of biological diagnostic reagents and vaccines, and was listed on the Shanghai stock exchange in 2020. The company's main business includes enzyme-linked immunity, chemiluminescence, colloidal gold immunity, nucleic acid, blood and supporting medical testing instruments, and its enzyme-immune products cover hepatitis, venereal diseases, respiratory diseases and digestive tract diseases, etc.

7.2.3 InTec PRODUCTS, INC

InTec PRODUCTS, INC was established in 1989, is a high-tech enterprise specializing in the research, development, production and sales of in vitro diagnostic products. The company's main business includes enzyme immunoassay, colloidal gold immunoassay and biochemistry. The enzyme immunoassay products mainly include hepatitis series and venereal disease series.

7.2.4 Shanghai Rongsheng Biotech Co., Ltd.

Shanghai Rongsheng Biotech Co., Ltd. (formerly Shanghai Rongsheng Biotechnology Co., Ltd.) was established in 1988. The company's products cover enzyme immunoassay, colloidal gold immunoassay, biochemical and vaccine, etc. The enzyme immune products mainly include hepatitis series, venereal disease series, and respiratory diseases.

7.2.5 BGI·GBI Biotech Co., Ltd.

GBI Biotechnology (Beijing) Co., Ltd. was established in 1994. In April 2003, the company officially changed its name to BGI·GBI Biotech Co., Ltd. Based on the complete series of enzyme immunoassay diagnostic reagents, the company developed nucleic acid diagnostic products and biochip products, and our enzyme immunoassay products mainly include hepatitis series, venereal diseases, and Epstein–Barr virus.

7.2.6 Beijing Kinghawk Pharmaceutical Co., Ltd.

Beijing Kinghawk Pharmaceutical Co., Ltd. established in 1993, is a high-tech enterprise specializing in biotechnology and product development. The company has six production lines of gold standard, enzyme immunoassay, fluorescence quantitative PCR, blood typing, medical equipment, and quality control products. The ELISA products mainly include hepatitis B series and venereal disease series.

7.3 ELISA Immunological Reagents Development Trend and Prospect

ELISA is a conventional detection technique with mature method, reliable technique, and simple operation. It has irreplaceable clinical application value. With the development of new techniques and methods, ELISA immunoassay system is developing rapidly toward automation and high efficiency.

7.3.1 Technology Upgrade Brings Application Expansion

Following the application of genetically engineered antibodies after monoclonal antibodies, the specificity of the assay and the accuracy of the analysis have been significantly improved, further enhancing the advantages of ELISA technology. ELISA has been developed in the continuous integration with modern technology, and through the progress of enzyme labeling technology, the application of labeled enzymes has been extended from horseradish peroxidase to alkaline phosphatase, β-galactosidase, urease, glucose 6 phosphate dehydrogenase, glucose oxidase and more than 20 other enzymes. In addition, the solid phase carriers for ELISA applications have developed from polyethylene or polystyrene microplates to nitrocellulose membranes, activated filter paper, silica sheets, nylon, various solid phase particles synthesized using polymeric materials, etc. At present, ELISA combined with other labeled immunoassays, new assays of ELISA have been carried out, such as fluorescent enzyme immunoassay, speckle enzyme-linked immunosorbent assay, magnetic particle ELISA, and chromatography-ELISA [2]. ELISA technology has stepped out of the pharmaceutical and clinical fields into the agriculture, fishery, animal husbandry, and food processing industries.

7.3.2 Increasing Number of ELISA Projects

According to incomplete statistics, there are more than a thousand test items established or developed by ELISA technology, and as many as 300 kinds of test kits can be purchased by commercial institutions, including nearly more than 100 kinds of commonly used test kits. In summary, all the substances corresponding to antigens and antibodies can be obtained, most of which can be established by ELISA.

7.3.3 Application of Blood Collection and Supply System Laboratory

According to the National Health Commission of China, the blood donation rate in China exceeded 12‰ in 2021, and the number of blood donations exceeded 16 million. At present, ELISA reagent is the first choice of in vitro diagnostic reagent for blood screening, which is widely used in blood collection and supply system. Most blood collection and supply institutions still adopt the detection mode of two ELISA + one nucleic acid detection (NAT), and chemiluminescent immunoassay (CLIA) blood detection is still in the stage of scientific research results comparison and testing. There are hundreds of blood stations and a larger number of plasma collection stations and biological products companies in China. ELISA reagents still have market development potential from the view of several diseases with large demand and mature development.

7.3.4 Application During the Novel Coronavirus Pandemic

In the special period of novel coronavirus outbreak, based on the mature ELISA technology platform, effective novel coronavirus serological antibody detection kits, and novel coronavirus nasopharyngeal swab and throat swab antigen detection kits were developed to meet the needs of epidemic control. The combined application of nucleic acid, antigen and antibody detection methods can shorten the detection window period and improve the positive detection rate, which is conducive to the detection, diagnosis, and prevention and control of cases.

7.3.5 ELISA Reagent Detection Mode Toward Full Automation, High-Throughput Development

With the growth of ELISA test volume, quality control and biosafety awareness in medical institutions, semi-automatic enzyme immunoassay analyzer can no longer meet the current demand for laboratory automation. There are fully automated ELISA analyzers that can combine the characteristics and parameters of reagents to introduce fully automated and high-throughput solutions to achieve full automation and high throughput of ELISA reagent detection mode while reducing costs. Full automation of ELISA reagent detection mode reduces the need for operators, reduces the work intensity of operators, and improves work efficiency. In addition, the full automation of ELISA reagent detection mode has a very big advantage in detecting infectious samples, which can effectively avoid the risk of infection due to misuse or accident.

In a word, with the development of science and technological innovation, ELISA technology will become more and more perfect, the degree of automation, accuracy and precision is getting better and better, will be better to serve mankind.

Declaration Chao Chen, Yuming Ji, Jianfang Liu and Haifeng Shi are employees of Shanghai Kehua Bio-Engineering Co., Ltd.

Wanhe Ding is an employee of Sinopharm Group Nanjing Medical Inspection Co., Ltd.

References

1. Wade D. The immunoassay handbook: theory and applications of ligand binding, ELISA and related techniques. 4th ed; 2013.
2. Tighe PJ, Ryder RR, Todd I, et al. ELISA in the multiplex era: potentials and pitfalls. Proteomics Clin Appl. 2015;9(3–4):406–22.

Part III

Clinical Chemistry

8 Instruments and Reagents for Biochemical Analysis

Zuojun Zou, Yanshang Ma, Dalei Li, Nengke Pan, and Yuanli Li

Biochemical diagnosis is often used for the testing of basic items such as liver function, kidney function, blood glucose, and blood lipid. By measuring the content (activity) of specific biochemical substances, people's physical conditions can be assessed and the relevant causes can be identified [1].

Biochemical diagnosis developed early in China and has always been a routine test item in hospitals for many years. Based on the statistical data of registration certificates of the China Food and Drug Administration, there are more than 200 enterprises related to clinical chemistry and more than 100 biochemical testing items in China. The data show that the market size of the biochemical diagnosis industry was about 16 billion CNY in China in 2019; however, as the domestic biochemical diagnosis market tends to mature, the overall import substitution rate has reached 55%. Moreover, partial technologies such as chemiluminescence have been substituted, and the growth rate will gradually slow down in the future, maintaining or even lower than 5%. The biochemical diagnosis industry has entered the Red Sea market.

In terms of the market structure, the market share of biochemical diagnosis ranks the second in the market segments of China's IVD industry; however, the biochemical diagnosis has the features of mature technology, simple operation, short analysis time, low-test cost, etc. For example, if the routine items such as blood glucose, blood lipid, cholesterol, and enzymes are tested by the chemiluminescence method, a series of preliminary preparations are required, such as cleaning the sample, to screen out the interfering factors. Therefore, the biochemical diagnosis will not be

Z. Zou · Y. Ma · D. Li (✉)
Beijing Strong Biotechnologies, Inc., Beijing, China
e-mail: lidalei@bsbe.com.cn

N. Pan · Y. Li
Zhong Yuan Bio-Technology Co., Ltd., Chongqing, China

H. Song, L. Dai (eds.), *In Vitro Diagnostic Industry in China*,
https://doi.org/10.1007/978-981-99-3110-1_8

replaced, although its market share had dropped from the first place to the second place in the in vitro diagnostic (IVD) market.

In terms of domestic substitution, biochemical diagnostic reagents have become the most mature segment of the IVD industry in China after more than 30 years of development, and the overall technical level is basically comparable to the international level of the same period. Although there is a gap in the detection accuracy and stability with the imported products for the biochemistry analyzers with relatively high technical requirements, the domestic products are still competitive. The domestic substitution of biochemical diagnosis takes the lead and the domestically produced chemical reagents account for more than 70%, which have entered Grade II Level A, and Grade III Level A hospitals. Presently, about 2/3 of the market share has been occupied by domestic brands. Meanwhile, some companies that can compete with international giants have emerged, including Beijing Strong Biotechnologies, Inc. (hereinafter referred to as BSBE), Medicalsystem Biotechnology Co., Ltd. (Medicalsystem), Beijing Leadman Biochemistry Co., Ltd. (hereinafter referred to as Leadman), BioSino Bio-Technology & Science Inc. (BioSino), Shanghai Kehua Bio-Engineering Co., Ltd. (hereinafter referred to as KHB), Maccura Biotechnology Co., Ltd., Zhong Yuan Bio-Technology Co., Ltd., etc.

In terms of the market situation, biochemistry analyzers with independent intellectual property rights have been developed in China since the mid-1970s, but their quality is not good enough and unsatisfactory. Even if it developed to the stage of R&D prototype, no product has been put on the market in the end; most of biochemistry analyzers used in China are imported. Since the 1990s, through unremitting efforts, various types of semi-automatic and automatic biochemistry analyzers have been independently developed in China. So far, a number of domestic enterprises have developed high-speed automatic biochemistry analyzers (for example, 2000T/H), which are comparable to the international level. However, we should be aware that there are still many deficiencies and "key & core technologies" in the industry and the domestic market is still occupied by the multinational giants, mainly because the biochemical instruments involve the optical, mechanical, electrical, soft, liquid circuit, temperature control and biochemical analysis technologies, the system structure is complicated, the control sequence is strict, the operational reliability and accuracy are high, etc. Currently, the domestic substitution rate of biochemical instruments is about 30%. The domestic biochemical instrument enterprises represented by Mindray, KHB, and Dirui mainly focus on the middle and low-end markets, while more domestic enterprises focus on the low-end markets.

Presently, the biochemical diagnosis market is close to the Red Sea market. Although the growth rate drops, the volume of the biochemical market cannot be ignored and is still in the second place in the IVD industry. In the future, the biochemical diagnosis market needs the integration capability of biochemical enterprises to form integrated supply. For example, BSBE, ZY Biotech, Medicalsystem with the biochemical diagnosis as the main business, will continue to work with foreign giants, and ultimately a high-end blue sea market will be formed in the biochemical industry.

8.1 Status Quo and Development of Biochemical Analysis Instruments

8.1.1 Overview

A biochemistry analyzer is an instrument that automatically completes the steps of sampling, adding reagents, removing interfering substances, mixing, constant temperature reaction, automatic monitoring, data processing, post-cleaning, etc. It can provide the clinical testing of biochemistry, hematology, and immunology items in the hospitals at all levels, including the clinical biochemical parameters for liver function, kidney function, blood lipid, diabetes, infection, rheumatism, immunity, etc., thereby providing an important scientific basis for the disease prevention, diagnosis, and treatment. The application of biochemistry analyzers has greatly improved the accuracy and precision and working efficiency of biochemical tests, and meets the requirements for the laboratory medicine. Presently, it has become one of the essential instruments for clinical diagnosis in medical institutions.

In recent years, the global market of biochemistry analyzers developed steadily, with a compound growth rate of approximately 4.30% from 2015 to 2020. The global market size of biochemistry analyzers reached 3.679 billion US dollars in 2019 and 3.790 billion US dollars in 2020. The Chinese market of biochemistry analyzers grew rapidly, with a compound growth rate of approximately 5.73% from 2015 to 2020. In 2019, the Chinese market size of biochemistry analyzers reached 582 million US dollars. Biochemistry analyzers include semi-automatic biochemistry analyzers and fully automatic biochemistry analyzers. Among them, the fully automatic biochemistry analyzers have a large market share, accounting for nearly 78.4% of total market in 2019. The biochemistry analyzer market is diversified; the top three enterprises, Roche, Danaher, and Hitachi, occupy nearly 50% of the total market share, they have possessed the key and core technologies and patents, and their products have been extensively recognized in the markets. The import and export trade and downstream industries will affect the needs for the biochemistry analyzers.

The Chinese biochemistry analyzers have experienced the technical progress from manual, semi-automatic to fully automatic biochemistry analyzers. A number of Chinese enterprises have produced fully automatic biochemistry analyzers. However, the domestic biochemistry analyzers started late, and the technology was weak. Presently, domestic companies represented by Mindray, KHB, and Dirui have successfully produced biochemistry analyzers that can compete with foreign companies. In terms of the market conditions, large hospitals and large laboratories prefer the fully automatic biochemistry analyzers of foreign brands because of high requirements on the technical parameters, performance, and brand of the equipment. The small- and medium-sized hospitals usually use small- and medium-sized biochemistry analyzers because of small sample size and cost consideration. Thus, the domestic high-end market is still dominated by foreign brands, and with the foreign brands entering the low-end markets, the competition in the markets of small- and medium-sized hospitals will become fiercer.

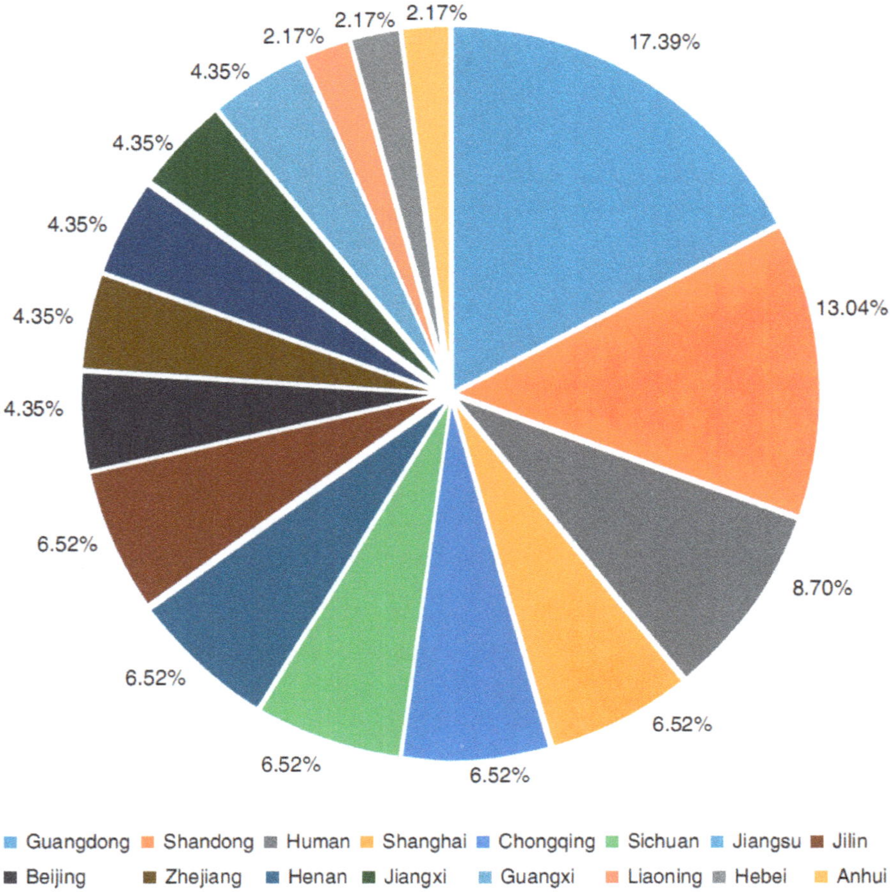

Fig. 8.1 Proportion of domestic manufacturers of biochemistry analyzers in different provinces and cities

Based on the data of CFDA, Fig. 8.1 shows that there are 90 new registration certificates for the production of fully biochemical analysis instruments in 2019–2020, covering 46 domestic manufacturers and 234 models of instruments. These manufacturers are mainly distributed in Guangdong, Shandong, Hunan, Shanghai, Chongqing, Sichuan, Jiangsu, Jilin, etc. Geographically, these manufacturers of biochemistry analyzers are mainly located in the eastern and southern coastal areas and the central area. The main market participants of domestic biochemistry analyzers are Mindray, Dirui, Medicalsystem, KHB, ZY Biotech, etc.

8.1.2 Status Quo of Domestic Biochemistry Analyzers

The fully automatic biochemistry analyzer, characterized by high technical content, high accuracy, high precision, high flexibility, and high working efficiency, has become one of the indispensable instruments in the modern clinical laboratory for the increasing testing work. According to the number of detected samples per hour, there are three types of fully automatic biochemistry analyzer, namely low speed, medium to high speed, and high-speed analyzers. Low speed: less than 800, including 200, 300, 400, 600; medium to high speed: 800, 1000, and 1200; high speed: 1600, 1800, and 2000.

Domestically produced chemical analyzers are in fierce competition at low speed, and mainly sold to the hospitals below Grade II. The imported biochemistry analyzers have occupied the high-quality customers such as large Grade II and Grade III hospitals for a long time. Especially in most Grade III hospitals, high-speed fully biochemical analysis instruments are required to complete the daily testing of samples, and these instruments are almost monopolized by foreign companies, since the domestic biochemistry analyzers, especially the domestic 2000-speed biochemistry analyzers have a big gap from the imported products in terms of the product quality, stability, and brand recognition. However, with the implementation of the hierarchical diagnosis and treatment policy, more and more patients are receiving treatment in the primary medical institutions, resulting in a surge in the demand for medical devices in the primary institutions. For the price-sensitive primary market, cost-effective domestic brands have obvious advantages. The Chinese government has continuously promulgated various policies, which have brought opportunities for the development of excellent and cost-effective domestic brands.

Since 2014, the China Association of Medical Equipment has been entrusted by the National Health and Family Planning Commission to carry out selections of excellent domestic medical devices for seven times. Table 8.1 shows the list of the seventh batch of excellent domestic biochemistry analyzers. The selection indicates the government support for the localization of domestic medical devices. This can facilitate to improve the quality of domestic medical devices and promote the development of domestic medical devices. With the reform of the medical insurance payment system that pays for the disease, when the diagnosis fee is no longer the source of the hospital's income but the hospital's cost, the cost-effective domestic products will be more favored. At the same time, domestic biochemistry analyzer manufacturers continue to increase investment in the R&D and improve product quality and performance; thus, the cost-effective domestic biochemistry analyzers will replace the imported brands gradually.

Table 8.1 List of biochemistry analyzers—the seventh batch of excellent domestic medical devices

Enterprise	Model
Fully automatic biochemistry analyzer (speed: 1600 and above)	
Dirui Medical Technology Co., Ltd.	CS-2000i, CSM-8000, CS-2000, CS-6400
Ningbo Medicalsystem Biotechnology Co., Ltd.	MS-2080
Jiangxi Tecom Science Corp.	TC9086
Shanghai Kehua Experimental System Co., Ltd.	Polarisc2000
Shenzhen Mindray Biomedical Electronics Co., Ltd.	BS-2000, BS-2200, BS-2000M, BS-2200M
	Fully automatic biochemistry analyzer (speed: 800 and above)
Dirui Medical Technology Co., Ltd.	CS-1600, CS-4000, CS-1300A, CS-1300B, CS-1200, CS-1400
Guilin Urit Medical Electronic Co., Ltd.	CA-800A/CA-800B/CA-800C, CA-801A, CA-801B, CA-801C
Jiangxi Tecom Science Corp.	TC9080
Ningbo Medicalsystem Biotechnology Co., Ltd.	MS-1280
Biobase Biodustry (Shandong), Co., Ltd.	BK-1200
Qingdao Hightop Biotechnology Co., Ltd.	HTSH-8000
Shanghai Kehua Experimental System Co., Ltd.	Polarisc1000, ZY-1250, ZY-1260, ZY-1200, ZY-1280
Shenzhen Rayto Life and Analytical Sciences Co., Ltd.	Chemray800 automatic biomedical analyzer
Shenzhen Mindray Biomedical Electronics Co., Ltd.	BS-800, BS-820, BS-800M, BS-820M, BS-830, BS-840, BS-830S, BS-850, BS-860
Zybio Inc.	EXC800, EXC810, EXC820, EXC830, EXC840, EXC850, EXC860, EXC870
Fully automatic biochemistry analyzer (speed: 400)	
Dirui Medical Technology Co., Ltd.	CS-450, CS-490, CS-650, CS-690, CS-480, CS-680, CS-380, CS-400B, CS-600B, CS-400
Guilin Urit Medical Electronic Co., Ltd.	URIT-8281, URIT-8280, URIT-8420/URIT-8460, URIT-8400
Jiangxi Tecom Science Corp.	TC6092L
Ningbo Medicalsystem Biotechnology Co., Ltd.	MS-680
Biobase Biodustry (Shandong), Co., Ltd.	BK-600
Qingdao Hightop Biotechnology Co., Ltd.	HTSH-4000
Shanghai Kehua Experimental System Co., Ltd.	ZY-680, ZY-690, ZY 400, ZY 450, ZY 460, ZY 480

(continued)

Table 8.1 (continued)

Enterprise	Model
Shenzhen Landwind Biological Engineering Co., Ltd.	LWC480, LWC400
Shenzhen Rayto Life and Analytical Sciences Co., Ltd.	Chemray420 automated chemistry analyzer, Chemray380 automated chemistry analyzer
Shenzhen Mindray Biomedical Electronics Co., Ltd.	BS-430, BS-450, BS-460, BS-600, BS-620
Zybio Inc.	EXC400, EXC420, EXC440, EXC450, EXC460, EXC470, EXC480, EXC490
Fully automatic biochemistry analyzer (speed: 200)	
Dirui Medical Technology Co., Ltd.	CS-T180, CS-T240, CS-T240Plus, CS-T300, CS-T300B, CS-300B
Guilin Urit Medical Electronic Co., Ltd.	URIT-8360
Qingdao Hightop Biotechnology Co., Ltd.	HTSH-2400
Shenzhen Landwind Biological Engineering Co., Ltd.	LWC200E
Shenzhen Rayto Life and Analytical Sciences Co., Ltd.	Chemray330, Chemray240
Shenzhen Mindray Biomedical Electronics Co., Ltd.	BS-360S, BS-350S, BS-370S, BS-360E, BS-370E, BS-230, BS-240, BS-350E
Zybio Inc.	EXC200, EXC220

8.2 Status Quo and Development of Biochemical Reagents

8.2.1 Overview

Biochemical diagnostic reagents, as one of the main categories of diagnostic reagents, are characterized by a large population coverage, a high proportion of services and service users and a huge market size. From 2015 to 2020, the market size of biochemical diagnostic reagents has increased year by year in China; in 2020, the market size of biochemical diagnostic reagents is about 16.1 billion CNY in China. The localization of biochemical reagents has been basically realized and they have been sold to Grade III Level A hospitals, and the import monopoly has been broken by domestic enterprises. Presently, about 70% of the market share has been occupied by domestic brands, and the rest is occupied by some powerful multinational corporations (such as Beckman, RANDOX, Toagosei). The domestic leaders of biochemical reagents mainly include BSBE, Medicalsystem, Leadman, Maccura, ZY Biotech, and other open reagent R&D manufacturers.

Taking homocysteine as an example, the abnormal blood homocysteine metabolism leads to the elevated concentration of homocysteine, which will greatly increase the risk of coronary heart disease, peripheral vascular disease, and cerebrovascular disease. Therefore, homocysteine is an important parameter of human health

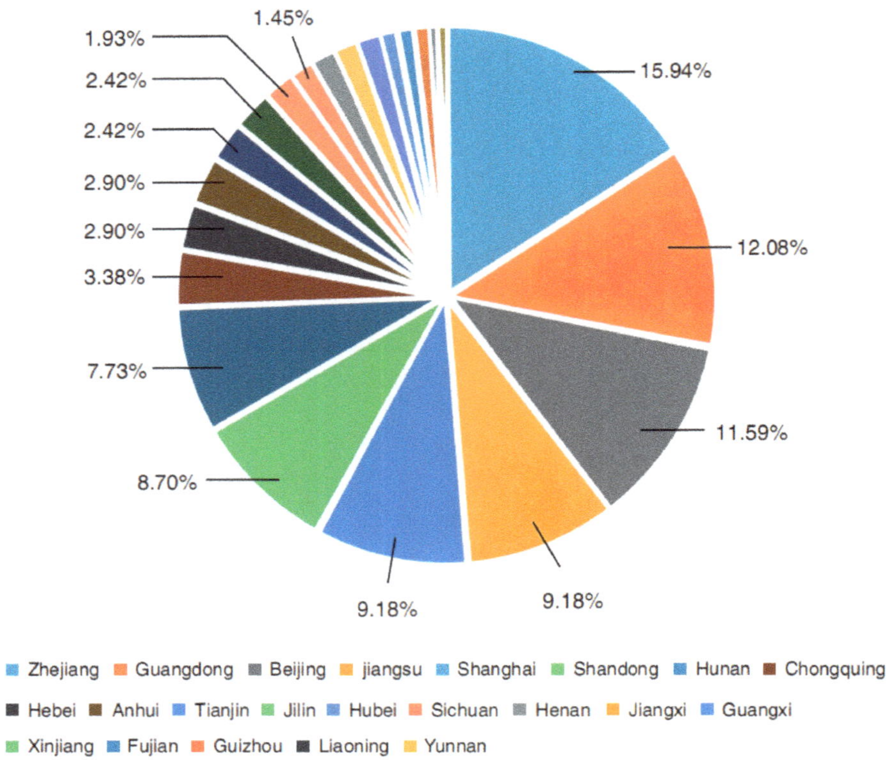

Fig. 8.2 Proportion of homocysteine kit (enzymatic cycling assay) manufacturers in different provinces and cities

condition. Based on the data of CFDA, there are 12 foreign enterprises and 207 domestic enterprises that produce the homocysteine kit (enzymatic cycling assay) in 2020. Figure 8.2 shows that the main manufacturers are distributed in Zhejiang, Guangdong, Beijing, Jiangsu, Shanghai, etc. Geographically, these manufacturers of biochemical reagents are mainly located in the eastern and southern coastal areas. The top 7 provinces and cities in terms of the number of enterprises account for more than 70% of the national market share, revealing a high degree of geographic concentration in the industry. The production and operation enterprises are mainly distributed in the Pearl River Delta, the Yangtze River Delta, and the Beijing-Tianjin-Hebei region, with the number of enterprises ranking the top nationwide.

8.2.2 Biochemical Reagent Products and Development of New Products and New Technologies in 2019–2020

Against the background of the current rapid development of life science and technology, with the development of clinical biochemical test technologies, there are more and more product categories and test items in the biochemical detection

Table 8.2 Some new products with registration certificates manufactured by BSBE in 2019–2020

Product	Category	Registration certificate
Carcinoembryonic Antigen Assay Kit (Latex Immunoturbidimetry)	Category III	Guo Xie Zhu Zhun 20203400704
α2-Macroglobulin Assay Kit (Immunoturbidimetry)	Category II	Jing Xie Zhu Zhun 20192400703
25-Hydroxyvitamin D Assay Kit (Latex Immunoturbidimetry)	Category II	Jing Xie Zhu Zhun 20192400436
Carbamazepine Assay Kit (Homogeneous Enzyme Immunoassay)	Category II	Jing Xie Zhu Zhun 20202400485
Glycocholic Acid Assay Kit (Homogeneous Enzyme Immunoassay)	Category II	Jing Xie Zhu Zhun 20202400488
Phenytoin Assay Kit (Homogeneous Enzyme Immunoassay)	Category II	Jing Xie Zhu Zhun 20202400486
Valproic Acid Assay Kit (Homogeneous Enzyme Immunoassay)	Category II	Jing Xie Zhu Zhun 20202400487
Serum Amyloid A Assay Kit (Latex Immunoturbidimetry)	Category II	Jing Xie Zhu Zhun 20192400696
Ammonia Assay Kit (Glutamate Dehydrogenase Assay)	Category II	Jing Xie Zhu Zhun 20192400700
Light Chain Kappa Assay Kit (Immunoturbidimetry)	Category II	Jing Xie Zhu Zhun 20192400704
Unsaturated Iron Binding Capacity Assay Kit (Ferene Method)	Category II	Jing Xie Zhu Zhun 20192400699
Ethanol Assay Kit (Alcohol Dehydrogenase Method)	Category II	Jing Xie Zhu Zhun 20192400701
α1-Antitrypsin Assay Kit (Immunoturbidimetry)	Category II	Jing Xie Zhu Zhun 20192400695
Inorganic Phosphorus Assay Kit (Phosphomolybdate Method)	Category II	Jing Xie Zhu Zhun 20202400190

platform. Moreover, in order to occupy the market, various biochemical diagnostic companies continuously improve the existing biochemical test menu and launch new test items, and develop new products with new methodologies to achieve cross-platform detection.

In 2019 and 2020, BSBE obtained a total of 18 new registration certificates; and some products are shown in Table 8.2.

As shown in Table 8.2, the BSBE's R&D of biochemical diagnostic products mainly focuses on the following two aspects in 2019–2020.

Firstly, the realization of other in vitro diagnosis in the biochemical platforms: Carcinoembryonic antigen assay kit is a product of tumor markers, and most of which follows the chemiluminescence detection method. BSBE has developed the biochemical products with the same sensitivity and accuracy as chemiluminescence. The α2-macroglobulin assay kit is a special protein product, which is detected by a special protein analyzer, or detected on a biochemistry analyzer. The 25-hydroxyvitamin D assay kit launched by BSBE has realized the transformation from three reagents to two reagents, and successfully realized the transformation from mass spectrometry to the detection on the biochemical platform.

Secondly, the development of new technologies based on the biochemical platforms: In recent years, with the increasing number of patients with major chronic diseases in China, more and more commonly used clinical drugs and new drugs have been used. However, a part of drugs will remain in the patient's blood after administration and metabolism. This part of drugs at a certain concentration will seriously affect the testing of various biochemical items of the patient's blood. The in vivo concentration of these drugs to be tested is extremely low. BSBE has realized the detection of low-concentration small molecule drugs on the biochemical platform, and developed the test kits of carbamazepine, glycocholic acid, phenytoin, valproic acid, etc.

In addition, the enterprises mainly engaging in the biochemical business work hard in the following two aspects: one is to enhance the product quality constantly in the original test items; and the other is to continuously develop new test items brought by the technological innovation. With the application of the latex-enhanced immunoturbidimetry and the enzyme immunoassay amplification, the sensitivity of biochemical test items is greatly improved. Representative products applied in the biochemical technology platform in 2019–2020 are as follows:

8.2.2.1 Creatine Kinase Isoenzyme Assay Kit (Latex Immunoturbidimetry)

BSBE is the first company that has obtained a registration certificate for the CK-MB mass determination on the biochemical platform and an invention patent at the end of 2018.

In principle, the CK-MB mass determination is to directly identify the CK-MB using the monoclonal antibody; the specificity of the antibody avoids the influence of giant CK and adenylate kinase on the test results, and solves the problem of the sample inversion in the immunosuppression method of the original biochemical platform. In addition, the antibody has better stability, which ensures the accuracy of the test results. All performance indexes can meet the clinical needs, and the performance is comparable to that of imported chemiluminescence products, which saves the user's cost and provides reliable quality assurance for laboratory testing.

8.2.2.2 Glutathione Reductase Assay Kit (Latex Immunoturbidimetric Assay)

Jiangxi Lecheng obtained the registration certificate for this product in 2017 and was granted an invention patent. Serum glutathione reductase is highly sensitive to the early stage of acute hepatitis. Clinical studies have shown that the Serum glutathione reductase reached the peak values earlier than the transaminase in the early stage of acute hepatitis, which can be used for the identification of early liver injury and the detection of malignant disease, nutritional assessment, and hereditary deficiency disease. The product adopts the dual liquid regent mode with a high accuracy, which can eliminate the influence of sample blanks (fat turbidity, hemolysis, jaundice, and other interfering substances), cuvette, etc., and the reagents are stored separately to improve the stability of the reagents.

8.2.2.3 Creatinine Assay Kit (Creatine Oxidase Method)

Maccura obtained the registration certificate of this product and was granted the invention patent in 2018. It is the first creatinine assay kit for anti-drug interference. Creatinine, as the most basic index for clinical evaluation of renal function, is widely used in the diagnosis and treatment monitoring of various chronic kidney diseases and acute kidney injury. However, for a diabetic patient, the administration of calcium dobesilate will produce serious negative interference to the subsequent creatinine test results, which generally exists in the testing products and methods of medical institutions at all levels, hides the actual condition of the patient, and delays the correct treatment of the patient, resulting in a very high medical safety risk. This product can guarantee the reliable and accurate results of the subsequent creatinine tests for the majority of patients who are taking calcium dobesilate.

8.2.2.4 Prostate-Specific Antigen Assay Kit (Latex Immunoturbidimetry)

BSBE obtained the registration certificates for PSA & fPSA assay kits in 2014 and 2020, respectively, which are the first domestic platform for rapid detection of PSA & fPSA. This product is used to quantitatively detect the content of total prostate-specific antigen in vitro in human serum for the dynamic monitoring of malignant tumor patients, so as to assist in assessing the disease progression or treatment effect. The detection sensitivity of fPSA reagent can reach the level of chemiluminescence, which is suitable for fully automatic biochemistry analyzers for fast testing in batches, effectively reducing the user costs.

8.2.2.5 Lipoprotein-Associated Phospholipase A2 (Lp-PLA2) Assay Kit (Rate Method)

ZY Biotech obtained the registration certificate and patent for the Lp-PLA2 assay kit (rate method) in 2015. The performance of the kit can reach the international leading level by using an innovative substrate design and reagent formula. The product is the first self-developed enzymatic assay kit that has been approved. Zybio continuously improves and optimizes product performance and stability, and is dedicated to better clinical application of Lp-PLA2. In 2018, ZY Biotech firstly reported the reason for the consistency of the results of enzymatic hydrolysis method and quality method, which was consistent with the conclusion published by Topbas C in Clinical Chemistry [2]. This further verified the scientificity of the Lp-PLA2 enzymatic determination method and it became the standard method for Lp-PLA2 detection.

The "inflection point of domestic products" is constantly approaching in the biochemical diagnosis industry. Although the in vitro diagnostic industry still needs continuous improvement in the field of raw materials, the process of domestic substitution has been accelerating for the midstream of the entire biochemical manufacturing industry. Particularly, the domestic biochemical reagents have replaced more than 70% of the imported reagents, and most Grade III Level A hospitals have used the domestic biochemical reagents. The domestic enterprises are constantly improving with the technological innovation.

8.3 Market Situation of Biochemical Diagnosis in China

Presently, the domestic biochemical diagnosis market is highly competitive, and some of domestic brands have occupied market shares that are close to or surpass that of the international brands. In 2019, China's IVD market size exceeded 71 billion CNY, with a year-on-year growth of 15%, of which, the biochemical diagnosis market accounted for 23%; in 2020, China's IVD market size exceeded 100 billion CNY, of which, the biochemical diagnosis market accounted for 18%. Although the biochemical market share in 2020 is lower than that in 2019, the market size in 2020 has increased by nearly two billion CNY compared with 2019.

8.3.1 Development of Biochemical Diagnostic Companies

8.3.1.1 Development of IVD Listed Companies (With Biochemical Business)

There were 10 and 9 newly added IVD listed companies nationwide in 2019 and 2020, respectively. Presently, there are 38 IVD listed companies nationwide. The domestic in vitro diagnostic industry giants have emerged, among which the representatives in the biochemical market include Mindray, BSBE, Medicalsystem, Maccura, Dirui, Leadman, Wantai, BioSino. The biochemical diagnostic reagents have a low technical threshold and there are many manufacturers, so the product homogeneity is high and the overall market structure is relatively dispersed. In the future, the leading enterprises will gradually build up the competitive advantages, and a large number of small- and medium-sized enterprises will develop longitudinally through innovation drive, and high-quality services and products.

In terms of the operating revenues, among 24 companies in Table 8.3, Mindray is the sole company with the operating revenue of more than ten billion CNY in 2019. Six companies have the operating revenues ranging from three billion to ten billion CNY, 11 companies ranging from one billion to three billion CNY, and 6 companies less than one billion CNY in 2019. In 2020, there are two companies (Mindray and DIAN Diagnosis) with the operating revenue of more than ten billion CNY, 9 companies with the operating revenues ranging from three billion to ten billion CNY, 8 companies ranging from one billion to three billion CNY, and 5 companies less than one billion CNY.

8.3.1.2 Development of Major Biochemical Diagnostic Companies

As companies developed with biochemical reagents, BSBE, Leadman, Medicalsystem, Maccura, Dirui, and ZY Biotech are still flourishing in the biochemistry field; they are also developing new products and expanding into other areas based on the biochemical diagnosis while maintaining the existing biochemical product lines. For example, the leading companies in the fields of immunity and chemiluminescence, such as Autobio, Snibe, Getein Biotech are continuously improving their product lines to enter the biochemical markets. The main businesses of the representative enterprises of biochemical products are shown in Table 8.4.

Table 8.3 Revenue of listed companies in the IVD industry in 2018–2020

Enterprise	Listing time	Securities category	2018 (100 million CNY)	2019 (100 million CNY)	Growth rate in 2019	Net profit in 2019 (100 million CNY)	2020 (100 million CNY)	Growth rate in 2020	Net profit in 2020 (100 million CNY)
Mindray	October 16, 2018	GEM	137.1	165.5	20.71%	46.85	210.3	27.07%	66.60
Health 100	May 18, 2005	SME Board	84.58	85.25	0.79%	−8.66	78.15	−8.33%	5.54
DIAN Diagnosis	July 19, 2011	GEM	69.67	84.53	21.33%	5.76	106.49	25.98%	10.70
Runda Medical	June 30, 2015	Shanghai A share market	59.64	70.52	18.24%	5.11	70.69	0.24%	5.04
KingMed Diagnostics	September 8, 2017	Shanghai A share market	45.25	52.69	16.44%	4.15	82.43	56.44%	15.73
BGI	July 14, 2017	GEM	25.36	28	10.41%	2.79	83.97	199.89%	21.02
Maccura	May 28, 2015	GEM	26.85	32.22	20.00%	5.66	37.03	14.93%	8.21
Medicalsystem	April 22. 2015	GEM	31.35	31.33	−0.06%	−5.77	23.02	−26.52%	2.94
KHB	July 21, 2004	SME Board	19.9	24.14	21.31%	2.73	41.55	72.12%	11.42
DAAN Gene	August 9, 2004	SME Board	14.79	10.98	−25.76%	−0.47	53.41	386.43%	24.50
Autobio	October 31, 2016	Shanghai A share market	19.3	26.79	38.81%	7.87	29.78	11.16%	7.57
Berry Genomics	July 5, 2017	Shenzhen A share market	14.4	16.17	12.29%	3.87	15.4	−4.76%	2.06
Wondfo	May 27, 2015	GEM	16.5	20.72	25.58%	4.27	28.11	35.67%	6.17
Sinocare	March 19, 2012	GEM	15.51	17.78	14.64%	2.51	20.15	13.33%	1.87

(continued)

Table 8.3 (continued)

Enterprise	Listing time	Securities category	2018 (100 million CNY)	2019 (100 million CNY)	Growth rate in 2019	Net profit in 2019 (100 million CNY)	2020 (100 million CNY)	Growth rate in 2020	Net profit in 2020 (100 million CNY)
Thalys Medical	October 1, 2016	Shanghai A share market	13.17	18.3	38.95%	1.42	21.25	16.12%	0.82
Dirui	September 10, 2014	GEM	9.33	10.09	8.15%	2.73	9.37	−7.14%	2.85
BSBE	October 30, 2014	GEM	7.74	8.41	8.66%	3.32	8.48	0.83%	1.22
Leadman	February 16, 2012	GEM	6.55	5.15	−21.37%	0.28	4.71	−8.54%	−0.29
Improve Medical	December 25, 2009	GEM	5.5	5.75	4.55%	0.26	9.19	59.83%	1.63
Getein Biotech	July 17, 2017	Shanghai A share market	6.86	9.68	41.11%	3.50	11.23	16.01%	3.30
Snibe Diagnostic	May 12, 2020	GEM	13.84	16.82	21.53%	7.73	21.95	30.50%	9.39
Sansure Biotech	August 28, 2020	GEM	0.62	3.65	444.78%	0.39	47.63	1204.93%	26.17
Tellgen	April 17, 2017	GEM	3.64	4.41	21.15%	1.57	4.9	11.11%	1.21
Wantai BioPharm	April 29, 2020	Shanghai A share market	0.98	11.83	110.71%	2.08	23.54	98.88%	6.77

Table 8.4 Main businesses of the representative enterprises of biochemical products

Enterprise	Main businesses
BSBE	Biochemistry, blood coagulation, blood type card, pathology
Leadman	Biochemistry
Mindray	Biochemistry, immunology, microbiological diagnosis
Medicalsystem	Biochemistry, immunology, POCT, mass spectrometry
Maccura	Biochemistry, immunology, molecular, POCT
Dirui	Biochemistry, urinalysis, blood cell analysis, immunology
ZY Biotech	Biochemistry, immunology, molecular, POCT, mass spectrometry, microbiological diagnosis
MC Bioengineering	Biochemistry, POCT, molecular
KHB	Biochemistry, immunology, molecular diagnosis
Autobio	Immunology, biochemistry, microbiological diagnosis
Snibe	Immunology, biochemistry
Getein Biotech	POCT, immunological diagnosis, biochemistry

Biochemical-Based IVD Companies

Since 2013, BSBE has successively established biochemical strategic cooperation with well-known domestic and foreign companies such as Abbott, Beckman, Roche, Hitachi, Mindray, and signed a *Technology Licensing and Transfer Cooperation Agreement* with Abbott, which has created the technology export of Chinese IVD companies.

In 2020, China National Pharmaceutical Investment Co., Ltd., a subsidiary of Sinopharm Group, invested in BSBE, and BSBE joined the Sinopharm, promoting the cooperation in the IVD field between the state-owned enterprises and privately owned enterprises.

As an established biochemical company, Leadman mainly engages in the biochemical diagnostic reagents, and actively researches and develops chemiluminescence products. Mindray has innovatively incorporated four independent testing systems (biochemistry, immunity, hematology, and coagulation) through the modular combination, forming a fully automatic detection module—the assembly line M6000.

Biochemistry line is the most traditional one of Medicalsystem. Medicalsystem has always focused on improving the innovation in the product raw material, reagents and instruments, and the diagnostic service levels.

Maccura self-produces and sells biochemical reagents. Its products are increasingly competitive against international brands in the domestic high-end markets such as Grade III and above hospitals, and have a broad space for substituting the imported products. In addition, Maccura is actively participating in the overall packaging of the laboratory tests to form an intensive service.

Dirui expands its business services to 8 major segments of IVD (biochemical analysis, urinalysis, blood cell analysis, chemiluminescence immunoassay, gynecological secretion analysis, coagulation analysis, molecular diagnosis, standardized laboratory) from its initial urinalysis test strips. It will continue to enter the fields of mass spectrometry, POCT, molecular diagnosis, etc., while enriching and improving the existing products, to complete the comprehensive development of the IVD market.

ZY Biotech started its business in biochemistry. It is also expanding its product lines in addition to focusing on the biological raw materials, chemical raw materials, and biochemical product series. Nowadays, its product lines cover multiple segments of IVD such as biochemical analysis system, chemiluminescence immunoassay system, POCT, molecular diagnostic system, mass spectrometry analysis system, coagulation analysis system. In addition, it carries out independent R&D and cooperation with well-known research institutions at home and abroad.

KHB is actively launching new products to the markets, covering the fields of biochemistry, immunity, chemiluminescence, dry chemistry, POCT and related instruments, etc.

IVD Companies That Enter the Biochemical Field Later

Autobio is a leader in China's immunodiagnosis industry. In order to accelerate the development of "product line + technology + channel," it acquired 75% of the equity of Beijing Bio-Top Biotechnology Co., Ltd. and quickly entered the biochemical diagnosis industry; meanwhile, it serves as the agent of Canon Medical's biochemistry analyzer series and forms a good synergistic effect with self-produced biochemical test reagents.

Snibe has been focusing on the research of chemiluminescence immunoassay and is the first-line company in the field of chemiluminescence in China. It also involves in the biochemical diagnosis and establishes the biochemical immune assembly lines with the independent intellectual property rights. By working with Thermo Fisher, it provides an overall solution of Satlas-TCA laboratory automation, and sells fully biochemical analysis instruments and supporting reagents across the world. Its supporting reagents cover numerous test items.

Getein Biotech focuses on the fields of POCT, radiation biochemistry, luminescence, etc. In order to meet the multi-dimensional needs of terminal hospitals for different testing items, Getein has continuously researched and developed biochemical testing reagents with its self-produced biochemistry analyzers.

8.3.1.3 Investment and Financing of Biochemical Companies and Cooperation Between Companies in the Past 2 Years

In 2019–2020, the industry consolidation has driven the "chain reaction" of IVD industry and becomes a mainstream. However, because of many segments of the IVD in China, the scale is still relatively limited in the short term despite the rapid growth; moreover, there are many domestic and foreign manufacturers competing with each other in each sub-industry, thus, it is very difficult to obtain an absolute market share in a sub-industry. Therefore, the active development and horizontal merger can allow enterprises to have multiple growth points, which is an important choice for the continuous development of enterprises.

In 2020, BSBE acquired MXB, and optimized the allocation of resources in terms of market, channels, R&D and management on the basis of its original businesses, to achieve mutual benefit and coordinated development.

Mindray has acquired HyTest, a world-renowned and first-class supplier of upstream raw materials for IVD. The company has original research and production capabilities in infectious diseases, inflammation, blood coagulation, etc. Through M&A, Mindray will strengthen the core R&D and construction of chemiluminescence products and raw materials, and promote the internationalization of in vitro diagnostic business.

In 2020, ZY Biotech acquired Jiangsu Skyray Instrument Co., Ltd., which owns the core team of former Xiamen Mass Spectrometry, all its assets and intellectual property rights in 2020. It has enhanced the competitiveness of product structure and brought a challenge to the international brands. This strong alliance will improve the level of mass spectrometry technology and make greater contributions to the cause of human health.

In 2020, after years of R&D and accumulation, the technology transfer income has become a new profit growth point for Wantai BioPharm, for example, technological cooperation with GSK and technology transfer to Pasteur. On March 31 of the same year, Wantai BioPharm and JSR signed the *Equity Transfer Agreement*. Through this equity acquisition, JHT became a wholly owned subsidiary of Beijing Wantai.

In recent years, a number of A-share listed companies (including related biochemical-based listed companies) have successively implemented equity transfers, and the actual controllers of some listed companies have changed to state-owned assets management departments, such as Leadman, Runda, Daan, BSBE, Dirui, Getein.

8.3.1.4 Acceleration of Localization for Foreign Companies

Under the current new situation, the localization is to encourage manufacturers of various brands to carry out manufacturing and promote the effective circulation of production factors within the territory of China rather than "protect the local brand products and expel the international brand products." With the improvement of Chinese manufacturing industry's contribution to the global economy in recent years, more and more international brands, such as Roche, Abbott, Siemens, Beckman, tend to establish the production bases and carry out production in China, to achieve the localization of imported brands. The four giants "Roche, Abbott, Siemens, Beckman" started the localization layout as early as 1985 in China.

1. *Beckman Coulter*: In 1997, Beckman Coulter established a reagent factory in Suzhou, Jiangsu Province, which was the first foreign IVD Company in China. Presently, it has carried out in-depth strategic cooperation with BSBE in the biochemical industry. As required by Beckman Coulter, BSBE will supply reagents suitable for the sales of Beckman Coulter biochemical equipment in China, to improve the biochemical reagent product line of Beckman Coulter in China.

2. *Roche*: In 2000, Roche Diagnostics officially entered China and established a production base in Suzhou. With the establishment of Roche Diagnostics (Suzhou) Co., Ltd., Roche Diagnostics has realized its localization layout. This is the first production base and R&D center established by Roche Diagnostics in the Asia-Pacific region as part of its global operation network, and presently China has become the second largest market of Roche Diagnostics in the world. In 2016, Roche Diagnostics China and BSBE held a contract signing ceremony for biochemical reagent cooperation in Shanghai, which officially opened a new chapter to work together in the Chinese market for new achievements between two sides. According to the requirements of Roche Diagnostics, BSBE would supply the biochemical reagents suitable for the instruments such as cobas c701/702, cobasc 501/502, cobasc 311, and Modular P for sales in China. Roche Diagnostics is committed to offering overall solutions for Chinese laboratory customers, including high-efficiency instrument testing platforms, comprehensive reagent testing menus, accurate and credible testing results, and professional full-process technical support services. In addition, Roche Diagnostics is actively seeking reliable partners to continuously improve the testing system and provide better services for customers. Through this cooperation, the two sides can further expand their market shares in the field of biochemical diagnosis, which is of positive and great significance to the enterprise development.
3. *Abbott*: Abbott, as a global diversified healthcare services company, has not yet established production base in China, but it actively acquired the domestic companies as its headquarters in China to provide various point-of-care testing (POCT) products and platforms in China. Its business services cover the diagnosis of cardiovascular diseases, diabetes and other chronic diseases and infectious diseases, toxicology diagnosis, women's health detection and tumor detection, etc., with a very complete localization layout. In 2016, Abbott and BSBE signed a strategic *Technology Licensing and Transfer Cooperation Agreement* on the biochemical diagnostic reagents. In accordance with the agreement, BSBE would provide Abbott with the production formula and process control flow of biochemical diagnostic reagents in the form of technology (including patent) licensing, and as consideration, Abbott would provide technology transfer fee and milestone payment in a lump sum, and the sales commissions of the transferred products in a certain period in the future. This cooperation has created a precedent for the technological output of Chinese IVD enterprises, and is of pioneering historical significance; in addition, it accords with Abbott's strategic plan as a global leader in biochemical diagnostics, strengthening Abbott's competitive advantage in the industry of biochemical reagents.
4. *Siemens*: Siemens started its layout in China as early as 1985. In this year, Siemens and the Chinese government signed a memorandum of cooperation and became the first foreign company to have in-depth cooperation with China. Siemens Healthineers has the ability to produce IVD reagents in China. The Shanghai Base, as the sole innovative base in the world for the integrated production of in vitro diagnostics and medical imaging, further assists Siemens Healthineers in promoting precision medicine and transforming the diagnosis and treatment model, and fully supporting the implementation of "Healthy China 2030" plan.

According to the layout and localization in China, the four giants have established offices, factories, and R&D centers in China and gradually expanded their scales, which are attributed to the comprehensive opening up of national policies and emphasis on innovation. Among them, Beckman Coulter (Suzhou) Co., Ltd. ranks the first in the number and types of approved IVD products, with 65 products registered for marketing, including the biochemistry analyzers, biochemical reagents, immunoassay reagents, flow cytometers, etc. Presently, Roche Diagnostics Suzhou factory has 3 products registered for marketing, including the biochemical reagent of γ-glutamyl transpeptidase assay kit (enzymatic colorimetry) (Su Xie Zhu Zhun 20202401213).

8.3.2 Influence of Policy and Environment on Biochemical Market

8.3.2.1 Support with Favorable National Policies

In 2019, the State Council successively promulgated three policy documents closely related to the biochemical analysis instruments and reagents, which laid an important policy foundation for the development of biochemical analysis instruments and reagents. The Office of the Central Cyberspace Affairs Commission issued the document on the management of biochemical analysis instruments and reagents, which played an important role in the related industry, and defined the relevant market management policies for the Internet resource collaboration service business regarding the business form of biochemical analysis instruments and reagents. The Ministry of Industry and Information Technology issued the *Three-Year Action Plan for the Development of Biochemical Analysis Instruments and Reagents (2019–2021)*, which proposed the guiding ideology, basic principles, development goals, and key tasks for the development of biochemical analysis instruments and reagents in China. In 2020, the *Thirteenth Five-Year Plan for the Development of Biochemical Analysis Instrument and Reagent Industry* issued by the central government unequivocally required that the scale of the biochemical analysis instrument and reagent industry would increase by 30% by 2020, and various local governments issued the local policies to increase the penetration rate of the industry.

In the recent 2 years, seven departments including the Ministry of Commerce have jointly formulated the *Special Action Plan for the Optimization and Upgrading of Commodity Markets (2021–2025)*, which explicitly proposes to promote the integration of domestic and foreign trade, and encourages the production and sales activities in the commodity market, and support export products to domestic sales according to the requirements of "same production line, same quality and same standard." Domestic enterprises are encouraged to complete the domestic substitution and sell their products abroad. The *Guiding Opinions of the General Office of the State Council on Promoting the Healthy Development of the Pharmaceutical Industry* stipulates that if the domestic drugs and medical devices can meet the requirements, domestic products must be procured for the government procurement projects in principle, and the allocation of domestic equipment must be gradually enhanced in public medical institutions.

8.3.2.2 Challenges and Opportunities in the Political and Economic Environment

Since the end of 2019, biochemical diagnosis companies have faced severe challenges due to the impact of the political and economic environment. All of the more than 280 operating companies were affected to different extents, especially for some small and micro-innovative companies, they have the problems of capital operation, raw material shortage, staff employment, and unsmooth supply chain, making them difficult to run. As an important part of the socialist market economy, the private enterprises are under unprecedented pressure. Affected by the political and economic environment in the past 2 years, the outpatient visits in hospitals dropped sharply, and the entire biochemical market has been in a downturn. Only a few companies have developed the diagnostic products for COVID-19 in time and achieved the rapid transformation to increase their operating incomes to a certain extent.

From 2019 to 2020, all people from the central government to general public have known in vitro diagnosis and its important roles, which will promote the healthy development of the in vitro diagnosis industry in the future, and has a practical significance for revitalizing the in vitro diagnosis industry and the far-reaching significance of creating a favorable development environment. The Chinese government has begun to increase the construction of public health, such as building and upgrading public health centers and infectious disease hospitals in various provinces, which will require a large amount of in vitro diagnostic equipment and testing reagents. In the future, people will pay more and more attention to their own health, and physical checkup will become people's daily needs. As the most important part of routine physical examination, biochemical diagnosis will become one of the important factors to increase the market share of biochemical products in the future.

8.3.2.3 Impact of Medical Insurance Cost Control, Centralized Procurement, and Online Bidding Through a Centralized Drug Procurement Platform

In terms of the pharmaceutical macro-political environment, the biomedical industry policies such as medical insurance cost control and target quantity procurement, are gradually implementing. The pilot of centralized procurement price reduction will face more difficulties, and the multi-modal procurement has continued to emerge. The centralized procurement of IVD reagents will be gradually implemented nationwide, and the biochemical reagents will face the pressure of price reduction. However, the centralized procurement will face challenges and opportunities. On the one hand, the centralized procurement will pose greater pressure on the imported biochemical reagents than the domestic biochemical reagents, which is conducive to achieving the import substitution in the biochemical diagnosis industry; and on the other hand, the government's centralized procurement is for the companies with high quality, large output, high market share and good distribution channels.

The online bidding procurement policy through a centralized procurement platform has been implemented in many provinces nationwide, and the centralized, open, and transparent procurement of reagents has become a mainstream. Since 2016, the sunlight procurement plan of in vitro diagnostic reagents has been successively issued in Sichuan, Shanxi, Anhui, Inner Mongolia, Hainan, Gansu, etc. According to the Plan, common medical consumables are purchased through online sunlight procurement, and the price is adjusted dynamically based on the variety and quality. For common medical consumables (including in vitro diagnostic reagents) that are used in large quantities and relatively stable, the quantity-based pricing, and target quantity procurement will be implemented gradually.

Under the overall idea of medical insurance cost control, with the policies of two-invoice system, target quantity procurement, Diagnosis Related Groups (DRG), regional inspection center model in the form of medical consortia, and the packaging, custody, and centralized procurement of medical institutions, etc., the distribution model of the biochemical diagnosis industry may encounter increasing challenges and pressures in the future. These policies will accelerate the promotion of the concentration ratio of the biochemical diagnosis industry, and the manufacturers will be required to establish their own marketing teams, reduce the dependence on the distributors and strengthen the terminal service capability. The accelerated implementation of DRG also proposes higher requirements for the reagent cost and quality of biochemical diagnostic manufacturers. In the face of complex policies and market environment, various companies should give full play to their existing technological brand and channel advantages, turn crises into opportunities, continuously seize opportunities in the competition, and consolidate their existing industry positions.

8.4 Future Development Trend

Presently, the biochemical diagnosis industry is facing fierce competitions in the price, policies, and development models (centralized procurement, rich production line). By sticking to the R&D route of high-quality products, increasing investment in high-end biochemistry analyzer R&D, the import substitution is completed; at the same time, by reducing the reagent costs and steadily advancing the market segments, the enterprise can maintain stable development and expand the market capacity, facilitating the industrial development.

8.4.1 "Intensive Cultivation"

For a long time, the domestic IVD market follows the imported brands and it is difficult to break the import monopoly. With the development of technology, the influence of fierce competition in the biochemical market has increased. Although the growth rate of the traditional biochemical diagnosis market has declined, the biochemical diagnosis has the natural advantages of time and cost for the testing of specific items and will not be replaced. By referring to the mature market structure of foreign countries, the biochemical diagnosis will occupy a certain market share.

After decades of extensive development, the key to the development of biochemical diagnosis is to adhere to the route of R&D of high-quality products, improve product stability, and master the core preparation technology of raw materials. The biochemical diagnosis should focus on the improvement of the product quality of the original testing items and the development of new testing items as a result of technological progress. For example, in the R&D of new products, with the application of latex-enhanced immunoturbidimetry and colloidal gold-enhanced immune technology, the detection sensitivity of the automatic biochemistry analyzers has been greatly improved, so that some items that are originally tested by the ELISA can be completed in the fully automatic biochemistry analyzer. The specific test items are based on the accuracy, cost and time, rather than only considering the advancement of technologies. Generally, companies should consider the product lines, marketing modes, and building high-quality items in making choices.

Through comprehensively sorting out the domestic biochemical industry chain, identifying the advantages and bottleneck in the industry chain, and making supplement, the stability of the supply chain is strengthened. In addition, the innovation chain of the industry is deployed around the industry chain in each stage of the entire life cycle of the product, to reasonably allocate the talents, funds and resources to each link of the product cycle. Moreover, the investment in R&D is increased, the combination of production, education, and research is further deepened, the platforms and human resources of universities and research institutions are utilized, favorable policies are issued, the income distribution of scientific researchers in research results is improved, the IP transformation efficiency is improved, and the refined quality services are implemented, which are important measures to boost the brand growth. A digital service platform will be built, to digitize offline entities online, integrate regional resources such as space, talent, capital, and policies, and expand the scope of services through virtual aggregation of online service resources. The needs of enterprises will be quickly responded to achieve precise resource matching. The industrial agglomeration is continuously promoted, the industrial innovation capability is enhanced, and the cost reduction and efficiency increase of the regional industrial development are promoted, to achieve the precise industrial governance.

8.4.2 Gradually Increasing Industry Concentration

In terms of the market share, the biochemical industry in the international market is highly concentrated. The "four giants" (Roche, Beckman, Siemens, and Abbott) have occupied more than 80% of the market share in the international market by virtue of their first-mover advantage. Domestically, many companies enter the IVD field due to low market entry barrier and high gross profit margins of biochemical reagents, so there are numerous enterprises. However, due to low technical barriers and serious homogeneity of related products, industry profits continue to decrease with the increasing number of companies.

In terms of the development trend of the biochemical diagnosis, it is mainly the competition in the stock market and an increasing market concentration is the development trend. After the intervention of the national administrative department and market governance, the industry has gradually improved, and the companies can improve the import substitution of fully automatic biochemistry analyzers and the coverage of biochemical diagnostic products in primary medical institutions through R&D advantages, brand effects and platform construction, to further promote the improvement of industry concentration. The listed companies take advantage of the financing and leverage advantages of the capital market to gradually open up the upstream and downstream chains of the industry and accelerate the pace of industrial integration through acquisitions and mergers, innovative technologies and capital combination, and the integration of channels, service providers, and suppliers. With industrial upgrading, standardized management and scientific and technological improvement, backward enterprises will be gradually eliminated in the industrial upgrading, and leading enterprises with core competitiveness will become the mainstream for the development of China's in vitro diagnostic industry. In the future, companies with high-cost performance and strong channel capabilities are expected to win and the market concentration will gradually increase.

8.4.3 Focusing on the Quality Control

As an important reference for clinical diagnosis and treatment, high sensitivities and accuracies are very important for the control over the error of test results. The metrological traceability can provide important support for the accuracy of test results by verifying the entire testing system, including reagents, instruments, personnel and operating procedures, so that the test results can be traced to international and domestic certified reference materials or reference methods, which is an important approach to standardize the medical testing [3–5].

The Clinical Laboratory Center of the National Health Commission of the PRC conducts external quality assessment (EQA) for various biochemical reagents every year. EQA is a process in which multiple laboratories analyze the same specimen, and the results reported by the laboratories are collected and fed back by an external independent organization to evaluate the laboratory operations [6, 7]. The interlaboratory comparisons can reflect the testing abilities of laboratories and monitor their continuity. The EQA program can provide objective evidence for assessing the data reliability and validity. BSBE's homocysteine is the product that is tested most by laboratories and ranks the first.

Presently, since no perfect testing process and standards have been established between different test institutions and the technicians have different levels, the test results cannot be mutually recognized among different medical institutions, so repeated testing is very common. With the continuous deepening of national medical reform and the gradual improvement of testing standardization, it is an inevitable trend for medical institutions to mutually recognize the test results. In the future, the establishment of a metrological traceability system will become an important competitive advantage for enterprises.

8.4.4 Development Switching from a Single Mode to a System Mode

Building a complete biochemical testing system is the future development trend in the biochemical industry. On the one hand, it can provide a relatively complete range of biochemical reagents to meet the needs of customers, to lay a solid foundation for the sales of closed-type instruments; on the other hand, when the production technology of biochemical reagents is relatively mature in most manufacturers, the advanced nature of the instrument has become an important factor to attract customers to purchase, to achieve the sales of reagents driven by the instrument.

8.4.5 Assembly Line

At present, various giants in the IVD market are competing the five mainstream market segments: biochemistry, immunity, molecular, POCT, and clinical testing. In the process of enterprise development, both endogenous growth and external mergers and acquisitions are important growth paths. However, because of many segments of the IVD in China, the scale is still relatively limited in the short term despite the rapid growth; moreover, there are many domestic and foreign manufacturers competing with each other in each segment, thus, it is very difficult to obtain an absolute market share in a segment. Therefore, the active development and horizontal merger can allow enterprises to have multiple growth points, which is an important choice for the continuous development of enterprises. In the current competition environment, many companies continue to expand product lines and create the second and third growth curves.

Biochemical immune cascade, also known as fully automatic biochemical immune analysis system or biochemical immunity integrated machine, has a high degree of automation and fast and accurate testing ability, mainly including control computer, data server, sample processing system, biochemical module, light-emitting module, and connection track [8]. Representative manufacturers include Roche, Abbott, Beckman, Siemens, Mindray, Snibe, and Autobio. At present, the domestic hospital clinical laboratories have a low automation level and most of them are still in the sage of modular assembly line. There are only more than 1000 modular assembly lines in stock nationwide. The Grade III hospitals are main markets of large-scale, fully automatic laboratory automation demands. The main application is the assembly line of foreign brands. There is a great room for the improvement of penetration rates of the whole laboratory automation system and other modular assembly lines, which provides an opportunity for the development of domestic automated assembly lines.

Mindray has innovatively integrated four independent testing systems of biochemistry, immunity, hematology, and coagulation through a modular combination. With China's first fully autonomous testing module-assembly line M6000, it brings a new era of the assembly line. Snibe works with Thermo Fisher to jointly build the overall solution of Satlas-TCA laboratory automation, and integrates the pre- and post-processing systems, and testing and analysis systems such as immunology and biochemistry, reflecting the strong integration capability and high expansibility. Autobio works with Toshiba to form the Autolas B-1 Series, a fully automatic biochemical immune assembly line, and based on the tailor-made design and services, to provide more flexible and efficient assembly line solutions for the medical laboratories. Other companies such as Runda Medical and Tellgen are actively promoting their own company's assembly line, and Maccura is actively deploying biochemical and luminescent instruments in recent years. It is expected to enter the biochemical immune cascade or the assembly line system in the future.

8.4.6 Improving the Comprehensive Service Capabilities

The reform of the circulating enterprises is imperative in the industrial chain, and the enterprises gradually begin to extend to service-oriented ones. Enterprises should improve their comprehensive service capabilities in terms of instrument automation, scientific research cooperation, quality control, logistics and distribution, daily services, etc.

The biochemical instruments require post-service installation and commissioning and subsequent continuous maintenance. The reagents have limitations on the validity period, and have high requirements for the cold chain transportation and inventory management; in addition, the hospital's warehouse area is limited and cannot meet sufficient inventory, so the requirement for the turnover efficiency of reagents is very high. Therefore, if the corresponding value-added services can be provided for the sold reagents and instruments, it will be able to obtain recognition from hospitals to a greater extent, thereby increasing the customer viscosity.

The application of the informatization tools can help medical institutions at all levels and the medical laboratory comprehensive service providers to simplify management processes and reduce comprehensive management costs, which is conducive to reducing the operating cost rate of laboratory service providers and other enterprises, and improving the operational efficiency of enterprises in the industry. The development and upgrade of the information service system can meet the customer informatization management requirements, accelerate the information transmission speed and information exchange efficiency between the company and the distributor, between the company and the customer, and between the company and the supplier, thereby providing services to the end hospital customers more efficiently. Through the construction of a high-quality, high-level, and highly intelligent information technology platform, the hospital's clinical laboratory management will be skilled, simplified, standardized, and refined, to help the hospitals to reduce the cost and increase the efficiency, and improve the hospital's service quality and patient satisfaction.

8.5 Summary

The technological innovation is the cornerstone of domestic substitution. At present, the upstream raw materials of biochemical reagents mainly rely on imports. For the long-term development of the industry, the preparation technology of raw materials must be mastered. The domestic listed companies have a large amount of cash flow, which can provide a solid support for the independent innovation. They have money to not only invest in R&D, but also to purchase core technologies, excellent enterprises and core supply chain of raw materials, etc., to achieve the accelerated improvement of the own strength. The performance of domestic biochemical instruments still needs to be improved. In the future, it is necessary to improve the sample storage capacity, detection versatility and detection efficiency. Biochemical diagnostic instruments will develop in the direction of automation, modularization and cascading. The large-scale automated assembly lines will be an important goal for the domestic biochemical enterprises to move towards the high end.

In addition, the enterprises should actively deploy the establishment of industry standards, the construction of a reference laboratory, FDA certification, etc., to enhance the enterprises' comprehensive competitiveness. With the accelerated entry of capital and the continuous integration and acceleration of mergers and acquisitions in the domestic biochemical diagnostic industry chain, a large number of products with domestic substitution capabilities will emerge. It is believed that the high-end biochemical market will be occupied by domestic products in the future!

Declaration Zuojun Zou, Yanshang Ma and Dalei Li are employees of Beijing Strong Biotechnologies, Inc.

Nengke Pan and Yuanli Li are employees of Zhong Yuan Bio-Technology Co., Ltd.

References

1. Büttner J. Clinical chemistry as scientific discipline: historical perspectives. Clin Chim Acta. 1994;232(1–2):1–9.
2. Topbas C, Swick A, Razavi M, Anderson NL, Pearson TW, Bystrom C. Measurement of lipoprotein-associated phospholipase A2 by use of 3 different methods: exploration of discordance between ELISA and Activity assays. Clin Chem. 2018;64(4):697–704.
3. Bons JA, Wodzig WK, van Dieijen-Visser MP. Protein profiling as a diagnostic tool in clinical chemistry: a review. Clin Chem Lab Med. 2005;3(12):1374–290.
4. Infusino I, Frusciante E, Braga F, Panteghini M. Progress and impact of enzyme measurement standardization. Clin Chem Lab Med. 2017;55(3):334–40.
5. Theodorsson E. Validation and verification of measurement methods in clinical chemistry. Bioanalysis. 2012;4(3):305–20.
6. Braga F, Panteghini M. Verification of in vitro medical diagnostics (IVD) metrological traceability: responsibilities and strategies. Clin Chim Acta. 2014;432(3):55–61.
7. Braga F, Pasqualetti S, Panteghini M. The role of external quality assessment in the verification of in vitro medical diagnostics in the traceability era. Clin Biochem. 2018;57(6):23–8.
8. Hawker CD. Laboratory automation: total and subtotal. Clin Lab Med. 2007;27(4):749–70.

Electrolyte Technologies 9

Jiandong Wang, Xiaolong Wang, Hui Xu, Dali Dai,
Lili Chen, Wenguang Tan, Meichen Jiang, and Min Yang

9.1 Introduction

The solutes of human body fluids can be chemically divided into electrolytes and non-electrolytes. Electrolytes usually refer to potassium (K^+), sodium (Na^+), chloride (Cl^-), calcium (Ca^{++}), lithium (Li^+), magnesium (Mg^{++}), and bicarbonate (HCO_3^-), noted that chemical valences are omitted in the following descriptions. Diseases of many organs of human body, some systemic pathological processes, certain changes in the external environment, and certain exogenous factors may cause or be accompanied by disturbances in electrolyte metabolism. For example, lithium ions are important in monitoring patients with mental disorders [1], while magnesium ion monitoring is important in patients with heart failure [2]. Therefore, electrolyte determination is an important part of the clinical laboratory testing.

Electrolyte determination is a routine analytical item in hospital laboratories and is also an emergency item, which requires rapid determination and accurate result. However, the traditional chemical and flame photometric methods used in the past fall far short of this requirement. Since the 1980s, ion-selective electrode technology (ISE) has developed rapidly [3]. Not only have various types of analyzers for the determination of electrolytes emerged, but many new electrode materials have also been developed, which greatly improving the specificity of the analysis. Ionized calcium and magnesium concentrations, which were difficult to determine accurately in the past, can now be determined with the new electrolyte analyzers, which has given a great boost to the study and monitoring of cardiovascular diseases.

J. Wang (✉) · X. Wang · H. Xu · D. Dai
Shenzhen Xilaiheng Medical Electronics Co., Ltd., Shenzhen, Guangdong, China
e-mail: Jack@horron.com

L. Chen · W. Tan · M. Jiang · M. Yang
Wuhan EasyDiagnosis Biomedicine Co., Ltd., Wuhan, Hubei, China

H. Song, L. Dai (eds.), *In Vitro Diagnostic Industry in China*,
https://doi.org/10.1007/978-981-99-3110-1_9

At present, the ISE method is the most used method in clinical testing and has been completely used in domestic instruments. Domestic instruments offer users more choices in terms of testing items, variety of consumables, and after-sales service, meanwhile they are gradually being accepted by clinical users worldwide.

9.2 Principle

Electrolyte analyzers have improved in recent years in terms of speed and accuracy, but the measurement principle of electrolyte analyzers remain the same, i.e., they are based on the Nernst equation. The relationship between the measured ion activity and the electrode potential can be expressed by the following equation [4]:

$$E = E_0 + \frac{2.303 \cdot RT}{nF} \lg a_x$$

where:

E is the potential of the ion-selective electrode in the measurement solution;
E_0 is the standard electrode potential of the ion-selective electrode, i.e., e.m.f. (electromotive force);
R is total gas constant;
T is absolute temperature;
n is the charge of the ion under test (valence of the chemical compound);
F is Faraday's constant;
a_x is activity of the ion under test.

For simplicity of calculation, the constant factors can be expressed as the slope "S" of the electrode, which can be determined by two kinds of standard solutions, the value of S is positive for cation-selective electrodes and negative for anions-selective electrodes.

It can be seen from the Nernst formula that the electrode potential is linearly related to the logarithm of the activity of the ion being measured under certain experimental conditions [5]. Therefore, the ion activity, which is a criterion for assessing the ability of an ion to interact with other ions, can be measured simply by measuring the electrode potential. The ion concentration can be calculated from its ionic activity.

There are eight common electrodes used in ion-selective electrode measurement instruments: potassium, sodium, chloride, calcium, lithium, magnesium, pH, and reference electrodes. Total carbon dioxide (TCO_2) can also be measured by using ion-selective electrodes, but many electrolyte analyzer manufacturers use the gas pressure method in recent years.

We define the electrodes other than reference electrode as working electrode. Each working electrode has an ion-selective membrane that reacts with the corresponding ion in the sample being measured. The difference ion concentration between either side of the membrane at the working electrode produces an electrochemical voltage, which is directly transmitted to the amplifier via the highly conductive internal electrode, at the same time the potential of the reference electrode is similarly directed to the amplifier, thus determination the ion concentration in the sample is transferred by detecting this potential difference and applying it on a calibration curve, which is obtained by detecting an accurate standard solution of known ion concentration previously. By combining various electrodes, the ion concentration of a sample can be determined simultaneously.

9.3 Electrodes

The core component of electrolyte measurement is the sensor, i.e., the ion-selective electrode. The principle of the PVC electrode can be simply described as follows: one side of the potentiometric circuit is the measuring electrode (i.e., the ion-selective electrode) and the other side is the reference electrode. When the selected ion in the solution reacts in contact with the ISE electrode membrane, the electric potential in the potentiometric circuit immediately changes, producing a potential difference. The magnitude of the potential difference is proportional to the activity of the measured ion in the solution, also proportional to the ion concentration.

The key part of the electrode is the ion-selective membrane, which is in contact with the sample on one side in response to changes in electrolyte concentration in the sample, and with the electrode's internal filling solution on the other side. The potential difference between two sides is then passed through an Ag/AgCl rod which is known as the internal conductive electrode to realize the transition from ionic to electronic conduction.

Different ion electrode membranes are only sensitive to their corresponding ions, the commercial ion-selective electrodes in the domestic market are K, Na, Cl, Ca, pH, Li, and Mg. More and more laboratories choose ISE method rather than traditional detection methods such as chemical methods for testing. The Mg electrode is the latest ion-selective electrode which can also be a good alternative to other methodologies in laboratory, Shenzhen Xilaiheng Medical Electronics Co. Ltd. holding the patent of Mg electrode and is the only manufacturer to provide the finished Mg electrode in domestic market.

Ion-selective electrodes are mainly divided into glass electrodes and polyvinyl chloride (PVC) electrodes depending on the material. Glass electrodes are mainly used to measure Na and pH [6], etc. The sensitive part in glass electrode is a glass spherical membrane, which is made by placing the components of the sensitive membrane in a platinum crucible and melting it at a high temperature above 1350 °C so that its solution becomes a transparent glass body without bubbles. Take a rod-like glass tube and preheated it at one end, then dipped it into the melted sensitive membrane glass body, blown it to a spherical shape, the pH buffer solution for the internal reference solution and an internal reference electrode Ag/AgCl added into this chamber.

The advantage of glass electrode is its large contact surface with sample but maintenance of glass electrode is not convenient, it is gradually replaced by PVC electrodes in the past few years. This article focuses on the main characteristics of PVC electrodes.

PVC electrodes are mainly composed of ion-selective membranes, electrode housing, Ag/AgCl internal conductive poles, electrode gold contacts, electrode internal liquid filling, and sealing rings. The electrode membrane is generally composed of three parts: ion active material, solvent, and PVC holder. The active material is an ion exchanger which must be able to combine with specific ions to form conjugates or complexes and is insoluble in water but soluble in organic solvents [3]. The solvent is generally an organic compound which is used to dissolve the electrode active material or holder. The holder, also known as the substrate, is an inert medium, an organic membrane that is insoluble in water.

Among those PVC electrodes, the K electrode is usually composed of a neutral carrier potassium ion-activated material with a selective response to K, PVC, etc. The inner side of this sensitive membrane is in contact with the inner filling of the electrode and the other side is in contact with the sample, the change in membrane potential which is a difference between the potassium electrode and the reference electrode is proportional to the logarithm of the K ion activity in the sample solution. Other ion-selective electrodes such as Na, Cl, Li, Mg follow a similar measurement procedure to that of K ion and will not be described further.

Calcium is the most abundant mineral in the human body. While most of the body's calcium is isolated in the skeleton, the free, hydrated cation in solution is a key physiologic mediator in a host of metabolic and regulatory processes [7]. Free calcium or ionized calcium (iCa) is the physiologically active form of calcium, many important physiological processes are related to the activity of iCa. iCa is a better indicator of the relationship between the patient's clinical symptoms and calcium metabolism than total calcium TCa [8]. However, since the sample for the electrolyte test is exposed to air and CO_2 dissolved in the sample may escape leading to the pH of sample rise, therefore the pH of the sample at this time is not the same as the pH in the patient's blood. As pH of sample increases, the complexation of Ca ion intensifies, resulting in a low measurement of iCa. Typically, iCa is negatively correlated with pH, i.e., an increase in pH results in a low iCa measurement and vice versa. Generally, for every 0.1 unit change in pH, the iCa change is approximately 4–5%. This relationship can be considered as linear within a certain range (pH in the range 7–8). It is usually assumed that results do not require correction when pH is 7.4 and that the pH at this value has no effect on the iCa of the solution to be measured, under this value of pH the iCa is considered to be the standardized calcium ion (nCa); if the pH is not 7.4, then a correction formula is required to convert the iCa to nCa for reporting. In general, nCa in the human body accounts for 40–50% of total calcium TCa.

As previously mentioned, pH of serum is unstable and no single meaning in clinical, it is usually used to correct iCa to nCa. The best way to measure the pH of a patient's blood is by using blood gas analyzer, which does not allow the blood sample to be contacted with air during the entire process from collection to analysis.

As for total carbon dioxide TCO_2, it exists in serum or plasma in three main forms [9]: the most abundant is the bicarbonate ion HCO_3^- which contributes to

64–65%, physically dissolved CO_2 accounts for about 3%, the aminoacyl derivatives of plasma proteins account for about 33%. There are many methods for the determination of TCO_2 in clinical tests, including the traditional enzymatic method, thermal conductivity method, gas-sensitive electrode method, carbonate ion-selective electrode method, and pressure sensor method; the pressure sensor method is used more and more in modern clinical applications.

There is a reference electrode which is used to provide a reference potential, thus forming a complete measurement circuit. As the concentration of electrolyte in the solution changes, the potential of the reference electrode remains constant, thus providing a reference point for measuring the potential difference. The potential difference can be fed into the input of the amplifier, the other input of the amplifier is connected to the reference electrode and grounded, since the reference electrode is grounded the electrode voltage can be further amplified.

The reference electrode connects the sample to the electrical signal ground, which consists of two parts: the reference electrode body and the reference electrode core. The reference fluid in the reference electrode body forms a salt bridge between the reference electrode core and the sample. The inner reference solution is injected into the reference electrode body before using the reference electrode. The reference electrode core in turn forms a circuit between the electrical signal ground and the inner reference solution.

In practice, the bias of the measurement comes from three aspects: (1) errors due to lack of selectivity of the ISE electrode, e.g., lack of specific selectivity of the Cl electrode for other halogen ions; (2) electrode multiple times used leading to protein covering the ion electrode membrane; (3) rupture or leak of the electrode membrane.

9.4 Reagents

As important as the electrodes to the measurement system is the electrolyte reagent, which require a stable pH and constant ion concentration, which are realized by adding specific components to the reagent, the reagent is mainly used for calibration and flushing pipeline of the electrolyte analyzer, the standard calibration solution is generally divided into two types, the first is the drift calibration solution, or low calibration solution, also known as an A standard, which is usually composed of an ionic solution with a human-like indicator plus a surfactant and a preservative. The other is the slope calibration solution, or high calibration solution, also known as a B standard, which is usually composed of an ionic solution with a difference from the human indicator plus a surfactant and a preservative, and each measurement sensor (electrode) builds its own internal measurement curve based on the two calibration reagents.

There are other reagents such as inner electrode filling solution to provide the electrode reaction environment; inner reference electrode filling solution (saturated potassium chloride solution) to provide a stable potential signal; electrode deproteinization solution to clean the residual proteins on the electrode membrane; cleaning solution to clean the instrument pipeline and TCO_2 reaction chamber, internal quality control solution to correct the instrument, activation electrode solution to fast stabilize the electrode, etc.

There are two methods in ISE measurement, one is direct method which means no need to dilute sample before testing, the other is indirect method which means the sample is needed to be diluted before testing. As mentioned before, reagents used in direct method include two standard calibration solutions, internal quality control solution, inner electrode filling solution, inner reference electrode filling solution, cleaning solution, electrode deproteinization solution, activation electrode solution, etc. The indirect method reagent includes not only the above solutions but also additional serum dilutions. Due to the high proportional dilution, the ionic activity can be considered as ionic concentration.

The reagent formulas of the various manufacturers are not fully disclosed, therefore reagents used in a measurement system should be provided by original manufacturers, we can understand the ion concentration of the high and low calibration solutions and the linear measurement range from these reagent instructions. The direct method does not require dilution of the sample, the result of this method is the relative ion activity. The indirect method has the advantage of providing faster and more stable results because the sample in the serum matrix is diluted at a high percentage to almost match the matrix of the calibrator solution. When electrolytes are in normal physiological concentrations, errors in ion concentration and activity are negligible. However, in the presence of pathological conditions, e.g., hyperlipidemia and hyperproteinemia, ion concentrations and activity will deviate considerably.

9.5 Latest Technologies of Electrolyte Device

Electrolyte analyzers have been developed in China for more than 30 years, the instrument hardware and software technologies have been basically mature, but in recent years there are some new development trends.

9.5.1 ISE Module

The one trend is an ISE module embedded in the biochemistry analyzer. The sample is drawn into the module by the biochemistry analyzer and the calibration solution is aspirated and discharged by control commands between the ISE module and the biochemistry analyzer. The ISE module generally tests three measurement parameters, K, Na, and Cl. The ISE module can also be used to build a stand-alone electrolyte analyzer.

The mainstream ISE modules currently used in biochemical analyzers are imported from abroad, they may adopt the direct method, which means that the sample is tested directly without dilution operations, or adopt the indirect method, which means that the sample needs to be diluted with diluent before testing. Both methods have their advantages and disadvantages. The direct method is simple to operate but cannot eliminate matrix effects fundamentally, while the indirect method is complicated to operate but the advantage is a small amount of sample needed and a faster overall testing process due to the less stable time of electrodes.

Major domestic manufacturers of electrolyte instruments have made different efforts on ISE module products, most of them are focusing on the technology based on direct method, such as the high-speed medical electrolyte analysis module based on flow injection technology, which is developed by Shenzhen University and Shenzhen New Industries Biomedical Engineering company. It adopts continuous dynamic sampling of sample and calibration solution, reducing the stable time of ion-selective electrodes. Shenzhen Xilaiheng Medical Electronics Company, Meizhou Cornley Company, Shenzhen Caretium Company, Nanjing Panshida Company, and other companies have designed their own different module products and tried to cooperate with biochemical analyzer manufacturers.

The electrolyte module is generally composed of a microprocessor, a sampling cell assembly, a peristaltic pump assembly, an ion-selective electrode assembly, etc. All operations are performed by means of communication with host analyzer. Typical technical parameters of electrolyte modules include.

1. Serum, plasma, whole blood, cerebrospinal fluid, or diluted urine can be tested on this module.
2. K, Na, Cl electrodes are usually used as measurement electrodes, other electrodes are optional.
3. The electrolyte module mainly uses two standard solutions to calibrate the measurement, which are drift calibration solution A and slope calibration solution B. Other reagents include reference inner electrode filling solution, inner reference electrode filling solution, pipeline cleaning solution, electrode activation solution, electrode deproteinized solution (protease), and quality control (QC) solution (for correction the instrument).
4. Electrolyte module can be connected to the biochemical analyzer to form an integrated machine, or can be connected to a PC to directly debug and check the module alone. The sample analysis speed is adjustable. Multiple modules can be combined in parallel mode to improve the overall testing speed to meet the requirements of high-throughput scenario.
5. The instrument can determine the calibration curve of each electrode and store it in the machine through calibration process. In this process, the millivolt value of each electrode can be compared by two calibrations cycles (A-B-A-B), by judging the stability of each electrode and calculation based on Nernst equation, the calibration curve of each electrode can be established automatically in the module.
6. Drift calibration solution A and slope calibration solution B are aspirated by independent peristaltic pumps, waste liquid is discharged by another peristaltic pump, this design improves the analysis speed while avoiding the carryover contamination caused by the traditional distribution valve.

At present, each company is optimizing their own module products and is trying to integrate the finished product in biochemical analyzer. We expect that these module products will eventually match the automatic biochemistry analyzer closely and work efficiently.

9.5.2 High-Speed Stand-Alone Analyzer

It is difficult to increase the testing speed in direct method because the time of electrodes stability cannot be greatly shortened. As mentioned before, one of the advantages of the indirect method is its faster electrode response due to the different electrode materials, so it is suitable as the main method for high-speed electrolytes. In addition, the indirect method can effectively eliminate the bias between the matrix effect of serum based sample and aqueous QC. The traditional direct method of ISE electrolyte does not thoroughly eliminate the matrix effect, i.e., there will be some deviation in measuring serum when the aqueous QC is accurate, or it will be less accurate when testing the aqueous QC in order to ensure the accuracy of measuring serum. Since quality control solution from many manufacturers are based on aqueous QC, so this problem can be effectively solved by using indirect method electrolyte instrument.

A typical high-speed electrolyte analyzer consists of sample racks loading/offloading system, a ZR rotating sample module, an electrode measurement module, a piping module, a circuit module, a data output module, a display module, etc. Typical technical parameters include:

1. Serum, plasma, whole blood, cerebrospinal fluid, or diluted urine can be tested on this module.
2. High-resolution touch color screen, user-defined interface, automatic fault alarm, and troubleshooting system.
3. Samples loading and offloading by sample racks, with automatic cup detecting function, automatic rotation of the testing tube, automatic barcode scanning, liquid surface detection function system. User only need to press the sample analysis key in each batch of tests, the instrument can automatically detect the sample location and perform sample analysis.
4. Automatic calibration function, sample analysis speed can be adjusted, test speed up to 200 samples/hour, 1400 T/hour (in the case of simultaneous test K, Na, Cl, Ca, pH, Li, Mg), built-in printer can print out the results, two-way LIS transmission.
5. The sample is diluted before entering the testing chamber. The dilution stirring tank is integrated into the instrument to avoid the impact of time-consuming and poor accuracy of manual dilution.
6. The calibration solution, buffer, cleaning solution and other reagents are degassed separately before entering the testing chamber.

7. Using precise plunger syringe, which achieves precise quantitative aspiration and discharge of liquid, the syringe is maintenance-free and can be used more than five million times in microliter (μL) level.

9.6 Major Domestic Manufacturers of Electrolyte Products

By the end of 1980s, the imported electrolyte products were dominant in the domestic market of China, these imported products with varieties of characteristics were specifically used to determine the ion concentration in serum, whole blood, or urine; the main customers of these stand-alone instruments were mostly secondary hospitals. Those imported ISE modular products based on direct method or indirect method were mainly installed in biochemical analyzers and used by high-end customers, such as tertiary hospitals.

From 1990s, domestic electrolyte industry in China has made rapid development, by now, the stand-alone electrolyte instruments have dominantly occupied many hospitals include township health centers, primary and secondary hospitals, following are introduction of major domestic electrolyte analyzer manufacturers which are active in China in recently years.

1. Shenzhen Xilaiheng Medical Electronics Co., Ltd.

   Xilaiheng, with a brand HORRON, focuses on the development and manufacture of clinical testing equipment and reagent, holding the electrolyte technologies covering all electrodes, ISE modules, reagents, and instruments; its products include: IMS-972Popular semi-automatic electrolyte analyzer; IMS-972/IMS-972Plus/H900 series full and semi-automatic electrolyte analyzer; H980 series high-speed electrolyte analyzer. It is the only manufacturer in the market that can determine 11 ionic parameters at the same time.
2. Meizhou Cornley Hi-Tech Co., Ltd.

   Cornley is one of the earliest companies that obtained CE certification for electrolyte products and blood gas electrolyte analyzers. Its blood gas and electrolyte analyzers include: BG-800 series, K-Lite8 series, K-Lite6 series, AFT800 series, AFT500 series, AFT400 series.
3. Caretium Medical Instruments Co., Ltd.

   Caretium is one of the earliest medical equipment enterprises specializing in the development and production of clinical tests, its electrolyte analyzers include: XI-1021 series, XI-931 series, XI-921 series.
4. Shanghai Xunda Medical Instrument Co., Ltd.

   Electrolyte analyzers of Xunda include; XD600 series, XD69 series, DIS-900 series. XD600, 69 series can be equipped with optional components to become fully automatic instruments.
5. Genrui Biotech Inc.

   Electrolyte analyzers of Genrui include: GE320, GE300, GE200 full or semi-automatic electrolyte analyzer.

6. Jiangsu Audicom Medical Technology Co., Ltd.
   Electrolyte analyzers of Audicom include: AC9100, AC9600, AC9800, AC9900 full or semi-automatic electrolyte analyzer.
7. Nanjing Panshida Electronic Instrument Co., Ltd.
   Electrolyte analyzers of Panshida include: PSD-11, PSD-15A, PSD-15B, PSD-16A, PSD-16B full or semi-automatic electrolyte analyzer series.
8. URIT MEDICAL Electronic Co., Ltd.
   URIT company is a manufacturer and service provider of medical diagnostic products. Electrolyte analyzers of URIT include: URIT-910, URIT-910C, URIT-910Plus electrolyte analyzer.
9. Shenzhen Histrong Medical Equipment Co., Ltd.
   Electrolyte analyzers of Histrong include: HC-9883, HC-9884, HC-9885, HC-9886 full or semi-automatic electrolyte analyzer.

9.7 Conclusions

In recent years, more and more core technologies have been mastered by domestic electrolyte analyzer manufacturers and the quality of devices and related products such as electrodes and reagents have been improving. By now, domestic products have occupied 90% market share of stand-alone machine, meanwhile, the major manufacturers have gone abroad and kept achieving good sales. However, information of the market analysis shows that the major profit is mainly from electrolyte modules which are embedded in the automatic biochemistry analyzers due to the large number of samples in the tertiary hospitals, these modules are monopolized by international brands and domestic manufacturers seldom involved.

We expect that the domestic manufacturers will continue to invest in R&D and launch high quality modular products and high-speed electrolyte instruments, with the help of national policies, these products can meet the requirements from high-end market customers to a greater extent and further enhance the influence of domestic electrolyte products all over the world.

Declaration Jiandong Wang, Xiaolong Wang, Hui Xu and Dali Dai are employees of Shenzhen Xilaiheng Medical Electronics Co., Ltd.

Lili Chen, Wenguang Tan, Meichen Jiang and Min Yang are employees of Wuhan EasyDiagnosis Biomedicine Co., Ltd.

References

1. Young A. More good news about the magic ion: Lithium may prevent dementia. Br J Psychiatry. 2011;198(5):336–7. https://doi.org/10.1192/bjp.bp.110.082875.
2. Wester PO. Electrolyte balance in heart failure and the role for magnesium ions. Am J Cardiol. 1992;70(10):44–9.
3. Akl ZF. Electrochemical selective determination of uranyl ions using PVC membrane sensor. Electroanalysis. 2017;29:1459. https://doi.org/10.1002/elan.201700007.

4. Helmenstine AM. Electrochemistry calculations using the Nernst equation. ThoughtCo. 2019. https://www.thoughtco.com/nernst-equation-electrochemistry-equations-606454. Accessed 27 Aug 2020.
5. Vidal-Iglesias FJ, Solla-Gullón J, Rodes A, Herrero E, Aldaz A. Understanding the Nernst equation and other electrochemical concepts: an easy experimental approach for students. J Chem Educ. 2012;89(7):936–9.
6. Mikhelson KN. Glass electrodes. In: Ion-selective electrodes. Lecture notes in chemistry, vol. 81. Berlin, Heidelberg: Springer; 2013. https://doi.org/10.1007/978-3-642-36886-8_5.
7. Baird GS. Ionized calcium. Clin Chim Acta. 2011;412(9–10):696–701, ISSN 0009-8981. https://doi.org/10.1016/j.cca.2011.01.004.
8. Sava L, Pillai S, More U. Dr Alka Sontakke, serum calcium measurement: total versus free (ionized) calcium. Indian J Clin Biochem. 2005;20(2):158–61.
9. Mikhelson KN. Ionophore-based ISEs. In: Ion-selective electrodes. Lecture notes in chemistry, vol. 81. Berlin, Heidelberg: Springer; 2013. https://doi.org/10.1007/978-3-642-36886-8_4.

Analysis of Blood Gas

10

Lili Chen, Wenguang Tan, Min Yang, Ziyan Luo, Jiandong Wang, Xiaolong Wang, Hui Xu, and Dali Dai

10.1 Introduction to Blood Gas Analysis Techniques

Analysis of blood gas has recently been a rapidly developed medical inspection technique. At the end of the 1950s, Poul Astrup, a Danish physician, and chemist, developed the first blood gas analyzer. Since then, blood gas analysis techniques have played an essential role in rescue and intensive care, diagnosis and treatment of acute respiratory failure, surgery, and other processes. Blood gas analyzers were manually operated in the early development and application stage from the end of the 1950s to the 1960s. They had an unwieldy structure (100 kg), required a large sample volume (about 2 mL), and could measure fewer values (only pH, pCO_2, and pO_2). From the 1970s to the 1980s, the rapid development of computer and electronic technologies pushed the development of blood gas analyzers into the fully automatic era. The integrated circuits were adopted to improve the structure and reduce the weight to below 30 kg. Besides, the menu was increasingly simple; users could conduct operations under the prompt and measure and calculate more parameters with the instrument. The continuous development also shortened the time required to preheat the instrument and measure the parameters. Since the 1990s, with the further application of computer technologies in the blood gas analysis sector, the advanced help mode and icon mode on the interface have made operations more intuitive. In addition, the blood gas analyzer has developed from a traditional device that can only judge the acid-base balance to a device that comprehensively monitors critical illness parameters according to the requirements of modern clinical medicine. The system can fully diagnose a

L. Chen · W. Tan (✉) · M. Yang · Z. Luo
Wuhan EasyDiagnosis Biomedicine Co., Ltd., Wuhan, Hubei, China
e-mail: tanwenguang@ediagnosis.cn

J. Wang · X. Wang · H. Xu · D. Dai
Horron XLH Medical Electronics, Shenzhen, Guangdong, China

H. Song, L. Dai (eds.), *In Vitro Diagnostic Industry in China*,
https://doi.org/10.1007/978-981-99-3110-1_10

patient's cardiopulmonary function, liver and kidney function, acid-base balance, oxygenation status, and metabolic function. Hospitals have put higher requirements on blood gas analysis techniques in patient care and cost management. Due to the particularity of its test parameters, blood gas analysis requires that samples are determined in the shortest time after sampling and that the data obtained is highly reliable, to help clinicians to make a rapid and accurate diagnosis and take timely and effective treatment. Therefore, blood gas analyzers have gradually developed to have the features such as portability, zero maintenance, easy operation, multi-parameter detection, fast detection, and accurate results. Thus, the point-of-care testing (POCT) blood gas analyzer has shown up. It has dramatically improved the efficiency of clinical diagnosis and treatment and has been accepted by an increasing number of hospitals and doctors. It has become an indispensable device for intensive care units, cardiac care units, operating rooms, emergency departments, respiratory departments, and other departments. Besides, it has become an excellent tool for laboratory diagnosis.

Due to the late start of blood gas analysis techniques in China, the market share of China-made blood gas analyzers is relatively low. However, considering the good performance close to foreign brands, relatively low price, and excellent after-sales services, China-made blood gas analyzers are a good choice for medical institutions. With the support of national policies and breakthroughs in crucial blood gas technologies, the turnover of cost-effective China-made blood gas analyzers has increased significantly. The China-made analyzers are expected to replace the expensive imported products. Currently, representative blood gas analyzer manufacturers in China include Wuhan EasyDiagnosis Biomedicine Co., Ltd., Shenzhen EDAN Instruments, Inc., Meizhou Cornley Hi-Tech Co., Ltd., Perlong Medical Equipment Co., Ltd. (Nanjing), and Guangzhou Wondfo Biotech Co., Ltd.

10.2 Principles and Key Techniques of Blood Gas Analyzer

10.2.1 Composition

A blood gas analyzer generally comprises an electrode system, a tubing system, a temperature control system, a computer system, and a data processing system. Its operating principles are as follows: The sample blood enters the electrode measurement chamber through the tubing system. The electrodes in the measurement chamber measure the sample and convert the measured values into corresponding electrical signals. After being amplified and converted from analog to digital values, the signals are sent to the microcomputer system of the instrument. Then, after computing and processing, the measurement results are displayed and printed.

10.2.2 Detection Principles

In the blood test results, pH, pCO_2, and pO_2 reflect the oxygen transport capacity and acid-base balance status of the human body; the test results of Na^+, K^+, Ca^{2+},

Cl^-, and other electrolytes are often used to diagnose diseases related to electrolyte imbalance; and the test results of Glu and Lac are used to diagnose diseases related to metabolic imbalance. Currently, China-made blood gas analyzers mainly focus on the detection of ten parameters, including three blood gas parameters (pH, pCO_2, pO_2), four electrolyte parameters (Na^+, K^+, Ca^{2+}, Cl^-), two metabolic parameters (Glu and Lac) and Hct. In principle, the analyzers mainly adopt electrochemical methods, involving ion-selective electrodes, gas electrodes, and biochemical sensors such as enzyme sensors.

10.2.2.1 Electrolyte Sensor

PH, pCO_2, Na^+, and other electrolytes are mainly determined by the potentiometric method. The pH sensor and electrolyte sensors (such as Na^+, K^+, Cl^-, and Ca^{2+}) operate based on the principle of ion-selective electrodes (also known as the membrane electrode). The membranes used in the sensors selectively respond to specific ions in the solution; therefore, potential differences are produced due to the different activity of the measured ions inside and outside the membranes [1, 2]. The potentiometric method is based on the Nernst equation, in which the exchange and diffusion of ions in the phase result in a potential difference. The potential difference is linear with the logarithm of the activity of the measured ions in the solution. Its equation is:

$$E = E_0 + \left(k \times \lg a_x\right)$$

where

E indicates the potential of the ion-selective electrode in the measured solution.
E_0 indicates the standard electrode potential of the ion-selective electrode.
k indicates sensitivity (electrode slope).
a_x indicates ionic activity.
E_0 and k can be determined by the sensor's response to the process control liquid. The activity of the measured ion in the solution can be obtained by simply measuring the voltage, and then the measured ion content can be obtained.

The measurement method for pCO_2 is slightly different from the measurement methods for pH and electrolytes. The pCO_2 electrode uses the H^+-sensitive membrane as the gas-permeable membrane. CO_2 in the sample diffuses into the internal bicarbonate buffer and dissolves and dissociates to release H^+. The transmembrane concentration gradient of H^+ results in the potential difference between the two sides of the membrane and such transmembrane potential change can be measured by the potentiometric method. According to the Henderson-Hasselbalch equation,

$$pH = pK_a + \lg \frac{\left[HCO_3^-\right]}{a \times pCO_2}$$

where

pK_a indicates the equilibrium constant for acid (also called acid dissociation constant).

$[HCO_3^-]$ indicates the concentration of bicarbonate ions.
a indicates the solubility coefficient.

The correlation between pCO_2 and pH: The difference between pCO_2 electrode potential and pH electrode potential is linearly correlated with $lgpCO_2$. Therefore, pCO_2 in the sample can be calculated according to the potential difference.

10.2.2.2 Amperometric Sensor

pO_2, Glu, and Lac are determined by the amperometric method. The pO_2 sensor operates based on the principle of the Clark measurement; that is, O_2 in the sample is reduced under the negative potential when it passes the diffusion-controlled membrane, and the response current is proportional to the concentration. pO_2 can also be determined through the optical method.

For a Glu sensor, its electrode structure includes a substrate electrode, an enzyme layer, and a glucose diffusion control layer. It uses glucose oxidase to catalyze the reaction between glucose and oxygen to produce gluconic acid and hydrogen peroxide (H_2O_2). The H_2O_2 produced is transported to the substrate electrode through the endometrium. An electrochemical reaction occurs at a constant positive potential, and the current is measured by a potentiostat. The current is proportional to the H_2O_2 concentration and the sample's glucose concentration [3].

For a Lac sensor, its electrode structure includes a substrate electrode, an enzyme layer, and a lactic acid diffusion control layer. It uses lactate oxidase to catalyze the reaction between lactic acid and oxygen to produce pyruvic acid and hydrogen peroxide (H_2O_2). The H_2O_2 produced is transported to the base electrode through the endometrium. An electrochemical reaction occurs at a constant positive potential, and the current is measured by a potentiostat. The current is proportional to the H_2O_2 concentration and the sample's lactic acid concentration.

10.2.2.3 Resistance Sensor

The Hct indicator is measured based on the conductivity method. The resistance of cell membranes is high, whereas the electric conductivity of the plasma is higher than the cell membrane. Therefore, the higher the cell concentration, the higher the blood resistivity. The corresponding Maxwell-Fricke equation:

$$r = R_p \times \frac{\left(1 + \frac{\text{Hct}}{100}\right)}{\left(1 - \frac{\text{Hct}}{100}\right)}$$

where

r indicates the resistivity of blood.
R_p indicates the resistivity of plasma.
Hct indicates hematocrit.

The Hct value mainly reflects the percentage of red blood cells in the total blood volume and is used to detect whether the blood is in a normal state. An abnormal Hct value is often related to anemia and polycythemia [4].

10.2.3 Key Techniques

1. Multi-parameter integrated electrochemical sensor chip.

To quickly detect acid-base balance status, blood oxygen level, electrolyte balance status, and metabolite level of patients, mainstream blood gas analyzer manufacturers integrate multiple measurement parameters such as blood gas/electrolyte/biochemistry on a test card and form an expandable chip platform.

2. Techniques of precision dispensing and biosensitive membrane preparation.

The multi-parameter integrated process realizes the measurement of multiple parameters on a chip. The chips are currently produced in automatic lines to improve capacity and productivity, thus supplying the market demands in and outside China.

3. High-precision weak signal acquisition and signal processing.

The high-precision weak signal acquisition hardware adopts the self-adaptive temporal logic software and intelligent signal acquisition, realizing accurate identification of weak signals.

4. Microfluidic tubing.

The accurate liquid path control system and timing sequence can realize the repeated and precise control of different liquid paths. Multiple sample injection modes reduce the volume of blood collected, alleviating patient pain.

5. Intelligent signal recognition, signal feedback, and system timing control.

The wet blood gas analyzer has a built-in self-diagnosis function. It can monitor the sensor signals and update the electrode status in real time. Besides, its automatic calibration and maintenance-free also simplify the operation.

6. Automatic pipetting, animation-guided operations, and user-friendly man-machine interaction.

The user-friendly man-machine interaction menu and simple menu navigation ensure that all operators can operate the instrument after a short training.

10.2.4 Basic Characteristics of POCT Blood Gas Analyzer

With the development of science and technology, higher requirements for blood gas analyzers are put forward. For POCT blood gas analyzers for rapid detection, the following requirements are raised:

1. Small volume of devices or reagents, portability, and preferably with built-in battery.
2. Fast detection speed: For dry blood gas analyzers, operators can obtain the test result within 2–3 minutes. For wet blood gas analyzers, operators can receive the test result within 1 minute.
3. Accurate test results to reliably support the clinical diagnosis.
4. Safe operation and sample recycling to avoid biological pollution.
5. Easy to use and maintenance-free.

10.3 Introduction to Blood Gas Analyzer Manufacturers in China

1. Wuhan EasyDiagnosis Biomedicine Co., Ltd.

Wuhan EasyDiagnosis Biomedicine Co., Ltd. has independent intellectual property rights for the PT1000 Blood Gas Analyzer. The instruments and reagents of the PT1000 passed the NMPA certification in 2019 and the CE certification in 2020. It is the first card-package integrated blood gas analysis system in China. Unlike the blood gas analysis platform of other manufacturers in China, it has achieved technological breakthroughs. PT1000 was awarded the Gold Medal in the Innovation Star Cup China Innovation Award of IVD product 2019.

2. Shenzhen EDAN Instruments, Inc.

The EDAN i15 Blood Gas and Chemistry Analysis System applies microfluidic design, microsensor multifunctional membrane preparation technology, and microsensor integrated liquid path control technology. With over 70 national and international patents, EDAN has won the "China Patent Excellence Award" and has produced the innovative high-performance dry rapid-detection blood gas analyzer in China.

3. Meizhou Cornley Hi-Tech Co., Ltd.

In 2006, Cornley launched its self-developed blood gas electrolyte analyzer BG-10, BG-20, and BG-30. Its representative blood gas analyzer models include BG-800E, Vitagas 8E, and Gaslite80E. Cornley is one of the earliest manufacturers of blood gas analyzers in China.

4. Perlong Medical Equipment Co., Ltd. (Nanjing).

Perlong is one of the earliest manufacturers of blood gas analyzers in China. Its representative blood gas product is PL2000 PLUS.

5. Guangzhou Wondfo Biotech Co., Ltd.

In early 2018, Wondfo successively launched its blood gas analyzer (BAG-101) and coagulation analyzer based on electrochemical platform technologies, supplementing its products applicable to the emergency and critical care medicine sector and enriching the company's product line.

Declaration Lili Chen, Wenguang Tan, Min Yang and Ziyan Luo are employees of Wuhan EasyDiagnosis Biomedicine Co., Ltd.

Jiandong Wang, Xiaolong Wang, Hui Xu and Dali Dai are employees of Horron XLH Medical Electronics.

References

1. Rechnitz G A, Kugler G C. Transient phenomena at glass electrodes[J]. Analytical Chemistry, 1967, 39(14):1682-1688.
2. Rechnitz G A. Special Report[J]. chem.eng.news, 1975, 53(4):29-35.
3. Updike S J, Hicks G P. The Enzyme Electrode[J]. Nature, 1967, 214-986.
4. Huehns ER, Beanen GH. Developmental changes in human hemoglobins. Clin Dev Med 1971; 37: 175-203.

Clinical Chemistry Laboratory Automation

11

Wei Qin, Jianmei Zhang, Ye Sheng, Jianer Yao, Yan Yang, Hongyun Zhao, and Zengli Yang

11.1 Overview

Total laboratory automation (TLA) refers to the integration of different testing platforms, pre-analysis, and post-analysis sample processing modules through automated transmission tracks and information networks in order to achieve integration within the laboratory, forming a fully automated assembly line operating environment, covering the entire inspection process, and forming large-scale automation of the whole inspection process, so it is often called an assembly line in China.

Clinical chemistry laboratory automation originated in Japan, and its original design was to liberate the test operators from the complicated and relatively low-tech daily work. At the beginning of the twenty-first century, the TLA was introduced in China and gradually became popular. At the same time, clinical laboratory testing with a high degree of automation, such as blood clotting and blood, has gradually developed corresponding TLAs. According to the classification of the samples tested, the TLA is divided into biochemical TLA, immune TLA, blood coagulation TLA, hematology TLA, and so on. The sample types and processing processes of biochemical and immunoassay items are the same, and most laboratories will synthesize them into a TLA. Of course, TLA is also on the market that integrates multiple clinical disciplines, connecting biochemical, immune, hemagglutinate, blood, and even molecular diagnostic instruments on the same line. It is more customary to separate the biochemical immunological TLA from other clinical disciplines to ensure the high quality of their sample testing and controllable TAT (sample turnaround time) while considering the number of specimens,

W. Qin · J. Zhang (✉) · Y. Sheng · J. Yao
Tellgen Corporation, Shanghai, China
e-mail: zhangjianmei@tellgen.com

Y. Yang · H. Zhao · Z. Yang
Autobio Diagnostics Co., Ltd, Zhengzhou, China

H. Song, L. Dai (eds.), *In Vitro Diagnostic Industry in China*,
https://doi.org/10.1007/978-981-99-3110-1_11

specimen type, processing flow, and the differentiation of subject groups. With the development of new technology and information intelligence, the ability of TLA to integrate different detection platforms will be more vital. In the future, more integrated TLA will emerge in the market.

Generally speaking, the standard procedure of biochemical immunological sample processing is as follows: after the samples arrive at the laboratory department, the samples are signed for and then classified into the corresponding group; after that, the samples are pre-processed, including centrifugation, capping, and classification to the corresponding detection instruments. If the same tube of blood is used for several items tested by different instruments, to ensure TAT, it is necessary to aliquot and then analyze the samples on corresponding instruments. After the completion of the test, the results should be reviewed and the samples should be archived. Generally, the samples should be stored for 7 days before being discarded. The scope of the biochemical immunological TLA covers all or part of the procedures after the sample is received.

Therefore, the composition of the general biochemical immunological TLA mainly includes a sample pre-processing system (composed of an input module, an automatic centrifugation module, an automatic de-caping module, an automatic aliquot module, and an output module), sample transportation system (to track and transfer module), sample detection system (with biochemical detection module and immunological detection module), and sample post-processing system (capable of recapping/add film module, online refrigerator, de-capping/de-film module, and output module). The laboratory can add or subtract part of the processing or testing module on the TLA according to the specific needs of the clinical testing project and the clinical testing process. At the same time, the TLA is an alternative to manual work of the above tasks and can also avoid errors caused by manual operation in some work links. In essence, the trend is replacing complicated repetitive manual work with automated and artificially intelligent TLA alongside the higher quality of analysis.

At the beginning of the twenty-first century, due to the gap between the Chinese medical level and manufacturing level and developed countries, all imported TLAs were introduced into and dominated the market at that time, among which the imported TLAs by brands such as Roche, Abbott, Beckman, Siemens, and Hitachi in the early Chinese medical market. With the rapid development of the Chinese medical level and industry chain, domestic manufacturers have launched production lines led by domestic manufacturers through independent research and development or cooperation with foreign manufacturers and officially entered the market that imported brands mainly covered. Many domestic brand TLAs have occupied a place in the domestic inspection market due to their stable performance, excellent inspection quality, and relatively reasonable prices. Nowadays, in some large tertiary hospitals, biochemical immunological TLAs of domestic brands are often seen. This phenomenon also proves that the domestic TLA can stand the test of the market and is gaining more recognition.

11.2 Common TLAs

Common TLAs have different characteristics due to their different design concepts. The following takes the brands such as Tellgen, Autobio, Mindray, and Dirui as examples to comprehensively analyze domestic brand assembly lines with different characteristics.

11.2.1 Tellgen: Particular Compatible TLA

At the end of 2018, Tellgen and Hitachi Diagnostics jointly launched Tellgen's particular compatible TLA, using Hitachi's high-speed and stable pre-processing, track and biochemical analysis systems, and access to Tellgen's unique immunological platform combining flow fluorescence and acridine ester chemiluminescence. At the same time, it is compatible with the mainstream immunological analyzers on the market, opening a new mode of domestic compatible TLA.

Tellgen's particular compatible TLA can customize to suit the laboratory's current and future development needs according to the customer's sample size and the number of tests. In the design concept of pre-processing system, biosafety is considered as much as possible, and sample processing and testing are all in a closed environment. There are two types of pre-processing systems, Sample Pre-Analytical Modular System (PAM) and Total Solution (TS). The TS line adopts a radio frequency identification system of single-sample management, the internal sample is more flexible, and the error sample is output separately. The five-hole rack is used for transportation, which reduces the part for changing racks in front of the instrument, facilitating the direct detection of the instrument and improving transportation efficiency.

Most TLAs on the market can only be connected to their brand of analyzers. However, customers want to retain the diversity of immunoassay brands because no one immunoassay brand can fully meet the hospital's needs. The compatible TLA can solve this problem very well. Combining multi-brand immunoassay instruments can achieve the effect of complete projects, quality selection, and reasonable cost performance. In the immunoassay instrument part by Tellgen, a combination of chemiluminescence analyzer and high-throughput multiplexed bead flow fluorescence immunoassay analyzer is used to realize the combination of joint assay and single assay, covering a broader menu of immunoassays. In conjunction with the joint assay kits, the advantages of the multiplexed bead flow fluorescence technology with the characteristics of Tellgen can be brought into full play. Only one consumable is used for one test; quantitative results of multiple indicators can be obtained, reducing the cost of consumables, storage, and transportation.

The machine intelligence of Tellgen's particular compatible TLA is at the forefront of domestic TLA. Tellgen's particular compatible TLA, based on intermediate software, independently developed various intelligent software functions, including automatic quality control, automatic audit, intelligent reagent recommendation, and intelligent data center. The automatic quality control function can automatically control the quality before sample detection, save the golden detection time, and optimize the TAT; the automatic audit function can standardize the audit plan based on multiple cross linkages such as patients' clinical information and historical results, saving labor on manual review; the intelligent reagent recommendation function can intelligently recommend the optimal amount of reagents according to the remaining amount of reagents and the estimation of the test amount, helping the stable operation of the laboratory; the intelligent data center function can perform real-time statistics of samples and test volumes, TAT timeout warning, reagent consumable monitoring, workload intelligent analysis, and AI gesture control.

11.2.2 Autobio: Single-Tube Magnetic Levitation Assembly Line

In 2017, Autobio launched the Autolas A-1 Series of magnetic levitation assembly line through independent research and development and international resource integration cooperation, becoming the first local enterprise in China to provide a fully automatic magnetic assembly laboratory line. The Autolas A-1 Series automatic assembly line of Autobio is an automatic assembly line that applied single-tube magnetic levitation base transportation technology under a contract between Autobio and Japanese assembly line manufacturer IDS; it can achieve functions such as automatic sample injection, centrifugation, capping, detection, storage, discarding, retest and classification, which replaces manual operations, reduces biological hazards, improves work efficiency, minimizes artificial error, and improves quality. The biochemical instrument connected to the Autolas A-1 Series assembly line is TBA-FX8, produced by Canon (formerly Toshiba). Moreover, the immune instrument AutoLumo A2000 Plus is self-developed and produced by Autobio, which is more flexible in connecting the instrument, and can flexibly choose the stand-alone on-orbit sampling mode or high-throughput connection mode according to the sample size, test number, and package distribution of the laboratory department. Since the biochemical immunization program is relatively comprehensive, and the carryover rate of biochemical samples can reach less than 0.1 ppm with the biochemical analyzer, the assembly line enables "shared biochemical immunodetection", which also means the realization of immunodetection after biochemical detection with one tube of blood and without dividing tubes or cups, effectively improving the detection efficiency of specimens on the track and reducing the workload and cost of blood collection and transportation. The overall solution of the Autolas A-1 Series assembly line covers automation solution, information solution, comprehensive service solution, and value-added service solution.

The automation solution has the characteristics of high-cost performance, a complete menu of inspection items, reliable quality, flexibility, and expansibility.

The information solution iLAS is a laboratory data management platform independently developed by Autobio, with B/S three-layer architecture as the main body and the whole laboratory automatic paperless as the construction goal, to provide customers with standardized products and standardized process solutions. iLAS has some basic functions, including TAT management, centralized control, reagent management, specimen statistics, equipment management, large-screen warning, and critical value reminder, as well as other functions such as automatic quality control, automatic check, assembly line load balancing, sample automatic retesting, and traceability. Moreover, iLAS can also be customized according to customer requirements.

Autobio technical service team provides professional, timely, and thoughtful technical services for users all over the country. Its remote intelligent service system Autolink can achieve intelligent warning, scanning to repair, remote assistance, regular maintenance reminder, and guaranteeing normal operation of the instrument.

Value-added service solution can provide assembly line users with AutoLean® lean management consulting services, including laboratory 6S management, laboratory layout design, workflow optimization, visual management, big data analysis, QCC and A3 project coaching, and laboratory satisfaction evaluation and analysis, as well as a complete set of laboratory lean management solutions from theory to practice. Apart from hereinabove mentioned, it also provides users with ISO15189 accreditation services with senior assessors as the core of the expert team, offering professional analysis of accreditation criteria and the whole process of on-site counseling, including laboratory ISO15189 system establishment, operation, and certification. It has served more than 50 customers in most provinces and has been highly recognized by customers.

Autobio laboratory automation assembly line Autolas A-1 Series registered and was put on record in China in 2018 and has been officially introduced to the market. It is highly welcomed and recognized by high-end users in the national biochemical immunization assembly line market. Up to now, Autobio has signed with more than 100 customers, covering 22 provinces in China.

11.2.3 Mindray: M6000, a Multidisciplinary Lab Automation System Incorporating Clinical Chemistry, Immunoassay, Coagulation, and Hematology

In 2019, Mindray launched M6000, an intelligent lab automation system with fully made-in-China detection modules. The system incorporates a range of technical capabilities across different disciplines. The three-track maglev track system is efficient, stable, quiet, eco-friendly, and can work intelligently for a much-enhanced user experience. Bringing together the One Tube of Blood lean management solution, Mindray Smart Lab digital solution, and many other beneficial solutions, M6000 has become a significant driver behind the automation, lean operation, digitalization, and intelligent development progress of clinical laboratories. Additionally, the track system for this lab automation system is also supplied by IDS. M6000 can achieve in-depth integration of four systems, namely, biochemistry, chemiluminescence, hematology, and coagulation. This is not about simply putting separate instruments together. Instead, it is about having analyzers for different areas of expertise deeply integrated together based on an underlying protocol, while offering shared visibility into the data on instrument statuses, device alarms, reagent consumption, measurement process, and others. With a three-track transfer mode, M6000 gives priority to emergency and retest samples and avoids repeated moving of samples in the track to greatly improve the sample transfer efficiency. The tracks are stacked together in a building block approach without requiring any reserved interface and can be scaled up as needed.

The biochemistry and immunoassay modules with which M6000 is connected are BS-2000 M/BS-2800 M and CL-6000i/CL-8000i. Mindray's BS-2000 M/BS-2800 M biochemistry analyzers are among the world's first to perform up to 2000 optical tests/hour, making them top performers among competing products in China. The CL-6000i/CL-8000i immunoassay analyzers can perform up to 480/500 tests/hour on a single module. The biochemistry and immunoassay analyzers are modularly scalable making adding more instruments easy. Samples can be intelligently scheduled by a scientific logic, in a way that prioritizes immunoassay reagents over biochemistry reagents to prevent the immunoassay reaction from being contaminated by the biochemistry reagents. M6000 can be integrated with Mindray's fully proprietary high-end hematology analysis line CAL8000 and brand-new coagulation module CX-9000 to support more test items and even the entire test package in the automation line of clinical laboratories. This gives M6000 a significant edge over other competing products. In general, M6000 provides a full-featured, intelligent solution that covers the entire workflow of the laboratory's automation line and allows for safe and flexible loading of samples, improved testing processes, and shortened TATs. Owing to the satisfactory detection speed and quality of the biochemistry and immunoassay analyzers as well as the stable and reliable pre-processing, track, and post-processing systems, many M6000 biochemistry and immunoassay automation lines have been installed and used in China.

Mindray has its unique advantages in laboratory intelligence. The M6000 middleware software can be remotely controlled and centrally managed. It integrates several personalized features that are ready for customization, such as sample path planning, automatic review, and dashboard visualization. The automated TLA interfaces with LIS software to conduct automated or parallel quality control, preventing delays in diagnostic test results. For automated QC, the system stores QC samples like calibrators, controls, and proficiency testing materials in connected refrigerators and analyzes them at pre-set intervals per regulations. For parallel QC with physician office labs lacking refrigerated connectivity, the system prioritizes running QC samples during peak test volumes, while simultaneously processing patient specimens loaded onto the modular conveyor line. This dual approach harnesses automation to analyze QC samples concurrently rather than sequentially, avoiding backlogs of patient samples awaiting quality control clearance. The streamlined workflow improves turnaround time for diagnostic test results. After the test results for the quality controls are reported, the peak-hour samples will be tested automatically to ensure the best performance and high efficiency. In addition, Mindray has built a "health cloud service platform" that provides remote diagnosis and intelligent warning services for laboratory instruments.

11.2.4 Dirui: Domestic TLA with Fully Independent Intellectual Property Rights

Dirui launched LA-60 in 2019, which is a domestic sample processing system with fully independent intellectual property rights. The detection module and the pre/

post-processing module are independently developed, designed, and produced by Dirui, realizing the real domestic production. LA-60 can be connected not only with biochemical and immunological analyzers but also with coagulation and blood analyzers, making it a perfect choice for laboratory convergence. Additionally, there is no external track connection in the middle of the pre-processing module; the floor area is smaller; and the overall operational efficiency of the pre-processing is high.

Dirui high-speed biochemical analyzer CS-2000 single-module detection speed can reach 2400 tests/h (including ISE); the assay menu covers 12 major categories of diseases with comprehensive assays; four detection modules can be connected simultaneously, with ultra-high detection speed and efficient process management. Dirui chemiluminescence immunoanalyzer CM-320 is based on the principle of avidin-acridine ester chemiluminescence principle with the throughput of 320 tests/hour. The front end of the analyzer can be equipped with a de-capping module to reduce aerosol hazards, and multiple modules can be connected. The biochemical and immunological platforms can be integrated into an all-in-one machine and connected to the LA-60, which is suitable for laboratories of different scales.

The LA-60 has complete processing modules, which can be flexibly configured for customers with different needs. The high speed of the LA-60 track ensures smooth sample transport. The software has an intelligent balance flow algorithm, which can reasonably allocate items, avoid sample congestion, ensure sample TAT and process integration, reduce labor input, and improve the overall efficiency of laboratory automation processes.

11.2.5 Other Domestic Brand Lines

See Table 11.1.

Table 11.1 Other domestic brand lines (not all included)

Company	Representative TLA
Maccura Bio Co., Ltd.	Hitachi-Maccura Compatible TLA
Shenzhen Snibe Biomedical Engineering Co., Ltd.	Snibe – Hitachi PAM-MAGLUMI X8-LST 008AS Snibe - Thermo Fisher SATLARS-TCA
Shenzhen YHLO Biotechnology Co., Ltd.	iTLA Hitachi - YHLO PAM
Sichuan Orienter Bioengineering Co., Ltd.	Lingyun TLA
Shanghai Runda Medical Technology Co., Ltd.	CLINILOG-RD
Beijing Wantai Bio-Pharmaceutical Co., Ltd.	Wan TLA
Ailex Technology Group Co., Ltd.	BRS
Biolihe Biomedical Engineering Co., Ltd.	BIOLIHE T6000
Bioscience (Tianjin) Biotechnology Co., Ltd.	CLIS beta CLIS alpha Axlas TCAutomation

11.3 Summary and Outlook

The domestic biochemical immune TLA has entered an era of rapid development in the twenty-first century. More and more domestic IVD companies have entered the TLA track, relying on the favorable domestic environment for rapid development, and there are no less than 17 domestic-brand TLAs. In addition to the biochemical immunological TLA brands mentioned above, many domestic TLAs are gradually entering the market. Fully automatic sample processing systems (pre/post-processing modules) are also being localized, such as Shanghai Trans-Age Medical Technology Co., Ltd., Changchun Sunostik Medical Technology Co., Ltd., and Shenzhen ReachGen Medical Technology Co., Ltd. Various domestic manufacturers have designed their own automation solution strategies and product layouts based on their characteristics and advantages. The laboratory automation solution is a system engineering and a system solution. It needs to cover the comprehensive needs of users in at least four aspects, namely, hardware, software, consumables, and services.

The trend in total laboratory automation (TLA) is toward greater integration and convergence of systems. There are common biochemical and immune TLAs in laboratories and separate blood coagulation and hematology TLAs. Only a few TLAs integrate related equipment platforms such as blood coagulation, hematology, urine, mass spectrometry, and molecular diagnostics. In the future, we will see more equipment from different clinical disciplines integrated into the same TLA. The intelligence of software functions will also become more and more powerful: data visualization, automatic audit log, automatic review, and automatic quality control will also become standard in the TLA, helping laboratories achieve artificial intelligent development.

On the other hand, domestically produced biochemical and immune TLA development marks the rapid development of the innovative Chinese manufacturing industry. Moreover, it also marks the improvement of the automation and intelligence of Chinese laboratory medicine. Of course, there is still much room for improvement in domestic TLAs. For example, the processing capacity of domestic TLAs is generally low, and the track speed and stability also need to be advanced; in the intelligent construction of TLAs, more must be done to try and improve. The future development trend of science and technology must be intelligence, automation, big data cloud computing, and the sharing and interconnection of all things. The future laboratory will 1 day achieve accurate artificial intelligent management.

Finally, the basic parameters of some types of TLAs mentioned above are sorted out in Table 11.2 for everyone to understand better and compare.

Table 11.2 Part of the basic parameters of the TLA

	Tellgen TS	Autobio Autolas A-1	Mindray M6000	Dirui LA-60
Input speed	800 tubes/h	750 tubes/h	750 tubes/h	700 tubes/h
Input capacity	400 tubes	400 tubes	400 tubes	500 tubes
Centrifuge speed	300 tubes/h	300 tubes/h	280 tubes/h	350 tubes/h
Centrifuge capacity	36 tubes	40 tubes	40 tubes	80 tubes
Decap speed	800 tubes/h	600 tubes/h	600 tubes/h	700 tubes/h
Aliquoter speed	800 tubes/h	550 tubes/h	550 tubes/h	400 tubes/h
Maximum number of dispensing cups	10	9	9	5
Output speed	800 tubes/h	750 tubes/h	750 tubes/h	700 tubes/h
Output capacity	400 tubes	400 tubes	400 tubes	500 tubes
Orbital speed	2400 tubes/h	7.7 m / min	7.7 m / min	2400 tubes/h
Biochemical analyzer brand	Hitachi	Canon (Toshiba)	Mindray	Dirui
Immunoassay analyzer brand	Tellgen + others	Autobio	Mindray	Dirui
Other discipline Analyzers	/	Can connect	Can connect	Can connect
Post-processing system speed	800 tubes/h	600 tubes/h	600 tubes/h	700 tubes/h
Post-processing system capacity	5000 tubes	3660 /5440 tubes	3660 /5440 tubes	6000 tubes

Declaration Wei Qin, Jianmei Zhang, Ye Sheng and Jianer Yao are employees of Tellgen Corporation.

Yan Yang, Hongyun Zhao and Zengli Yang are employees of Autobio Diagnostics Co., Ltd.

Part IV

Molecular Diagnosis

12 Molecular Diagnosis of Novel Coronavirus

Lizhong Dai, Zhongping Deng, Jia Liu, Xiaomei Ren, Kang Wu, Deyong Tan, Hongjian Zhang, Yong Deng, Yingjuan Ai, Bozhi Ji, Yaping Xie, Jack Shao, and Qiang Li

12.1 Etiology of the Novel Coronavirus and its Variation

12.1.1 Etiology and Epidemiological Characteristics of the Novel Coronavirus

12.1.1.1 The Novel Coronavirus and Severe Acute Respiratory Syndrome Coronavirus (SARS-CoV) Belong to the Same Virus Species

The novel coronavirus is a positive-strand RNA virus, which is the seventh coronavirus known to infect humans [1] and is the thirteenth β-CoV. It can be directly translated to generate RNA polymerase for RNA transcription and replication and the translation and synthesis of protein. There is no correction mechanism in the whole process; as a result, it is characterized by rapid variation, multiple hosts, and strong host adaptation [2].

The consistency of the whole genome sequences between the bat coronavirus (BatCoV RaTG13) and the novel coronavirus is 96.2% [3]. The bat coronavirus and the novel coronavirus are closely related. Studies have found that the SARS-like coronavirus of bat origin is most closely related to the novel coronavirus, with the nucleotide similarity reaching 89.1% [1].

L. Dai (✉) · Z. Deng · J. Liu · X. Ren · K. Wu · D. Tan · H. Zhang · Y. Deng · Y. Ai · B. Ji · Y. Xie
Sansure Biotech Inc., Changsha, Hunan, China
e-mail: lizhongd@sansure.com.cn

J. Shao · Q. Li

Key Laboratory of Medical Molecular Virology, Shanghai Medical College, Fudan University, Shanghai, China

Shanghai ZJ Bio-Tech Co., Ltd, Shanghai, China

H. Song, L. Dai (eds.), *In Vitro Diagnostic Industry in China*,
https://doi.org/10.1007/978-981-99-3110-1_12

Compared with the bat coronavirus, the genome similarity between the novel coronavirus and the SARS-CoV is low, and the difference between the genome similarity of the two is as high as 21% [4]; at the same time, in terms of the genome similarity between the bat coronavirus and the novel coronavirus and that between the MERS-CoV and the novel coronavirus, it exhibits a difference of 50% [4]; therefore, the novel coronavirus is genetically closely related to the bat coronavirus.

However, according to the virus classification method, the classification of coronaviruses mainly depends on the conserved replicase domain on the non-structural proteins. The amino acid sequences of the seven replicase domains of two kinds of coronaviruses, that is, nsp3 (ADRP, adenosine diphosphate ribose-1′-phosphatase), nsp5 (3CLpro, 3C main protease), nsp12 (RdRp, RNA-dependent RNA polymerase), nsp13 (Hel, helicase), nsp14 (ExoN, exonuclease), nsp15 (NendoU, uridylate-specific endoribonuclease), and nsp16 (O-MT, O-methyltransferase), are connected in series. If the consistency of sequence between the two coronaviruses is greater than 90%, it means that the two coronaviruses belong to the same species [5].

Therefore, although the whole genome sequences of the novel coronavirus and SARS-CoV differ by 21%, the ORF1b conserved region of the two is highly stable and similar, and the similarity between the two in the above-mentioned seven domains reaches 94%. Therefore, the novel coronavirus and SARS-CoV belong to the same virus species, that is, the SARS-related coronavirus species, but they are not the same virus.

12.1.1.2 Ways for the Novel Coronavirus to Infect Cells

Studies have found that the overall structure of the novel coronavirus is similar to SARS-CoV, with raised spike glycoprotein (spike glycoprotein, S-glycoprotein, S protein) on the surface, the S protein of the virus binds to the angiotensin converting enzyme 2(ACE2) of the receptor cell [6], the TMPRSS2 protein in the molecules of the host cells will cleave the S protein, and the exposed part allows the outer membrane of the virus to fuse with the host cell membrane; the viral RNA inside the cell is translated into non-structural proteins (NSPs); these NSPs can rapidly inhibit the translation of host messenger RNA (mRNA) while facilitating the translation of the mRNA of the virus. After virus infection, the cell's endoplasmic reticulum will be remodeled into a vesicular structure of double-membrane vesicles (DMVs), which allows more viral RNA to replicate and translate safely. Once the newly produced molecule is assembled into a complete viral particle, it leaves the cell through the organelles of the Golgi or lysosome. The host cell's furin makes a critical cleavage at five amino acid sites on the virus's spike protein, which prepares the virus to invade the next cell. It causes cell lesions and death, thereby causing tissue and organ lesions. However, the infectivity of the novel coronavirus and the degree of damage to tissues and organs after infection are not necessarily related to the level of ACE2 expression of the cells. Therefore, the way the novel coronavirus infects cells needs further exploration and research.

12.1.1.3 Infectivity of the Novel Coronavirus

Both the novel coronavirus and the SARS-CoV enter cells by contacting the ACE2 receptor on the cell surface via the S protein. Some studies have found that the structure of the receptor-binding domain (RBD) of the novel coronavirus is closer to the central part of the tripolymer, and one of the three RBDs will protrude upward. This special spatial conformation makes it easier for the S protein of the virus to bind to the host's ACE2, and the result of this easy binding is that the affinity of the novel coronavirus to ACE2 is about 10–20 times higher than that of SARS-CoV to ACE2, which serves as one of the strong evidences that the infectivity of the novel coronavirus is higher than that of the SARS-CoV [7].

12.1.2 Virus Variation

The simple biological structure of the virus—nucleic acid and protein—results in the characteristics of fast reproduction speed, poor gene stability, and high susceptibility to the external environment. The novel coronavirus is a positive-strand RNA virus. Compared to DNA viruses, RNA viruses lack error-correcting polymerases; as a result, they cannot be repaired in case of replication errors and, at the same time, lead to errors in downstream protein synthesis. Therefore, RNA virus has lower stability, faster variation, and higher mutation rate. The direction of virus variation is difficult to predict, and not every variant strain causes a threat to humans. However, only variant strains that are more infectious can survive environmental selection and spread widely among people, thereby further accelerating the production of more infectious variant strains. Up to now, variant strains that spread more rapidly have appeared in some countries one after another. Accordingly, the World Health Organization (WHO) has been monitoring and evaluating the variation of the novel coronavirus around the globe since January 2020, and based on the pathogenicity and transmission risk, the variants are divided into three categories: variants of concern (VOC), variants of interest (VOI), and variants that need further monitoring.

Among them, the variants of interest refer to those with a genetic mutation that has been confirmed or predicted to increase the infectivity of the virus and the severity of the disease and make diagnosis difficult (for example, the mutation happens to be in the position of the primers used in the Polymerase Chain Reaction (PCR) test, which will affect the PCR results), affecting the effectiveness of existing medical treatment methods (mainly refers to the occurrence of immune escape, resulting in the decreased therapeutic effect of monoclonal antibodies, or an impact on the effectiveness of vaccines); from an epidemiological point of view, such variant strains cause obvious community transmission or there may be multiple concentrated outbreak points, and the number of associated cases and their proportions in all infected cases are increasing in multiple countries.

Variants of concern refer to those with greater threat and impact than VOI. First, they must meet the standard characteristics of VOI, and secondly, there is solid evidence that the variant causes a huge impact on global public health in one or more of the following aspects: increased transmissibility and pathogenicity, and decreased effectiveness of public health response measures, treatments, or vaccines.

The spike protein in the novel coronavirus is an important structure for the immune system to recognize the virus and neutralize the virus with antibodies. It is because of the mutations in critical sites that the affinity of the variant strains to cell

Table 12.1 Mutation Sites and Transmissibility of the Novel Coronavirus Variant Strains

Name	Discovery time	Main mutation site	Effects on infectivity, pathogenicity, and immune escape
B.1.1.7	Cases were found in the UK as early as September 2020 and confirmed on December 18, 2020	69del, 70del, N501Y, D614G, P681H	• Transmission rate increased by about 50%. • According to reports on hospitalization rate and case fatality rate, the probability of severe illness increases after infection.
B.1.351	Cases were found in South Africa as early as May 2020 and confirmed on December 18, 2020	K417N, E484K, N501Y, D614G	Transmission rate increased by about 50%

receptors or to neutralizing antibodies changes significantly, which further led to the two variant strains in the United Kingdom and South Africa are more infectious and being included in the VOC category.

- B.1.1.7 variation appeared in England in September 2020 (Table 12.1).
- B.1.351 appeared in South Africa in May 2020 (Table 12.1).

12.1.3 Development of COVID-19 Diagnostic Products

At present, the detection of novel coronavirus mainly includes nucleic acid detection and immunoassay method (antigen or antibody). Nucleic acid detection is to detect the specific nucleic acid target sequences. The technical principle is that first conduct the reverse transcription of the novel coronavirus RNA into DNA and then amplify the specific nucleic acid sequence in the specimen for detection. Nucleic acid detection is currently the "gold standard" for novel coronavirus detection. It has been recommended by the National Health Commission and written into the coronavirus disease 2019 (COVID-19) prevention and control plan. It has the characteristics of early diagnosis, high sensitivity, and specificity. Based on the principle of specific reaction between antibody and antigen, immunoassay detects the viral proteins (antigens) in vivo or antibodies specific to viral proteins in vivo. Antibody detection is convenient to operate and the quality of the specimens is guaranteed. It greatly reduces the risk of infection for medical staff in the process of specimen collection and detection and the detection is rapid. It can be used as a supplementary method for nucleic acid diagnosis. When the nucleic acid test is negative, IgM and IgG antibody detection can make up for the shortcomings of nucleic acid detection that are prone to missed detections. Compared with nucleic acid diagnosis, immunoassay kits can be used to quickly screen asymptomatic virus carriers and can be used for distributed screening in high-traffic public places such as airports, stations, and wharves, providing technical support for comprehensive prevention and control and thorough investigation of the pandemic. It is more suitable for the screening of people with fever in primary medical institutions and community and township hospitals.

The technical guidelines of China for laboratory detection of pneumonia caused by the novel coronavirus infection pointed out that nucleic acid detection methods are mainly targeted at *ORF1ab* and *N* genes in the novel coronavirus genome. In terms of genetic sequence similarity, the genome-wide similarity between the novel coronavirus and the SARS is about 79% [7]. The homology of *1ab*, *1a*, *1b*, *S*, *E*, *M*, and *N* protein gene sequences are, respectively, 79.5%, 75.4%, 86.3%,72.7%, 93.5%, 85.1%, and 88.1%.

For the real-time fluorescent quantitative PCR kits approved in China, the primers are mainly designed for the conserved regions of the open reading frames *ORF1ab*, *N* gene, and *E* gene of the novel coronavirus genome. Because an important feature of the novel coronavirus is its unique transcription strategy, the subgenomic RNA is further synthesized from genome RNA using the negative-strand RNA as the template. *The ORF1ab* gene is transcribed from the full-length viral genome, so it exists only in the complete viral genome, while the *N* gene exists in both the full-length genome and other subgenomic RNA. Then, during the transcription process of the novel coronavirus, the transcription and synthesis amount of the *N* gene is more than that of *ORF1ab*. At present, most of the molecular diagnostic products are designed for dual-target detection (*ORF1ab* and *N*), and a small part are single-target detection (*ORF1ab*) and triple-target detection (*ORF1ab*, *N* and *E*).

For all the novel coronavirus molecular diagnostic kits approved in China, the sensitivity is <1000 copies/mL. On December 28, 2020, the "Workbook for the Novel Coronavirus Nucleic Acid Detection in Medical Institutions (Trial Version 2)" issued by the National Health Commission put forward the requirements of selecting highly sensitive nucleic acid detection reagents (detection limit ≤500 copies/mL) in the "Performance Verification" and "Other Requirements" sections. In fact, a number of previous technical specifications and work notices have clearly put forward similar suggestions (selecting detection reagents with high sensitivity), but it is clearly stated for the first time in this document that the threshold value for the highly sensitive detection reagent should be 500 copies/mL. For the novel coronavirus RT-PCR detection reagents currently approved by the National Medical Products Administration (NMPA), the detection sensitivity claimed in most of the reagent instructions meets this requirement.

12.2 The Certification at Home and Abroad of the Novel Coronavirus Nucleic Acid Detection Reagents and Instruments

12.2.1 Certification of the Novel Coronavirus Nucleic Acid Detection Reagents

As of the end of December 2020, the National Medical Products Administration (NMPA) approved a total of 54 novel coronavirus detection reagent products, and a total of 25 nucleic acid detection reagents were approved (Table 12.2), of which the fluorescent PCR is the main method with a total of 17 products certified, including

Table 12.2 Performance and domestic registration of domestic novel coronavirus molecular diagnostic products

No.	Product name	Enterprises	Detection method	Covered gene locus	Sensitivity	Certification status
1	Novel Coronavirus 2019-nCoV Nucleic Acid Detection Kit (fluorescent PCR method)	Shanghai ZJ Bio - Tech Co., Ltd.	Fluorescent PCR Method	*ORF1ab*, *N* and *E* genes	200 copies/mL	NMPA CE EUL
2	Novel Coronavirus 2019 - nCoV Nucleic Acid Detection Kit (Fluorescent PCR Method)	Shanghai GeneoDx Biotechnology Co., Ltd	Fluorescent PCR Method	*ORF1ab* and *N* genes	500 copies/mL	NMPA CE EUL
3	Novel Coronavirus 2019 -nCoV Nucleic Acid Detection Kit (Combinatorial Probe-Anchor Polymerization Sequencing)	BGI Biotechnology (Wuhan) Co., Ltd. (Holding Company: BGI PathoGenesis Pharmaceutical Technology Co., Ltd.)	Sequencing Method	/	/	NMPA CE
4	Novel Coronavirus 2019 - nCoV Nucleic Acid Detection Kit (Fluorescent PCR Method)	BGI Biotechnology (Wuhan) Co., Ltd. (Holding Company: BGI PathoGenesis Pharmaceutical Technology Co., Ltd.) (EUL holding company: BGI Europe A/S)	Fluorescent PCR Method	ORF1ab gene	100 copies/mL	NMPA CE FDA EUA EUL
5	Novel Coronavirus 2019 - nCoV Nucleic Acid Detection Kit (Fluorescent PCR Method)	Da An Gene Co., Ltd. of Sun Yat-sen University	Fluorescent PCR Method	*ORF1ab* and *N* genes	500 copies/mL	NMPA CE EUL
6	Novel Coronavirus 2019 - nCoV Nucleic Acid Detection Kit (Fluorescent PCR Method)	Sansure Biotech Inc.	Fluorescent PCR Method	*ORF1ab* and *N* genes	200 copies/mL	NMPA CE FDA EUA
7	Novel Coronavirus 2019 - nCoV Nucleic Acid Detection Kit (Fluorescent PCR Method)	Shanghai BioGerm Medical Technology Co., Ltd	Fluorescent PCR Method	*ORF1ab* and *N* genes	500 copies/mL	NMPA CE

8	Six Respiratory Viruses Nucleic Acid Detection Kit (Isothermal Amplification Chip Method)	Chengdu CapitalBio Biochemical Technology Co., Ltd.	Isothermal Amplification	*S* and *N* genes	150 copies/mL	NMPA
9	Novel Coronavirus 2019 - nCoV Nucleic Acid Detection Kit (Fluorescent PCR Method)	Beijing Applied Biological Technologies Co., Ltd.	Fluorescent PCR Method	*ORF1ab*, *N* and *E* genes	200 copies/mL	NMPA CE EUL
10	Novel Coronavirus 2019 - nCoV Nucleic Acid Detection Kit (Fluorescent PCR Method)	Maccura Biotechnology Co., Ltd. (Holding Company: Maccura Biotechnology (USA) LLC)	Fluorescent PCR Method	*ORF1ab*, *E* and *N* genes	450 copies/mL	NMPA CE FDA EUA
11	Novel Coronavirus 2019 - nCoV Nucleic Acid Detection Kit (Fluorescent PCR Method)	Wuhan EasyDiagnosis Biomedicine Co., Ltd.	Fluorescent PCR Method	*ORF1ab* and *N* genes	500 copies/mL	NMPA CE
12	Novel Coronavirus 2019 - nCoV Nucleic Acid Detection Kit (Real-time Isothermal Amplifcation)	Ustar Biotechnologies (Hangzhou) Ltd.	Isothermal Amplication-Real-time Fluorescence Method	*ORF1ab* and *N* genes	200 copies/mL	NMPA CE
13	Novel Coronavirus 2019 - nCoV Nucleic Acid Detection Kit (Hybrid Capture Immunofluorescence Method)	Anbio (Xiamen) Biotechnology Co., Ltd.	Hybrid Capture Immunofluorescence Method	*ORF1ab*, *N* and *E* genes	100 copies/mL	NMPA CE
14	Novel Coronavirus 2019 - nCoV Nucleic Acid Detection Kit (Fluorescent PCR Method)	The name of Shanghai Fosun Long March Medical Science Co., Ltd. was changed to: Fosun Diagnostics (Shanghai) Co., Ltd. (Holding Company: Fosun Pharma USA Inc.)	Fluorescent PCR Method	*ORF1ab*, *N* and *E* genes	300 copies/mL	NMPA CE FDA EUA EUL
15	Novel Coronavirus 2019 - nCoV Nucleic Acid Detection Kit (RNA Capture Probe Method)	Shanghai Rendu Biotechnology Co., Ltd.	RNA Capture Probe Method	*ORF1ab* gene	250 copies/mL	NMPA CE
16	Novel Coronavirus 2019 - nCoV Nucleic Acid Detection Kit (RNA Isothermal Amplification - Gold Probe Chromatography)	Wuhan Zhongzhi Biotechnologies Inc.	RNA Isothermal Amplification - Gold Probe Chromatography	*ORF1ab* and *E* genes	100 copies/mL	NMPA

(continued)

Table 12.2 (continued)

No.	Product name	Enterprises	Detection method	Covered gene locus	Sensitivity	Certification status
17	Novel Coronavirus 2019 - nCoV Nucleic Acid Detection Kit (Dual Amplification Method)	Wuhan Zhongzhi Biotechnologies Inc.	Dual Amplification Method	*ORF1ab* and *E* genes	100 copies/mL	NMPA
18	Novel Coronavirus 2019 - nCoV Nucleic Acid Detection Kit (Fluorescent PCR Method)	Beijing Kinghawk Pharmaceutical Co., Ltd.	Fluorescent PCR Method	*ORF1ab* and *N* genes	500 copies/mL	NMPA CE
19	Novel Coronavirus 2019 - nCoV Nucleic Acid Detection Kit (Fluorescent PCR Method)	Jiangsu Bioperfectus Technologies Co., Ltd.	Fluorescent PCR Method	*ORF1ab* and *N* genes	350 copies/mL	NMPA CE FDA EUA EUL
20	Novel Coronavirus 2019 - nCoV Nucleic Acid Detection Kit (Fluorescent PCR Method)	Zhejiang Orient Gene Biotech Co., Ltd.	Fluorescent PCR Method	*ORF1ab* and *N* genes	300 copies/mL	NMPA CE
21	Novel Coronavirus 2019 - nCoV Nucleic Acid Detection Kit (Fluorescent PCR Method)	Shenzhen Uni-medica Technology Co., Ltd.	Fluorescent PCR Method	*ORF1ab* gene	200 copies/mL	NMPA CE
22	Novel Coronavirus 2019 - nCoV Nucleic Acid Detection Kit (Fluorescent PCR Method)	Beijing Nagene Diagnosis Reagent Co., Ltd.	Fluorescent PCR Method	*ORF1ab* and *N* genes	200 copies/mL	NMPA CE
23	Novel Coronavirus 2019 - nCoV Nucleic Acid Detection Kit (Fluorescent PCR Method)	Coyote Bioscience Co., Ltd.	Fluorescent PCR Method	*ORF1ab* and *N* genes	400 copies/mL	NMPA CE
24	Novel Coronavirus 2019 - nCoV Nucleic Acid Detection Kit (Fluorescent PCR Method)	Da An Gene Co., Ltd. of Sun Yat-sen University	Fluorescent PCR Method	*ORF1ab* and *N* genes	500 copies/mL	NMPA CE
25	Novel Coronavirus 2019 - nCoV Nucleic Acid Detection Kit (CRISPR Immunochromatography)	Hang zhou Zhongce Biotechnology Co., Ltd.	CRISPR Immunochromatography	*N* gene	1000 copies/mL	NMPA CE

combinatorial probe-anchored polymerization sequencing method, isothermal amplification chip method, hybrid capture immunofluorescence method, and RNA capture probe method; 26 antibody detection reagents were approved, among which colloidal gold method and magnetic particle chemiluminescence method are the main ones; 3 antigen detection reagents were approved.

As of December 2020, the World Health Organization (WHO) has received a total of 55 EUL expressions of interest (EOI) for the novel coronavirus nucleic acid detection products: 23 products from 23 enterprises have been approved, of which there are 13 Chinese enterprises; 19 products are still under examination and approval, and there are 8 Chinese manufacturers.

From March 15, 2020 to December 30, 2020, a total of 125 entities in the world have applied for the FDA EUA nucleic acid diagnostic test of the United States, involving 133 kinds of products, and there are a total of 7 domestic companies, accounting for 5.6%.

According to the statistics, as of December 2020, a total of 292 novel coronavirus detection reagents have obtained EU CE standard certification or registration across China. The fluorescent PCR method is adopted as the main detection method, also including internationally recognized and mature molecular detection technologies such as isothermal amplification, digital PCR, and sequencing and CRISPR.

12.2.2 Instruments

12.2.2.1 Approval of Novel Coronavirus-Related Instruments in Domestic Enterprises (Table 12.3)

From January to December 2020, there were seven types of IVD instruments and one IVD software product that obtained emergency approval from NMPA. Among the eight products, a sequencing device and sequencing software are included, and the remaining six are nucleic acid analyzers.

As of December 30, 2020, a total of 34 domestic enterprises in China have obtained registration certificates for instruments such as PCR analyzers, with a total of 56 certificates obtained. The product names mainly included real-time fluorescence quantitative PCR analyzer, PCR amplifier, fully automated medical PCR analysis system, and nucleic acid amplification analyzer. Based on the fact that PCR analyzers are classified as Others under the EU IVDD directive, most instruments have CE certification.

Table 12.3 Details of Instruments and Software Products that Have Obtained Emergency Approval

Product name	Manufacturer	Approval date
Gene Sequencing System	Wuhan MGI Tech Co., Ltd.	2020.01.26
Novel Coronavirus 2019 - nCoV Nucleic Acid Analysis Software	BGI Biotechnology (Wuhan) Co., Ltd.	2020.01.26
Isothermal Amplification Nucleic Acid Analyzer	Chengdu CapitalBio Biochemical Technology Co., Ltd.	2020.02.22
Isothermal Amplification Microfluidic Chip Nucleic Acid Analyzer	Chengdu CapitalBio Biochemical Technology Co., Ltd.	2020.02.22
Nucleic Acid Amplification and Detection Analyzer	Ustar Biotechnologies (Hangzhou) Co., Ltd.	2020.03.16
Nucleic Acid Detection Analyzer	Sansure Biotech Co., Ltd.	2020.04.23
Real-time Fluorescence Quantitative PCR Instrument	Coyote Bioscience(Beijing) Co., Ltd.	2020.07.13
Real-time Fluorescence Quantitative PCR Instrument	Hangzhou AnYu Technologies Co., Ltd	2020.09.21

12.3 Novel Coronavirus Nucleic Acid Detection Technology Platform

Novel coronavirus detection methods include nucleic acid testing, serological testing, and antigen testing, all of which play different roles in hospitals, point-of-care, and large-scale population testing. In terms of nucleic acid detection, viral RNA is reverse transcribed into DNA and then amplified via the polymerase chain reaction (PCR) or other amplification methods for amplification. Nucleic acid detection is the most widely used to detect the novel coronavirus, and it more and more tends to be automated, and the running time is reduced to less than 2 hours. This testing method is also promoted and recognized by the World Health Organization (WHO). As of the end of 2020, NMPA has approved a total of 25 novel coronavirus nucleic acid detection reagents. The proportion of detection products by methodologies is shown in Fig. 12.1.

12.3.1 Fluorescent PCR Method

PCR method refers to the polymerase chain reaction, which can greatly increase the amount of DNA. To detect the novel coronavirus, as the novel coronavirus is an RNA virus, the viral RNA needs to be reverse transcribed into DNA first for PCR detection. At present, the nucleic acid detection reagents used are mainly based on fluorescent PCR detection technology using TaqMan probes. With the progress of the PCR process, the reaction products continue to accumulate, and the fluorescence signal intensity also increases proportionally. Finally, the change in the product amount is monitored by the change of the fluorescence intensity,

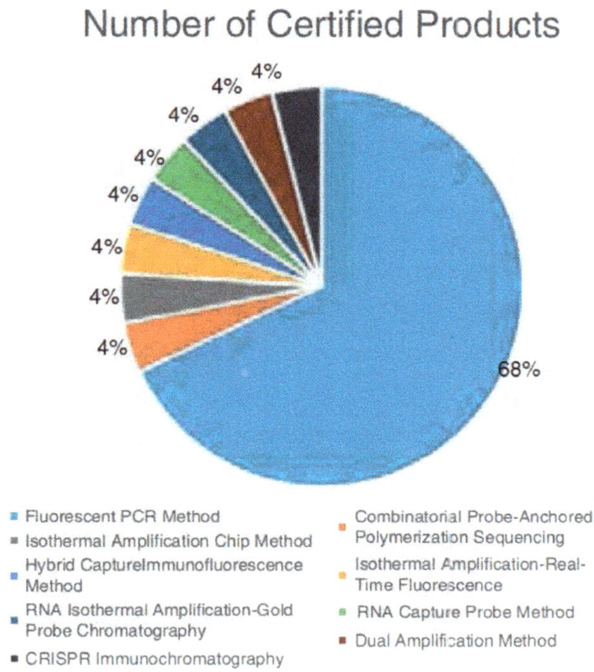

Fig. 12.1 Methods adopted by domestic novel coronavirus nucleic acid detection products

thereby obtaining a fluorescence amplification curve. During the outbreak period of the novel coronavirus, fluorescent PCR has been developed rapidly and applied in the field of rapid amplification and detection technology, the traditional amplification time of 100–120 minutes is also reduced to 30–60 minutes, and some ultra-fast PCR can be completed in minutes with 40 cycles of amplification and detection.

12.3.2 Combinatorial Probe-Anchored Polymerization Sequencing Method

The combinatorial probe-anchored polymerization sequencing technology can test the base sequence carried by the DNA nanoball (DNB) loaded on the slide. The experimental process is mainly divided into three parts, namely, DNB preparation, DNB loading, and sequencing. Specifically, the DNA library is first cyclized, then DNB is prepared by rolling circle replication, and finally the DNB is loaded onto a sequencing slide. During the sequencing process, the specially modified bases at the ends are labeled with different fluorescent probes, the DNA molecular anchors and the fluorescent probes are polymerized on the nanoballs, and then the high-resolution imaging system collects the optical signals. The sequence to be tested can be obtained after the optical signals undergo digital processing.

12.3.3 Isothermal Amplification Chip Method

The chip system adopts isothermal amplification technology and microfluidic chip technology. The microfluidic disc chip has the characteristics of multi-index parallel detection and less sample and reagent consumption. This chip adopts isothermal amplification technology, as the isothermal amplification reaction does not require a high-temperature denaturation process at above 90 °C, but only between 60 °C and 70 °C, and the structure of the microfluidic chip is designed to have a liquid sealing effect. The volatilization of the reaction mix is not serious; therefore, it has the characteristics of uniform reaction in each detection hole and controllable results.

12.3.4 Hybrid Capture Immunofluorescence Method

This system is a novel rapid molecular diagnostic technology based on the combination of nucleic acid hybrid and immunofluorescence capture, namely, hybrid capture immunofluorescence. The average sample detection time is 45 minutes. Its technical characteristics are that it can quickly detect pathogenic nucleic acid in one step, with no need for nucleic acid extraction or purification and with no need for PCR amplification; the pathogen is directly lysed by the treatment solution and the target nucleic acid is released. The target nucleic acid and the probe form DNA/RNA hybrids; fluorescent particles identify the DNA/RNA hybrids by fluorescent signals and realize the qualitative judgment of the target nucleic acid in the sample.

12.3.5 RNA Capture Probe Method

This method combines RNA-specific target capture technology and isothermal amplification real-time detection technology, completes nucleic acid extraction and amplification in one reaction tube, and can realize continuous and parallel detection. Its detection sensitivity and specificity can reach that of the PCR method.

12.3.6 Isothermal Amplification—Real-Time Fluorescence Method

This method combines the new generation nucleic acid isothermal amplification technology and real-time fluorescence detection technology and has the advantages of high sensitivity, high specificity, low contamination, and stable reaction. Under isothermal conditions, the viral RNA is first reverse transcribed into DNA, the T7 promoter is introduced through primers, and then multiple RNAs are transcribed from the DNA by the T7 RNA polymerase. Each RNA starts from reverse transcription and enters the next amplification cycle. The fluorescently labeled probe specifically binds to RNA, and the generated fluorescence is captured by the fluorescence detection instrument, which reflects the amplification cycle in real time.

12.3.7 RNA Isothermal Amplification—Gold Probe Chromatography

This technology adopts the method of lysing the exfoliated cells in the specimen, and the pathogenic RNA released from the lysis undergoes reverse transcription and transcription process under the action of reverse transcriptase and T7 RNA polymerase to achieve T7 nucleic acid amplification of viral RNA. Relying on the action of the nfo enzyme, specific molecular probes designed according to the template are added, and the final result can be obtained using the colloidal gold technology (sandwich method).

12.3.8 Dual Amplification Method

The dual amplification method has the following three characteristics: (i) No PCR amplification of the target molecule is required, and the signal of the target molecule to be detected is amplified by the polybiotin molecule polymer, which improves the detection sensitivity to several target molecules. (ii) It is not necessary to perform exponential amplification of the template on nucleic acid molecules to reduce the false positive rate. (iii) It is not necessary to extract the nucleic acid, and analysis can be performed directly after the cell lysis. Therefore, the method is simple and convenient.

12.3.9 CRISPR Immunochromatography

By this method, first extract the target nucleic acid (such as viral DNA or RNA) from human samples. The Cas is guided via a guide RNA (gRNA, guide RNA) to be paired to the target nucleic acid sequence position, and then it is amplified by RPA (recombinase polymerase amplification) amplification (an isothermal amplification technology; the optimal reaction temperature is 37 °C) to increase the concentration of the target gene. It is cleaved by gene editing technology to release the fluorescent signal, and then the fluorescent signal is detected.

12.4 Introduction to Key Extraction Technologies and Products of COVID-19 Detection Systems

Nucleic acid extraction and purification, as the first step in the basic steps of nucleic acid detection, plays an extremely important role in clinical molecular diagnosis. Whether or not high-quality nucleic acid can be obtained is the key to the subsequent correct diagnostic result. The quality of nucleic acid extraction directly affects the follow-up PCR process, sequencing, and other analyses. With the continuous development of medical research, clinical molecular diagnosis has derived different application scenarios and detection requirements, so the requirements for nucleic acid extraction are also different, which further promotes the development of nucleic acid extraction and purification technology.

The traditional nucleic acid extraction methods include phenol extraction, alkaline lysis, CTAB extraction, and boiling. Since Vogelstein and Gillespie first used glass fibers (the main component is SiO2) to recover DNA fragments from agarose gels in 1979, new nucleic acid extraction methods based on solid-phase carriers have been developed, including spin column extraction, glass bead adsorption, and micro-nano magnetic bead extraction. In addition, with the development of technology, in order to meet the needs of clinical molecular diagnosis, some unconventional nucleic acid extraction technologies have emerged, such as nucleic acid release agents, which are based on a simple and fast nucleic acid extraction technology.

Although nucleic acid extraction technology is constantly iterating and developing, its purpose of serving clinical molecular diagnosis remains unchanged, and different technologies have their own advantages in clinical application. The detection of the novel coronavirus nucleic acid by the real-time fluorescent reverse transcription polymerase chain reaction is an important method for the screening and diagnosis of COVID-19. The sample types are mainly nasopharyngeal swabs and oropharyngeal swabs. In the face of sudden pandemics, high-throughput and automated equipment and methods are needed to monitor and control the pandemic more effectively and accurately. Therefore, the sample processing technologies such as the magnetic bead extraction method and nucleic acid release agents have played an important role during the COVID-19 pandemic.

12.4.1 Magnetic Bead Extraction Method

According to the principle similar to the adsorption membrane, the specific functional groups that can adsorb nucleic acid are modified on the surface of the magnetic beads, then different solution environments are provided to achieve the purposes of lysis, binding, washing, and elution. At the same time, by using the magnetic property of the magnetic beads, directional movement and enrichment can be easily achieved under the action of an external magnetic field, so as to achieve the purpose of separating nucleic acids from impurities, thereby realizing the separation and purification of target substances and obtaining purified nucleic acids. Magnetic bead nucleic acid extraction technology has become the mainstream method for the extraction of novel coronavirus samples because of its high degree of automation, large sample throughput, high product concentration and purity, and especially high safety. Representative products include nucleic acid extraction or purification reagents from Sansure Biotech Co., Ltd., nucleic acid extraction reagents (magnetic bead method) from Shanghai ZJ Bio-Tech Co., Ltd., nucleic acid extraction kits

(Virus) from Zybio Inc., nucleic acid extraction or purification reagents from Xi'an Tianlong Technology Co., Ltd., and nucleic acid extraction kits (magnetic bead method) from Jiangsu Bioperfectus Technologies Co., Ltd.

12.4.2 Nucleic Acid Release Agents

Use protein denaturants and biochemical reagents to quickly destroy the structure of the viral coat protein and release the nucleic acid into the liquid for detection using the nucleic acid detection reagents. It only needs to add an efficient nucleic acid release agent (RNA nucleic acid release agent) to quickly destroy the structure of the pathogen coat protein to release the nucleic acid of the sample and then use the PCR amplification reagent with high amplification efficiency and high anti-interference ability to achieve rapid molecular detection. It is characterized by the rapid lysis of pathogens at room temperature or a low heating temperature to release the nucleic acid, with no need for boiling, centrifugation or tube changing, reducing biological safety hazards, and realizing rapid release of nucleic acid through simple operations. The entire sample processing process takes a very short time, greatly saves the operation time compared with column extraction and magnetic bead extraction technologies, and therefore it is easier to popularize. Amplification detection after direct treatment is suitable for detection reagents with lower requirements for nucleic acid purity. Representative products include a nucleic acid release agent from Sansure Biotech Co., Ltd. and a sample release agent from Da An Gene Co., Ltd. of Sun Yat-sen University.

12.4.3 Automated Nucleic Acid Extraction Instruments

Due to the characteristics of magnetic nanoparticles, when they are used as carriers for nucleic acid extraction and purification, automated operations can be achieved very well, manpower can be saved to the greatest extent, and errors caused by manual operations can also be reduced. At the same time, during the outbreak of the novel coronavirus pandemic and the follow-up screening work, it can also reduce the frequency of the frontline inspection personnel being exposed to positive samples and thus reduce the risk of being infected. The current mainstream automated extraction instruments, according to their operating modes, can be mainly divided into three types: pipetting type, magnetic rod type, and a combination of the two. After the outbreak of the novel coronavirus pandemic, due to the great increase in the number of tests and the need for centralized screening in the later sporadic outbreaks, new requirements have been raised on the throughput and speed of nucleic acid extraction. In order to improve the screening efficiency and shorten the detection cycle, various domestic manufacturers have launched a series of nucleic acid extraction equipment, such as ZJ Bio-Tech, Xi'an Tianlong, Sansure Biotech, Chongqing Zybio, Da An Gene, and Shanghai BioGerm. It not only increases the number of samples processed in a single time but also shortens the nucleic acid extraction time to 10–25 minutes, which greatly shortens the detection cycle. There is also a fully automated nucleic acid extraction, purification, and real-time fluorescent PCR analysis system that integrates sample aliquoting, nucleic acid extraction, purification, amplification, and detection in the pipeline, which can realize "sample in and results out". In the process of novel coronavirus screening, automated nucleic acid extraction equipment has played a huge role in different detection scenarios such as central laboratories, air dome laboratories, mobile cabin hospitals, and mobile detection vehicles.

12.5 Progress and Application of Molecular Instrument Detection Technology during the COVID-19 Pandemic

The global pandemic of the novel coronavirus has pushed society's attention to life sciences and medicine to an unprecedented level. During this period, the genome sequence determination and traceability of the novel coronavirus based on gene sequencing technology and the research and development of virus nucleic acid detection products based on gene detection technology have helped to quickly form a response system for this public health emergency, which played a key role in the prevention and control of the global novel coronavirus pandemic.

In the gene technology industry, from the technical perspective, sequencing technologies related to the detection and identification of nucleic acid sequence (NGS, single-molecule sequencing, etc.), amplification technologies (PCR, qPCR, dPCR, and isothermal amplification) and multiplex detection technologies (microarrays, biochips, biosensors, etc.), and related products occupy the mainstream of the market. In recent years, microfluidic technology, which is closely related to functional integration, has also been applied more and more, and the development of new technologies such as nucleic acid mass spectrometry has also attracted attention.

From the development trend of equipment platformization, the value of automation, especially integrated solutions, is becoming more and more obvious in reducing the difficulty of the operation and human intervention, and especially the increased requirements on pollution, biosafety, and protection caused by the novel coronavirus have accelerated this trend. At the same time, great importance has been attached to improving processing speed and adapting to multiple testing modes (such as rapid establishment of large-scale centralized processing capacity, decentralized testing and even home/self-testing) to shorten sample turnaround time and increase testing accessibility to finally curb the spread of the pandemic. On the other hand, the need for multi-target detection to improve the data throughput in a single detection is also considered a development direction in a specific field.

Nucleic acid detection is a common method for clinical etiological diagnosis with the advantages of high sensitivity and strong specificity. A variety of nucleic acid detection technologies have been applied to the clinical diagnosis of novel coronavirus infection. The following is an overview of the application of several common nucleic acid detection technologies in novel coronavirus detection.

12.5.1 Real-Time Fluorescent PCR Technology and Instruments

By real-time fuorescent PCR technology, fuorescent probes or fuorescent dyes are added to the PCR reaction system to detect the fuorescent signals of each cycling product from PCR amplifcation reaction in real-time, to achieve the quantitative and qualitative analysis of the initial template. The technology is characterized by strong specificity, high sensitivity, short detection period, quantitative detection, and closed detection process and solves the PCR contamination problems well and has been widely used in scientific research and clinical disease diagnosis.

At present, real-time fluorescent PCR instruments have been domestically made to a large extent, and domestic manufacturers mainly include Shanghai Hongshi Medical Technology Co., Ltd., ZJ Bio-Tech, and Ares. During the COVID-19 pandemic, Da An Gene's AGS series of miniaturized real-time fluorescent PCR instruments have received great attention for the improvement in the speed of heating and cooling.

12.5.2 Next-Generation Sequencing Technology and Sequencer

Next-generation sequencing (NGS) has the main advantages of high throughput, large amount of information, and high accuracy. It can detect and identify unknown pathogens in specimens, confirm the genome information of pathogens, and provide powerful means for pathogen identification of emerging infectious diseases, the diagnosis and differential diagnosis of complex and critical infections, and the study of genetic variation.

Driven by pandemic demand, the long-read Oxford nanopores (ONT) platform has made great progress in clinical application and promotion. The Wuhan University joint team developed a nanopore targeted sequencing method based on the ONT platform, which can detect the novel coronavirus and more than 40 kinds of respiratory viruses of ten categories at the same time within 4 h with high sensitivity and accuracy after sequencing. The pandemic has accelerated the birth of complete solutions for nucleic acid detection. The DNBSEQ-T7 made by the MGI has become the world's first ultra-high-throughput gene sequencing platform that has obtained both CE-IVD certification of the EU and China medical device registration certificate. In the direction of small throughput, MGI's MGISEQ-200 has completed the upgrade in 2020. On the basis of retaining the original compactness, flexibility, and efficiency, it has upgraded the slides and read lengths, with higher sequencing quality and wider applications.

Considering the need for miniaturization and convenience of operation, Qitan Tech launched China's first independently researched and developed nanopore gene sequencer QNome-9604 in September 2020. It has the advantages of ultra-long read length, fast sequencing speed, direct detection of nucleic acid, low sequencing cost, and compactness and portability of the instrument.

12.5.3 Isothermal Amplification Technology and Isothermal Amplification Instruments

By isothermal nucleic acid amplification technology, amplification can be performed under isothermal conditions, and it has the characteristics of fast speed, high specificity, and high sensitivity. Its requirement for hardware equipment is low, so it fits the detection work conducted in primary hospitals. Among the existing isothermal amplification technologies, loop-mediated isothermal amplification (LAMP) is widely used in clinical molecular diagnosis and other fields.

The typical representative of the industrialization of isothermal amplification technology in domestic applications is CapitalBio. Its isothermal amplification microfluidic chip nucleic acid analyzer, based on loop-mediated isothermal amplification technology, is used in conjunction with its detection reagents for the qualitative detection of nucleic acids in human sputum samples in clinical use.

12.5.4 Nucleic Acid POCT Technology and POCT Instrument

Point of care testing (POCT) is a testing method that uses portable analytical instruments and supporting reagents to quickly obtain test results at the sampling site. This technology integrates the functional modules of nucleic acid extraction, amplification, and detection and pre-seals the reagents required for the reaction in the detection cartridge. Operators only need to add the samples such as swabs or blood, then the nucleic acid amplification, signal collection, and result analysis can be automatically completed in a short time.

Nearly 30 types of POCT products at home and abroad have been put into the efforts against the novel coronavirus pandemic. In China, a representative is the Sansure iPonatic mobile molecular diagnostic system. iPonatic nucleic acid detection analyzer is the latest mobile portable nucleic acid detection analyzer developed by Sansure Biotech Co., Ltd. It is equipped with the core technology of Sansure Biotech – one-step nucleic acid extraction-free technology – and is equipped with a rapid nucleic acid detection system, one-stop completion of sample lysis, nucleic acid extraction, PCR amplification, and result analysis; it is easy to operate and is able to accurately detect a variety of pathogens and gene targets; it is suitable for a wide range of scenarios.

12.6 Situation of the Novel Coronavirus Nucleic Acid Emergency Testing Laboratory during the Novel Coronavirus Pandemic

12.6.1 Emergency Mobile Testing Laboratory—Air Dome Laboratory

The air dome laboratory consists of four air dome lab rooms, with each covering an area of about 210 m^2. The air dome laboratory is divided into reagent preparation area, sample processing area, and amplification area. The interior is equipped with fully automated detection equipment for automatic cap opening and sample adding, fully automated nucleic acid extraction, fully automated sampling, etc., as well as a PCR amplifier. Each air dome laboratory operates around the clock, and the daily testing capacity can reach 30,000 tubes to ensure the results can be obtained within 24 hours. The air dome mobile cabin lab is represented by the "Falcon" air dome laboratory and the Fire Eye laboratory. The "Falcon" air dome laboratory receives technical guidance from the Guangzhou Laboratory, the National Respiratory Center, and the Guangzhou Respiratory Health Research Institute, and KingMed Diagnostics is responsible for the operation. The Fire Eye Laboratory is operated by BGI and has been put into use in many cities across the country. After the outbreak of the global pandemic, the Fire Eye laboratory model has become a Chinese example and established and operated overseas such as in the United Arab Emirates, Brunei, and Serbia to export Chinese solutions for the international anti-pandemic efforts.

12.6.2 Mobile Cabin Laboratory

The mobile cabin laboratory adopts a mobile model room design, which is equipped with water and electricity, air conditioner, negative pressure facilities and sewage treatment facilities, etc. After the installation is completed, it is a standardized laboratory. As the assembling time is short, it can quickly respond to the needs of the fight against the pandemic. The mobile cabin laboratory is divided into reagent preparation area, sample preparation area, amplification area, and sterilization area. It is equipped with a sample aliquoting system, a fully automated pipetting workstation and a fully automated nucleic acid extraction system, etc. After the test sample enters the laboratory, there is "zero contact" with the lab staff, which can prevent infection and biosafety risks. The mobile cabin laboratories, represented by Sansure Biotech, Labway, and Nucleus Gene, have played a huge role in the fight against the pandemic in 2020.

12.6.3 Mobile Detection Vehicle

The mobile detection vehicle is composed of a high-mobility vehicle and a cabin laboratory. It adopts a modular design and integrates a mechanical direct-flow conditioning system, a high-efficiency air filtration system for air supply and exhaust, a negative pressure control system, an information system, and a vibration isolation for onboard equipment. The mobile cabin lab is composed of a core experiment room and a buffer room, and a variety of key protective equipment and instruments are integrated inside. The core experiment room has high negative pressure, and the air is safely discharged after high-efficiency filtration, providing good biological safety protection to effectively protect the safety of medical staff and the surrounding environment. Compared with fixed labs, mobile labs provide better mobility.

The mobile vehicle can directly reach the test site. It helps a lot to provide PCR detection in all regions. Mobile detection is of great significance for regional control/on-site detection under emergencies and timely prevention and control of pandemics in inconvenient areas.

12.7 Summary

During the COVID-19 pandemic, China's IVD industry has made great progress, and a large number of outstanding enterprises such as Mindray, Sansure Biotech, ZJ Bio-Tech, Autobio, Da An, Wondfo, BGI, and KingMed have gained significant development. In the fight against the novel coronavirus pandemic, China's IVD industry has fully demonstrated world-leading innovation efficiency and speed. According to the result report of the national novel coronavirus nucleic acid detection laboratory external quality assessment by the Clinical Laboratory Center of the Ministry of Health, all participating laboratories used domestic novel coronavirus reagents, and the laboratories included the Center for Disease Control and Prevention, secondary or tertiary public medical institutions (including general hospitals, specialized medical institutions, and maternal and child health care institutions), independent medical laboratories, international travel health care centers affiliated to the customs, reagent research and development manufacturers, and scientific research institutes.

At the same time, Chinese IVD products have played a vital role in the global fight against the pandemic. According to the data from a press conference held by the State Council Information Office, China exported 1.08 billion novel coronavirus test kits in 2020. According to the information released by the China Chamber of Commerce of Medicines and Health Products Importers and Exporters, there are more than 500 manufacturers whose novel coronavirus detection reagents have obtained export qualifications and foreign standard certification or registration and are on the white list. China's anti-pandemic practice has fully demonstrated that China's IVD industry is not only fully capable of replacing imports but can also go international and even provide global leading solutions. Through the efforts against the novel coronavirus pandemic, the international market has a deeper understanding of China's medical products, and the recognition of "Intelligent Manufacturing of China" has also been greatly improved. There will be great demand from the global market for high price-quality ratio medical products that are both affordable and easy to use. More and more IVD enterprises will speed up to "go out" and export more "Chinese solutions" in the medical and health field. We must be confident in our science and technology, take the initiative to undertake the industrial mission of China, further increase investment in scientific and technological innovation, more actively integrate into the global innovation system, grasp the high-end links of the industrial chain and value chain, and cultivate more global industry leaders with international competitiveness.

Declaration Lizhong Dai, Zhongping Deng, Jia Liu, Xiaomei Ren, Kang Wu, Deyong Tan, Hongjian Zhang, Yong Deng, Yingjuan Ai, Bozhi Ji and Yaping Xie are employees of Sansure Biotech Inc.

Jack Shao and Qiang Li are employees of Shanghai ZJ Bio-Tech Co., Ltd.

References

1. Wu F, Zhao S, Yu B, et al. A new coronavirus associated with human respiratory disease in China[J]. Nature. 2020;579(7798):265–9. https://doi.org/10.1038/s41586-020-2008-3.
2. Na Z, Dingyu Z, Wenling W, et al. A Novel Coronavirus from Patients with Pneumonia in China, 2019[J]. N Engl J Med. 2020;382(8):727–33. https://doi.org/10.1056/NEJMoa2001017.
3. Zhou P, Yang XL, Wang XG, et al. A pneumonia outbreak associated with a new Coronavirus of probable batorigin[J]. Nature. 2020;579(7798):270–3. https://doi.org/10.1038/s41586-020-2012-7.
4. Lu R, Zhao X, Li J, et al. Genomic characterisation and epidemiology of 2019 novel coronavirus: implications for virus origins and receptor binding[J]. Lancet. 2020;395(10224):565–74. https://doi.org/10.1016/S0140-6736(20)30251-8.
5. Coronaviridae study group of the international committee on taxonomy of viruse. The species severe acute respiratory syndrome-related coronavirus: classifying 2019-nCoV and naming it SARS-CoV-2[J]. Nat Microbiol. 2020;5:536–44. https://doi.org/10.1038/s41564-020-0695.
6. Zou X, Chen K, Zou J, et al. Single-cell RNA-seq data analysis on the receptor ACE2 expression reveals the potential risk of different human organs vulnerable to 2019-nCoV infection[J]. FrontMed. 2020;14(2):185–92. https://doi.org/10.1007/s11684-020-0754-0.
7. Wrapp D, Wang N, Corbett KS, et al. Cryo-EM structure of the 2019-nCoV spike in the prefusion conformation [J]. Science. 2020;367(6483):1260–3. https://doi.org/10.1126/science.abb2507.

Molecular Diagnostic Analyzers and Reagents

13

Jack Shao, Qiang Li, Jie Zhang, Zhongping Deng, and Xiaomei Ren

13.1 Introduction

Molecular diagnostics uses human saliva, tissue, blood, feces, urine, and other samples to detect disease-related markers and provides experimental diagnostic results for medical professionals in disease prevention, screening, diagnosis, stratification, prognosis, and efficacy monitoring. Affected by coronavirus disease 2019 (COVID-19), the molecular diagnosis market witnessed explosive growth in 2020. The global sales of molecular diagnosis products reached US$14.97 billion, and it is expected to reach US$32.08 billion by 2027, with a compound annual growth rate of 11.5% [1].

Infectious diseases, genetic diseases, and tumors are the most widely used types of diseases in molecular diagnosis because these three kinds of diseases are related to changes in nucleic acid levels [2].

Infectious diseases are diseases caused by pathogens that invade human tissues and begin to multiply and damage human cells and tissues. The reproduction of pathogens is bound to be accompanied by the amplification of their genomes in the body. As the invasion of exogenous nucleic acids, the pathogen genome is the best marker to distinguish between disease and health [3]. Because the sensitivity and specificity of molecular diagnostic technology are higher than traditional immunological methods and culture methods, it has become a diagnostic method for some infectious diseases and is more and more widely used in clinical practice.

J. Shao · Q. Li (✉) · J. Zhang

Key Laboratory of Medical Molecular Virology, Shanghai Medical College, Fudan University, Shanghai, China

Shanghai ZJ Bio-Tech Co., Ltd, Shanghai, China
e-mail: qiang_li@liferiver.com.cn

Z. Deng · X. Ren
Sansure Biotech Inc., Changsha, Hunan, China

H. Song, L. Dai (eds.), *In Vitro Diagnostic Industry in China*,
https://doi.org/10.1007/978-981-99-3110-1_13

Genetic diseases are caused by congenital endogenous nucleic acid mutation, including monogenic genetic diseases, chromosomal diseases, polygenic genetic diseases, and mitochondrial diseases. The diagnosis of genetic diseases mainly depends on clarifying the correlation between pathogenic gene mutations and diseases. At present, molecular diagnostic reagents are often used in the field of genetic diseases if the association of the analyte to a clinical condition or physiological state is well established. At present, ClinVar, a genetic disease genotype, and phenotype database have collected more than 825,000 records, but most of them need to be verified by further clinical studies.

The occurrence of tumors is often related to the mutations of human susceptibility genes. The application of molecular diagnosis in the field of tumors is mainly due to the emergence of a large number of tumor-targeted drugs. The targeted drugs mainly target the mutated tumor-driving genes. Due to the variation of driving gene mutations in different populations, the use of targeted drugs must be accompanied by the diagnosis of driving gene mutation to identify patients who are most likely to benefit from the corresponding drugs. At the same time, the research results of some tumor markers also promote the application of molecular diagnosis in the field of tumor screening and diagnosis, such as the correlation between human papillomavirus and cervical cancer [4].

In addition, molecular diagnosis can be used to detect drug metabolic enzymes and drug target genes including the metabolism, transport, and action of drugs in vivo. The genetic mutation and expression level of target-related genes can affect the concentration and target sensitivity of drugs, resulting in differences in individual drug responsiveness. Pharmacogenomics has become an important tool to guide clinical individualized drug use, assess the risk of serious adverse reactions, guide new drug research and development, and evaluate new drugs [5]. The Food and Drug Administration (FDA) has approved the addition of drug genome information to the drug labels of more than 140 drugs. Molecular detection of drug response-related genes and their expression products is the premise of individualized drug therapy [6].

In addition to the study of disease and drug-related nucleic acid markers, the rapid development of molecular diagnosis also benefits from the rapid development of molecular biotechnology. At present, fluorescent PCR is still the most commonly used technology for molecular diagnosis. It has high sensitivity and specificity, relatively simple operation, and short detection time. The use of other technologies has also enriched the application scenarios of molecular diagnosis. For example, high-throughput sequencing technology is applicable for the simultaneous detection of hundreds to thousands of targets, digital PCR technology can meet the needs of accurate quantification, isothermal amplification technology can be used in point-of-care testing (POCT) [7] and non-laboratory environments, capillary electrophoresis technology can distinguish the length of fragments, and fluorescence in situ hybridization (FISH) technology can realize in situ detection on tissues [8].

13.2 Research and Development of Molecular Diagnostic Products

The clinical application of molecular diagnostic technology is mainly in the form of detecting nucleic acid markers, including reagents and instruments, which are regulated by the National Medical Product Administration (hereinafter referred to as NMPA).

13.2.1 Molecular Diagnostic Reagents

According to the statistics published on the website of NMPA, as of December 31, 2021, NMPA has approved a total of 951 domestic (excluding Hong Kong, Macao, and Taiwan) molecular diagnostic reagents (class III), and 79, 71, and 67 were approved in 2019, 2020, and 2021, respectively (Fig. 13.1). The number of approved reagents were stable in the past 3 years.

From the classification of applications, most of the approved reagents in 2020 and 2021 focused on the field of infectious diseases, accounting for 54% in 2021 (Fig. 13.2) with a slight decrease from 61% in 2020. In 2020, the proportion of infectious diseases reagents rose to 61% due to the approval of a large number of novel coronavirus detection reagents (Fig. 13.2).

From the technical platform adopted by the approved detection reagents, fluorescent PCR is the most used technology, accounting for 62% in 2020 and 76% in 2021 (Fig. 13.3), which is slightly higher than 56% in 2019, indicating that the products were developed based on the need for rapid testing PCR technology for infectious diseases.

Fig. 13.1 Number of molecular diagnostic reagents approved by NMPA annually during 2019–2021

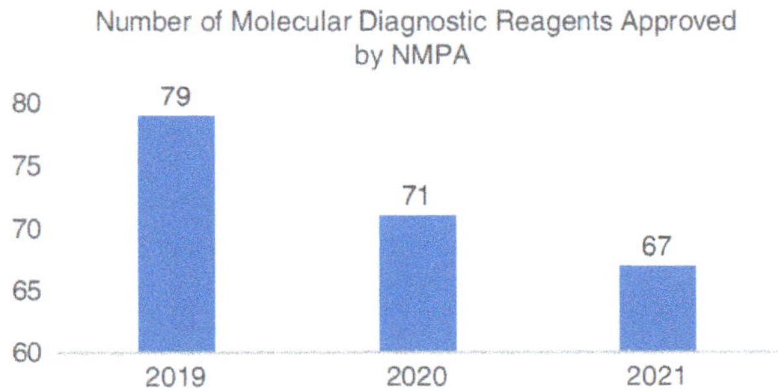

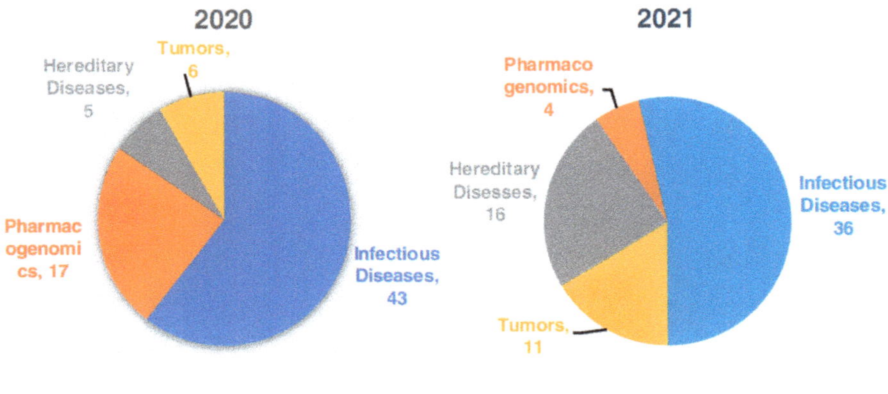

Fig. 13.2 Number of molecular diagnostic reagents approved by NMPA for each application field in 2020 and 2021

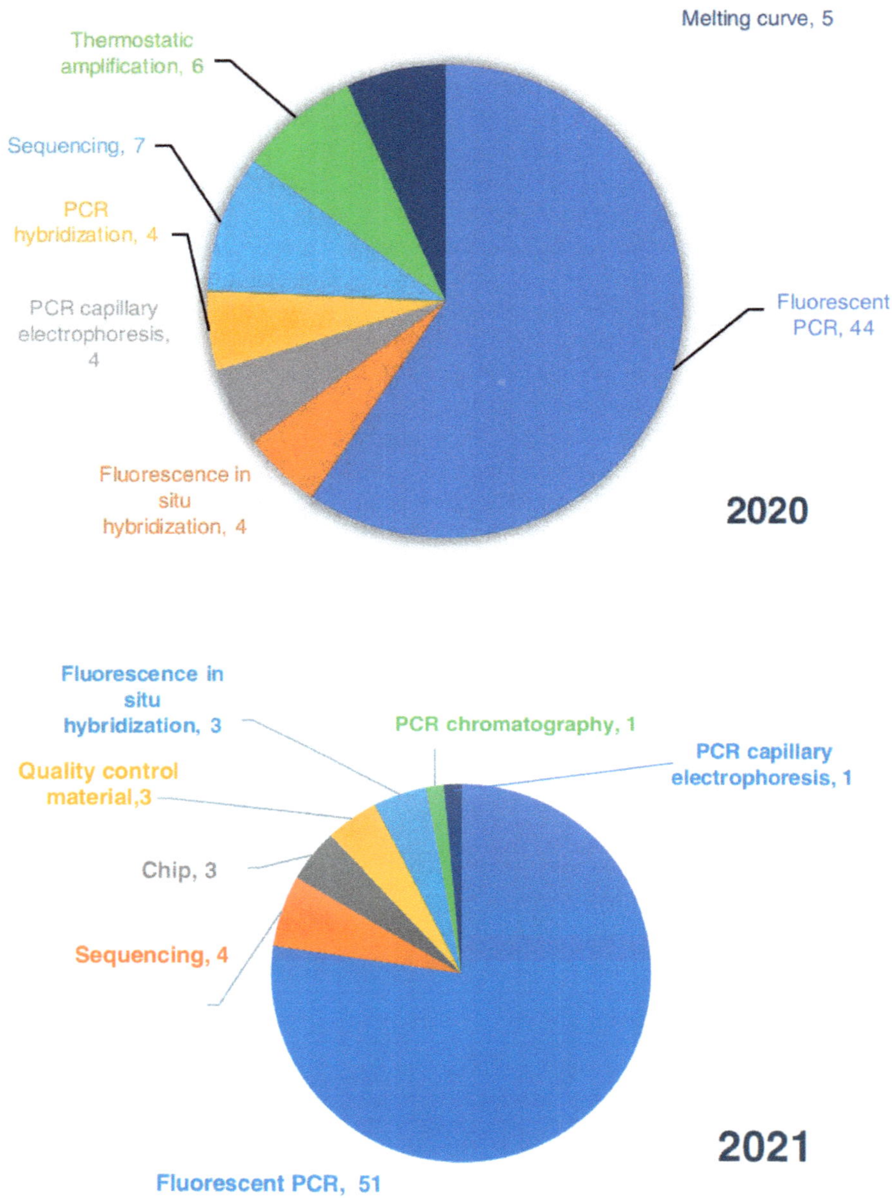

Fig. 13.3 Number of molecular diagnostic reagents based on various technical platforms approved by NMPA in 2020 and 2021

13.2.2 Molecular Diagnostic Instruments

In 2020, NMPA approved 18 types of class III molecular diagnostic instruments, and the provincial medical product administration approved 11 types of class II molecular diagnostic instruments, a total of 29. In 2021, 19 types of class III molecular diagnostic instruments were approved, and 25 types of class II molecular diagnostic instruments were approved by the provincial medical product administration, with a total of 44 types (Fig. 13.4). The obvious increase in 2021 compared with 2020 may be the result of the NMPA's accelerated approval in response to the epidemic.

The above instruments are classified according to their uses. In 2020, seven fluorescent PCR instruments, three PCR amplification instruments, one nucleic acid extraction and detection system, three nucleic acid extraction and PCR set-up systems, one chip analyzer, three hybridization instruments, six sequencing instruments, two isothermal amplification instruments, one capillary electrophoresis gene analyzer, and three POCT instruments were approved. In 2021, 10 fluorescent PCR instruments, seven PCR amplification instruments, one sequencing sample preparation system, two nucleic acid extraction and amplification system, four nucleic acid extraction and PCR set-up system, 11 chip analyzers, two hybridizers, two sequencers, four isothermal amplification instruments, and one microfluidic nucleic acid amplification instrument were approved (Fig. 13.5). Compared with 2020, more types of instruments were added in 2021, including fluorescent PCR instruments, PCR amplification instrument, nucleic acid extraction, PCR set-up system, isothermal amplification instrument, and chip analyzers.

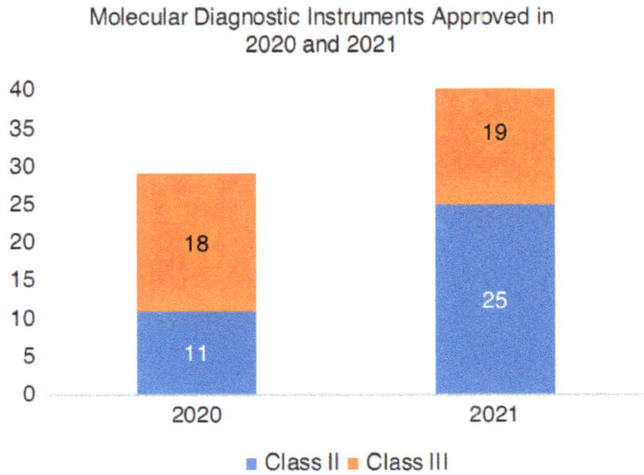

Fig. 13.4 Molecular Diagnostic Instruments Approved by NMPA in 2020 and 2021

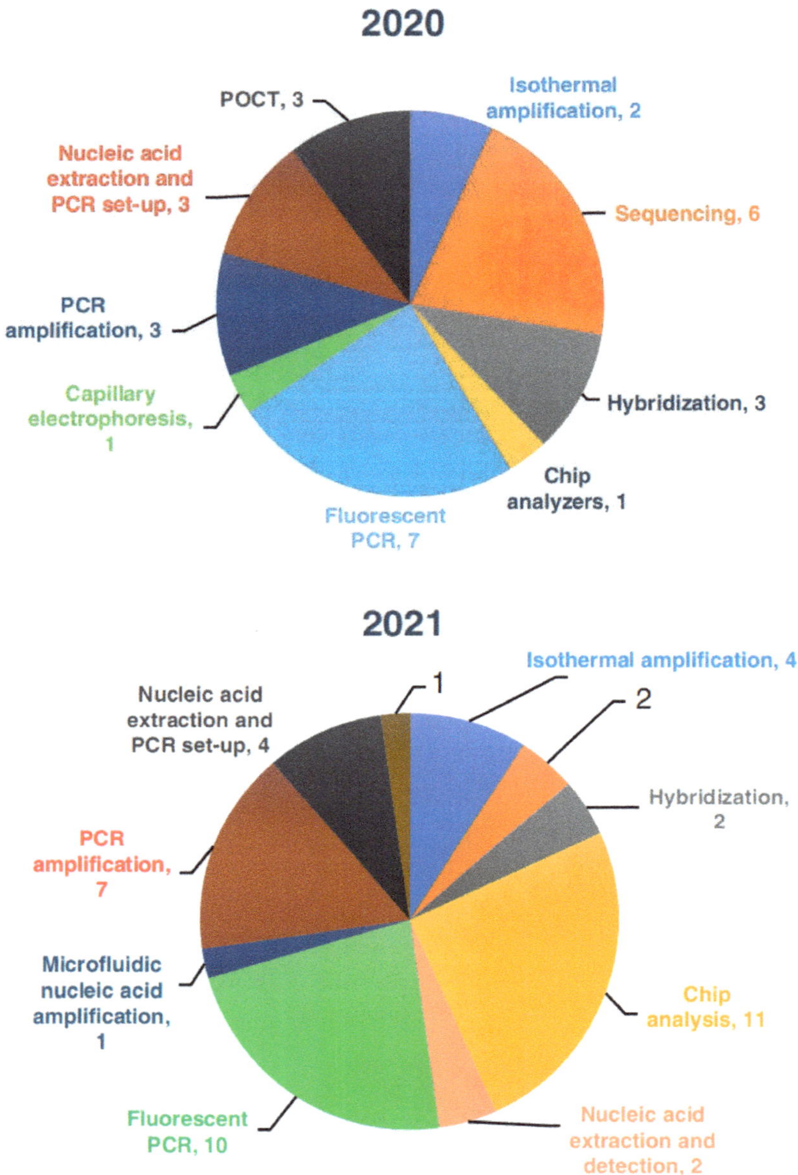

Fig. 13.5 Number of Molecular Diagnostic Devices Approved by NMPA for Different Uses in 2020 and 2021

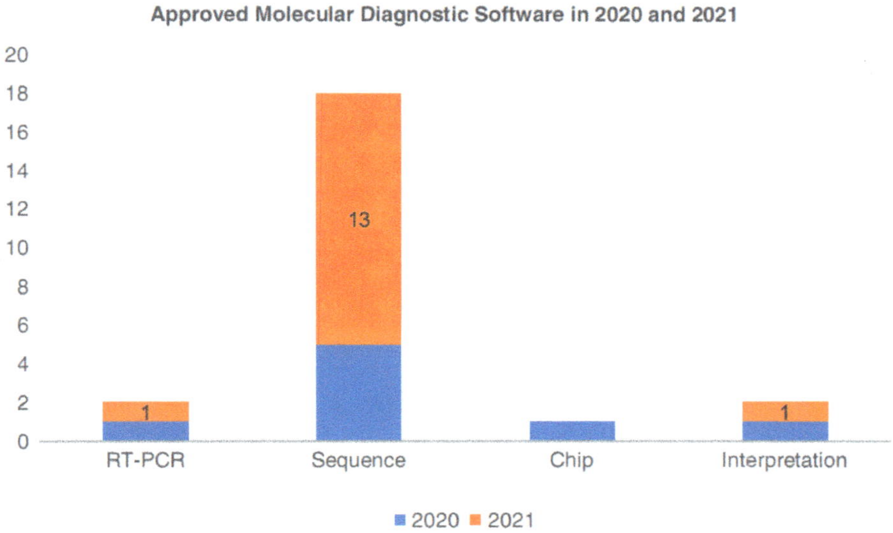

Fig. 13.6 Number of Molecular Diagnostic Software Approved by NMPA for Different Uses in 2020 and 2021

13.2.3 Molecular Diagnostic Software

According to the statistics published on the website of the NMPA, in 2020, NMPA approved eight models, one is for fluorescent PCR data analysis, one is for chip data analysis, five are for sequencing data analysis, and one is for interpretation of tumor and genetic disease gene detection results. The NMPA approved a total of 15 software for molecular diagnostics in 2021, one of which is for fluorescence PCR data analysis, one is for pharmaco genomics data interpretation, and the other 13 are for sequencing data analysis (Fig. 13.6). It can be seen that the amount of data obtained by sequencing is large, and special software is required for analysis. These softwares are used in conjunction with molecular diagnostic reagents.

13.2.4 Consumables for Molecular Diagnostics

According to the data published on the NMPA website, a special collection vessel for nucleic acid testing was approved in 2020 and 2021.

13.3 Innovative Products

The following innovative products have obtained the registration certificate of regulatory authorities for the first time in the industry based on the technology platform, and are open to the whole market as the benchmark. Only some representative products are listed.

13.3.1 Molecular Diagnostic Instruments

13.3.1.1 Nucleic Acid POCT

The UC0102 Nucleic Acid amplification and detection system (Certificate No.: G.X.Z.Z. 20,193,221,026) of Ustar Biotechnology (Hangzhou) Ltd. (hereinafter referred to as "Ustar") is the first approved instrument for point-of-care testing (POCT) in China. At present, the reagents supporting the instrument are all based on crossing priming amplification (CPA). Independent detection reaction, which can effectively avoid cross-contamination between samples, and the operation is sample. Just add the sample to the reaction tube after pretreatment, and the subsequent detection process can be completed automatically in this instrument.

The reaction tube is divided into three segments: the lysis zone, the elution zone, and the amplification zone. When the tube is inserted into the instrument, the instrument first heats the lysis zone of the tube, so that the nucleic acid in the sample is released into the solution, and then adsorbed by the magnetic beads. The magnetic beads and nucleic acid are dragged from the lysis zone by the magnet through the hydrophobic layer to the cleaning area. The impurities on the magnetic beads in the cleaning area are removed by the elution solution, and the magnetic beads and nucleic acids are dragged by the magnetic steel through the hydrophobic layer to reach the large-scale system for nucleic acid extraction and PCR tests; the extraction, system preparation, and amplification are completed in one amplification zone. The nucleic acid in the amplification zone is eluted by the elution buffer, and the eluted nucleic acid and reagent start to react at the amplification zone by temperature control. At the same time, the fluorescent probe binds to the specific amplification zone to produce a fluorescent signal. After detecting the signal, the instrument generates an amplification curve, CT value, and detection result.

In 2020, the NMPA approved additional four nucleic acid real-time detection instruments, namely, Galaxy Nano PCR cycler (Registration No.: G.X.Z.Z. 20,203,220,597), Universal Nano PCR cycler (Registration No.: G.X.Z.Z. 20,203,220,012) of igenesis Biotechnology (Shanghai) Co., Ltd. (hereinafter referred to as "igenesis"), the iponatic Portable Molecule Workstation of Sansure Biotech Inc. (Registration No.: G.X.Z.Z. 20,203,220,419), and Universal Pro automatic PCR analysis system (Registration No.: G.X.Z.Z. 20,203,220,825). These instruments need to be used with fluorescent PCR reagents. The amplification reaction of igenesis Galaxy nano is carried out in the Galaxy smart box. The smart box contains nucleic acid extraction reagents, and the PCR reagents need to be added separately.

13.3.1.2 Portable Fluorescence PCR Cycler

The miniaturization of fluorescent PCR instruments is also a trend. Small PCR cyclers are portable and realize mobile detection. The detection can be carried out on-site, or put into biosafety cabinets to reduce the infection risk of operators, and it saves space so that more instruments can be placed in the same space. From 2019 to 2021, the NMPA approved several portable fluorescent PCR systems, among which the Mic POC DX 48 real-time fluorescent quantitative PCR cycler (Registration No.: G.X.Z.Z. 20,203,220,013) of Shanghai ZJ Bio-Tech Co., Ltd. (hereinafter referred to as "Liferiver") has a size of only 13 cm × 15 cm × 15 cm, weighing only 2.1 kg, 48 samples can be detected at one time, and 4 fluorescent channels can be detected at the same time. It can be completed in 30 mins at the fastest.

13.3.1.3 Automatic Nucleic Acid Extractor Paraffin Sample

With a large number of tumor-targeted drugs on the market, companion diagnosis is increasingly used in the process of tumor treatment. The results of using tissue samples for tumor companion diagnosis are more accurate than selecting plasma-free DNA (cell-free DNA, cfDNA). Formalin-fixed paraffin-embedded (FFPE) tissue samples are the most commonly used type of tissue samples in pathology, so the nucleic acid extraction of FFPE samples has become a necessary step for the companion diagnosis of most tumors. However, it is more difficult to realize an automatic extraction of nucleic acid from FFPE samples than that of liquid samples, and most FFPE samples need to undergo manual dewaxing, digestion, and cross-linking steps before subsequent automatic extraction. Liferiver iMagNext automatic nucleic acid extractor (Record No.: H.M.X.B. 20,190,065) can automatically complete the steps of sample dewaxing, digestion, and cross-linking in the instrument, and the whole process takes only 2.5 h.

13.3.1.4 Automatic Database Building

Database building is a link to high-throughput sequencing. Manual database building is cumbersome and time-consuming; it requires multiple labs, and it is difficult to meet the requirements for hospital labs with limited space. The ANDiS 400 PCR cycler (Registration No.: H.X.Z.Z. 20,192,220,494 of 3D Medicines) (hereinafter referred to as "3D Med") is a domestic approved instrument with the function of automatically closed sequencing library preparation, which can shorten the database construction time from the previous 6–9 h to at least 3.5 h and the manual operation time from 2.5 h to 3 min. And the process of building a sample database is completed in a closed cassette, which reduces the risk of cross-contamination between samples.

13.3.1.5 Sequencer with the Highest Throughput

In 2020, the DNBSEQ-T7 Gene Sequencer of Wuhan MGI Technology Co., Ltd. (hereinafter referred to as "MGI") was approved (Registration No.: G.X.Z.Z. 20,203,220,061). It uses DNA nanosphere sequencing technology (DNBSEQTM) to build a database. The amount of data sequenced at one time can reach 1.5 ~ 6 T, Q30 > 80%, and the running time is 24 ~ 30 h.

13.3.2 Molecular Diagnostic Reagents for Infectious Diseases

13.3.2.1 Latent Tuberculosis Infection Detection Reagents

Latent tuberculosis infection (LTBI) is defined as a state of persistent immune response to stimulation by *Mycobacterium tuberculosis* antigens with no evidence of clinically manifested active TB. There is no gold standard test for LTBI, and thus only a rough estimate of the number of infections can be made. One-third of the world's population is estimated to be infected with *M. tuberculosis*. Many studies have shown that 5–10% of people with LTBI will subsequently develop active TB disease. Treating LTBI to prevent active TB disease has become a very important part to achieve the targets of the WHO's End TB Strategy.

Testing LTBI is the first step in the treatment. Interferon-γ release assay (IGRA) and tuberculin skin test (TST) are the most commonly used methods to detect LTBI. The ability of these two methods to predict active TB is approximately equivalent. TST is an in vivo diagnostic method that detects hypersensitivity by intradermal injection of *Mycobacterium* antigen, with the disadvantage of cross-reactivity with BCG and environmental mycobacteria. IGRA is an in vitro diagnostic method that stimulates peripheral blood T-lymphocytes with *M. tuberculosis*-specific antigens. It will not produce false positive results when people have been vaccinated with BCG or encounter environmental mycobacteria. However, both IGRA and TST have low diagnostic sensitivity in young children and immunocompromised patients, such as those with HIV infection, corticosteroid treatment, and other immunosuppressive drugs. As a result, researchers have been searching for new markers for the detection of LTBI.

IFN-γ-induced protein 10 (IP-10) mRNA is a potential marker that has been studied in recent years. Its expression level is 100-fold higher than that of interferon-γ after antigen stimulation. The Mycobacterium Tuberculosis Specific Cellular Immunoreaction Detection Kit (PCR-Fluorescence) (Registration No.: G.X.Z.Z 20203400334) of Suzhou Chuanglan Bio-Tech Co., Ltd. is a qualitative kit that uses IP-10 mRNA as the target of the test and detects IP-10 mRNA levels before and after stimulating with TB-specific antigen by using an anticoagulated peripheral blood sample. This reagent will be used for the detection of LTBI.

13.3.2.2 Tuberculosis Diagnostic Reagents

In 2019, there were about ten million TB patients worldwide and 1.5 million deaths, and China ranks third in the world with 895,000 new cases of TB each year, most of which are pulmonary TB. The diagnosis of pulmonary TB is based on pathogen detection. Molecular diagnostic is one of the methods of pathogen detection, and the target of the test is the *Mycobacterium tuberculosis* complex (MTBC). Most of the molecular diagnostic reagents for tuberculosis are based on fluorescent PCR technology. In 2019, NMPA approved two Mycobacterium Tuberculosis Complex Detection Kits based on Isothermal Amplification Technologies, which are products of Guangzhou Deaou Bio-technology Co., Ltd. ("Deaou") (Registration No.: G.X.Z.Z 20193400313) and Ustar Biotechnologies (Hangzhou) Ltd. ("Ustar") (Registration No.: G.X.Z.Z 20193401027).

Deaou's kit is developed based on the nucleic acid strand displacement reactions technology, and the detection target is *M. tuberculosis* insertion sequence IS6110. The LoD is 100 bacteria/mL. Since the copy number of the IS6110 reference strain H37Rv is 16, it can be deduced that the LoD of the kit is 1600 copies/mL, which is roughly the same as the LoD of fluorescent PCR reagents in the market. Ustar's kit uses crossing priming amplification (CPA) technology to detect the IS6110 insertion sequence specific to the *M. tuberculosis* complex.

13.3.2.3 Pathogen Diagnosis of Gastroenteritis

Gastroenteritis is a common disease in infants and young children. The treatment of mild cases is based on the prevention and correction of dehydration, electrolyte disturbance, and acid-base imbalance, while anti-infective treatment should be considered for infants and young children with gastroenteritis that has obvious toxic symptoms and cannot be completely explained by dehydration. The common pathogens include viruses, bacteria, parasites, and fungi, and there are appropriate drugs for bacterial, parasitic, and fungal infections. Viruses are the most common pathogens, with Rotavirus and Adenovirus being the main types of viruses that cause gastroenteritis in infants and young children. Rotavirus causes up to 36% of all gastroenteritis deaths in infants and children. There is a lack of specific antiviral drugs, and antibacterial drugs should not be used. Since different pathogens are treated in different ways, pathogen testing is helpful to identify the causative agent and implement precise treatment.

The diagnostic criteria for Rotavirus and Adenovirus gastroenteritis recommended in the *Infectious Diarrhea Diagnostic Guidelines* include electron microscopy, polyacrylamide gel electrophoresis, agarose gel electrophoresis, enzyme-linked immunosorbent assay (ELISA), reverse transcription-polymerase chain reaction (RT-PCR)/polymerase chain reaction (PCR), and virus isolation. NMPA has approved 59 single test or multiplex test kits with immunochromatographic or ELISA methods. The detection targets are viral antigens. In 2020, Chongqing Wecan Bio-Tech Co., Ltd. launched Group A Rotavirus, Group F Enteric Adenovirus Type 40/41 Nucleic Acid Detection Kit (PCR-Fluorescence) (Registration No.: G.X.Z.Z 20203400618), which is the first Rotavirus and Adenovirus nucleic acid test kit. The sensitivity of fluorescence RT-PCR is better than that of immunochromatography and ELISA, so it will be better for the detection of low-concentration samples.

13.3.2.4 Pertussis Diagnosis

Pertussis is a highly contagious acute respiratory disease that can last for several months and often causes epidemics. In recent years, the incidence of pertussis in children has increased yearly. For the diagnosis of pertussis, the *Chinese Guidelines for the Diagnosis and Treatment of Pertussis in Children* recommends using nucleic acid tests for laboratory confirmation of pertussis. In 2020, NMPA approved the Pertussis Bacteria Nucleic Acid Detection Kit (PCR-Fluorescence) (Registration No.: G.X.Z.Z 20203400152) of Shenzhen Yilifang Biotechnology Co., Ltd., which is the first pertussis bacteria molecular diagnostic kit. It is more sensitive than serological methods and allows an earlier diagnosis of pertussis.

13.3.3 Molecular Diagnostic Reagents for Tumor

13.3.3.1 Tumor Screening Reagents

Colorectal Cancer Screening Test

The U.S. Preventive Services Task Force (USPSTF) recommends four types of screening for cancers: lung cancer, colorectal cancer, breast cancer, and cervical cancer. All screening methods are based on imaging tests, except for cervical cancer, which can be screened by using the human papillomavirus (HPV) molecular diagnostic method. In November 2020, NMPA approved the KRAS Gene Mutation BMP3/NDRG4 Methylation and Stool Occult Blood Combination Test Kit (PCR-Fluorescence - Colloidal Gold method) (Registration No.: G.X.Z.Z 20203400845) of Shenzhen New Horizon Health Ltd., which is a colorectal cancer screening kit based on fluorescent PCR and colloidal gold technology. The kit detects KRAS gene mutations (including G12D, G12A, G12V, G12S, G12R, G12C, and G13D), BMP3, and NDRG4 gene methylation and hemoglobin in human stool samples in vitro. The test values will be calculated by KRAS Gene Mutation, BMP3/NDRG4 Gene Methylation, and Stool Occult Blood Combination Analysis Software (Registration No.: Z.X.Z.Z 20202210848) and used for the screening of colorectal cancer high-risk group (40–74 years old) with poor colonoscopy compliance.

Gastric Cancer Detection Test

Gastric cancer is a common gastrointestinal carcinoid tumor, with the sixth highest incidence and second highest mortality rate among tumors. The recommended screening method in the *Expert Consensus on Early Gastric Cancer Screening Process in China (Draft)* is based on age, gender, serum gastrin-17 concentration, *H. pylori* antibody results, and pepsinogen ratio, giving a separate gastroscopy screening protocol by differentiating between high-, intermediate-, and low-risk groups. In 2020, when the screening program for gastric cancer based on molecular diagnostic methods was available, NMPA approved the Diagnostic Kit for RNF180/Spetin9 Gene Methylation (Real Time PCR) (Registration No.: G.X.Z.Z 20203400447) of Biochain (Beijing) Science-Technology Inc. This product is designed for the in vitro qualitative detection of methylation RNF180 and Septin9 genes in human plasma. It is indicated for patients who have been diagnosed by a clinician and recommended for gastroscopy and who refuse to undergo gastroscopy for personal reasons.

13.3.3.2 Tumor Diagnostic Reagents

Lymphoma, also known as malignant lymphoma, is a general term for a group of malignant tumors originating from the lymphopoietic system. It is one of the most common tumors in China. In 2020, there were 544,352 new cases of non-Hodgkin lymphoma (NHL) worldwide, ranking 13th among all new cases of malignancies. The immunoglobulin gene rearrangement test is one of the methods for the pathological diagnosis of lymphoma, but there has been a long-standing lack of approved products. Immunoglobulin Gene Rearrangement Detection Kit (Capillary

Electrophoresis method) (Registration No.: G.X.Z.Z. 20,203,400,736) of Suzhou Yuntai Bio-Tech Ltd. is the first in vitro immunoglobulin gene rearrangement detection molecular diagnostic product approved in China, which can qualitatively in vitro detect clonal immunoglobulin gene rearrangement status in human formalin-fixed paraffin-embedded sections (FFPE) samples. It is used for the auxiliary diagnosis of B-cell non-Hodgkin lymphoma.

13.3.3.3 Tumor Companion Diagnostic Reagents

Non-small Cell Lung Cancer Companion Diagnostic Tests

High-throughput sequencing (HTS) has started to be applied in tumor companion diagnosis in recent years. NMPA approved two test kits based on HTS in 2020. Human EGFR/KRAS/BRAF/HER-2/ALK/ROS1 Gene Mutation Detection Kit (Semiconductor Sequencing Method) (Registration No.: G.X.Z.Z. 20,203,400,094) of Xiamen Spacegen Co., Ltd. ("Spacegen") uses a PCR platform combining specific modified primers and RingCap® Ring-Link Capture Library technology (Patent No.: 201510496049.5) for library construction. Compared to other targeted sequencing library preparation, RingCap® technology simplifies the manual process with two steps of sample-adding and two steps of purification in 3.5 h.

The other test is the Eight-Gene Mutations Screening Kit (Semiconductor Sequencing Method) (Registration No.: G.X.Z.Z. 20,203,400,072) of Beijing Genetron Holdings Limited. It is based on the "One-Step Method" technology (Patent No.: 201710218529.4), which contains target-specific sequences, junction, and label on a pair of primers, and completes the steps of specific fragment amplification, the addition of junction, and the addition of label in one step of PCR amplification. Compared to the traditional "two-step" method, one amplification and one purification step are reduced. As a result, the total time for library construction and manual operation is reduced.

Ovarian Cancer Companion Diagnostic Tests

In 2019, the BRCA1 and BRCA2 Gene Mutation Detection Kit (Reversible Terminator Sequencing) of Xiamen Amoy Diagnostics Co., Ltd. was approved. It is intended for the qualitative detection of point mutations and insertion-deletion mutations using DNA isolated from peripheral whole blood, which contains full and uniform coverage of both BRCA1 and BRCA2 genes, covering all coding exons, exon/intron junctions, some introns, and UTR regions. This kit is used for the Olaparib dosage guidance, filling the gap of approved reagents for the BRCA1/2 gene test in China.

Breast Cancer Companion Diagnostic Tests

Human epidermal growth factor receptor 2 (HER-2) is an important driver gene and prognostic indicator for breast cancer. It is also a major predictor of anti-HER-2 therapy. The clinical application of the anti-HER-2 drug Trastuzumab has changed the diagnosis and treatment of breast cancer and greatly improved the prognosis for HER-2-positive breast cancer patients. It is an important breakthrough in targeted breast cancer therapy. In recent years, new anti-HER-2 drugs such as Pertuzumab, Lapatinib, Pyrotinib, and Ado-trastuzumab emtansine (T-DM1) have been developed and successfully marketed, achieving good effects in the treatment of HER-2 positive breast cancer and changing clinical practice.

The gold standard for detecting HER-2 amplification is fluorescent in situ hybridization (FISH) and immunohistochemistry (IHC). HER-2 Gene Amplification Kit (Digital PCR Method) (Registration No.: G.X.Z.Z. 20,193,400,770) of Nanjing Questgenomics Biotechnology Co., Ltd. is based on the digital PCR method. Compared with FISH and IHC, digital PCR requires less tissue sampling, and the results are more objective. Moreover, the results of digital PCR are in good conformity with the gold standard.

13.3.4 Genetic Disease Molecular Diagnostic Reagents

13.3.4.1 Preimplantation Screening Reagent

In vitro fertilization embryos are prone to chromosomal aneuploidy abnormalities. Chromosome aneuploidy refers to the increase or decrease in the number of a single chromosome or multiple chromosomes. It is the most common chromosome number abnormality in clinical practice. The implantation of embryos with abnormal chromosomes into a woman's uterus can lead to implantation failure, abortion, birth defects, and other problems. Preimplantation genetic testing for aneuploidies (PGT-A) reduces the probability of implantation of embryos with chromosomal abnormalities. Thus, it reduces the number of repeated implantation failures, repeated abortions, birth defects, and other problems caused by the implantation of embryos with chromosomal abnormalities. Common techniques for detecting chromosomal aneuploidy include fluorescence in situ hybridization (FISH) and comparative genomic hybridization (Array-CGH) and single nucleotide polymorphism (SNP array).

Suzhou Basecare Medical Co. Ltd. developed a preimplantation genetic testing kit for aneuploidies (Registration Number: G.X.Z.Z. 20,203,400,181) using high-throughput sequencing technology to analyze whether there is an abnormal number of aneuploidies in the embryo chromosome. DNA detection of some cells of this embryo can assist clinicians to judge whether the embryo is implanted.

13.3.4.2 Abortion-Related Chromosome Testing

Recurrent spontaneous abortion (RSA) refers to the loss of the fetus 3 or more times before 28 weeks of gestation according to the usual definition in China, but it is also believed that the second consecutive procedure should be valued and evaluated. Chromosomal abnormalities in embryos are the most common cause of recurrent abortion. Chromosomal abnormalities are reported in about 45% of embryos in accidental early spontaneous abortion. Both Chinese Experts' Consensus on The Diagnosis and Treatment of Recurrent Spontaneous Abortion and European Guidelines for the Diagnosis and Treatment of Recurrent Loss suggest chromosome karyotype analysis of peripheral blood and its flow products in couples with recurrent abortion, and the use of assisted reproductive technology for abortions caused by chromosomal abnormalities is recommended to solve their fertility problems.

Karyotype analysis is the gold standard for the detection of chromosomal abnormalities, but its operation process is complicated, and cells need to be interpreted manually under the microscope after culture and treatment, which requires a long-time cycle, is highly dependent on personnel skills, provides low test flux, is limited by aseptic conditions, and has the possibility of maternal contamination. The villus cells required for karyotype analysis developed well in the early stage of pregnancy, but after 11 weeks, metamorphosis villi increased, resulting in reduced mitotic phase and poor chromosome morphology, which increased the difficulty of karyotype analysis. If the embryo dies for a long time in the mother or the uterine clearance operation is carried out late, and the success rate of culture will be reduced.

The Abortive Tissue Chromosome Aneuploidy Detection Kit developed by Genesky Bio-Tech Co., Ltd. (Registration Number: G.X.Z.Z. 20,193,400,107) was used for in vitro qualitative detection of six chromosome aneuploidy of human genomic DNA in abortion villous tissue, including trisomy 13, trisomy 16, trisomy 18, trisomy 21, trisomy 22, and X monomer. The test results need to be combined with the special abortion tissue chromosome aneuploidy detection and analysis software (Registration Number: S.X.Z.Z. 20,202,210,756). This is the first application of multiplex Ligation-dependent Probe Amplification (MLPA) technology in China (Patent Number: 201010180551.2) and obtained the registration approval for class III in vitro molecular diagnostic medical device product. It is also the first molecular diagnostic product to obtain the registration approval of a class III medical device product in the field of abortive tissue chromosome aneuploidy detection.

Compared with karyotype analysis, the samples used for MLPA detection do not need to be cultured, so the detection time is short, the operation is relatively simple, the equipment is highly automated, and the detection flux is high. Two studies comparing MLPA with traditional karyotype analysis showed a higher detection success rate with MLPA. The clinical application of MLPA detection products of Genesky Bio-Tech will help improve the ability of hospitals to detect chromosomal abnormalities in abortion tissues.

13.3.5 Pharmacogenomics Molecular Diagnostic Reagent

Systemic lupus erythematosus (SLE) is the most common systemic autoimmune disease in China, with an incidence of 30.13–70.41/100000 population. The kidney is the most commonly involved organ in SLE, and 40% ~ 60% of SLE patients have lupus nephritis (LN). In China, nearly half of SLE patients are complicated with lupus nephritis. There is increasing evidence showing that tacrolimus (also known as FK506) has good efficacy and safety in lupus nephritis.

In 2015, the Clinical Pharmacogenomics Implementation Consortium published guidelines on the CYP3A5 genotype and tacrolimus dose for patients with

CYP3A5*1/CYP3A5*1, CYP3A5*1/CYP3A5*3, CYP3A5*1/CYP3A5*6, and CYP3A5*1/CYP3A5*7 genotype; it is recommended to use 1.5–2 times of the standard dose as the initial dose. The main alleles in the Asian population are CYP3A5*1 (25.8%) and CYP3A5*3 (74.2%). Therefore, the Outline of Technical Guidelines for Gene Detection of Drug Metabolism Enzymes and Drug Action Targets (Trial) also recommends reducing the dose of tacrolimus in CYP3A5*3/*3 genotype patients to avoid adverse reactions.

Although there is a slight difference in methodology, both CYP3A5 (A6986G) Gene Detection Kit (Registration No.: G.X.Z.Z. 20,193,400,286) developed by Shanghai BaiO Technology Co., Ltd. and Human CYP3A5 Genotyping Detection Kit (Fluorescence-PCR Method) (Registration No.: G.X.Z.Z. 20,203,400,784) developed by Hangzhou KBM Life sciences Co., Ltd. will play a role in the precise drug use of tacrolimus in the treatment of lupus nephritis.

13.4 Top Manufacturers in China

The top 15 companies with the most approved molecular diagnostic kits in China are listed in The Blue Book of In Vitro Diagnosis Industry Development in China (Volume 2018 · Total Volume 4) [9]. In 2018, the combined number of approved kits from these companies accounted for 44% of the total, but this proportion fell to 21% in 2020 (Table 13.1). The molecular diagnostic industry is a sunrise industry. COVID-19 has further accelerated the enlargement of market capacity, and the proportion of approved kits from leading companies has decreased, indicating that more companies have entered this field and the competition will be fiercer in the future.

Table 13.1 Top manufacturers in China

Serial number	Manufacturer name	Number of approved reagents				
		2018	2019	2020	2021	Total
1	Daan Gene Co., Ltd.	50	3	2	5	60
2	Shanghai ZJ Bio-Tech Co., Ltd	34	2	1	1	38
3	Sansure Biotech Inc.	26	5	2	3	36
4	Shanghai Kehua Bio-Engineering Co., Ltd.	28	0	0	0	28
5	Wuhan Biotech Gene Engineering Co., Ltd.	24	0	0	0	24
6	Triplex International Biosciences (China) Co., Ltd.	23	0	0	0	23
7	ACON Biotech (Hangzhou) Co., Ltd.	21	0	0	1	22
8	Xiamen Amplly Biotechnology Co., Ltd.	16	2	3	0	21
9	Suzhou Tianlong Biotechnology Co., Ltd.	16	1	3	1	20
10	Shenzhen Puruikang Biotechnology Co., Ltd.	15	2	1	0	18
11	BGI Genomics Co., Ltd.	13	0	1	3	17
12	Jiangsu Bioperfectus Technologies Co., Ltd.	15	0	1	0	16
13	Shanghai Rendu Biotechnology Co., Ltd.	13	1	0	0	14
14	SinoMD Gene Technology Co, Ltd.	12	0	1	1	14
15	Guangdong Hybribio Biotech Co., Ltd.	12	0	0	1	13

Declaration Jack Shao, Qiang Li and Jie Zhang are employees of Shanghai ZJ Bio-Tech Co., Ltd. Zhongping Deng and Xiaomei Ren are employees of Sansure Biotech Inc.

References

1. Chu D K W, Pan Y, Cheng S M S, et al. Molecular diagnosis of a novel coronavirus (2019-nCoV) causing an outbreak of pneumonia[J]. Clin Chem, 2020, 66(4): 549-555.
2. Girod, S.D., Giraud, S., Decullier, E., Lesca, G., Cottin, V., Faure, F., Merrot, O., Saurin, J.C., Cordier, J.F. and Plauchu, H. Hemorrhagic hereditary telangiectasia (Rendu-Osler Disease) and infectious diseases: an underestimated association[J]. Clin Infect Diseases, 2007, 44(6):841-845.
3. Feng W, Newbigging A M, Le C, et al. Molecular diagnosis of COVID-19: challenges and research needs[J]. Anal Chem, 2020, 92(15): 10196-10209.
4. Walter W, Pfarr N, Meggendorfer M, et al. Next-generation diagnostics for precision oncology: preanalytical considerations, technical challenges, and available technologies[C]Seminars in cancer biology. Academic Press, 2020.
5. Taylor C, Crosby I, Yip V, et al. A review of the important role of CYP2D6 in pharmacogenomics[J]. Genes, 2020, 11(11): 1295.
6. Bhutani P, Joshi G, Raja N, et al. US FDA approved drugs from 2015–June 2020: a perspective[J]. J Med Chem, 2021, 64(5): 2339-2381.
7. Kost G J. Molecular and point-of-care diagnostics for Ebola and new threats: National POCT policy and guidelines will stop epidemics[J]. Expert Rev Mol Diagnostics, 2018, 18(7): 657-673.
8. Prudent E, Raoult D. Fluorescence in situ hybridization, a complementary molecular tool for the clinical diagnosis of infectious diseases by intracellular and fastidious bacteria[J]. FEMS Microbiol Rev, 2019, 43(1): 88-107.
9. Haibo Song, Jiańer Yao, In vitro diagnostic industry in China[M]. Shanghai Scientific & Technical Publishers, 2020.

Part V

POCT

14 Review

Yaping Zhao, Xiaofang Wang, Jiaqi Zou, Li Tian, and Shan Guo

14.1 Introduction

Point-of-care testing (POCT) is a subfield of in vitro diagnostics (IVD), where portable analytical instruments and supporting reagents are used to obtain test results quickly at the sampling site. POCT is a dynamically developing category of testing methods. Its core goal is to meet the diagnostic requirements to realize clinical treatment or home monitoring, with rapid and reliable diagnostic results. POCT is defined by the National Academy of Clinical Biochemistry (NACB) as "Clinical laboratory testing performed in close proximity to a patient's treatment by clinical personnel or patients (self-monitoring, testing) not trained in clinical laboratory science." In other words, POCT refers to all tests performed outside the traditional, core laboratory.

POCT dates back to 1500 BC, when doctors observed that ants were attracted to the urine of a patient with a "wasting disease." Physicians inferred that the urine contained sugar; thus, they were able to diagnose diabetes. The second scientific and technological revolution, which took place between the 1870s to the early twentieth century, was mainly marked by the invention and application of atomic energy, electronic computers, space technology, and biological engineering. These factors accelerated the rapid development of POCT detection technology.

As POCT technology has developed, it has achieved complete quantification, automation, as well as improved precision. While POCT detection technology itself has developed, more information technology, intelligence, big data, and other "Internet+" elements have been integrated. POCT has become an essential link in

Y. Zhao (✉) · X. Wang · J. Zou
Guangzhou Wondfo Biotech Co., Ltd., Guangzhou, Guangdong, China
e-mail: ypzhao@wondfo.com.cn

L. Tian · S. Guo
Wuhan EasyDiagnosis Biomedicine Co., Ltd, Wuhan, Hubei, China

H. Song, L. Dai (eds.), *In Vitro Diagnostic Industry in China*,
https://doi.org/10.1007/978-981-99-3110-1_14

the clinical diagnosis and treatment of critical diseases and in other fields, making it a key support for most primary institutions seeking to establish detection, diagnosis, and treatment capabilities. As POCT technology has improved, it is expected that the detection index range and performance will be further improved. POCT has also been gradually extended from an exclusively in vitro detection technology to include multidimensional detection technologies, such as mobile ultrasound and electrocardiography. POCT enables more convenient information collection platforms, such as implementing convenient rapid monitoring for a target population. It can be combined with traditional hospital information collection and third-party lab omics information, both in hospitals and in large data centers for disease control. By connecting this rapidly acquired information with artificial intelligence (AI)-based auxiliary analysis, it can provide comprehensive and accurate assessments of health. It can also provide early warning and management reference for public health emergencies, chronic disease management, and early tumor screening. POCT can become an important starting point for improving global public health management.

14.2 Technical Platform

POCT technology has gradually evolved from classical immunochromatography to more sensitive platforms hosting multiple detection technologies, such as luminescence and molecular detection. Classical technologies, such as colloidal gold immunochromatography, have improved and multiple technologies become integrated. POCT does not refer to a single detection technology; rather, it has become a technology that can be adapted to different scenarios.

14.2.1 Immunochromatographic Techniques

Depending on the marker used, immunochromatography includes colloidal gold immunochromatography, fluorescence immunochromatography, and others. In recent years, with the emergence of new markers such as colored latex, aptamers, nanoenzymes, and carbon nanotubes, the performance of immunochromatography has improved. Among these novel markers, fluorescent substances, such as fluorescein, quantum dots, and up-conversion nanoparticles, not only retain the advantages of on-site rapid detection by immunochromatography but also allow highly sensitive fluorescence detection; thus, they are widely applied to the detection of cardiac markers and infectious disease indicators.

Colloidal gold immunochromatographic techniques use gold as a marker to qualitatively detect or semiquantitatively analyze a target object through band color development. This does not need to be matched with special equipment, can be used to detect many kinds of samples, and can be performed by a single person. This method is mainly used for pregnancy testing and rapid detection of infectious diseases. It is particularly suitable for emergency, on-site, and home self-testing. Future directions of colloidal gold immunochromatography include quantification, improved sensitivity, multi-assay, and lessening the environmental impact.

14.2.2 Dry Chemical Technology

The biggest difference between "dry chemistry" and traditional "wet chemistry" (i.e., solution chemistry) is the media involved in the chemical reactions. In this method, the liquid in the sample to be tested is used as the solvent, which directly reacts with the dry powder reagent solidified on the carrier. Dry chemical technology has the advantages of requiring no reagent preparation and calibration, long-term stability, and usefulness for whole blood tests. It is widely used for the check of myocardial enzymes, liver function, kidney function, and routine blood tests.

14.2.3 Electrochemistry and Biosensor Technology

A biosensor is an analytical tool composed of a biometric element, a signal converter, and a signal amplification device. The new generation of POCT instruments uses biosensors, such as ion-selective electrodes, substrate-specific electrodes, and conductivity sensors. These sensors combine enzyme chemistry, immunochemistry, electrochemistry, and computer technology, to perform ultra-microanalysis of biological fluids, such as for the detection of basic blood gases, electrolytes, and metabolites. Biosensor technology is fast, sensitive, inexpensive, and easy to automate, and its detection equipment can be miniaturized. Since the advent of smartphones and other mobile devices, wearable biosensors have received considerable attention because of their potential to provide continuous, real-time physiological information through dynamic, non-invasive, or minimally invasive measurements. Simultaneously, multiple biosensing, microfluidic sampling, and delivery systems have been integrated, miniaturized, and combined with flexible materials to improve wear resistance and ease of operation.

14.2.4 Biochip Technology

Biochips enable the accurate, rapid, and high-throughput detection of DNA, RNA, polypeptides, proteins, cells, tissues, and other biological components, with great advantages in disease screening and early diagnosis. Biochip research has become a hot topic in laboratory medicine. It allows many items to be simultaneously measured on a small chip, thereby significantly improving the efficiency of analysis. Currently, biochips can be divided into gene, protein, or cell chips, as well as the lab-on-a-chip. They have the advantages of high sensitivity, short analysis time, and the ability to analyze many items simultaneously. Many analysis steps involved in life science research use microelectronics, micromechanics, physical technology, sensor technology, and computer technology to realize continuous, integrated, and miniaturized sample detection and analysis processes. They also have obvious advantages for the detection of infectious diseases, such as the integration of a portable low-cost customized detector and a novel detection platform with microporous array biochips.

14.2.5 Chemiluminescence Immunoassay Technology

Chemiluminescence immunoassays use specific immune responses. Combined with the high sensitivity of chemiluminescence, it has the advantages of high sensitivity, strong specificity, good precision, and a wide linear range. This has become an important non-isotope-labeled immunoassay method. This traditional test method has been greatly expanded and enriched by the miniaturization and portability concepts of POCT. Chemiluminescence POCTs can be used in some clinical application fields that demand high accuracy and quick turnaround, such as hospital ICU, emergency department, cardiology department, and chest pain centers. Furthermore, it can also be used in small and medium-sized hospitals, social health centers, and clinics to improve the efficiency of diagnosis. Chemiluminescent POCT products are well suited for use in the initial diagnosis of severe inflammatory infections, cardiovascular and cerebrovascular diseases, and rapidly monitoring changes in the clinical course. Domestic POCT manufacturers have also successively introduced chemiluminescent POCT instruments and reagents, which will become the key development direction of POCT detection technology in the future.

14.2.6 Microfluidic Technology

Microfluidic chip technology integrates basic operational units such as sample preparation, reaction, analysis, and detection, harnessing techniques from the fields of chemistry and biology into a chip of several square centimeters, automatically completing the entire analysis process. POCT instruments based on microfluidic technology have allowed further miniaturization and refinement, allowing quick, accurate, and high-throughput detection. Microfluidic technology has been applied in blood gas, biochemical diagnosis, immune diagnosis, molecular diagnosis, and other fields. Microfluidic chips have controllable liquid flow, consume minimal samples, and reagents, and offer from ten up to one hundred times faster analyses. Microfluidic technology allows simultaneous analysis of hundreds of samples in a few minutes or less, and online sample pretreatment and whole-process analysis can be realized, such as in the POCT detection of urinary tract infections (UTIs). Each chip can be used for multiple detection of bacteria to accelerate the diagnosis of UTIs. The entire process of chemical cell lysis, solid-phase DNA extraction, secondary washing, DNA elution, multiple loop-mediated isothermal amplification (LAMP), and real-time fluorescence detection can be completed in 100 min, and the concordance rate of bacterial detection can reach as much as 100% [1].

14.2.7 Infrared and Near-Infrared Spectrophotometry

Infrared and far-infrared spectrophotometries are commonly used in the manufacture of percutaneous detection instruments. They are convenient, rapid, noninvasive, nonpolluting, and inexpensive. Thus, they show great potential for application in medical tests. Within POCT, these technologies are commonly used for noninvasive blood glucose detection. Using near-infrared spectroscopy for blood glucose detection can avoid cross-infection and blood sample pollution caused by blood draw, reduce the cost of each test, and shorten the reporting time. However, its stability, accuracy, and sensitivity still require improvement.

14.2.8 Molecular POCT Technology

Molecular diagnosis is performed at the gene level with nucleic acids as the object for detection, with high sensitivity and accuracy. However, traditional nucleic acid detection processes are complex to operate and take a long time. Further, it needs to be partitioned independently in clinical laboratories to establish a standard molecular diagnostic laboratory, which is costly. As the technology has developed and clinical needs have been promoted, fully automatic and integrated molecular detection POCT platforms, based on a “sample in – result out” paradigm has emerged. Since 2020, molecular diagnostic POCT has received significant attention. Related products are mainly based on polymerase chain reaction (PCR), isothermal amplification, and other technologies that integrate complex nucleic acid detection steps into a system, greatly simplifying the process to hasten nucleic acid detection. For example, the US Food and Drug Administration (FDA) has approved the first CRISPR-based COVID-19 detection kit, which provides results in approximately 1 h, greatly shortening the detection time and improving the detection efficiency. Therefore, with the advantages of rapidity and convenience, molecular POCT has great application potential in screening, auxiliary diagnosis, and treatment guidance of infectious diseases, tumors, and other diseases.

14.2.9 POCT Mass Spectrometry Technology

Mass spectrometric analysis first ionizes substances, separates them according to the mass-to-charge ratio (m/z) of ions, and then measures the intensities of various ion peaks to achieve the purpose of analysis. Mass spectrometry is very suitable for qualitative and quantitative analyses of substances and it is one of the most powerful tools for the identification of pure substances. At present, most mass spectrometers used in China are large, expensive, and difficult to upgrade and maintain. In addition, the entire process, from sample pretreatment to mass spectrometric determination, is completed in the laboratory, which means that it cannot be used for clinical bedside detection. To meet the needs of mobile detection, on-site rapid detection, and cost reduction, the development of portable miniaturized mass spectrometers with on-site analysis and emergency detection capabilities has become a hot topic in the field of mass spectrometry. Multiple layers of filter paper have been used for liquid chromatography with LC-MS/MS to separate hormones and biological matrices, and mass spectrometry has been used for qualitative and quantitative analysis of three hormones: testosterone (T), androsterone (ADT), and androstenedione (4-AD). The multilayer PS-MS established by this method realizes rapid, simple, and reliable quantitative analysis of various hormones and provides a broad prospect for clinical analysis of small molecules in different biological samples [2].

Declaration Yaping Zhao, Xiaofang Wang and Jiaqi Zou are employees of Guangzhou Wondfo Biotech Co., Ltd.

Li Tian and Shan Guo are employees of Wuhan EasyDiagnosis Biomedicine Co., Ltd.

References

1. Li N, Lu Y, Cheng J et al. A self-contained and fully integrated fluidic cassette system for multiplex nucleic acid detection of bacteriuria[J]. Lab Chip. 2020; 20(2):384-393.
2. Wu T, Sun G, Ma M et al. Rapid quantitative analysis of serum hormones by multilayer paper spray MS: Free MS from HPLC. Talanta. 2022; 237:122900.

The POCT Market 15

Yaping Zhao, Xiaofang Wang, Jiaqi Zou, Li Tian, and Shan Guo

15.1 International Market Conditions

The POCT market is large and has enjoyed sound growth. From 2008 to 2018, the sales volume of the global POCT market doubled, with an average annual compound growth rate of 7.5%. The global POCT sales volume in 2019 was $24.3 billion. In 2020, the global POCT sales volume reached $29.32 billion. In 2021, the global POCT sales volume reached $31.5 billion. POCT testing worldwide can be divided into professional testing and self-testing. By 2025, the global market for POCT testing is expected to reach $45 billion (Fig. 15.1). For each segment, infectious disease testing accounts for the highest share of the market, excluding blood glucose testing. Simultaneously, an increase in new technology and demand also promotes market growth.

At present, there are large regional differences in the global POCT market. Developed countries, such as Germany, America, and Japan, are still the main battlefields of POCT. However, with economic growth and improvement in medical and health conditions, emerging countries such as China, Brazil, and India have further promoted the application of POCT in recent years. These countries have gradually become potential powers for the growth of the POCT market.

Y. Zhao · X. Wang (✉) · J. Zou
Guangzhou Wondfo Biotech Co., Ltd., Guangzhou, Guangdong, China
e-mail: xiaofang.wang@wondfo.com.cn

L. Tian · S. Guo
Wuhan EasyDiagnosis Biomedicine Co., Ltd, Wuhan, Hubei, China

H. Song, L. Dai (eds.), *In Vitro Diagnostic Industry in China*,
https://doi.org/10.1007/978-981-99-3110-1_15

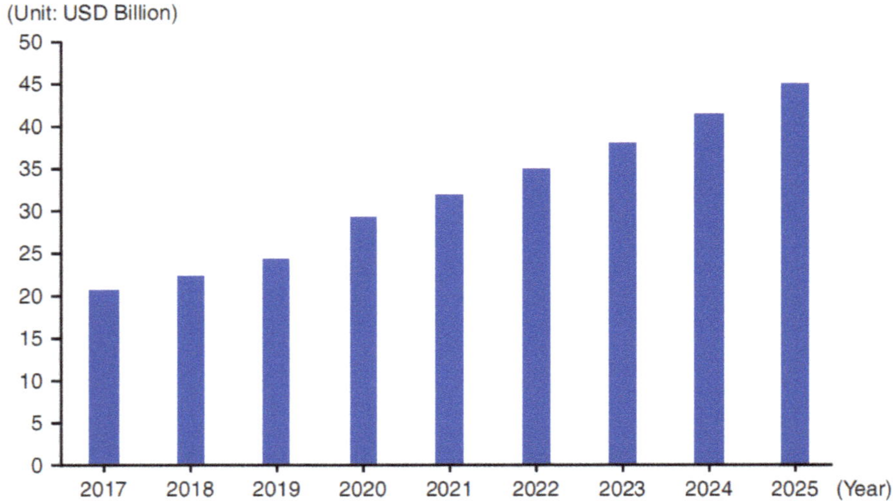

Fig. 15.1 POCT Sales in Global Markets (Unit: USD Billion)

15.1.1 Blood Glucose

The International Diabetes Federation (IDF) estimates that diabetes affects 536.6 million people worldwide, and the global prevalence of diabetes among people aged 20–79 is estimated to be 10.5% (536.6 million people) in 2021. Twenty years ago, there were only 30 million people worldwide suffering from diabetes. Due to the increase in unhealthy habits among people in developing countries, the prevalence of diabetes is expected to rise to 12.2% in 2045 (783.2 million people). In 2021, the global health expenditure related to diabetes was estimated at 966 billion US dollars and is expected to reach 105.4 billion US dollars by 2045 [1]. Diabetes is becoming a major public health challenge of the twenty-first century, particularly in developing countries. With the steady growth of patients with type 2 diabetes, increased public awareness of the disease, and the tilt of the health insurance reimbursement policy, blood glucose testing has continued to grow at a relatively high rate in recent years. In 2019, the global market capacity of POCT blood glucose tests was $13.42 billion, which increased by 15% in 2020. It is now estimated to be worth $15.434 billion in 2020, mainly due to the growth of the dynamic blood glucose test. Meanwhile, the market value of France, Russia, and other European countries is growing rapidly. The global POCT blood glucose test market is estimated to be worth $15.62 billion in 2021 and is expected to grow by $6.77 billion from 2021 to 2025—a growth of nearly 10%.

15.1.2 Cardiovascular Diseases (Cardiac Markers)

Cardiovascular disease remains the leading cause of death worldwide. Approximately 423 million adults worldwide suffer from cardiovascular diseases, of whom 18 million die each year. This causes cardiovascular disease to account for approximately 31% of annual global deaths [2]. More importantly, many cardiovascular events are not fatal but may be sufficient to reduce body function and seriously affect the quality of life. The global market for POCT for the detection of cardiac markers (CK-MB, troponin, myoglobin, and BNP) is estimated to be $686 million in 2019 and $731 million in 2020. At present, cardiac marker POCT is widely carried out in the medical systems of developed countries and is currently the main source of sales, with a relatively stable overall growth trend. Simultaneously, developing countries are a potential source of growth point that is expected to reach $955 million in 2025, with an annual growth rate of 5.5%.

15.1.3 Infectious Diseases

Infectious disease detection products include influenza, AIDS, syphilis, viral hepatitis, malaria, and *Helicobacter pylori*. The global market for infectious disease POCT testing is expected to reach $1.3 billion in 2019, with the largest numbers tested for influenza, hepatitis, HIV, Streptococcus A, and respiratory viruses. The global infectious disease POCT market is expected to reach $6025 million in 2020, and influenza testing is significantly affected by the demand for testing during the influenza season. From 2019 to 2020, the professional infectious disease detection market grew by approximately 368%. While the scale of household self-testing remains small, it is expected to experience rapid growth in 2021, making the POCT infectious disease self-testing market achieve a compound annual growth rate of 8.8% from 2020 to 2025.

15.1.4 Blood and Electrolytes/Coagulation

The boundaries between the POCT and laboratory-based systems for blood and electrolyte testing are somewhat blurred, and instruments can be used in multiple scenarios. The global blood and electrolyte market was $1956 million in 2019, compared to $2025 million in 2020 for blood and electrolyte testing. In the coagulation field, the global POCT coagulation test market in 2019 was $1026 million, while it was $845 million in 2020, with activated clotting time of whole blood (ACT) accounting for approximately $100 million. Routine blood tests and other non-life-threatening assessments are limited because of lockdowns, limited doctor/patient access, and patients' reluctance to seek medical treatment. Market growth is expected to be driven by the increased use of automated hematology instruments, increased penetration of the POCT testing market, and the introduction of innovative hematology instruments. However, market growth has slowed over the past few years because of economic difficulties in Europe and the highly cost-conscious US market.

15.1.5 Gestation Category

The most widely used professional and over the counter (OTC) patient self-tests for women's health are pregnancy and ovulation tests. OTC includes tests offered by pharmacies and other retail outlets. This field of POCT is relatively mature. The demand for pregnancy-related POCT products depends on the number of women with childbearing potential and the number of births. At present, the global population is approximately 7.7 billion, and the global birth rate is approximately 18.66‰, that is, the number of new births worldwide is approximately 140 million per year. According to the Kalarama Information, the global POCT pregnancy and childbirth test market generated $968 million in revenue in 2019. The global POCT pregnancy and fertility testing market generated $917 million in revenue in 2020 and is expected to grow to approximately $1025 million over the 2020–2025 forecast period, with a Compound Annual Growth Rate (CAGR) of 2.3%. The United States is the largest market for POCT pregnancy and fertility testing with 45%, Europe with 32%, Japan with 7.0%, and the rest of the world with 16.0%. POCT pregnancy and fertility self-testing are by far the largest source of sales with $795 million in 2020 with an average annual growth rate of 2.4%.

15.1.6 Substance Abuse Categories

Millions of dollars are spent annually on drug abuse testing worldwide. In 2019, POCT sales for drug abuse testing reached $3015 million, and a major factor contributing to the growth was the continued growth in illicit drug use worldwide, the emergence of new drugs of abuse, and the availability of high-quality, cost-effective drug abuse testing products. POCT sales for drug abuse testing reached $1351 million in 2020. The US market is the world's largest, accounting for approximately 56%. In the rest of the world, market conditions differ, with some countries, such as Australia and Japan, increasing drug abuse testing in the workplace, while others are experiencing an increase in illicit drug use, such as ecstasy use in South Africa, and increased injecting drug use in Pakistan, Egypt, and other African countries.

15.2 Market Status and Trends of Domestic Biochemistry Analyzers in China

The POCT industry in China started late. Currently, the industry is still in the early stages of development, with a small market size. Its permeation of clinical departments in hospitals is still low, especially in primary hospitals, where the occupancy of personal test equipment is still relatively small compared with the overall market size in developed countries such as Europe and America. However, benefiting from the rapid development of the domestic economy and continuous innovation in the medical system, the overall medical device market in China is rapidly developed. At present, three structural factors in China are expected to present opportunities to

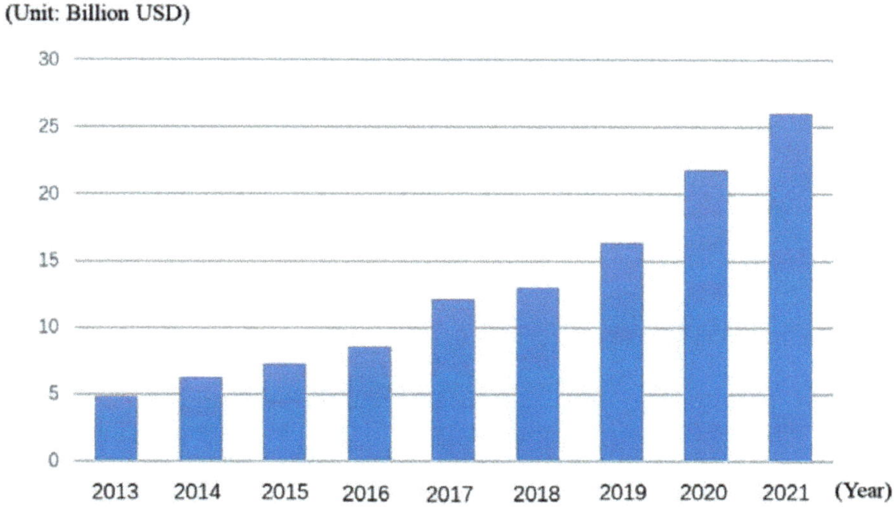

Fig. 15.2 China POCT market scale (Unit: Billion USD)

promote the increasing demands of the POCT industry. First, with the continuous deepening of medical reform, the number of primary medical institutions has increased, owing to the hierarchical diagnosis and treatment system, bringing about a large demand for rapid testing. Second, the population structure is gradually aging, and the increase in the number of patients with chronic diseases such as diabetes increases the demand for self-examination. Third, China is currently upgrading medical services overall, from simple medical care to accurate diagnosis, with personalized care as the core. Simultaneously, the domestic medical system has paid more attention to IVD since 2020, which also provides an opportunity for the development of domestic POCT enterprises. According to Frost & SullivanFrost's report, the market size of POCT in China was only $0.483 billion in 2013. With the progress of health reform and the increase in government investment in POCT products and technologies in primary healthcare, the market size in China reached $2.18 billion (¥14.4 billion) in 2020 and $2.6 billion (¥17.6 billion) in 2021 in China (Fig. 15.2).

At present, POCT is applicable to multiple kinds of detection, such as blood glucose, blood gas/electrolyte classification, cardiovascular, infectious disease, drug abuse, pregnancy, and other forms of detection. Considering growth rates from the perspective of subsectors, cardiac markers, and infectious disease POCT products are experiencing rapid growth, with rapid growth in demand and substantial potential for development in the future. This is because the timely rescue of cardiovascular patients is more important than for many other diseases, and POCT meets this requirement by offering fast detection speeds. Therefore, cardiovascular detection has become the fastest-developing application of POCT.

Infectious disease POCT is mainly a product for primary hospital on-site screening and rapid detection of various common and major infectious diseases, including HIV, syphilis, viral hepatitis, malaria, and influenza. Infectious diseases have attracted varying degrees of attention worldwide owing to their infectious, epidemic, regional, and seasonal characteristics. China has gradually strengthened the prevention and monitoring of major infectious diseases. POCT products have become important tools in related studies. Judging from the current market share, infectious and cardiac marker POCT accounts for the highest share of total products (except for blood glucose), followed by blood gas, pregnancy, and other rapid tests.

15.2.1 Blood Glucose

Currently, blood glucose detection is the largest and most mature segment of the domestic market. Glucose meters are widely used in clinical departments and families as the main detection instrument for blood glucose POCT. At present, the overall market for blood glucose monitoring systems in China is about ¥5 billion, but the market permeability is only 20%; compared with the 90% market permeability in developed countries, there remains huge potential for growth, even compared with the average global permeability level of 60%, and there is still great development potential. After preliminary estimation, the annual compound growth rate of the blood glucose POCT market in China will reach 18.72% from 2021 to 2026, and the market capacity will exceed $1.7 billion in 2026 according to the EqualOcean Forward-looking Industry Institute. Blood glucose POCT shows an increasing trend in China, which is mainly related to the increase in the number of diabetic patients in China and the increasingly improved management of patients with diabetes in China.

In 2019, the number of patients aged 20–79 years with diabetes in China reached 116 million, accounting for 25.1% of the global patient population, ranking first in the world for diabetes. The number of deaths due to diabetes has reached 834,000 per year, and the market size of glucometers in China reached ¥4.18 billion in 2019. According to the predictions of the IDF, by 2030 and 2045, there will be 141 million and 147 million patients with diabetes patients in China, accounting for 24.3% and 21.0% of the total number of patients in the world, respectively. According to Medii Research, the domestic market for blood glucose testing will reach ¥8.6 billion by 2025.

15.2.2 Cardiovascular Testing

According to the China Cardiovascular Report 2018, 290 million patients have cardiovascular disease in China. Since 2015, cardiovascular disease has remained the main cause of mortality, which is higher than tumors and other diseases. The age of onset of patients with heart failure also decreases annually. According to the China Cardiovascular Health and Disease Report 2019, the prevalence of cardiovascular disease is increasing, and cardiovascular disease has become a serious threat to human life and health. On November 1, 2017, the original National Health Committee Office issued the chest pain center construction and management guidelines (Trial) notice, requiring secondary general hospitals or related specialized hospitals to construct chest pain centers. The emergency department must simultaneously be able to carry out 24-h bedside electrocardiogram and echocardiography, troponin, D-dimer, and other rapid tests to issue medical quality control indicators for chest pain center. These indicators can be divided into basic and classification indicators. Basic indicators are applicable to all chest pain centers, including "time from blood draw to report acquisition for instant detection items such as troponin, D-dimer, brain natriuretic peptide, and blood gas analysis" and "proportion of combined detection of D-dimer and troponin." The establishment of chest pain centers has greatly increased the demand for POCT for the detection of cardiovascular diseases, prompting POCT manufacturers to launch solutions for chest pain centers.

According to the data of Intelligent Research Consulting, the domestic market size of cardiovascular POCT was ¥3.7 billion in 2019, and it is estimated that the market size will reach ¥4.8 billion in 2020, with a high-speed growth of approximately 30% within five years. The domestic cardiovascular POCT market grew faster than the global market, mainly because of the implementation of the domestic grading diagnosis and treatment policy, increased equipment procurement for primary hospitals, and accelerated construction of chest pain centers.

15.2.3 Infectious Diseases

With the increase in the frequency and harm of outbreaks of major infectious diseases, many countries have strengthened their prevention and monitoring efforts. POCT products have become powerful tools for the prevention and monitoring of infectious diseases. According to the Industry Survey of Infectious and Infective POCT in China in 2019, the market size of infectious POCT in China reached ¥3818 million in 2019, which is estimated to reach ¥4573 million in 2020.

The reasons for the rapid growth in the market size of the infectious POCT industry in China can be attributed to the following three aspects: the country has strengthened its emphasis on major infectious diseases, strengthened prevention and control efforts, and the need for emergency response time. Simultaneously, factors such as technological upgrades, graded diagnosis and treatment, and marketing channel integration also promote the development of the industry. In response to sudden infectious diseases, the POCT allows tests to be completed rapidly in different scenarios, providing the basis for clinical decision-making and epidemic prevention and control over time. In addition, POCT detection of inflammatory factors (such as PCT and CRP) can facilitate timely monitoring of the patient's condition and optimization of patient treatment plans, in addition to the differential diagnosis of the disease.

15.2.4 Blood Gas and Coagulation

Blood gas and electrolyte POCTs are mainly used in the diagnosis and treatment of acute respiratory failure, surgery, rescue, and monitoring processes. It is mainly used in critical care units, cardiac care units, operating rooms, and emergency rooms, meaning it has a very broad market. However, because it is mainly aimed at critically ill patients, tests arterial blood samples, and has high technical requirements, it has been monopolized by foreign brands such as Denmark's Redoubt, Abbott, Wolfen, and Roche, which limits the development of these products in China. As medical insurance cost control, graded diagnosis and treatment, and the core technological research of domestic manufacturers have developed in recent years, the share of domestic blood gas electrolyte POCT products has gradually increased. In 2019, the market size of blood gas POCT in China was approximately ¥1.4 billion, and it was estimated to be about ¥1.8 billion in 2020. Four coagulation items must be checked before surgery, as well as thrombotic examination items. Patients also need to be monitored for clinical oral anticoagulant drugs when undergoing important procedures, especially for critical illnesses, such as myocardial infarction (acute coronary syndrome) and stroke. The hemagglutination market is an IVD segment that has undergone rapid development in recent years, with a compound growth rate of up to 30%. Foreign-funded enterprises also have an absolute advantage in this field and are expected to account for more than 90% of the market share.

15.2.5 Gestation Category

Pregnancy detection products are mainly used for the prenatal and postnatal care of the population, including human chorionic gonadotropin (HCG), sex hormone, and thyroid-stimulating hormone detection methods.

The demand for pregnancy-related POCT products depends on the number of women with childbearing potential and the number of births. In 2019, the domestic birth rate was 10.5‰, i.e., the number of new births per year was 14.65 million, while the number of new births in 2020 was about 12 million, which had an impact on the pregnancy POCT market. With the promotion of the national maternity policy and women's increasing attention to their health and privacy protection needs, the home market of pregnancy POCT is expected to develop further.

15.2.6 Drug Testing Category

POCT products for drug (drug abuse) detection are mainly qualitative and used for urine or saliva detection. It is widely used in drug rehabilitation centers, hospitals, military conscription, customs border checks, highway traffic safety in areas with high-risk populations, special industries, and recruitment for physical examination screening work. According to the 2019 China Drug Situation Report, the drug abuse situation in China continued to improve in 2019. By the end of 2019, China had 2.148 million drug addicts, accounting for 0.16% of the country's total population, which is a decrease of 10.6% for the second consecutive year. The number of abusers of the three main drugs of abuse, namely, heroin, methamphetamine, and ketamine, decreased. However, with increasingly stringent drug testing in China, the demand for POCT products will increase in the future.

Declaration Yaping Zhao, Xiaofang Wang and Jiaqi Zou are employees of Guangzhou Wondfo Biotech Co., Ltd.

Li Tian and Shan Guo are employees of Wuhan EasyDiagnosis Biomedicine Co., Ltd.

References

1. Sun H, Saeedi P, Karuranga S, et al. IDF Diabetes Atlas: Global, regional and country-level diabetes prevalence estimates for 2021 and projections for 2045. Diabetes Res Clin Pract. 2022 183:109119.
2. Dr Gregory Roth et al, "Global, regional and national burden of cardiovascular diseases for 10 causes, 1990 to 2015", J Am Coll Cardiol. 2017; 70(1):1-25.

Major Manufacturers in China

16

Yaping Zhao, Xiaofang Wang, Jiaqi Zou, Li Tian,
and Shan Guo

16.1 Guangzhou Wondfo Biotech Co., Ltd.

Wondfo is one of the leading POCT enterprises in China and specializes in R&D, manufacturing, marketing, and services for rapid diagnostic reagents and supporting instruments. Wondfo currently has platforms such as immune colloidal gold, immunofluorescence, electrochemical, dry biochemical, chemiluminescence, molecular diagnosis, pathological diagnosis, instrument, and biological raw material. Relying on these nine technology platforms, there have formed a rich product line in the fields of cardiovascular and cerebrovascular diseases, inflammation, cancer, infectious diseases, drug abuse, genetic screening, and other testing fields. Their products are sold to more than 140 countries and regions worldwide. They are widely used in clinical laboratories, critical illnesses, primary medical care, epidemic surveillance, disaster rescue, on-site law enforcement, family and personal health management, and other fields.

16.2 Wuhan EasyDiagnosis Biomedicine Co., Ltd.

This is a national high-tech enterprise specializing in providing IVD reagents and supporting instruments, including POCT, molecular diagnosis, chemiluminescence, and blood gas analysis products. Further, they provide medical services such as emergency and critical treatment integration (including chest pain, stroke, and trauma centers), PCR laboratories, the construction of intelligent fever outpatient services. Mingde Biology has successively passed the European Union CE and

Y. Zhao (✉) · X. Wang · J. Zou
Guangzhou Wondfo Biotech Co., Ltd., Guangzhou, Guangdong, China
e-mail: ypzhao@wondfo.com.cn

L. Tian · S. Guo
Wuhan EasyDiagnosis Biomedicine Co., Ltd., Wuhan, Hubei, China

H. Song, L. Dai (eds.), *In Vitro Diagnostic Industry in China*,
https://doi.org/10.1007/978-981-99-3110-1_16

ISO13485 quality management system certifications and has more than 30 POCT rapid diagnostic reagent products registered with NMPA (National Medical Products Administration). They have also realized the rapid bedside detection of procalcitonin and S100-β protein in whole blood. Their projects cover many fields, such as cardiovascular and cerebrovascular diseases, infectious diseases, nephropathy, diabetes, physical examination, and obstetrics and gynecology, making them an enterprise with rich POCT product lines in China.

16.3 Getein Biotech, Inc.

This company focuses on research and development, production, sales, and service of IVD products. It has a professional diagnostic product research and development team; and has successively established seven technological platforms, including colloidal gold immunochromatography, fluorescence immunochromatography, biochemistry, chemiluminescence, and diagnostic raw materials.

16.4 Shanghai Upper Biotech Co., Ltd.

Upper Biotech was the first to publish two industry-academic monographs in China: real-time and intelligent real-time inspections. They promoted the introduction of the national standard GB/T29790–2013 Requirements for Instant Detection Quality and Capability, and have built five core technology platforms with nearly 100 independent intellectual property rights, including "digital biological information image detection, automatic batch loading for multitype samples, micro-blood quantitative inspection, time-resolved fluorescence, and ion homogeneous phase calibration technologies." This led to the development of effective identification of bacterial and viral serum amyloid A protein quantitative real-time detection kits.

16.5 ReLIA Biotech (Shenzhen) Co., Ltd.

The company has two series of bedside rapid detection systems: a multifunctional immune detection system and an immunofluorescence rapid detection system. The detection areas include rapid cardiovascular disease, acute kidney injury, and inflammatory response rapid detection series.

16.6 Shanghai Chemtron Biotech Co., Ltd.

With monoclonal antibody technology, immunofluorescence, and microfluidic technology, there are committed to research the localization of IVD. At present, they have more than 40 products in seven series, including drug, tumor, infectious disease, cardiovascular disease, and hormone detection, and equipment such as gold standard quantitative instrument, immunofluorescence analyzer, and reagent integration, which are registered trademarks of "Kaichuang Biology" and "Chemtrue®."

16.7 ACON Biotech (Hangzhou) Co., Ltd.

This company has successfully developed more than 100 kinds of rapid diagnosis products, such as the AICO series blood glucose meter, urine analyzer, dry biochemical analyzer, hemoglobin analyzer, blood lipid analyzer, and other medical devices and corresponding detection reagents, such as PCR detection, enzyme-linked immunosorbent assay, or colloidal gold detection reagents.

16.8 Blue Cross Bio-Medical (Beijing) Co. Co., Ltd.

In 1990, Blue Cross first proposed and introduced the concept and method of "*in vitro* rapid detection." From 1991 to 1995, it established a practical model of first- and second-generation rapid detection products in China, introduced the first standardized commercial batch-produced product, namely, early pregnancy detection reagents, and created the first rapid detection product in China, namely "Verification Regulation for Early Pregnancy Manufacturing." In recent years, the company has expanded its product field rapidly, and successfully occult blood, developed and produced more than 20 products with nearly 100 specifications in six series, including reproduction, drugs, infectious diseases, tumor markers, venereal diseases, and food safety transgenesis, obtaining four new drug certificates from the China SFDA and 11 medical device certificates.

16.9 Beijing Hotgen Biotech Co., Ltd.

Beijing Hotgen has constructed eight technological platforms: an IVD reagent bioactive raw material, sugar chain abnormal protein detection (sugar capture), magnetic particle chemiluminescence, up-conversion luminescence, colloidal gold immunochromatography, enzyme-linked immunosorbent assay, molecular diagnosis, and instrument research and development technology platforms, forming a closed-loop system for IVD research, development, and production.

16.10 W.H.P.M Bioresearch & Technology Co., Ltd.

This company has passed the ISO 9001 and ISO 13485 international quality management system certifications. Its main products, pregnancy, ovulation, and mock drug test strips, have been certified by CE in Europe and the FDA in the United States.

16.11 InTec PRODUCTS, Inc. (Xiamen)

InTec has successfully developed diagnostic products such as enzyme-linked immunosorbent assay, colloidal gold, clinical biochemical, and blood type detection reagents, as well as medical devices and corresponding reagents, such as Yi Jie series blood glucose meters, dry biochemical analyzers, and hemoglobin analyzers.

16.12 Goldsite Diagnostics Inc.

This company offers products including immune-specific protein detection reagents (IgA, IgG, IgM, anti-streptococcal hemolysin O, rheumatoid factor, complement C3, complement C4, C1 inactivation factor, KAP light chain, and LAM light chain assay kits), and cardiovascular disease assay kits (D-dimer, apolipoprotein A1, apolipoprotein B, N1AT3 antithrombin III, N1 PAB prealbumin, ALB albumin, and lipoprotein (a) assay kits).

16.13 Micropoint Diagnostics Inc.

This company offers products including its Ngabs dry fluorescent immunoassay analyzer (D-Dimer, BNP, NT-proBNP, PCT, TNI, and Cardiac Panel 3), qLabs PT/INR monitoring system (with Bluetooth function) (Microfluidic POCT rapid detection expert), and mLabs Immunofluorescence platform.

16.14 Hipro Biotechnology Corp.

The main products of this company are an automatic detection platform and 48 projects that support diagnostic reagents. The company's products have passed the European Union CE certification and obtained 70 authorized patents, including more than 10 invention patents, 51 NMPA registration certificates, and 26 registered items.

16.15 Guangzhou Tebsun Bio-Tech Development Co., Ltd.

The products developed by the company cover immune tests for cardiovascular disease, infectious inflammation, renal function, gynecology, and pediatrics.

16.16 Lifotronic Technology Co., Ltd. (Macau)

This company has developed clinical department treatment solutions such as bedding for major surgery, internal medicines, obstetrics and gynecology, skin beauty, and home treatment products and solutions.

16.17 Zhejiang Orient Gene Biotech Co., Ltd.

At present, Orient Gene primary products are instant diagnostic reagents for POCT, which are mainly used in the fields of infectious disease, drug, prenatal and postnatal care, tumor markers, and myocardial marker detection. Among these, infectious disease and drug detection are their two core product lines.

Declaration Yaping Zhao, Xiaofang Wang and Jiaqi Zou are employees of Guangzhou Wondfo Biotech Co., Ltd.

Li Tian and Shan Guo are employees of Wuhan EasyDiagnosis Biomedicine Co., Ltd.

Part VI

Diagnosis of Blood and Body Fluids

Blood Coagulation Analyzer and Reagents

17

Zuojun Zou, Yanshang Ma, Qifan Tian, Hai Wang, Chonghui Ding, and Jiahong Zhang

17.1 Overview of Domestic Blood Coagulation Market

Conventional thrombosis and hemostasis diagnostic applications are mainly concentrated on screening for bleeding disorders and diagnosis of bleeding origins, with a relatively narrow scope of application and relatively poor accuracy. Modern in vitro thrombosis and hemostasis diagnostic technology can be applied in multiple aspects, such as screening, monitoring, diagnosis, and treatment, with greater targeting and accuracy, and can remind patients to take preventive treatment in advance based on their conditions, meanwhile, it can also assist physicians in formulating more accurate diagnosis and treatment plans for patients, thereby improving the level of thrombosis diagnosis and treatment in hospitals and reducing treatment expenses for patients.

As indicated in the *Feasibility Study Report on* in Vitro *Thrombosis and Hemostasis Diagnostic Market in China 2020–2024* released by NewSijie Industry Research Center, compared with developed countries such as Europe and the United States, the in vitro thrombosis and hemostasis diagnostic market in China has been developed for a relatively short period of time with low penetration rate and is now in a period of rapid growth. During 2015–2019, the average compound annual growth rate of the in vitro diagnostic market size of thrombosis and hemostasis in China was 24.8%; in 2019, the in vitro diagnostic market size of thrombosis and hemostasis in China was RMB 6.47 billion, an increase of 17.4%; it is expected that by 2024, the in vitro diagnostic market size of thrombosis and hemostasis in China will reach about RMB 13.65 billion [1].

Z. Zou · Y. Ma · Q. Tian (✉)
Beijing Strong Biotechnologies, Inc., Beijing, China
e-mail: tianqifan@bsbe.com.cn

H. Wang · C. Ding · J. Zhang
Beijing Succeeder Technology, Inc., Beijing, China

H. Song, L. Dai (eds.), *In Vitro Diagnostic Industry in China*,
https://doi.org/10.1007/978-981-99-3110-1_17

The coagulation test accounts for over 95% of the domestic thrombosis and hemostasis in vitro diagnostic market share, with major overseas manufacturers such as Stago, Werfen, and Sysmex holding over 80% of the domestic market share. The three giants in the thrombosis and hemostasis diagnostics market, Sysmex from Japan (Sysmex Group), Instrumentation Laboratory (IL, Werfen Group), and Stago from France (Stago Group), have a total market share of about 66%. The coagulation instruments used in the domestic grade III market are still mainly imported, besides the above three, there are also Sekisui from Japan, BE from Germany, etc. Among domestic thrombosis and hemostasis diagnostic companies in China, Shanghai Sunbio, Succeeder, and Mindray as well as new entrants in the field of blood coagulation such as BSBE (BEIJING MDC) hold a relatively small but increasing market share year by year.

In the domestic in vitro thrombosis and hemostasis diagnostic market, foreign companies such as Sysmex, Stago, and IL have taken the absolute lead with their technology and first-mover advantage, and cover most of the Grade III hospitals in China. Domestic brands are primarily targeting Grade II hospitals while covering primary care institutions, private hospitals, and continuously breaking through to Grade III hospitals.

To sum up, in the future, with the increase in the number of installed domestic coagulation instruments, the localization rate of in vitro thrombosis and hemostasis diagnostic instruments in China will further rise and boost the sales of domestic in vitro thrombosis and hemostasis diagnostic reagents and consumables. The share of domestic brands in the in vitro thrombosis and hemostasis diagnosis market in China is also expected to increase gradually.

17.2 Current Conditions of Blood Coagulation Analyzers and Reagents in China

As indicated by the release of the *China Cardiovascular Health and Disease Report 2019*, the current number of cardiovascular patients is 330 million and is still on the rise [2]. Moreover, cardiovascular disease continues to be the leading factor in mortality, with two out of every five deaths resulting from cardiovascular disease. Thrombosis is the most critical factor resulting in cardiac, cerebral and peripheral vascular events, as well as a direct cause of death or disability. In terms of prevention, diagnosis, and prognosis of thrombotic disorders, testing of coagulation items is particularly important.

To better understand the current market use of coagulation at all levels in China, a study has been performed at hospitals of different levels. The study mainly consists of two parts: The first part is to research the use of instruments at medical institutions of different levels (mainly Grade II hospitals) (hereinafter referred to as "basic research"), with the aim of understanding the preferences of hospitals at different levels in terms of instrument selection. In the basic research, a total of 80

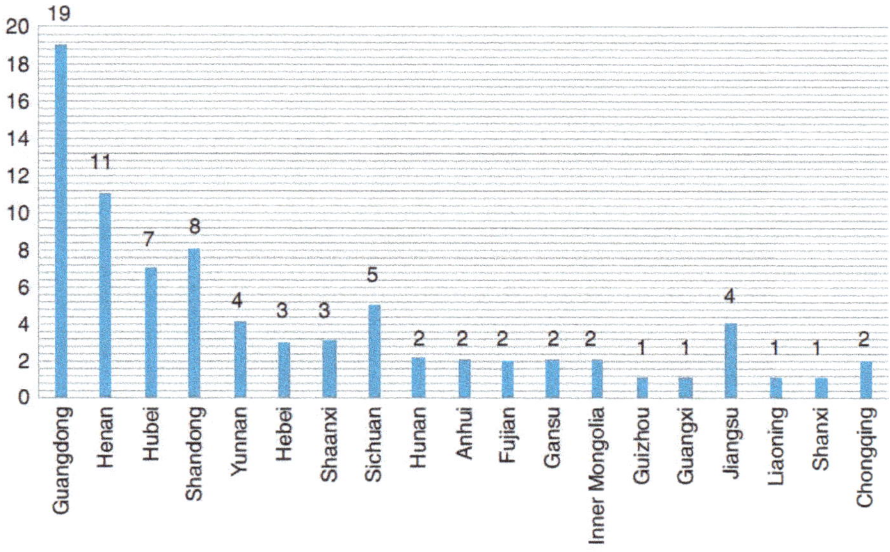

Fig. 17.1 Number of hospitals participating in the study by provincial regions

hospitals were surveyed, with 65% of the hospitals below Grade III Level A, from 19 provincial regions, including Guangdong, Henan, and Hubei (Fig. 17.1), including 28 Grade III Level A hospitals, 11 Grade III Level B hospitals, 2 Grade III Level C hospitals, 33 Grade II Level B hospitals, and 6 Grade I Level A hospitals.

The second part mainly focuses on large domestic Grade III Level A hospitals. Given that routine coagulation programs are now relatively common in China, and there may be significant differences in terms of the implementation of some new programs, a total of 13 top Grade III Level A hospitals in China were selected for the study of other coagulation programs (hereinafter referred to as "new program study"), involving Beijing, Shanghai, Tianjin, etc.

17.2.1 Blood Coagulation Analyzers

Coagulation analyzers are mainly applied for laboratory tests of thrombosis and hemostasis, which can provide valuable indicators for the diagnosis and differential diagnosis of hemorrhagic and thrombotic diseases, detection, and efficacy of thrombolytic and anticoagulant therapy [3]. To date, the development of coagulation analyzers has undergone five major stages: initial manual method, current method, dual magnetic circuit magnetic bead method, optical turbidimetric method, and optical electromagnetic bead method. Currently, different types of coagulation devices available on the market employ different principles. The mainstream detection methods include coagulation, substrate chromogenesis, immunoassay, latex agglutination, etc.

17.2.1.1 Brand Research and Analysis on the Use of Blood Coagulation Analyzers in Different Medical Institutions

According to the results of the basic research (Fig. 17.2), different medical institutions have selected different imported and domestic brand instruments: 38 domestic and 58 imported. The general trend is still dominated by imports; however, it is gratifying to note that the gap between domestic and import ratios is gradually decreasing. Among the medical institutions studied (Fig. 17.3), it has been found that the proportion of domestic production in Grade III Level A hospitals is also on the rise. The reasons for this include: On one hand, the progress of domestic instruments and the enhanced marketing efforts brought about by the optimistic market, while the state also encourages the use of domestic instruments; on the other hand, the higher quality of operation of medical and nursing staff in Grade III Level A hospitals and the ability to control the quality.

The instruments employed by hospitals participating in the basic study were mainly from various manufacturers such as Sysmex, Stago, Werfen, Sekisui, Beckman, Mindray, Succeeder, BSBE (BEIJING MDC), and Rayto, involving 96 instruments, of which 11 hospitals used instruments from two manufacturers, with

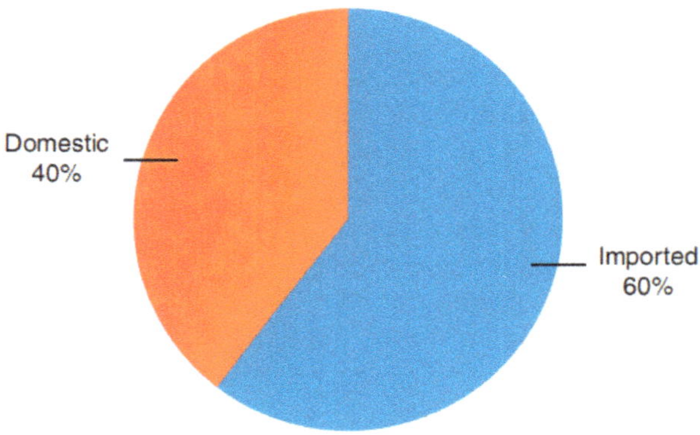

Fig. 17.2 Ratio of domestic and import products at hospitals of different levels

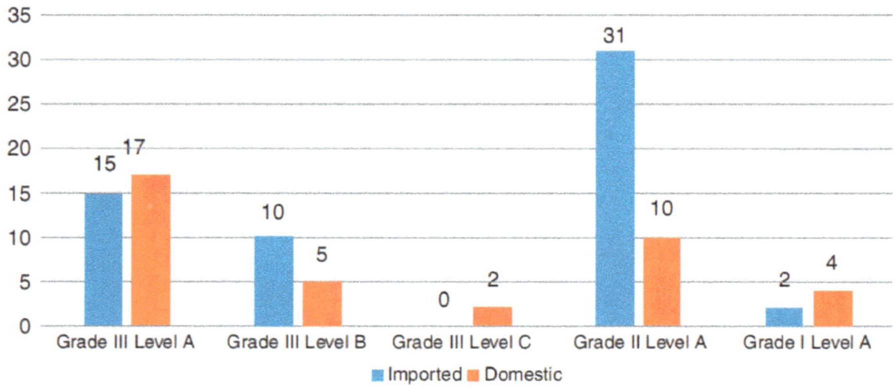

Fig. 17.3 Preferences of hospitals at different levels in selecting instruments

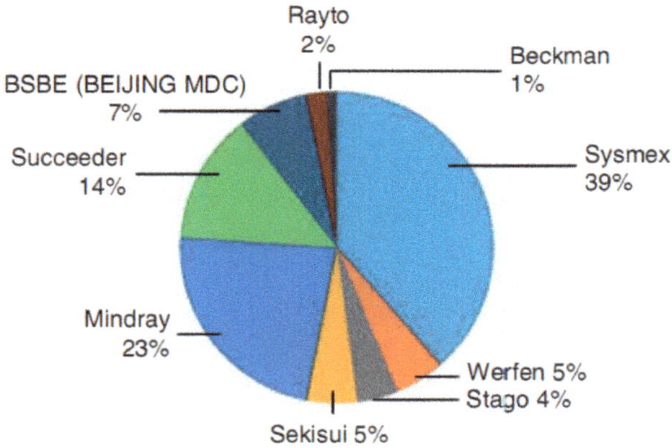

Fig. 17.4 Research on use of blood coagulation analyzers in hospitals

the use of each brand of blood coagulation analyzers shown in Fig. 17.4. As shown from the figure, among the hospitals participating in the study, the proportion of hospitals using Sysmex instruments was 39%, the proportion of those using Mindray was 23%, followed by 14% for Succeeder and 7% for BSBE (BEIJING MDC), indicating that the domestic instruments have been recognized by hospitals to a certain extent. Among the 80 hospitals participating in the study, 75 hospitals had used the corresponding matching reagents, while 5 hospitals had chosen reagents of noninstrument brands; in terms of the selection of consumables, 74 hospitals used matching consumables, indicating that these hospitals preferred to choose the original matching reagents and consumables, with the reason being that the selection of matching reagents and consumables could largely ensure the suitability between the items and the instruments. However, the use of noninstrument brand reagents and consumables signifies that due to the cost pressure of imported reagents and the advocacy of national policies, some hospitals are prepared to choose manufacturers with reliable quality and cost advantages, such as Shanghai Sunbio and BSBE.

17.2.1.2 Registration of Instruments in Recent 2 Years

China has been engaged in the R&D and manufacturing of semi-automatic coagulation analyzers for nearly 10 years, and based on the data from the website of the National Medical Products Administration (hereinafter referred to as the NMPA), in 2019 and 2020, a total of 11 instruments from 6 manufacturers have obtained registration certificates for semi-automatic coagulation analyzers (Table 17.1).

With the development of science and technology, domestic manufacturers have gradually progressed toward fully automated coagulation analyzers. Since 2010, domestic manufacturers in China have been continuously applying for approval of the registration certificate for fully automated coagulation analyzers. According to the latest NMPA data, by the end of 2020, over 30 instruments by 18 manufacturers had obtained registration certificates for fully automated coagulation analyzers (Table 17.2), basically covering coagulation, chromogenic substrate, and immunoturbidimetric methods. The R&D and production of fully

Table 17.1 New semi-automatic coagulation analyzers in 2019 and 2020

Serial No.	Enterprise name	Instrument registration certificate	Instrument model	Approval time
1	Shenzhen Rayto Life and Analytical Sciences Co., Ltd.	Yue Xie Zhu Zhun 20,192,220,959	RT-2204C, RT-2202C	September 2019
2	Jinan Hanfang Medical Devices Co., Ltd.	Lu Xie Zhu Zhun 20,192,220,877	HF6000–4	December 2019
3	Nanjing Ruimai Technology Development Co., Ltd.	Su Xie Zhu Zhun 20,202,220,129	AY8001, AYW8002, AYW8003	January 2020
4	Taizhou Steellex Biological Technology Co., Ltd.	Su Xie Zhu Zhun 20,202,220,327	SC20	March 2020
5	Shenzhen Caretium Medical Instruments Co., Ltd.	Yue Xie Zhu Zhun 20,152,220,866	XN-2	October 2020
6	Shenzhen Sinothinker Technology Co., Ltd.	Yue Xie Zhu Zhun 20,172,400,490	SK5001, SK5002, SK5004	November 2020

Table 17.2 New automatic coagulation analyzers in 2019 and 2020

Serial No.	Enterprise name	Instrument registration certificate	Instrument model	Approval time
1	Shandong Accurdx Biological Technology Co., Ltd.	Lu Xie Zhu Zhun 20,192,220,031	GW-3000	January 2019
2	Ningbo Reebio Biological Technology Co., Ltd.	Zhe Xie Zhu Zhun 20,192,220,077	ACA-1000	February 2019
3	Wuhan King Diagnostic Technology Co., Ltd.	E Xie Zhu Zhun 20,192,222,690	BCA-700, BCA-710	June 2019
4	Beijing Strong Biotechnologies, Inc.	Jing Xie Zhu Zhun 20,192,220,555	MDC3500	September 2019
5	Hunan Housheng Medical Devices Co., Ltd.	Xiang Xie Zhu Zhun 20,192,220,848	MRX-auto 400	September 2019
6	Hunan Housheng Medical Devices Co., Ltd.	Xiang Xie Zhu Zhun 20,192,220,859	MRX-auto 500	October 2019
7	Zhongshan Biogentech Co., Ltd.	Yue Xie Zhu Zhun20182400655	S2000, S1000	February 2020
8	Hunan Hailu Biological Technological Co., Ltd.	Xiang Xie Zhu Zhun 20,202,220,657	HL660	March 2020
9	SysCan Medical Technology Co, Ltd.	Su Xie Zhu Zhun 20,202,220,314	Ci-120i, ci-120n, ci-120x, Ci-120	March 2020
10	Wuhu 3H Biotechnology Co., Ltd.	Wan Xie Zhu Zhun 20,202,220,127	TH-7022, TH-7011	March 2020
11	Chengdu Excelen Medical Technology Co., Ltd.	Chuan Xie Zhu Zhun 20,152,220,052	EC6800, EC6800P	April 2020
12	Taizhou Steellex Biological Technology Co., Ltd.	Su Xie Zhu Zhun 20,192,220,876	AC800, AC200, AC100	June 2020

Table 17.2 (continued)

Serial No.	Enterprise name	Instrument registration certificate	Instrument model	Approval time
13	Medicalsystem Biotechnology Co., Ltd.	Su Xie Zhu Zhun 20,202,220,907	MS-T1550, MS-T1560, MS-T1580	July 2020
14	Maccura Biotechnology Co., Ltd.	Chuan Xie Zhu Zhun 20,152,220,117	H2600	July 2020
15	Changde Pushkang Biotechnology Co., Ltd.	Xiang Xie Zhu Zhun 20,202,221,399	HMC500	August 2020
16	Dirui Medical Technology Co., Ltd.	Ji Xie Zhu Zhun 20,202,220,318	BCA-3000	August 2020
17	Hunan Ultra-Diagnostics Biotec. Co., Ltd.	Xiang Xie Zhu Zhun 20,202,221,682	UD-C2000, UD-C2100	November 2020
18	Zhejiang Pushkang Biological Technology Co., Ltd.	Zhe Xie Zhu Zhun 20,182,400,151	MC500	December 2020
19	Zhejiang Pushkang Biological Technology Co., Ltd.	Zhe Xie Zhu Zhun 20,202,220,770	MC510, MC550	December 2020
20	MD Pacific (Tianjin) Biotechnology Co., Ltd.	Jin Xie Zhu Zhun 20,192,220,115	TSA8000, TSA9000C	December 2020

automated coagulation devices signify that China has made significant progress in automation and is actively catching up with the pace of mainstream manufacturers.

17.2.1.3 Opportunities and Challenges for the Development of Domestic Blood Coagulation Analyzers

In 2019–2020, restrictions on import and export have affected the use of imported devices to a certain extent, making them unavailable in a timely manner. At this point, the advantages of the supply chain of national brands have emerged. Regardless of instruments, reagents, or consumables, domestic manufacturers are able to satisfy the demands of users and supply them in a timely manner, providing great convenience to users and bringing new opportunities for the development of domestic blood coagulation analyzers.

Meanwhile, however, certain challenges have been posed to the development of domestic blood coagulation analyzers in the recent 2 years. Due to the specificity of the testing methodology, the construction, optical and mechanical components of the instrument are relatively demanding, and the quality of domestic brand instruments is still subject to improvement. Furthermore, there is still a gap between domestic supporting testing reagents in terms of the variety of testing items, the rate of self-production, etc. of raw materials, and imports. This has posed new requirements for manufacturers and suppliers of domestic blood coagulation analyzers.

17.2.2 Blood Coagulation Reagents

Thrombotic diseases, in particular cardiovascular and cerebrovascular thrombotic diseases, have become the top cause of death in the population of China, and their incidence has increased, seriously endangering human health [4]. The rapid advances in thrombosis and hemostasis research have contributed to an improved understanding of the pathogenesis of thrombotic disorders, thereby promoting advances in experimental diagnostic techniques for thrombotic disorders [5]. Coagulation testing is a process in which a series of enzymatic reactions are performed in vitro to simulate the transformation of fibrinogen into fibrin in vivo, with the aim of assessing the systemic functions of coagulation, fibrinolysis and anticoagulation in humans.

17.2.2.1 Test Methods

The current test methods for blood coagulation reagents include coagulation, chromogenic substrate, and immunoassay.

Coagulation: Coagulation refers to the conversion of soluble fibrinogen into insoluble fibrin by activating or mimicking the human coagulation system, so as to complete plasma coagulation, a process that causes changes in optical or mechanical properties. The routine four items (PT, APTT, TT, and FIB) are representative items of the coagulation assay.

Chromogenic Substrate Method: Chromogenic substrate method, also known as a biochemical method, aims to calculate the content or activity of the measured substance by measuring the change in absorbance of the color-producing substrate. AT, PC, t-PA, PAI, etc. are representative items of the chromogenic substrate method.

Immunoassay method involves latex agglutination, immunoturbidimetric method, enzyme-linked immunosorbent assay, colloidal gold colorimetric assay, etc.

1. Latex agglutination method: Latex agglutination method refers to an indirect agglutination test using latex particles as the carrier, in which the antigen in the sample being examined interacts with the monoclonal antibody encapsulated on the latex particles to produce a flocculent precipitation reaction for qualitative or semi-quantitative determination. The method features simple operation, short detection time and is suitable for POCT, which is often applied as a screening test.
2. Immunoturbidimetric method: Immunoturbidimetric method consists of direct turbidimetric method and latex immunoturbidimetric method, however, the direct turbidimetric method features weak response signal and low sensitivity, and the latex turbidimetric method is being applied increasingly. The colloidal immunoturbidimetric method refers to the reaction of the antigen in the sample with monoclonal antibodies encapsulated on colloidal particles, which produces an increase in turbidity by agglutination, the rate of change of turbidity being proportional to the concentration of the antigen. The method features simple operation, fast response, high precision, and high interference resistance, and is widely used in D-dimer (D-D) and fibrin (pro) degradation products (FDP) applications.

3. Enzyme-linked immunosorbent assay (ELISA): ELISA refers to the combination of antigen and antibody in the samples, the addition of enzyme-labeled antibodies to constitute a complex, and then adding the substrate to show a color reaction, with the absorbance measured proportional to the amount of antigen in the samples. The method features high sensitivity and accurate quantification; however, the process is complicated and time-consuming and is not suitable for emergency use.
4. Colloidal gold colorimetric reaction method: Colloidal gold method refers to the monoclonal antibody adsorbed in a porous film and adhered to a plastic disk with a multilayer absorbent pad, and the specimen being examined is incorporated and combined with the antibody, and then the colloidal gold-labeled antibody is added to produce red intensity, and the red intensity is proportional to the antigen in the plasma. The method is convenient and rapid; however, the specificity of clinical application is not strong and the anti-interference ability is weak.

17.2.2.2 Clinical Test Items

Overview of Routine Coagulation Function Items

At present, the coagulation tests are mainly applied for the screening of thrombotic diseases and hemorrhagic diseases, and the routine six items are relatively common in clinical practice (Table 17.3), mainly including prothrombin time (PT), activated partial thromboplastin time (APTT), thrombin time (TT), fibrinogen (FIB), D-dimer (D-D), and fibrin (pro) degradation products (FDP) [6].

Coagulation tests are essential in the examination of patients prior to surgery. Understanding whether the coagulation function of the patient is defective or not can enable the surgeon to prepare accordingly in advance before the operation and avoid accidents as much as possible. Failure to perform the appropriate preoperative tests to identify coagulation deficiencies in patients is likely to result in intraoperative hemorrhage leading to surgical accidents and even death.

Based on the results of the basic study (Table 17.4), for the routine four items, the implementation rate of hospitals is greater than 93.75%, indicating that the routine four items are very common in China. The number of surgeries performed in Grade I as well as below Grade I hospitals is relatively low; therefore, coagulation testing is mostly applied for drug monitoring of thrombotic diseases. The huge base of elderly people and high cardiovascular and cerebrovascular morbidity in rural areas of China enables Grade I and below hospitals to obtain a relatively low market as well. In contrast, the other two of the conventional six items, D-D and FDP, exhibited some differences. Among them, 93.75% of the hospitals have performed D-D and only 32.50% of them have performed FDP, indicating that there is still a lack of knowledge of the clinical significance and application of FDP in these hospitals. The main manufacturers within the industry of the above items basically produce and sell or distribute the corresponding products, and the market competition is relatively intensive. Besides the regular six items, some hospitals have also performed other tests such as thromboelastography (TEG) (33.75%), corrective test (17.5%), hematology rheology (27.50%), and coagulation factors (3.75%).

Table 17.3 Profile of the six routine items

Item	Concept	Extend/raise	Shorten/lower
PT	All conditions of exogenous coagulation in vitro are simulated in vivo, and the time required for plasma clotting is measured. It is a common screening test for the exogenous coagulation system, and is also applied to the monitoring of oral anticoagulants such as oral warfarin.	• Congenital factor FII, FV, FVII, FX deficiency and hypofibrinogenemia/afibrinogenemia. • Acquired liver disease, vitamin K deficiency. • The presence of anticoagulant substances, oral anticoagulants, etc. in the blood circulation. • Primary hyperfibrinolysis, DIC, etc.	• Congenital FV hyperplasia. • Long-term use of oral contraceptives. • Hypercoagulable states and thrombotic disorders.
APTT	All conditions of endogenous coagulation are simulated in vitro, and the time required for plasma clotting is measured, so as to reflect whether the coagulation factors in the endogenous coagulation pathway are abnormal. It is one of the common screening indicators for the endogenous coagulation system, and is also serve as a monitoring indicator for heparin anticoagulation therapy	• Hemophilia A, B and FXI deficiencies with decreased levels of FVII, FIX, and partial vascular hemophilia. • Severe deficiencies of FI, FII, FV, FX, for example, severe liver disease, vitamin K deficiency, etc. • Primary or secondary hyperfibrinolysis. • Oral anticoagulants, heparin, etc. • Presence of pathological anticoagulants in the circulation, for example, anti-FVIII, FIX antibodies, lupus anticoagulants, etc.	• Hypercoagulable and thrombotic diseases, for example, DIC hypercoagulable phase (dynamic observation of APTT changes is conducive to the diagnosis of DIC), myocardial infarction, deep vein thrombosis, diabetic vasculopathy, nephrotic syndrome and hypertensive syndrome of pregnancy, etc.
TT	It serves as a screening indicator to reflect the abnormal conversion of plasma fibrinogen to fibrin and as a monitoring indicator for thrombolytic therapy	• Hypofibrinogenemia/afibrinogenemia, abnormal fibrinogenemia, acquired hypofibrinogenemia. • Increase in heparin or the presence of heparin-like anticoagulants, for example, heparin therapy, tumors, systemic lupus erythematosus, etc. • Primary or secondary hyperfibrinolysis (for example, DIC).	–

Table 17.3 (continued)

Item	Concept	Extend/raise	Shorten/lower
FIB	It reflects the presence of anticoagulation or hyperfibrinolysis in the common pathway and may be available as an indicator for monitoring thrombolytic therapy	A type of acute temporal protein, an increase of which is mostly a non-specific response: • Infections: Toxemia, pneumonia, subacute bacterial endocarditis, etc. • Aseptic inflammation: Nephrotic syndrome, rheumatic fever, rheumatoid arthritis, etc. • Pre-thrombotic status and thrombotic diseases: Diabetes, myocardial infarction, etc. • Malignant tumors. • Trauma, burns, surgical procedures, post-radiation therapy. • Others: Late pregnancy, gestational hypertension syndrome, etc.	• Primary fibrinogen reduction or structural abnormalities, for example, hypofibrinogenemia/ afibrinogenemia, abnormal fibrinogenemia, etc. • Advanced DIC, hyperfibrinolysis, fibrinogen reduction secondary to severe hepatitis and cirrhosis.
D-D [7]	It serves as an important indicator for screening for secondary hyperfibrinolysis, a specific molecular marker for active thrombosis in the body, as well as the most commonly used item for screening and aiding in the diagnosis of thrombophilia	• Pre-thrombotic status and thrombotic diseases: Plasma D-D is significantly elevated in active deep vein thrombosis and pulmonary embolism. • It serves as an important basis for early diagnosis of DIC and is a specific marker for secondary fibrinolysis. • Thrombolytic therapy monitoring: Increased plasma D-D within 2 days of thrombolysis following effective thrombolytic therapy for deep vein thrombosis. • D-D may also increase in cases of malignant tumors, severe hepatitis, etc.	–

(continued)

Table 17.3 (continued)

Item	Concept	Extend/raise	Shorten/lower
FDP	Increased plasma FDP is indirectly associated with hyperfibrinolytic activity and can serve as a screening indicator for fibrinolytic activity	• Prominent elevation: DIC, deep vein thrombosis, pulmonary infarction, acute promyelocytic leukemia, primary hyperfibrinolysis, thrombolytic therapy. • Mild elevation: Certain malignant tumors, kidney disease, liver disease, acute infections, post-traumatic and surgical procedures.	–

Table 17.4 Study on implementation of s coagulation items in hospitals

Item	PT	APTT	TT	FIB	D-D	FDP	TEG	Correction test	Blood rheology	Blood coagulation factor
Number of participating hospitals	78	79	76	75	75	26	27	14	22	3
Proportion (%)	97.50	98.75	95.00	93.75	93.75	32.50	33.75	17.50	27.50	3.75

17.2.2.3 Some Domestic Emerging Products

Emerging Blood Coagulation Products

The routine four items are usually used for preoperative examination, but they cannot specifically determine the cause of thrombosis and bleeding in patients [8]. With the continuous in-depth studies in the hemostasis and thrombosis, there is increasing demand for the testing of coagulation items. The existing six routine items cannot meet the clinical diagnosis of various thrombotic diseases, and there is an urgent need for new test items to supplement the existing testing menu. As a result, more and more new and valuable test indexes have been found (Table 17.5), which can escort the testing and diagnosis of thrombosis and hemostatic diseases [6].

New Blood Coagulation Items

In terms of the domestic IVD markets of hemostasis and thrombosis, the special testing items are gradually promoted and popularized in domestic medical institutions. The Grade III hospitals are carrying out test items selectively according to their professional needs. In order to understand the current implementation of new blood coagulation items, a survey is conducted in large Grade III Level A hospitals

Table 17.5 New indexes for detection of thrombosis and hemostasis

Item	English name	Concept	Clinical significance
Antithrombin	Antithrombin, AT	• AT is the most important anticoagulant in the plasma physiological inhibitor, which has an important role in maintaining the dynamic balance between coagulation and anticoagulation.	• Increased AT level: It occurs in the acute bleeding phases of hemophilia, leukemia, and aplastic anemia, requiring treatment with oral anticoagulants and progesterone. • AT deficiency: Acquired AT deficiency occurs in liver disease, nephrotic syndrome, prethrombotic and thrombotic diseases, cardiovascular and cerebrovascular diseases, DIC, sepsis, preeclampsia, major surgery, and drug effect (such as heparin therapy), etc.; hereditary AT deficiency.
Protein C	Protein C, PC	• PC is an important vitamin K-dependent physiological anticoagulant protein; after being converted into APC, it can inactivate FVa and FVIIa and inhibit blood coagulation.	• Hereditary PC deficiency. • Acquired PC deficiency: DIC, liver disease, malignancy, vitamin K deficiency, and acute respiratory distress syndrome. • Effects of oral anticoagulants. • PC: Ag and increased activity: Coronary heart disease, diabetes, nephrotic syndrome.
Protein S	Protein S, PS	• PS is a glycoprotein produced in the liver; it is dependent on vitamin K and can synergistically activate protein C to become activated APC, eliminate the protective effect of FXa on FVa and of FIXa on FVIIa and hydrolyze them, thereby exerting an anticoagulant effect.	• Acquired PS deficiency: Liver disease, vitamin K deficiency, acute respiratory distress syndrome, oral anticoagulants, oral contraceptives. • Hereditary PS deficiency.
Lupus anticoagulant	Lupus anticoagulant, LA	• LA is an immunoglobulin, most of which is IgG, and a few of which is IgM or a mixture of them. It mainly exerts its anticoagulation effect by binding to phospholipid complexes and inhibiting the coagulation reaction that occurs on the surface of phospholipids, and interfering with the phospholipid-dependent coagulation process.	Positive reactions often occur under the following circumstances: • Systemic lupus erythematosus, antiphospholipid syndrome, autoimmune disease, thrombotic disease, malignancy, immune thrombocytopenia, DIC. • Oral anticoagulants, heparin therapy.

(continued)

Table 17.5 (continued)

Item	English name	Concept	Clinical significance
Von Willebrand factor	Von Willebrand factor, vWF	• vWF is a multimeric macromolecule protein with multiple functional domains that bind to collagen, heparin, FVIII light chain, GPIb and GPIIb-IIIa, ristocetin, etc. it is used as a molecular marker of vascular injury.	• Diagnosis and classification of von Willebrand disease. • Thrombotic diseases: Ischemic cardiovascular and cerebrovascular disease, peripheral vascular disease, glomerular disease, uremia, diabetes, pregnancy-induced hypertension syndrome, etc. may cause a remarkable rise in vWF: Ag. • Acute phase reaction: vWF may rise significantly when suffering from rheumatoid disease, vasculitis, malignancy, and after organ transplantation and major surgery, etc.; it may also rise in pregnant women and newborns.
Thrombin-antithrombin complex	Thrombin-antithrombin complex, TAT	• The generated thrombin can quickly bind to AT in the plasma at 1:1, to produce inactive TAT complex, thereby regulating the intensity of blood coagulation reaction. The elevated plasma TAT concentration indicates that the thrombin concentration increases and AT is consumed in large quantities, the blood presents a hypercoagulable state, and the risk of thrombosis increases. TAT is one of the molecular markers of coagulation activation.	• Slightly elevated TAT: Prothrombotic state, acute myocardial infarction. • Dramatically elevated TAT: Thrombotic diseases, such as deep vein thrombosis, pulmonary embolism, acute leukemia, and some malignant tumors (for example, lung cancer, ovarian cancer, etc.) • Monitoring of thrombolytic therapy: If TAT is <6 μg/L 2 hours after thrombolytic therapy, it indicates successful thrombolytic therapy; and if TAT is >6 μg/L 36 hours after thrombolytic therapy, it indicates possible occurrence of coronary infarction.
Plasmin-antiplasmin complex	Plasmin-antiplasmin complex, PAP	• PAP is a complex formed by binding the generated plasmin to $\alpha 2$ anti-plasmin in a ratio of 1:1. It is an index reflecting the activation of fibrinolysis and the actual level of in vivo fibrinolysis more sensitively.	The increase in plasma PAP concentration suggests hyperfibrinolysis and increased risk of bleeding, which mainly occurs in: • DIC. • Monitoring of thrombolytic therapy. • Rheumatic immune diseases: Systemic lupus erythematosus, nephrotic syndrome, etc.

Thrombomodulin	Thrombomodulin, TM	• TM is synthesized and secreted by endothelial cells and has an important anticoagulant effect. The binding of TM to thrombin can accelerate the activation of PC greatly.	• Elevated TM: It may be caused by a variety of diseases involving vascular endothelial damage, such as diabetes, glomerular disease, systemic lupus erythematosus, disseminated intravascular coagulation, acute myocardial infarction, cerebral infarction, etc. • Decreased TM: TM deficiency.
Tissue plasminogen activator inhibitor complex (tPAIC)	Tissue plasminogen activator inhibitor complex, tPAIC	• tPAIC is a complex formed by t-PA (tissue plasminogen activator) and PAI-1 (plasminogen activator inhibitor-1) in a ratio of 1:1, which can comprehensively reflect the damages to the fibrinolytic system and vascular endothelial cells and is an important marker in the process of venous thrombosis to reflect the occurrence of fibrinolytic inhibition in the early stage.	The elevated tPAIC occurs under the following conditions: • DIC. • Vascular endothelial injury. • Various arterial thrombosis and venous thrombosis.

Table 17.6 Implementation of new items

Serial No.	Item	Implementation rate
1	vWF: Ag	100%
2	Anti-Xa	60%
3	PC/PS/fPS	80%
4	LA	80%
5	Four new test items for thrombosis (TAT, PAP, TM, and tPAIC)	40%
6	Coagulation factors (FVII, FIX, FXIII, etc.)	80%

in Beijing, Shanghai, Wuhan, Sichuan, Tianjin, etc., which involves the items such as vWF, anti-Xa, LA, PC, PS, fPS, etc. The survey mainly involves these items, the sample size, and the testing dosage forms, etc. in each hospital. The items are shown in Table 17.6.

According to the project survey results, the Sysmex and Werfen blood coagulation analyzers are mainly utilized in the hospitals, which are used together with their original reagents. For the surveyed project, the testing of von Willebrand factor has been carried out in all hospitals, and other test items are carried out in most hospitals. Since the target populations are different in the survey Grade III Level A hospitals, the test items are different; in addition, it also indicates that some test items of coagulation are not popularized in large hospitals, let alone in Grade II and below hospitals. In the future, they should be popularized clinically to further promote the development of the blood coagulation industry.

17.2.2.4 Domestic Substitution Trend

In the future, with the increasing aging population, the increasing incidence of chronic diseases such as cardiovascular and cerebrovascular diseases, the increasing number of operating tables, and the improvement of various diagnostic technologies, the expansion of thrombosis and hemostasis diagnostic markets will be jointly promoted. In recent years, with the implementation of the hierarchical diagnosis and treatment policy and the continuous promotion of related concepts such as community hospitals, the markets of medium and low-end blood coagulation analyzers will increase significantly. For a long time, the domestic brands are mainly used in Grade II and below hospitals; while the imported brands are mainly used in public Grade III hospitals. Since the end users are not sensitive to price, some excellent domestic brands that have met the clinical requirements with the performance even surpassing the imported brands have not thrown away the "domestic hat" and have no chance to compete fairly in the market. With the support of national policies and the technological progress of domestic brands, it will be conducive to the development and growth of domestic brands, and promote the import substitution of blood coagulation testing in Grade III hospitals.

17.2.3 Development of Domestic Coagulation Enterprises

17.2.3.1 Leading Domestic IVD Companies Have Paid More Attention to the Development of Blood Coagulation and Actively Expanded the Blood Coagulation Business Services

With the development of the blood coagulation industry, more and more IVD companies have joined it and actively expanded the related services.

- In 2006, Succeeder started to enter the coagulation testing market and launched the first set of domestic fully automated coagulation analyzer SF-8000, breaking the monopoly of imported products on the Chinese market.
- In 2012, Maccura began to enter the blood coagulation market and successively launched semi-automated and fully automated coagulation analyzers.
- On October 31, 2012, Mindray became the dominating shareholding company of Prismlab. On January 9, 2014, Mindray and Long Island Biotech reached an equity transfer to control Long Island. With the joining of Prismlab and Long Island Biotech, Mindray has owned a platform for the R&D, production and sales of thrombosis and hemostasis business, and expanded its IVD channels, catering to the ever-growing market trend for the detection of cardiovascular-related diseases.
- In 2016, Shenzhen Ultra-Diagnostics Biotec. Co., Ltd. was founded, specializing in the research and development, manufacturing, and sales of IVD instruments and supporting reagents, and dedicated to providing overall solutions for the thrombus and hemostasis diagnostic products.
- On October 31, 2016, Thalys, which owns the coagulation business, was listed on the Shanghai Stock Exchange.
- On May 2, 2017, BSBE acquired 100% equity in Beijing MDC. After Beijing MDC's joining, BSBE has a complete production line of coagulation analysis instruments and reagents, which is a supplement to the existing IVD system and forms a more complete production line, thereby offering better services to customers.
- In 2018, Wondfo launched an instant coagulation analyzer, which can detect routine four items plus ACT.
- In 2019, BSBE successfully launched the first set of domestic fully automated coagulation analyzer MDC3500, taking a solid step into the blood coagulation market.
- In 2019, Dirui successfully launched its first set of coagulation analyzer and supporting reagents, officially entering the coagulation analysis market.
- On July 24, 2020, Getein Biotech officially released the *Progress Announcement on the Proposed Acquisition of Partial Shares of Wuhan King Diagnostic Technology Co., Ltd. and Capital Increase*, to enter the segment of blood coagulation testing industry and start its business segment of coagulation testing.
- On August 6, 2020, Succeeder was officially listed on the Shanghai Stock Exchange STAR Market and became the first listed company of the coagulation industry in China.

17.2.3.2 Key Companies

According to the statistics of CACLP, there are more than 40 domestic manufacturers related to coagulation testing, some of which are shown in Table 17.7.

17.2.4 Existing Problems in the Blood Coagulation Industry and Influencing Factors

17.2.4.1 Implementation of in Vitro Diagnosis of Thrombosis and Hemostasis in the Chinese Market

After 2000, more and more hospitals are equipped with the blood coagulation analyzers, and carry out testing of four screening items (PT/APTT/FIB/TT) in the clinical laboratory, which are mainly used for screening and diagnosis of clinical bleeding risk, etc. to dramatically reduce the occurrence of intraoperative bleeding and postoperative complications. This brings the first round of rapid development of the in vitro diagnostic market for thrombosis and hemostasis in China.

After 2007, with the improvement of clinical academic awareness of thrombotic diseases, some test items of fibrinolysis and anticoagulation (D-D/FDP/AT) are gradually carried in Grade III hospitals; after 2012, these test items were gradually popularized in Grade II and below hospitals. The above diagnostic items can help doctors to control the risk of thrombosis in the diagnosis and treatment, reduce the risk of thrombosis in the post-operative populations, pregnant women, and patients with cardiovascular and cerebrovascular diseases, and promote the second development of the IVD market for thrombosis and hemostasis. After 2015, Grade III Level

Table 17.7 Some Chinese companies in the blood coagulation industry

Serial no.	Enterprise name	Instrument	Reagent
1	Beijing Strong Biotechnologies, Inc.	MDC3500, MDC7500, Teco5000, Teco3000, Teco1800	Four routine test items, D-D, FDP, AT, etc.
2	Shenzhen Mindray Biomedical Electronics Co., Ltd.	ExC810, ExC800, C3510, C3280, C3200, C3100, C2000-A, etc.	Four routine test items, D-D, FDP, AT
3	Beijing Succeeder Technology Co., Ltd.	SF8200, SF8100, SF8050, SF8000, SF400	Four routine test items, D-D, FDP
4	Rayto Life and Analytical Sciences Co., Ltd.	RAC-2800, RAC1800, RAC120, RAC050, RAT-2204C, RAT-2202	Four routine test items, D-D, FDP, AT
5	Beijing Zonci Technology Development Co., Ltd.	XL3690, XL3600, XL3200, XL1000e, XL1000	Four routine test items, D-D, FDP
6	Shandong Accurdx Biological Technology Co., Ltd.	GW3000, GW6000, ADX-E1, ADX-X1	Four routine test items, D-D, FDP, AT, anti-Xa, etc.
7	Shanghai Sunbio Biotechnology Co., Ltd.	UP1500, UP3000, UP5000, UP5500	Four routine test items, D-D, FDP, AT

A hospitals began to carry out more testing projects, such as monitoring of new oral anticoagulants, diagnosis of thrombophilia, and diagnosis of antiphospholipid syndrome, etc., together with the development trend of clinical targeted monitoring and precision treatment, the level of individualized diagnosis and treatment is enhanced, allowing doctors to accurately formulate diagnosis and treatment protocol for thrombosis and hemorrhage and promoting the development of the diagnosis of thrombosis and hemostasis. Since China has the largest population, with the development of the aging process, there will be an increasing number of patients with thrombotic diseases year by year. In the future, with the development of research and technologies, thrombosis and hemostasis diagnosis will develop dramatically in the Chinese market.

17.2.4.2 Existing Problems of Blood Coagulation Testing

According to basic survey results, the existing main problems for coagulation testing include nonunified standardization, insufficient academic knowledge of blood coagulation, less equipment, few testing items, insufficient sample size, insufficient clinical communication, etc. These factors have restricted the development of blood coagulation to a great extent, especially in primary hospitals. Although there are many academic associations, industry reports and lectures, etc., doctors in primary hospitals may not have access to these contents and the latest blood coagulation knowledge, and cannot keep up with the trend of blood coagulation development.

For the above problems, the respondents generally believe that the most urgent issues to be solved for the blood coagulation testing are standardization and quality control, communication with clinical department, improvement of professional skills of personnel, and interpretation of abnormal results, etc. They also expect to obtain corresponding assistance, for example, standardized coagulation testing, quality control, professional technical guidance of coagulation, continuous quality improvement, report interpretation, etc. All these issues need to be studied and improved in the future.

17.2.4.3 Factors Affecting the Development of Blood Coagulation

Domestic Policies

The mortality rate of cardiovascular and cerebrovascular diseases has ranked first in China in recent years, and thrombosis is always one of the main causes of its occurrence. Seventy percent of deaths are caused by venous thrombosis and there are no signs before the onset of the disease; therefore, there will be increased demand for screening for thrombosis diseases, which will promote the growth of the coagulation testing market.

In addition, since China has the largest population, with the development of the aging process, there will be an increasing number of patients with thrombotic diseases year by year. In the future, with the development of research and technologies, thrombosis and hemostasis diagnosis will develop dramatically in the Chinese market.

Opportunities for Domestic Demand in the Secondary Market

In the high-end market, due to the large sample size, there is low price elasticity of demand for patients; in addition, with the strong strength and comprehensive academic promotion of foreign companies, customers prefer to choose imported instruments and reagents, which causes a low penetration rate of domestic coagulation brands in the high-end market. However, the imported products have the disadvantages of high cost, high price, and inflexible services, which promote the domestic substitution of Grade II hospitals to a certain extent. Since the sample size of Grade II hospitals is smaller than the throughput of imported instruments, there is a waste of throughput; in addition, the academic promotion of foreign companies is rarely popular in the low-end markets. Therefore, Grade II hospitals tend to choose domestic products with higher cost performance, allowing the secondary market to become a main battlefield for domestic substitution of imports.

Positive Guidance of Domestic Academic Environment

The Chinese Society of Laboratory Medicine, China Society of medical laboratory equipment, and Chinese Medical Doctor Association Laboratory Doctor Branch, and other national main secondary testing branches set up special committees or coagulation forums respectively and invite famous domestic and foreign researchers to give special speeches on the relevant progress in the bleeding and coagulation diseases, and conduct academic exchanges in the form of special academic reports and conference speeches, etc., to promote the academic progress of coagulation and the development of the whole coagulation industry.

On July 2, 2019, the preparatory meeting for the establishment of the Thrombosis and Hemostasis Professional Committee of the Chinese Research Hospital Association (hereinafter referred to as the "Association") was successfully held in Haikou. The initiators of the professional committee, Professor Cong Yulong, a famous expert in the field of thrombosis and hemostasis, and Professor Zhou Zhou, a talent of "Thousand Talents Program," jointly applied to the Chinese Research Hospital Association to establish a secondary branch of "Thrombosis and Hemostasis," and it was approved on June 5, 2019. The establishment of the Association marks the establishment of the first secondary branch in the field of thrombosis and hemostasis in China, which is of great significance in promoting the development of thrombosis and hemostasis in China. *The Basic Follow-up Course of Coagulation Experiment* is actively organized by the society and jointly implemented by Beijing Strong Biotechnologies, Inc. Through the society, the domestic laboratory experts in the field of thrombosis and hemostasis are convened to compile a series of basic follow-up courses for coagulation experiments, which is mainly used in the primary hospitals, including clinicians in the township hospitals, community hospitals, Grade I and Grade II hospitals and doctors in the clinical laboratory, etc. It is expected that the standardization of coagulation testing items in grass-roots laboratories can be promoted in China through a series of training courses, to promote the progress and discipline development of coagulation laboratory diagnosis.

17.3 Future Development Trend of Blood Coagulation Industry

Presently, the domestic IVD market shows a slow overall growth rate, but with the emergence of new projects, the improvement of industry concentration, and the emergence of assembly line trends, etc., the blood coagulation market will become thriving.

17.3.1 The Improvement of Academic Cognition Drives the Growth of Demand for Blood Coagulation Testing

Clinically, bleeding and thrombosis are common in various departments of medical institutions. In the past, the in vitro diagnosis of thrombosis and hemostasis in domestic clinical departments is applied in the screening of bleeding causes and bleeding diseases. With the deepening of domestic clinical cognition, the applications of in vitro diagnosis of thrombosis and hemostasis for screening, diagnosis, treatment, and monitoring of thrombosis and thrombotic diseases are continuously developing. Therefore, in recent years, various discipline associations such as cardiology, orthopedics, vascular surgery, respiratory, and oncology have successively issued guidelines and expert consensuses related to the prevention and treatment of various thrombotic diseases, promoting the clinicians' recognition of thrombotic diseases-related diagnostic items.

At present, in the Chinese market, the clinical applications of thrombosis and hemostasis testing technologies tend to disease prevention, disease diagnosis, and drug monitoring from the screening of thrombotic diseases and bleeding diseases. With the development of novel direct oral anticoagulants (DOACs), numerous clinical validations have shown that single-target anticoagulation therapy also requires the targeted monitoring.

Therefore, the implementation of the special test items for bleeding and coagulation (including PC/PS/LA/vWF/Anti-Xa/FVIII/FIX, etc.) not only makes up for the blank of traditional laboratory monitoring but also continuously advances the diagnostic level to precise treatment and individualized treatment, conforming to the development trend of the clinical technology applications. Under the guidance of clinical needs, the above special test items for bleeding and coagulation also follow the law of gradually developing from Grade III hospitals to Grade II and below hospitals and finally are applied and popularized in the domestic market, bringing the development of a new round of blood coagulation testing.

17.3.2 The Growing Importance of Blood Coagulation Testing

Against the background of an increasingly aging global population, the incidence of thrombotic and hemostatic diseases, including cardiovascular diseases, remains high. The coagulation testing can not only provide guidance for the safe use of antithrombotic drugs for cardiovascular diseases but also play an indispensable role in the diagnosis of bleeding disorders. Accurate diagnosis of bleeding disorders requires a comprehensive assessment of the patient's bleeding history, family history, physical examination, and laboratory tests. As one of the three routines of laboratory tests, coagulation testing can provide an important basis for clinical diagnosis and treatment of bleeding and thrombotic diseases, with increasing medical value. Clinically, a high requirement for the quality and efficiency of coagulation test is proposed.

17.3.3 From Decentralization to Centralization

As one of the segments of in vitro diagnostics, the blood coagulation testing is faster than other industries in terms of the growth rate. In the capital market, there are frequent mergers and acquisitions in the coagulation diagnosis industry. Mindray, BSBE, Maccura, and other listed companies of IVD started their business in the coagulation; and Succeeder, whose main business is blood coagulation, has also been listed. The R&D and production capacity and capital advantages of leading IVD companies will inevitably promote the centralization of the coagulation market, and the demand for mergers and acquisitions is strong. On the one hand, the mergers and acquisitions of these listed companies can increase the coverage of testing business, enhance the ability to negotiate prices of the downstream of the industry, and obtain more comprehensive business coverage, consolidate and improve their own business strength, and increase overall competitiveness. On the other hand, with the introduction of a series of national policies and the continuous improvement of the regulatory system, some small enterprises will gradually withdraw from the field under the pressure of competition and supervision, while the large leading enterprises will dominate the market and greatly increase the degree of concentration of the blood coagulation industry, ultimately prompting the development of the entire industry.

17.3.4 Assembly Line Trend

With the in-depth study of the hemostasis and thrombosis, the hemostasis and coagulation testing has become increasingly important. With the increasingly abundant coagulation test items, increasing number of blood coagulation specimens, and rising requirements for testing quality and efficiency, how to build an automated and intelligentized coagulation automation assembly line has become a key concern of the coagulation laboratory. First of all, the assembly line can greatly improve the testing efficiency, especially for large-scale Grade III Level A hospitals, there are so many patients and samples that the conventional single-module measurement cannot meet the huge testing needs. Therefore, the assembly line can help the department to solve this problem. In addition, the automated assembly line can make the medical staff to get rid of tedious manual operations, so that they can spend more time in more valuable work such as interpretation of reports, academic research, etc., to provide better services for patients.

17.3.5 Quality Improvement to Promote Domestic Substitution

In terms of instruments, there is a huge domestic substitution potential for imported instruments. Although imported instruments have a first-mover advantage, it has a longer development history and experiences than domestic equipment regarding the performance and doctor education. However, in recent years, under the policy of high fees of services and consumables for imported equipment, as well as the policy of controlling medical insurance costs, domestic high-quality medical devices are gradually substituting the imported devices, with a promising growth potential.

In addition, more and more domestic manufacturers have developed reagents that can be used on imported brands, such as Sunbio and BSBE (BEIJING MDC). With the improvement of blood coagulation research and development, the quality of reagents has increased greatly. Through the continuous updating of blood coagulation technology and products, the main technical indexes or performance parameters of many domestic companies' blood coagulation testing systems have been close to or even reached the international advanced level. In addition to the price advantage, the domestic reagents can be comparable to or even superior to the imported reagents in terms of measurement accuracy, precision, and anti-interference ability.

Although the foreign companies occupy a high proportion, with the release of several national policies and support for domestic substitution, it provides space for the development of China's local IVD companies. The domestic substitution in China's medical device stock market will present changes qualitatively.

17.3.6 Continuous Research and Development of New Blood Coagulation Test Items

There is a huge gap between the development and popularity of coagulation test items in China and developed countries, with a huge room for growth in the coagulation testing industry. Chinese coagulation testing industry is still in the early stage; in terms of the abundance of test items, more than 150 test items of coagulation have been carried out in developed countries such as the United States, accounting for 1/3 of the routine tests. However, due to starting late, only four to eight test items are popularized in China, with a huge difference in the test items from the developed countries. Therefore, there is a huge growth potential in the test field [9]. In terms of the IVD consumption, the per capita IVD expenditure in China is less than half of the global average, and far behind the developed countries such as Europe and the United States [9].

In the Chinese thrombus and hemostasis diagnostic market, seven items (PT/APTT/TT/FIB/D-D/FDP/AT) are the mainstream test items, with the revenue from reagents accounting for more than 90%; special test items (items other than PT/APTT/TT/FIB/ D-D/FDP/AT) are still very limited nationwide, and the revenue from reagents accounts for not more than 10%.

At present, the in vitro diagnosis of thrombosis and hemostasis in China tends to be disease prevention, disease diagnosis, and drug monitoring from the screening of thrombotic diseases and bleeding diseases. The types of thrombosis and hemostasis testing items carried out in Grade III hospitals will also continue to increase (including PC/PS/LA/vWF/Anti-Xa/FVIII/FIX, etc.). More and more thrombus molecular markers such as TAT, PAP, TM, and tPAIC will be popularized in clinical practices, which are close to the testing quality of imported reagents.

17.3.7 Construction of Quality System

The standardization and quality control of thrombus and hemostasis testing methods is to perform reasonable management, testing, and assessment of the quality level of the techniques, operations, instruments, reagents, and specimens of thrombus and hemostasis experiments by using standardized physical, chemical, and biological methods according to the statistical principles, so as to eliminate errors and improve the precision, accuracy, and reliability of experiments. The purpose of standardization and quality control is to provide a reliable basis for clinical diagnosis and treatment, improve the efficiency and value of basic research on thrombosis and hemostasis, and contribute to population health surveys and the establishment of a normal reference range of hematology testing [10]. It can reflect the medical and research levels of thrombosis and hemostasis in a country, a region, and a research institution.

Factors affecting hemostasis testing mainly include specimens (collection method, storage method, and transportation method), reagents (anticoagulant ratio, detection reagent type), equipment (semi-automated, fully automated), and technology (proficiency, interference factors), etc. [11]. Due to the particularity of thrombosis and hemostasis tests, there is still no mature standardized protocol for the detection of platelet function, anticoagulation factors, and fibrinolytic components. There are clear specifications in only three test items of prothrombin time (PT) and activated partial thromboplastin time (APTT) by the International Committee for Standardization of Hematology (ICSH), the International Committee on Thrombosis and Hemostasis (ISTH), or the National Committee for Clinical Laboratory Standards (NCCLS) [12]. The standardization of coagulation testing is conducive to improving the accuracy and scientificity of coagulation testing [13] and establishing the coagulation item traceability system. However, for the particularity of coagulation items, researchers should work hard in the future.

In conclusion, although foreign-funded companies occupy a large market advantage in the blood coagulation industry, one of the fastest-growing segments of IVD, with the emergence of domestic enterprises, they will overcome the difficulties and occupy a certain market share in the blood coagulation industry.

Declaration Zuojun Zou, Yanshang Ma and Qifan Tian are employees of Beijing Strong Biotechnologies, Inc.

Hai Wang, Chonghui Ding and Jiahong Zhang are employees of Beijing Succeeder Technology, Inc.

References

1. Xinsi Industry. Xinsi industry: the thrombus and hemostasis in vitro diagnostics market is growing rapidly. Domestic enterprises occupy a relatively small share [R/OL]. (2020-09-16[2021-10-16]. https://www.163.com/dy/article/FMIDMGUQ0514E30D.html.
2. China Cardiovascular Health and Disease Report Group. China Cardiovascular Health and Disease Report 2019 Summary [J]. Chin J Circul. 2020;35(9):833–54.
3. Chen BS. Where is the import alternative space of hemagglutinometer [J]. J Med Econ. 2014;003:1–2.
4. Riley RS, Gilbert AR, Dalton JB, et al. Widely used types and clinical applications of D-dimer assay[J]. Lab Med. 2016;47:90–102.
5. Weitz JI, Eikelboom JW. Advances in thrombosis and hemostasis: An introduction to the compendium [J]. Circul Res. 2016;118(9):1337–9.
6. Wei X, Tingmei C. Clinical hematology test technology [M]. Beijing: People's Medical Publishing House; 2019. p. 57–65.
7. Olson JD. D-dimer: an overview of hemostasis and fibrinolysis, assays, and clinical applications [J]. Adv Clin Chem. 2015;69:1–46.
8. Ning T. Development status and trend of coagulation test [R/OL]. (2020-01-02) [2021-10-22]. https://www.sohu.com/a/364246867_668702.
9. Yao X. Analysis on market characteristics and M&A driving factors of coagulation testing industry [J]. Zhifu Times. 2019;004:1–5.
10. Mike Bio. Standard delivery: the standardization of blood coagulation experiment [R/OL]. (2019-09-18) [2021-9-16]. https://www.sohu.com/a/341718576_326142.
11. Mingting P. Quality control of coagulation test [J]. Zhejiang Lab Med. 2004;04(29):5–7.
12. Yulong C. The present situation and development of thrombosis and hemostasis test diagnosis [J]. Chin J Lab Med. 2001;01:4–6.
13. Yunying L. Analysis and discussion on standardization of coagulation test [J]. Contemporary Med J. 2013;19(28):39–40.

Blood Typing Instruments and Reagents 18

Pengfei Lai, Nan Sun, Tao Zhao, Rongbang Xia, Yunqi Li, Yanshang Ma, Xiaoyan Yang, and Boping Dong

18.1 Overview

Blood typing has become a routine test item of clinical blood transfusion department and clinical laboratory, which includes ABO blood group, Rh blood group, and cross-matching of blood test. At present, tests are mainly conducted against ABO and Rh blood group system of the greatest clinical significance [1], Kell, Duffy, Kidd, MNS, P, and Lewis blood group system of certain clinical significance and irregular antibodies, that is, detect unknown antibodies with known antigens or detect unknown antigens with known antibodies through immunological techniques, and identify blood group based on agglutination [2]. Genetic detection techniques directly targeting on carrier of genetic information—base sequence of DNA or RNA—are still subject to certain limitations, and not extensively used in clinical blood grouping tests.

Blood typing technique has experienced development from glass way (include ceramic plate test and paper method), tube method to microcolumn gel method (henceforth referred to as MGT) [3]. In 1985, Dr. Yves Lappierre in Lyons, France, developed MGT who attempted to capture agglutinator at precipitation and centrifugation step through study on gelatin, acrylamide gel, and glass bead. He cooperated with Switzerland-based DiaMed A.G. in 1988 for commercialized production of blood group gel cards; MGT boasts of high sensitivity, high specificity, excellent test repeatability, and easy standardization. At present, most clinical blood transfusion departments take gel technique as blood typing and cross-matching of blood method [4].

P. Lai (✉) · N. Sun · T. Zhao · R. Xia · Y. Li
Aikang MedTech Co., Ltd, Shenzhen, Guangdong, China
e-mail: laipengfei@aikang-medical.com

Y. Ma · X. Yang · B. Dong
Beijing Strong Biotechnologies, Inc., Beijing, China

H. Song, L. Dai (eds.), *In Vitro Diagnostic Industry in China*,
https://doi.org/10.1007/978-981-99-3110-1_18

18.2 Blood Typing Instruments and Reagents

Blood typing-related products mainly include two sectors of blood typing instruments and blood typing reagents.

18.2.1 Blood Typing Instruments

Accompanied with scientific and technological progress of domestic industry and improvement of enterprises' independent R&D and production capacity, blood grouping analyzer has gone through the journey from small semi-automatic instruments at early stage to large fully automated device. Automatic blood grouping analyzer can finish whole process of blood typing in a fully automated manner, and all test steps are controlled by PC to make sure every sample is tested under the same conditions, which boast of higher precision, more accurate test results, reduced operators' workload, higher test efficiency, and reduced risk of hazardous biological matters of laboratory. Meanwhile, intelligent information management system can realize real-time dynamic test, and original test images are saved permanently to ensure traceability of test process. Accompanied with blood transfusion industry's standardization of management and government's focus and support on safety of blood transfusion, automatic blood grouping analyzer has been used extensively in recent years.

Automatic blood grouping analyzer is an analyzer that can forward and reverse ABO blood group, Rh (D) blood group test, irregular antibody screening and cross-matching of blood test. It mainly consists of liquid handling system, incubator, centrifuge, interpretoscope, and microcomputer system. It realizes distribution and transfer of samples and reagents by liquid handling system, conducts incubation of microcolumn gel card by incubator, carries out centrifugation of microcolumn gel card by centrifuge, finishes digital imaging of microcolumn gel card by interpretoscope, and completes comparative analysis of images of the microcolumn gel card by microcomputer, which allow it to achieve full automation and intellectualization of blood typing, irregular antibody screening, and cross-matching of blood test.

1. Automatic blood grouping analyzer based on MGT: MGT is the combined product of gel filtration technology and immunoreaction, and gap of gel plays the role of molecular sieve that only allows free erythrocytes to pass. Upon centrifugation by centrifuge, if erythrocytes without agglutination in micro-column gel are deposited at the bottom of agglutinatior, then it indicates negative reaction. It shall be deemed as agglutination if erythrocytes are agglutinated at upper or middle part of agglutinatior, which indicates positive reaction. The instrument is used in combination with suitable microcolumn gel card for automatic completion of the whole process of scanning, sample and reagent distribution, blood grouping cards handling, puncture, pipetting, incubation, centrifugation, image acquisition, and automatic interpretation [5].

2. Automatic blood grouping analyzer based on microplate technique: take microplate or a transparent 96-well plate as carrier, it shall be deemed as non-agglutination if erythrocytes are laid on bottom of micro-pores, and it shall be deemed as agglutination if erythrocytes deposit to the bottom of micro-pores and form concentrated dots. Microplate can be divided into two types of trapezoidal microplate and 96-well U-shaped microplate. Trapezoidal microplate uses Japan-based Olympus's trapezoidal microplate for antigen-antibody immunoreaction, and uses core components of digital camera and digital camcorder (CCD) imaging technique for judgment of agglutination. U-shaped microplate uses microplate reader for scanning of transmittance within diameter of U-shaped pores, and then calculates relative transmittance by microplate reader software to get blood typing results.
3. Tube method-based automatic blood grouping analyzer: in recent years, domestic enterprises take blank reaction card (6-well card) as test carrier for blood cell antigen and antibody agglutination test pursuant to test principles and operations of classic blood group and serum test method of manual test tube method, test agglutination strength through changes in curve of transmitted flux, and automatically interpret test results. Such technique further enriched blood typing instruments, and provided users with new use experiences.

18.2.2 Blood Typing Reagents

Blood typing reagents mainly refer to reagents and kits used separately or in combination with blood grouping analyzer, which belong to a segment of in vitro diagnostic (IVD) reagent industry. Blood typing reagents can be mainly divided into forward and reverse blood ABO blood group, Rh (D) blood group test, irregular antibody test, anti-human globulin test, platelet antibody test, and other reagents. In clinical transfusion test, importance of Rh blood group system is only next to ABO blood group system. RhD has the strongest antigenicity in Rh blood group system, which is a main factor that gives rise to adverse reactions in clinical blood transfusion. Hence, screening of Rh blood group is very necessary before blood transfusion. C, c, E, and e antigens are several antigens of significant clinical significance in addition to D antigen of Rh blood group system, which test method's basically the same to that of RhD antigen test. Anti-human globulin test is the most reliable method for the identification of irregular antibodies, and it is also the "gold standard" for antibody identification and cross-matching of blood at the moment. Surface of platelet contains Human Leukocyfe Antigen (HLA), Human Platelet Antigen (HPA), and other antigens; hence, test of HLA and HPA antigen on the surface of platelet is also of great clinical significance.

Blood typing reagents mainly include ABO test erythrocyte, anti-A (anti-B or anti-D) blood typing reagents, irregular antibody screening erythrocyte, forward and reverse ABO blood grouping card, Rh blood grouping card, anti-human globulin card, and erythrocyte cross matching kit. Both microplate and microcolumn gel card methods need to add specific blood group antibodies (such as anti-A, anti-B and anti-D reagent), erythrocyte, and other reagents to carrier medium. Quality and stability of specific blood group antibodies, erythrocyte, and other reagents will have direct impact on accuracy of test results to a certain extent; hence, blood typing reagents as supporting products of automatic blood grouping analyzer are of great significance to blood typing as well. Microcolumn gel card technique has been extensively used in blood typing; the regent card has been added various blood group antibodies to gel, and it only needs to add samples to realize typing during the test. The technique boasts of high sensitivity, easy standardization, easy observation and retention, and it has become the first choice for clinical ABO and Rh (D) blood typing and cross-matching of blood.

18.3 Blood Typing Instruments and Its Technology Development Direction and Status of Market Development

18.3.1 Main Brands and Manufacturers of Domestic Automatic Blood Grouping Analyzers

Microplate-based automatic blood grouping analyzer Metis of Aikang MedTech Co., Ltd. (henceforth referred to as Aikang) received approval for marketing in 2015; and its MGT-based automatic blood grouping analyzer Aigel received approval for marketing in 2016. Both products can conduct the test of forward and reverse human blood ABO, Rh (D) blood typing, irregular antibody screening, and cross-matching of blood. Aikang became the only domestic enterprise in possession of microplate-based and MGT-based automatic blood grouping analyzers.

Subsequently, MG12 automatic blood grouping analyzer of Zhongshan Bio-Tech Co., Ltd.(henceforth referred to as Zhongshan Bio-Tech), SA-120 automatic blood grouping analyzer of Suzhou Hybiome Biomedical Engineering Co., Ltd. (henceforth referred to as Suzhou Hybiome), Aretha automatic blood grouping analyzer of Shinva Medical Instrument Co.,Ltd.(henceforth referred to as Shinva), and other excellent domestic enterprises' MGT-based automatic blood grouping analyzer received approval for marketing successively. Manual tube method-based BG-Optics-II automatic blood grouping analyzer of Baso Zhuhai Bio-Tech Co., Ltd.(henceforth referred to as Baso) received approval for marketing in 2020, which further enriched categories of domestic blood typing instruments and brought new experiences to users. See details of partial domestic automatic blood grouping analyzer brands and manufacturers in Table 18.1.

At present, application method of domestic brands of automatic blood grouping analyzer has covered MGT, microplate and tube method, and their basic functions involve automatic barcode scanning, sampling, reagent injection, incubation, centrifugation, oscillation, and result interpretation. They can conduct the test of forward and reverse human blood ABO blood group, Rh (D) blood typing, irregular antibody screening and cross-matching of blood, and meet requirements of clinical blood typing and analysis. Domestic brands of automatic blood grouping analyzer have received excellent feedbacks from users in terms of functional practicability, operational simplicity, and maintenance convenience.

Table 18.1 Domestic automatic blood grouping analyzer brands and manufacturers

Brand/model	Place of origin	Application method	Manufacturer	Date of approval
Metis	Domestic	Microplate	Aikang MedTech Co., Ltd.	29-Oct-15
Aigel	Domestic	MGT	Aikang MedTech Co., Ltd.	19-Aug-16
MG12	Domestic	MGT	Zhongshan Bio-Tech Co., Ltd.	30-Sep-16
SA-120	Domestic	MGT	Suzhou Hybiome Biomedical Engineering Co., Ltd.	26-Jul-18
Aretha	Domestic	MGT	Shinva Medical Instrument Co.,Ltd.	18-Mar-19
BG-Optics-II	Domestic	Tube method	Baso Zhuhai Bio-Tech Co., Ltd.	17-Apr-20
Blozer	Domestic	MGT	Yantai Addcare Bio-Tech Limited Company	28-Apr-21

Note: See National Medical Products Administration's Medical Device Database for reference

18.3.2 Technology Development Direction of Blood Typing Instruments

18.3.2.1 Current Status of Technical Development of Blood Typing Instruments

At present, domestic blood typing instruments have covered microplate, MGT, tube method, and other international mainstream test methods, and they can provide highly automatic and standardized blood typing process, which play an important role in clinical transfusion. Current status of domestic blood typing instruments is mainly characterized by normative, standard and convenient operation; high sensitivity and excellent accuracy; high test efficiency; open reagent; intuitive, stable, reliable, clear and easy to save results; and data management by PC.

Demands for individualized clinical blood transfusion treatment have increased substantially accompanied with rapid development of blood transfusion techniques, which led to increased blood transfusion risks and increasingly more precise requirements on blood transfusion-related test techniques. Fully automatic blood grouping analyzer mainly includes: Computer, Pipetting Arm, Robotic Arm, Incubator, Centrifuge and Reader. Because of these independent modules, The Fully automatic blood grouping analyzer can complete all the processes of blood grouping tests. It can improve results accuracy, improve the traceability of the test processes, reduce the intensity of labor, reduce user errors and reduce the risk of contamination by using fully automatic blood grouping analyzer. Because of these advantages, it can increase the safety of blood transfusion.

Domestic enterprises have made numerous innovations of blood typing instruments. It can be learned from research of domestic patents in the field that related patent applications in China have been continuously active, number of patent applications have maintained the growth momentum, and innovation awareness has been continuously increasing. According to incomplete statistics, as indicated in Fig. 18.1, the number of domestic blood typing instruments-related patent applications was relatively low before 2008; the number of patent applications experienced certain

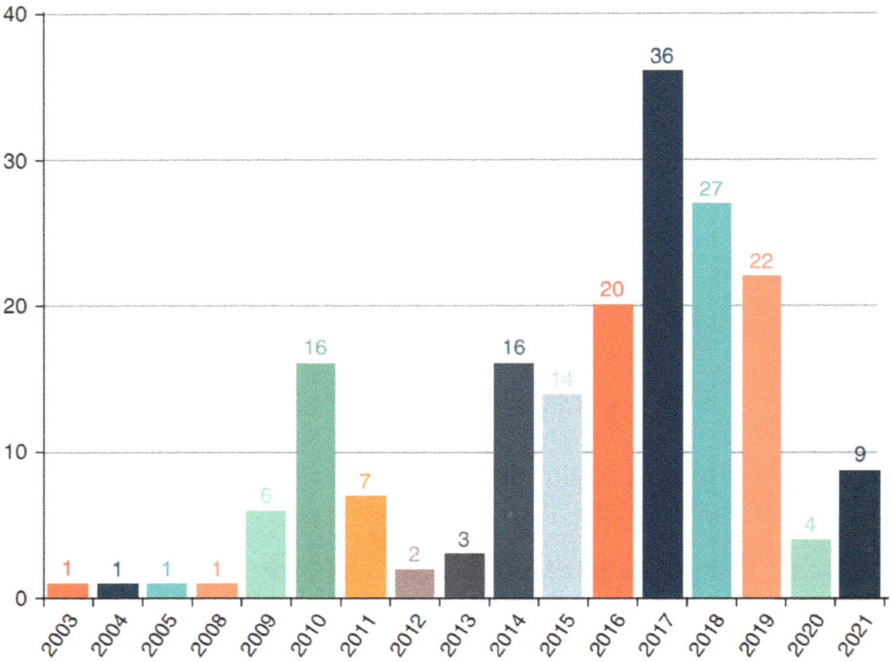

Fig. 18.1 Tendency diagram of blood typing instruments-related patent applications in China

growth between 2009 and 2012, which indicates domestic enterprises started technological R&D and deployment in the field; it entered the stage of rapid growth from 2014 to 2017, and related domestic products were already introduced to the market for distribution; the number of patent applications reached the peak in 2017 with total number of 36 applications in the whole year; and number of applications reduced somewhat in 2018 and 2019, but the number remained above 20 a year. Hence, it can be seen that our country's technological studies on automatic blood grouping analyzers are still at the stage of active development; despite the relative reduction, there was still a certain number of applications in 2020 and 2021. Therefore, China's technological research and development is still at development stage, which is expected to experience a new round of development at the next stage (Fig. 18.1).

Aikang and Suzhou Hybiome already started technological research on automatic blood grouping analyzer between 2012 and 2014, which allowed them to become relatively early market entrants. In recent years, many excellent domestic device manufacturers made deployment in the field successively and carried out technical researches and innovations, such as Shinva, Zhongshan Bio-Tech and Baso. Technical innovations based on blood grouping analyzer have been put into use, new automatic blood grouping analyzer have been introduced to the market continually, and those products not only covered MG and microplate method, but also included unique product form of test tube-based automatic blood grouping analyzer, which further enriched blood typing instruments and provided users with new experiences.

18.3.2.2 Future Development Trend of Blood Typing Instruments

It can be seen from analysis on major blood grouping analyzer-related patent applications published in the 3 years from 2018 to 2021 that benefited from the basically stable original technologies of the industry; domestic enterprises have continuously increased R&D inputs, constantly improved technical innovation capability, made breakthroughs in many technologies, and developed a batch of core components of instruments with independent intellectual property rights through follow-on R&D strategy. Technical researches on automated blood group typing instruments mainly focus on transfer control techniques, grasp control techniques, image processing techniques, interpretation system techniques, module compatibility and coupling, intensification and other aspects at the moment, and it is foreseeable that blood typing instruments will develop towards the direction of further increase in degree of automation of blood typing, improvement of blood typing efficiency, and enhancement of blood typing accuracy.

On the other hand, accompanied with continuous social and economic development and acceleration of aging population, laboratories' workload along with requirements on accuracy and timeliness has been increasing, and laboratory departments of hospitals have been increasingly relied on test results in terms of monitoring of diagnosis and treatment. Therefore, laboratories of large general hospitals have strong demands for provision of precise and highly efficient test analyzers and automatic comprehensive solutions for laboratories, and integrated pipeline, intellectualization, and bio-safety guarantee will become future trend for technical development of blood typing instruments.

1. Integrated pipeline: high speed and high throughput instrument's rigid demand of high-end hospitals and laboratories will develop towards the direction of integrated pipeline to meet high-end hospitals' test requirements. Laboratories may deploy instruments flexibly based on current devices and layout, and different modules in the pipeline all support multi-module operation, which allows continuous upgrade of automation process accompanied with development of laboratories' automation requirements. Intermediate software of modular design can be gradually expanded from basic modules like connection and sample management to advanced modules like automated audit, samplestorage, and retrieval as well as intelligent laboratory management, which gradually enrich laboratory information system.
2. Intellectualization: accompanied with continuous development of artificial intelligence (henceforth referred to as AI) technology, AI software played an increasingly important role in development journey of laboratory automation. The construction of intelligent laboratory is not only reflected by convenient operation management but also reflected by in-depth analysis and understanding of

mass data of test. Intelligent management and decision aids support are realized by automatic audit, analysis, and interpretation of those data. AI has great potential for improvement in operating efficiency and workflow of laboratory as well as patient prognosis.

3. Biosafety guarantee: from sample entry upon centrifugation to lid opening and completion of test, the whole process upon entry of sample into the system is in an enclosed environment, which can reduce operator's sample contact and possibility of infection, and thus ensure biosafety.

18.3.3 Market Conditions of Blood Typing Instruments

18.3.3.1 Market Size of China's Blood Typing Instruments between 2014 and 2020

Blood typing is closely associated with surgical operation volume, number of blood donors and other factors, and main application scenarios of blood typing instruments include hospitals and blood banks at the moment. According to network data analysis, market size of China's blood grouping analyzer was RMB 0.366 billion in 2021, and the compound growth rate is predicted to be 6.1% from 2021 to 2025. Market size of blood grouping analyzer will maintain a steady growth trend in the future. (Fig. 18.2).

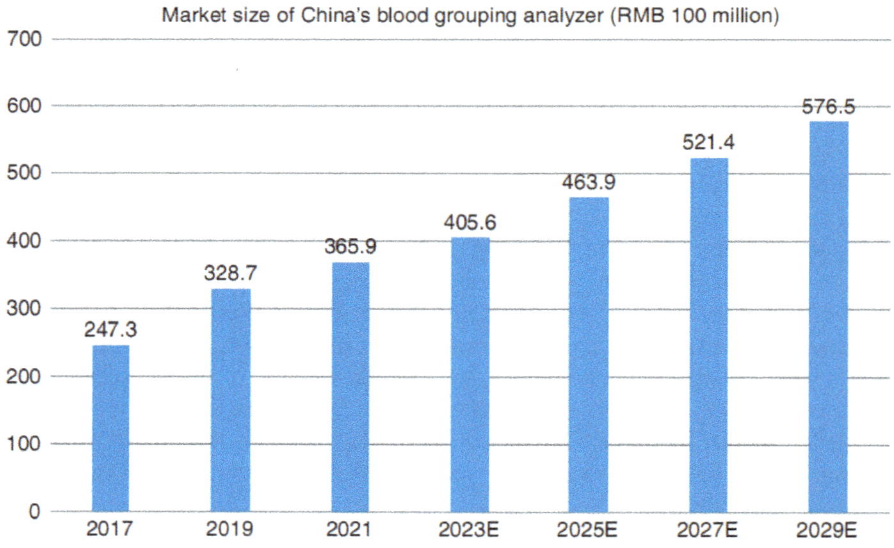

Fig. 18.2 Diagram of market size trend of China's blood grouping analyzer between 2017 and 2029 (Data source: research on network data collation)

18.3.3.2 Future Development of Blood Typing Instruments

Working Party on Clinical Transfusion Management, Chinese Society of Blood Transfusion investigated blood transfusion departments of 2309 hospitals in different provinces and cities throughout the country through "Internet Plus"; proportion of blood transfusion departments taken as an independent administrative unit is 45% at the moment, proportion of blood transfusion departments under management of laboratory department is 32%, proportion of blood transfusion departments taken as a professional group of laboratory department is 23%, utilization ratio of Automatic blood grouping analyzer is only 40%, while utilization ratio of manual/semi-automatic test instruments is still 60%. Accompanied with promotion and application of fully automated test devices, market size of Automatic blood grouping analyzer is expected surpass manual/semi-automatic test instrument in the next 3–5 years. Besides, accompanied with facilitation of the trend towards administrative independence of blood transfusion department of medical institutions and acceleration of domestic replacement, domestic automatic blood grouping analyzers are expected to achieve greater market coverage.

According to National Health and Family Planning Commission's statistics, the number of Grade III and Grade II hospitals with blood transfusion department isover 2000 and over 7000 respectively. It is foreseeable that Grade II hospitals and township grassroots hospitals still have relatively large automated blood typing demands in the future. In addition, accompanied with promotion of hierarchical medical system, blood typing instruments of small throughput will future penetrate into county markets with low cost and flexible application scenarios, which will become new growth points that drive market share of blood typing instruments. In the future blood typing sector, whole series of reagents and instruments for Blood typing will be provided to offer all-round blood transfusion test solutions for clinical applications, and satisfaction of use requirements of different clinical units will become the trend. Enterprises in the industry shall stay close to users' requirements; strengthen their technological innovation efforts in integrated automation, stability, intellectualization, safety and other aspects of products; maintain core competence, achieve growth in competition and realize optimization in growth; and jointly facilitate long-term development of blood typing industry.

18.4 Blood Typing Reagents and its Technology Development Direction and Status of Market Development

18.4.1 Main Products and Manufacturers of Domestic Blood Typing Reagents

At present, domestic blood typing reagent-related products already covered ABO blood typing, test of Rh and other irregular antibodies, and anti-human globulin test. They can conduct forward and reverse human blood ABO blood group typing, Rh (D/C/E) blood group typing, irregular antibody screening, and cross-matching of blood test, which can meet requirements of clinical blood typing. MGT has been extensively used in blood typing; the regent card has been added various blood group antibodies to gel, and it only needs to add samples to realize typing during the test. The technique boasts of high sensitivity, easy standardization, easy observation and retention, and it has become the first choice for clinical ABO and Rh (D) Blood typing and cross-matching of blood test.

Domestic blood typing reagents have come into were introduced to the market successively in the recent three years, which opened up a new prospect for Blood typing reagents and enriched Blood typing reagent market. New items and new methods mainly include anti-human globulin test, irregular antibody test, newborn blood typing, and erythrocyte genotyping. It can be seen that domestic blood typing reagent manufacturer kept up with the pace of R&D of imported product manufacturers, actively engaged in innovation and creation, and made breakthroughs in genotyping methods. Human erythrocyte ABO blood group genotyping kit polymerase chain reaction-sequence specific primer (PCR-SSP) and human erythrocyte RhD genotyping kit (PCR-SSP) products already received approval for marketing, and they are used for test of ABO and RhD alleles in DNA of human erythrocyte genome, which can identify rare blood groups and help doctors acquiring more accurate and more comprehensive blood group results. See partial domestic Blood typing reagents in Table 18.2.

18.4.2 Direction of Technical Development of Blood Typing Reagents

18.4.2.1 Current Status of Technical Development of Blood Typing Reagents

In recent years, in vitro diagnostic (henceforth referred to as IVD) reagents have been playing an increasingly greater role in disease prevention, diagnosis, prognostic judgment, screening and test of therapeutic drug, health status evaluation, estimation of heritability and other aspects, and IVD industry has become one of China's industries with rapid development and promising future.

It can be learned from research and analysis of domestic blood typing reagent patents that most blood typing reagents belong to optimized, improved, or supplementary products at the moment. Trend of domestic blood typing reagent patent applications can be seen from Diagram 18.3, number of domestic Blood typing reagent-related patent applications increased rapidly between 2014 and 2017, which reached the peak of 38 applications for the whole year of 2017. The number of patent applications dropped somewhat in 2018 and 2019, but remained above 20. Therefore, trend of blood typing reagent patent application's basically similar to that of blood typing instruments, and China's technical researches on blood typing reagents are currently at the stage of active development; the number of patent applications comparatively reduced in 2020 and 2021, but there were still certain number of applications. Besides, the number of patent applications in 2021 increased to a certain extent in comparison with that in 2020, so technical R&D of China's

Table 18.2 Partial domestic blood typing reagents

Product name	Registrant	Date of approval
ABO and rh (CDE) blood group typing test card	Zhong Shan Shengke Pragent Instruments Co., Ltd.	16-Jan-17
Human Rh system typing test card (MGT)	Tianjin Dexiang Biotech Co., Ltd.	23-Mar-18
ABO forward and reverse typing and Rh (D/C/E) blood group test card (MGT)	Aikang Diagnostics Co., Ltd.	02-Apr-18
ABO/RhD blood group antibody test card (MGT)	Aikang Diagnostics Co., Ltd.	02-Apr-18
Newborn ABO and RhD blood group test card (MGT)	JiangYin LIBO Medicine Biotechnology Co., Ltd.	09-Oct-17
ABO blood group forward typing and RhD blood group typing kit (solid-phase)	InTec PRODUCTS, INC.	16-Mar-16
ABO forward and reverse typing and RhD blood group test card (MGT)	Beijing Strong Biotechnologies, Inc.	02-Mar-18
RBC kit for human ABO blood group reverse typing	SHPBC	04-Jun-19
ABO blood group reverse typing kit (human erythrocyte)	Lepu Medical Technology (Beijing) Co., Ltd.	25-Sep-17
ABO blood group reverse typing test card (MGT)	Bioxun Biotech Co., Ltd.	15-Aug-16
ABO blood group reverse typing kit (human erythrocyte)	Bioxun Biotech Co., Ltd.	24-Nov-16
Product name	Registrant	Date of approval
Irregular antibody test reagent (human erythrocyte)	Bioxun Biotech Co., Ltd.	29-Jun-17
Anti-human globulin (anti-IgG) test card (MGT)	JiangYin LIBO Medicine Biotechnology Co., Ltd.	03-May-16
ABO and RhD blood group antigen test card (MGT)	Suzhou Suda Saier Immune Biotechnology Co., Ltd.	18-Sep-18
ABODE blood group test card (MGT)	Bioxun Biotech Co., Ltd.	02-Feb-18
Anti-human globulin reagent (anti-IgG + anti-C3d)	Bioxun Biotech Co., Ltd.	12-Mar-18
Anti-human globulin (anti-IgG + C3d) test card	Maccura Biotechnology cCo., Ltd.	07-Nov-18
Anti-human globulin test card	Baso Zhuhai Bio-Tech Co., Ltd.	16-Jan-17
Anti-human globulin test card	Bioxun Biotech Co., Ltd.	22-Mar-19
Anti-human globulin test card (IgG+C3d) (MGT)	Aikang Diagnostics Co., Ltd.	31-May-19
Irregular antibody test kit (human erythrocyte)	Changchun Brother Bio-Tech Co., Ltd.	14-Feb-20
Human RBC ABO blood group genotyping kit (PCR-SSP)	Tianjin Super Biotechnology Development Co., Ltd.	19-May-20
Human RBC RhD genotyping kit (PCR-SSP)	Tianjin Super Biotechnology Development Co., Ltd.	18-May-20

Note: See National Medical Products Administration's Medical Device Database for reference

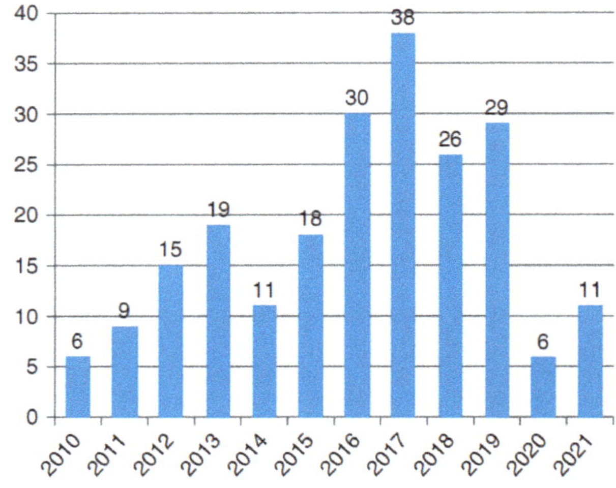

Fig. 18.3 Tendency diagram of number of Blood typing reagent related patent applications in China

Blood typing reagent sector is still at development stage, which is expected to experience a new round of development at the next stage (Fig. 18.3).

At present, MGT-based blood group test card has been used extensively in the field of blood typing, and MGT boasts of easy operation, high sensitivity, accurate results that can be saved and other strengthens, which allowed it to become method recommended by American Association of Blood Banks (AABB), technique recognized by FDA and internationally recognized blood group analysis test technique. Domestic MGT-based blood group test card entered into the market successively, which gradually changed the situation of medical institutions' long-term use of imported MGT-based blood group test cards. The MGT-based blood group test cards and their reagent products provided by Bioxun Biotech Co., Ltd., SHPBC, JiangYin LIBO Medicine Biotechnology Co., Ltd., Aikang Diagnostics Co., Ltd. and other excellent domestic enterprises have been recognized and praised by medical institutions.

Solid-phase blood typing reagent created by InTec PRODUCTS, INC. uses the principle of antibody and antigen immunosorbent assay to bond anti-A, anti-B, and anti-D monoclonal antibodies to solid phase carrier respectively; erythrocytes will be intercepted by carrier and displayed in red during immunoreaction of antigen on erythrocytes of samples to be tested and solid-phase antibodies, which indicates positive reaction. Solid-phase blood typing reagent can be used for point-of-care testing of blood group, it boasts of convenient operation and accurate results, and it has been extensively used in numerous fields at the moment.

18.4.2.2 Development Trend of Blood Typing Reagent Technologies

It can be seen from analysis on major Blood typing reagents-related patent applications published in the 3 years between 2018 and 2021 that directions of technical researches mainly focused on rare specific antigen test, PCR genotyping test technique and improvement of existing test methods. It is foreseeable that development trend of Blood typing reagent technologies is mainly reflected by improvement of Blood typing accuracy, increase in Blood typing efficiency and reduction of test time; improvement of Blood typing sensitivity and prevention of missed test; evaluation of antibody titer determination and other aspects.

In terms of improvement of Blood typing accuracy, different techniques mainly focus on provision of genotyping-based ABO blood typing, and acquirement of target segments through design of specific primers and use of single-tube multiplex PCR amplified reaction, which allow doctors to acquire more precise and comprehensive blood group results; in respect of reduction of test time and improvement of test efficiency, multiplex PCR method is introduced to ABO blood group genotyping, which can reduce number of PCR reactions of a single person-time in ABO antigen genotyping, reduce human and reagent cost of test, and increase test throughput; as for evaluation of antibody titer test capability, blood group antibody titer test capability of different laboratories engaged in test are judged, and accuracy of blood group antibody test capability verification results are improved based on media and methods used by them; in case of improvement of sensitivity and prevention of missed test, technologies are mainly distributed in the fields of use of antigen and antibody immunoreaction for high strength adsorption and bonding of erythrocytes as well as use of freeze-drying technique and two-step indication system, which can solve existing clinical difficulties.

18.4.3 Market Conditions of Blood Typing Reagents

18.4.3.1 Market Size of China's Blood Typing Reagent between 2019 and 2020

According to Medii Research's investigation and statistics, market size of China's blood group reagent consumable was RMB 1.04 billion in 2019, which grew to RMB 1.15 billion in 2020 with growth rate of 10.57%. While market size of China's Blood typing instrument was RMB 0.335 billion in 2020, and the market size of Blood typing reagent consumables was far higher than that of Blood typing instruments.

18.4.3.2 Market Size of Different Test Items of Blood Typing Reagents in China between 2019 and 2020

According Medii Research's investigation and statistics, size of China's ABO Blood typing reagent consumable market was RMB 0.468 billion in 2019, which is higher than that of RhD Blood typing of RMB 0.312 billion and that of antibody screening test of RMB 0.177 billion; market size of China's ABO blood typing reagent consumable was RMB 0.517 billion in 2020, which is higher than that of RhD blood typing of RMB 0.345 billion and that of antibody screening test of RMB 0.195 billion.

18.4.3.3 Future Status of Blood Typing Reagent Market

Accompanied with further expansion of coverage of automated blood typing instrument market, promotion of newborn test, genotyping, and other new test items will also facilitate further expansion of blood typing reagent market. According to Medii Research's estimate, market size of China's Blood typing reagent consumable market will reach RMB 1.848 billion in 2025, which still has huge development potentials. Enterprises in the industry shall meet clinical requirements, increase R&D inputs, continuously develop series test reagent products compatible with instruments, and provide all-round blood transfusion test solutions for clinical applications to meet use requirements of clinical units of different levels.

In recent years, the country has promulgated centralized bulk-buying policy for high value medical consumables in the field of medical devices. For instance, centralized procurement in the fields of chemiluminescent detection reagents for coronary stent, joint prosthesis, and chemiluminescence detection reagents for IVD and SARS-CoV-2 detection reagents have been conducted, while blood typing reagents have not been included in centralized procurement yet. Accompanied with gradual expansion of scope of centralized procurement, it is possible for blood typing reagents to be included in the scope of centralized procurement, and concentration ratio is expected to further increase by then. Enterprises in the industry of blood typing instruments and reagents shall seize opportunities, strengthen their technical innovations, use advanced diagnostic techniques to realize more efficient, precise and safe analysis and test, and offer more advanced products and better services for the field of blood typing to benefit the public.

Declaration Pengfei Lai, Tao Zhao, Rongbang Xia and Yunqi Li are employees of Aikang MedTech Co., Ltd.

Yanshang Ma, Xiaoyan Yang and Boping Dong are employees of Beijing Strong Biotechnologies, Inc.

References

1. Skaik, AM Younis. Further considerations in investigating the association of ABO and Rh (D) blood groups with glaucoma (Association of ABO blood groups with glaucoma in the Pakistani population [J]). Canadian J Ophthalmol, 2010, 45(2):177
2. STICHTING SANQUIN BLOEDVOORZIENING. Solid-phase method for antigen and antibody determinations in bloodgroup serology, and test kit: AU3059499A[P] .1999-10-18.
3. Noiphung Julaluk, Talalak Kwanrutai, Hongwarittorrn Inn, et al. A novel paper-based assay for the simultaneous determination of Rh typing and forward and reverse ABO blood groups [J]. Biosensors Bioelectron,2015, 67: 485-489. .
4. Technical manual, 16th edition [M]. American Association of Blood Banks, Betheda, 2008.
5. Langston M M, Procter J L, Cipolone K M, et al. Evaluation of the gel system for ABO grouping and D typing [J]. Transfusion, 1999,39(3):300-305.

Urine

19

Jun Jiang, Chuanjun Su, Kun Wang, and Yongqing Zhou

19.1 Status Quo of China's Urinalysis Market

The major brands in China's urinalysis market are URIT, DIRUI, AVE, etc. URIT produced China's first urine analyzer in 1984. And after nearly 40 years' strenuous cultivation, it pioneered the modular urine analysis workflow using deep learning artificial intelligence (AI) image recognition technology. Combined with urine-specific protein detection technology, the workflow of urine full detection chain has been realized. The company has a perfect urinalysis traceability system, and has participated in the drafting of a number of industry standards in the field of urinalysis. DIRUI is the first company to develop a urine formed element analyzer using flow digital image shooting technology, the pioneer of integrated urinalysis system, has won a number of national invention patents, and participated in the drafting of two industry standards for urine analyzer and urinalysis quality control solution. AVE has been deeply cultivated in the field of urine morphology for many years, and its key common technologies such as "machine vision technology" and "automation of medical microscope morphology examination" have filled a number of technical gaps at home and abroad.

J. Jiang (✉) · C. Su · K. Wang · Y. Zhou
URIT Medical Electronic Co., Ltd., Guilin, Guangxi, China
e-mail: jiangjun@uritest.com.cn

H. Song, L. Dai (eds.), *In Vitro Diagnostic Industry in China*,
https://doi.org/10.1007/978-981-99-3110-1_19

19.2 Product and Technology Innovation of Urinalysis in China

19.2.1 Overview

Urinalysis is the basic routine item of clinical laboratory, which is usually based on urine dry chemistry analysis and urine formed element analysis.

Urine dry chemistry analyzer generally uses reflectance photoelectric colorimetry to qualitatively or semi-quantitatively analyze the urine chemical composition of urine. In recent years, there are also instruments that use imaging colorimetry to do qualitative or semi-quantitative analysis. The feature of this method is that it can also provide the original image of the test strip for convenient review.

According to the technical principles, the urine formed element analyzers are mainly divided into static digital imaging shooting technology, flow digital image imaging technology, and flow nucleic acid fluorescence staining technology. At present, the main brands of urine formed element analyzers in the domestic market use flow digital imaging shooting technology or static digital imaging shooting technology. With the development of artificial intelligence technology, it plays an important role in laboratory medicine, especially in the automatic identification of cell morphology. The new generation of AI technology shows the characteristics of deep learning, autonomous learning, human-machine collaboration, and so on. All these technologies have been introduced into urine formed element analyzers. Through continuous training of massive image databases and autonomous deep learning, the automatic identification ability of intelligent equipment for urine formed elements has been continuously improved, and the burden of manual review has been gradually reduced, which takes digital image shooting technology in urine formed elements instruments to a higher level.

Only taking urine dry chemistry and urine formed element as the basic detection of urine routine is still insufficient in the diagnosis and differential diagnosis of urinary system diseases. At present, the new combining scheme of urinalysis workflow consisting of dedicated urine-specific protein analyzer and biochemical analyzer has been launched. In addition to urine routine analysis and urine formed element analysis, it can also quantitatively analyze specific proteins, enzymes and other chemical components in urine, realizing one-stop detection of multiple dimensions and multi-methods of clinicopathological urine specimens, providing accurate, timely and rich diagnostic information for clinical practice. At the same time, with the continuous development of chromatography tandem mass spectrometry, polymerase chain reaction (PCR), and other testing technologies, the detection of proteomics, metabolomics, and genomics of urine will become the future development trend.

At present, the main manufacturers leading urine routine test products in China are URIT, AVE, DIRUI, Mindray, Mejer, etc. The main manufacturers of other urine test products such as urine-specific protein or dedicated equipment for biochemical detection are Biostec, Goldsite Biology, Sinocare, and so on.

19.2.2 Products and Technology Innovation of Urine Dry Chemical Analysis

19.2.2.1 UC-1800 Automatic Urine Analyzer

It is a new generation of products produced by URIT, which has fast testing speed, stable, and reliable test results, and can complete the continuous sample test with one key.

1. **Structure:** It consists of automatic sample feeding device, automatic strip selection device, test strip transfer device, liquid circuit device, optical system, central processor, waste collection device, analysis and processing software, display, and printer.
2. **Test principle:** Use contact image scanning analysis technology to obtain the content of the substance to be tested by judging the reaction color of the test strips. The specific gravity, turbidity, and color of urine are tested by refraction/transmission method and red, green and blue (RGB) color method.
3. **Parameters:** The testing speed is 480 T/H. It can test 14 items of dry chemistry and 3 items of physical parameter, and provide Albumin-to-Creatinine Ratio (ACR) and PCR.
4. **Technological innovation:** (1) Liquid level sensing function combines with closed puncture sampling to block the transmission of urine aerosol. The test trip cabin is sealed with magnetic strips and has built-in desiccants, which ensures the quality of the test strips. (2) Matrix high-speed sample dropping and accurately quantitative sample dropping can avoid cross contamination between test items. (3) Temperature control function keeps the temperature of test area constant, and ensures that the dry chemistry reaction is carried out at the optimal temperature; (4) The image display function of urine test strip can capture, display, and store the images of urine test strips after dropping samples, so as to facilitate review and traceability.

19.2.2.2 H-1600 Automatic Urine Dry Chemistry Analyzer

Produced by DIRUI, it can meet the needs of intelligent, automated, and high-throughput urine dry chemical test in hospitals.

1. Structure: It consists of mechanical module, liquid circuit module, circuit module, prestore tray, and reclaiming tray (optional) and software.
2. Test principle: Multiwavelength photoelectric colorimetry.
3. Parameters: The testing speed is 240 T/H. It can test 14 items of dry chemistry and four physical items and provide ACR.
4. Technological innovation: (1) Exact volume dropping technology can eliminate cross interference between test items. (2) The reaction time is precisely controlled to ensure the accuracy of test results. (3) High brightness cold light source and multi-wavelength detection can reduce ambient light interference.

19.2.2.3 AVE-752 Full Automated Urine Analyzer

Produced by AVE, it has a high degree of automation, and the front end is equipped with automatic sample delivery device.

1. Structure: It consists of automatic sample delivery device, sample processing device, test strip convey device, dry chemical analysis device, physical test device, and central control unit.
2. Test principle: Charge coupled device (CCD) detecting technique.
3. Parameters: The testing speed is 240 T/H. It can test 14 items of dry chemistry and five items of physical parameter, and provide ACR.
4. Technological innovation: (1) It adopts innovative cassette strip loading system, so as to ensure that the test strips are clean and free of pollution, and to avoid the interference with the test results caused by direct manual contact. (2) The patented strip distribution technology and device ensure that it outputs test strips automatically and singly on front side, place test strips accurately without jamming. (3) It adds unique sample sprinkling technology. (4) The test results are photographed and stored by CCD to facilitate manual review and traceability.

19.2.2.4 UA-5800 Automatic Dry Chemistry Urine Analyzer

Produced by Mindray, it can detect all routine physical and chemical items in urine and provide complete urine dry chemical analysis. The instrument has advantages of compact structure and simple operation.

1. Structure: It consists of mechanical system, detecting unit, liquid circuit system, and circuit system.
2. Test principle: It uses the principle of multi-wavelength reflection colorimetry and the interference is eliminated by color compensation. As the accepted reference method, the reflective refractive index method is used to determine specific gravity.
3. Parameters: The testing speed is 240 T/H. It can test 14 items of dry chemistry and three items of physical parameters, and provide ACR.
4. Technological innovation: (1) Automatic dot matrix sampling technique improves the analysis accuracy and avoids cross interference between items. (2) The test strip cabin can hold no less than 200 test strips at a time, has good sealing performance, can inhibit accompanying substances, so that the quality of test trips during storage is ensured. (3) It adopts mature hardware technology. The syringe and solenoid valve use the same platform and technology as the hematology products, so that the stability and reliability of the whole machine are ensured.

19.2.3 Products and Technology Innovation of Urine Formed Element Analysis

19.2.3.1 UD-1320 Auto Urine Sediment Analyzer

Produced by URIT, it upgraded and optimized the AI deep learning recognition algorithm in 2019, has greatly improved the ability of rapid and intelligent analysis and identification of urine formed elements, which can meet the requirements of medical institutions for intelligence, automation, and rapid processing of large quantities of specimens.

1. Structure: The analyzer is composed of microscope shooting system, liquid circuit system, control system, identification software, mechanical device, input and output parts.
2. Test principle: The formed elements are identified by digital imaging identification, planar flow cytometry, and deep learning AI technology. For physical test, it adopts electrical impedance method.
3. Parameters: The testing speed is 240 T/H. It can test 38 items of formed element, two items of physical parameter, and four items of RBC morphology.
4. Technological innovation: (1) Using AI deep learning technology, a large number of particle pictures reviewed and classified by experts are used to train the instrument, from which it summed up a set of recognition rules covering the majority of particle variation, and its comprehensive recognition rate of urine formed elements has increased from the industry average of 80% to more than 95%. (2) It supports biosafety test tubes, which are made of sealing plastic complex films and can be punctured; At the same time, it can prevent damage, leakage and spillage, and reduce the biohazard of urine aerosol to inspection personnel. (3) It cooperated with Huawei Cloud to realize AI training and cloud computing, so that the AI recognition rate and recognition items continues to improve.

19.2.3.2 FUS-360 Urine Sediment Analyzer

Produced by DIRUI, it can detect urine formed elements with high automation and high throughput.

1. Structure: The analyzer is composed of microscopic imaging module, automatic sample injection module, liquid circuit mechanism, and data processing module.
2. Test principle: It is based on the principle of flow digital image shooting. The hydrodynamic system consists of a specially made flow cell with a thin layer structure. After sampling, sample enters the flow cell. Under the action of the laminar flow fluid used for urinalysis, the sample flows through the thin layer structure of the flow cell as thick as a single layer of cells, and then is shot at high speed.
3. Parameters: The testing speed is 120 T/H. It can test 25 items of formed element.

4. Technological innovation: (1) Flow cytometry technology is used to ensure that within the focal range of the microscope lens, each formed element flows in front of the microscope lens and the high-speed camera, and is photographed at high speed. In addition, the diffusive flow of urine can also effectively avoid the accumulation of formed elements. (2) AI recognition technology, automatic formed element recognition software, and highly trained intelligent recognition technology can quickly extract the images of formed element particles, and then identify and classify them according to the morphology, texture, and frequency domain characteristics of the photographed "particles." After automatic identification and classification, the concentration of formed elements is calculated based on the number of "particle" images taken and the volume of urine samples scanned.

19.2.3.3 AVE-766 Formed Element Analyzer

Produced by AVE, it is a new serial of product with machine vision technology, low power screening, positioning, and high-power tracking recognition.

1. Structure: It is composed of automatic sample delivery device, sample processing mechanism, visual transmission processing device, physical detection device, and central control system.
2. Test principle: Machine vision technology, microscope fast autofocus technology, low power negative screening technology, low power target positioning technology, and high-power target tracking and recognition technology.
3. Parameters: The testing speed is 100–200 T/H. It can test more than 30 items of formed element and four items of RBC morphology.
4. Technological innovation: (1) The matched urine sample collector adopts a fully sealed design, so that the sample is closed in the whole process of conveying. Pneumatic transmission is available. After the machine is started, the cover is closed and sampling is performed by means of puncture so as to avoid environmental pollution and the risk of aerosol infection, economize on manpower, and shorten sample turnaround time. (2) The function of negative sample screening is realized by using full-field rapid scanning technology under low power lens. For positive samples, positioning and tracking technology are used to locate the target under low power lens, automatically track and enlarge the target under high-power lens, and then identify and classify the fine structures. (3) The high-speed Advanced RISC Machines (ARM) microscope control technology and fast autofocus technology are used to quickly collect images of formed element to ensure image clarity and image quality stability. (4) Relying on AI technology, the recognition algorithm is continuously optimized, and it is continuously trained based on the massive database of 5000 users.

19.2.3.4 EH-2080 Fully Automatic Urinary Sediment Analysis System

Produced by Mindray, it can automatically adjust the focal length of the microscope, and its patented technologies improve the image clarity and stability.

1. Structure: It is composed of automatic sampler, automatic digital microscope, sample injector, multi-channel counting cell, and computer control processing system.
2. Test principle: Dynamic intelligent focusing technology(DIF), coordinate positioning and tracking technology, and machine vision technology.
3. Parameters: The testing speed is 100 T/H. It can test 16 items of parameter including RBC morphology.
4. Technological innovation: (1) The patented DIF technology, combined with flow counting cell, machine vision technology and coordinate positioning tracking and identification technology, realizes the quantitative detection of various urine formed elements without the need for fixed focus fluid, and greatly reduces the cost of laboratory testing. (2) The problem of focal length control in the detection process is solved, the backhaul difference caused by environmental factors is eliminated, and the stability of focal plane is effectively maintained.

19.2.3.5 Mejer-1800 Urine Sediment Analyzer

Produced by Mejer, it is the first instrument in China that uses S-M staining method combined with AI technology to automatically identify urine formed elements.

1. Structure: It is composed of automatic injection device, sampling device, staining pool, and micrograph device.
2. Test principle: Machine vision imaging technology is used to automatically locate, focus, identify, classify, and count the formed elements in urine.
3. Parameters: The testing speed is(90–150)T/H. It can test 39 items of urine formed elements.
4. Technological innovation: (1) Urine formed elements are stained and counted by using a 16-bore disposable quantitative counting plate. According to the physiological characteristics of different types of cells in the urine sediment, the pigments in the staining solution are attached to the cell surface to different degrees, the contour edge is clearer, and the contrast is higher. (2) Different kinds of cells also showed large differences in color. After staining, the overall image contrast is enhanced and the cell edge is clear, which improves the precision of focusing and the accuracy of recognition. (3) The thick samples are automatically diluted to ensure the accuracy of the results. (4) Multithreaded AI recognition models make high cell recognition rate.

19.2.4 Product and Technology Innovation of Urinalysis System (Workflow)

19.2.4.1 US-3000/US-1680 Urinalysis Workflow

It is a product of URIT. On the basis of the original urine routine analysis workflow, US-3000 series has added urine-specific protein module and urine biochemistry detection module to realize one-stop detection of urine physics, dry chemistry, formed element, specific protein, and biochemical quantification. On the basis of all-in-one machine, US-1680 series adds online functions to meet the needs of different markets.

1. Structure: US-3000 series is composed of dry chemistry test module, urine formed elements test module, specific protein test module, biochemical test module, and fully automatic sample processing module. It supports a variety of combinations of five layout: "I," "L-90," "L-270," "U," and "Z." US-1680 series is composed of one or more dry chemistry and formed elements test modules, and automatic sample processing modules connected. The system integrates the dry chemistry test module, the formed elements test module, and the physical test module, combined with ST pre-processing device, SS conveying device, YC post-storage device, and SZ transition device of automatic sample processing system, to form urinalysis workflow.
2. Test principle: For physical test, the specific gravity, turbidity, color, electrical conductivity, and osmotic pressure of urine are measured by refraction/transmission method, RGB color method, and impedance method. For dry chemistry, it adopts contact image scanning analysis technology to judge the reaction color of the test strips and output test results. For urine formed elements, digital imaging automatic identification, planar flow cytometry, and deep learning AI technology are used to automatically identify the morphology of formed particles and classify them correctly. Immune scatter turbidimetry is used to quantify each specific protein index. For biochemistry, colorimetry and transmission turbidimetry are used to quantify each trace proteins, enzymes, and other indexes.
3. Parameters: The testing speed of US-3000 series is up to 800 samples/hour. US-1680 series system is divided into dry chemistry and formed element combined mode, single mode of dry chemistry, and single mode of formed element. When two US-1680 are online, the testing speed is up to 240 samples/hour. Up to 87 comprehensive items can be measured, including 38 items of formed elements, 14 items of dry chemistry, 4 items of red blood cell morphology, 5 items of physical parameter, 10 items of specific protein, 14 items of biochemistry, and 2 items of research parameter.

    Formed element items: Normal RBC, Acanthocyte, Humped spherocyte, Humped spherocyte, WBC, Macrophage, Urothelial Cells, Renal Tubular Epithelium Cell, Cell Cast, Blood Cast, Broad Cast, CAOX, Uric Acid Crystal, Amorphous Phosphate, Coccus, Bacillus, Yeast, Fusarium, etc.

    Dry chemistry items: VC, WBC, KET, NIT, URO, BIL,PRO, GLU, SG, BLD, pH, CR, Ca, and Ma.

    RBC morphology: MCV, MCV-CV, R-RATE, RBC volume distribution histogram.

    Physical items: Physical items: color, SG, turbidity, COND and OS.

    Specific protein quantitative test items: mALB, TRF, IgG, A1M, BMG, CRE, ACR, etc.

    Urine biochemical quantitative test items: mALB, UTP,α-AMY, TRF, IgG, RBP, NGAL, CRE, etc.

    Research parameter: ACR and PCR.

4. Technological innovation and clinical significance: (1) The sheath fluid wraps and compresses the formed particles into a single layer to pass through a high-power microscope lens, avoiding accumulation and overlap. (2) Upgraded and optimized deep learning AI recognition technology, perfect expert database of formed particles, and AI autonomous learning, training and automatic iteration in the cloud, truly solve the fuzzy identification problem of urine formed elements in complex environments. (3) Five erythrocyte subclasses are provided, which can effectively help clinical judgment of the source of hematuria. (4) It can accurately identify macrophages, renal tubular epithelium cells and cell casts, and provide laboratory evidence for clinical differentiation of urinary tract inflammation and tubulointerstitial nephritis. (5) ACR/PCR can provide important basis for early diagnosis, treatment, and prognosis of renal diseases. (6) High-definition pictures of the original particles and test strips reaction are retained, and the results can be traced. (7) The specific protein and biochemical module can quantitatively detect more than 20 items and accurately locate the protein source, which is helpful for clinical judgment of the damaged kidney parts.

19.2.4.2 MUS-3600/ MUS-9600 Urinalysis System

It is a modular urinalysis workflow launched by DIRUI, which can meet the realistic needs of clinical laboratories for automated and high-throughput urine testing.

1. Structure: MUS-3600 series is composed of FUS-360 urine sediment analyzer and H-1600 automatic urine dry chemistry analyzer online, supporting 11 combinations of linear layout, and can realize the maximum combination mode of 2 + 4. MUS-9600 series is composed of a new all-in-one module. The test modules are connected together by a pre-storage device, a recycle device and a delivery device, supporting a maximum of four modules for joint detection.
2. Test principle: Using multi-wavelength photoelectric colorimetric method, the dry chemical test results are obtained by measuring the color value of the test strip after reaction. Using planar flow cytometry + high-speed shooting technology + AI recognition technology, the formed element images are segmented by software, converted into digital information, and then classified.
3. Parameters: MUS-3600/ MUS-9600 can load up to 520 samples at a time. The testing speed is 480 T/H. A total of 44 parameters could be completed by one-key test, including 25 items of urine formed elements, 14 items of dry chemistry, four items of physical parameter, and 1 research parameter.

   25 items of formed element: NRBC, Micro RBC, Acanthocyte, Ghost cell, Other Poikilocyte, WBC, WBCC, Squamous Epithelial Cell, Renal Tubular Epithelium Cell, Transitional epithelial cell, Hyaline Cast, Granular Cast, Waxy Cast, Broad Cast, Other cast, Bacillus, Suspicious coccus, Pseudohypha yeast, Yeast, Calcium Oxalate Crystal, Uric Acid Crystal, Ammonium Magnesium Phosphate Crystal, Other crystal, Spermatozoa, MUCS, etc.

   10–14 items of dry chemistry can be selected: URO, BIL, KRT, BLD, PRO, NIT, WBC, GLU, pH, SG, VC (optional), MA (optional), CR (optional), Ca (optional).

Physical items: Colour, SG, turbidity and COND.
Research parameter: ACR.

4. Technological innovation and clinical significance: (1) Urine sample is wrapped in the sheath fluid and enters the detection system, which ensures that the formed elements of the urine always pass through the microscope lens in a single layer and independent way to avoid particle overlap and aggregation. More than 2500 pictures of each sample are taken by using high-speed photograph technology and 40x objective magnification to avoid missing detection. (2) Based on massive clinical samples, a large image database of urine formed elements is established by using AI recognition technology. Artificial neural network technology is used to accurately extract image feature information and automatically complete the recognition and classification of formed elements. (3) The system provides red blood cell morphology information (phase prompts), prompting homogeneous red blood cells, heterogeneous red blood cells and mixed red blood cells, assisting in the diagnosis of renal diseases and bleeding parts, and showing abnormal red blood cell morphology in detail. The subclassification of cast is rich, which can effectively assist in clinical diagnosis and monitoring of renal parenchymal lesions and the process of nephropathy. (4) It can distinguish the pathogenic bacteria, indicate the information of urine culture, and provide reference for the diagnosis and treatment of urinary tract infection. Also, it provides ACR parameters, which is a basis for early screening of nephropathy. (5) Review condition is settable. The instrument prompts microscopic examination automatically when review condition is satisfied.

19.2.4.3 EU 8000 Fully Automated Urine Analysis Line

Mindray blood cell analysis research and development team launched this product based on stable, accurate and reliable quality.

1. Structure: The system is composed of UA-6800/5800 automatic dry chemical urine analyzer and EH-2080 B/C fully automatic urinary sediment analyzer.
2. Test principle: Photoelectric colorimetry + dot matrix sampling technology is adopted to avoid cross-contamination between items and achieve dry chemical results output. DIF technology, combined with flow counting pool, machine vision technology, coordinate positioning tracking and identification technology, to achieve the quantitative detection of urine formed elements.
3. Parameters: In 1 + 2 online mode, the testing speed is 200 T/H. 40 comprehensive items can be measured, including 20 items of urine formed elements, 14 items of dry chemistry, one item of red blood cell morphology, three items of physical parameter, and 1 research parameter.

   Formed element items: Normal RBC, Ghost cell, WBC, WBCC, Urothelial Cells, Cast, Calcium Oxalate Crystal, Coccus, Bacillus, Yeast, Spermatozoa, etc.

   Dry chemistry items: VC, WBC, KET, NIT, PRO, GLU, SG, BLD, pH, CR, MA and so on.

   RBC morphology items: RBC volume distribution histogram.

Physical items: Color, SG and turbidity.

Research parameter: ACR.

4. Technological innovation and clinical significance: (1) DIF focusing technology is adopted in the system, which does not require consumables such as fixed focus fluid, so the use cost reduces. (2) Use morphological gold standard, combined with flow counting pool, machine vision technology, coordinate positioning tracking and identification technology, to achieve the quantitative detection of urine formed elements.

19.2.4.4 AVE-772 Integrated Urinalysis Analyzer

Produced by AVE, it uses integrated design, easy to operate, and saves laboratory space. The physical, dry chemical, and formed elements test can be completed in one sample aspiration.

1. Structure: The analyzer is composed of dry chemical test module, formed elements test module, physical test module, sample injection module, sampling module, and so on.
2. Test principle: The charge-coupled device (CCD) technique is used to realize the automatic detection of urine physical items and dry chemical indexes. AI machine vision technology is used to simulate the classical microscope examination, and the real images of formed elements are collected under high and low power lens, and the images are automatically identified and classified and counted.
3. Parameters: The testing speed is up to 240 T/H. More than 50 comprehensive items can be measured, including more than 30 items of urine formed elements, 14 items of dry chemistry, five items of physical parameter, and 1 research parameter.

   Formed element items: Normal RBC, Ghost cell, WBC, WBCC, Renal Tubular Epithelium Cell, Transitional epithelial cell, Cell Cast, Blood Cast, Calcium Oxalate Crystal, Uric Acid Crystal, Coccus, Bacillus, Yeast, Fusarium, Spermatozoa, MUCS.

   4–14 items of dry chemistry can be selected according to clinical needs: URO, BIL, KET, CR, BLD, PRO, MA, NIT, WBC, GLU, SG, pH, VC, CA and so on.

   Physical items: Color, SG, turbidity, COND, and OS.

   Research parameters: ACR.
4. Technological innovation and clinical significance: (1) The system can complete the urine physical, dry chemistry and formed elements test at one time, and provide the parameters of RBC morphology, conductivity and osmotic pressure, ACR, etc., which can provide reference for the clinical diagnosis of urinary system and endocrine system diseases, and renal concentration and dilution function. (2) The system has perfect review rules. Automatic and intelligent comprehensive analysis of dry chemical and microscopic examination results can improve audit efficiency and reduce work burden. (3) The test results are objective and true. It provides pictures of dry chemical test strips and realistic

pictures of formed elements, and the confirmatory report can be issued. It has a perfect quality control system, providing original reagents, test strips, quality control products, calibration products, AAA traceability system, to ensure the quality of detection. (4) Equipped with a remote intelligent service platform, the system can know the running status of the equipment in the first time, provide online fault diagnosis, real-time technical support, remote diagnosis and guidance and other services, so as to improve the service efficiency and quality.

19.2.5 Urine-Specific Protein Analysis and Biochemical Analysis Products

19.2.5.1 Specific Protein Analyzer

It is a highly automated specific protein analysis system launched by Biostec in 2020.

1. Structure: The system matches bar code identification and sample pre-processing module, is compatible with track and turntable injection, also electrolyte module is optional. The instrument can be connected with multiple modules to form a specific protein detection workflow. It can also be connected with urine routine analysis workflow and biochemical immune workflow to form the urine full detection workflow.
2. Test principle: The system adopts the double optical path detection technology of scattering turbidimetry, compatible with biochemical immunoturbidimetry and enzymatic method, to quantitatively determine the specific proteins and routine biochemical items of the samples.
3. Parameters: The testing speed of single machine is 300 T/H, and more than 20 comprehensive items can be measured, including more than 4 glomerular proteins, more than 6 renal tubular proteins, and more than 10 routine urine biochemical items. The ACR value can be quantitatively output.
   Glomerular proteins items: mALB, TRF and G(IgG).
   Renal tubular proteins items: A1M, BMG and RBP, etc.
   Routine biochemical items: More than 10 items such as CRE, UTP, UUA, etc.
4. Clinical significance: The detection of specific proteins can realize the screening of chronic kidney disease and provide a possibility for the detection of early renal injury. It is helpful for the early monitoring and pathological localization of renal injury before the parenchymal damage caused by various nephropathy (before the appearance of dominant proteinuria). It provides a more comprehensive auxiliary diagnostic basis for clinical intervention to treat various kidney diseases and protect the kidney. It helps prevent various complications of kidney disease.

19.2.5.2 Aristo-Specific Protein Analyzer

It is a urine-specific protein detection instrument launched by Goldsite Biology.

1. Structure: The instrument consists of continuous injection track, sampling device, reagent adding device, reagent refrigeration device, and reaction detection device. It can be connected with the urine routine analysis workflow to form the urine full detection workflow.
2. Test principle: It adopts immune scatter turbidimetry, equipped with reagents with high sensitivity and wide linear range, to realize the quantitative detection of specific proteins in samples.
3. Parameters: The testing speed of single machine is 300 T/H. There are 10 comprehensive items for urine test, including mALB, TRF, IgG, A1M, BMG, AMG, KAP, LAM, CRE, and ACR.
4. Clinical significance: Determination of mALB, TRF, IgG, and A1M (or BMG) in urine can effectively exclude individual differences, locate protein sources, and determine the site of renal damage. Quantification of ACR is helpful for early detection and diagnosis of nephritis and nephropathy. Monitoring the change of microalbumin at 20 mg/L-200 mg/L can effectively evaluate the severity of renal injury. The urine detection instrument is for dedicated purpose, avoiding cross detection of blood samples and urine samples on biochemical analyzer; specific protein detection can be carried out in the urine test group, forming a urine routine + urine formed element + urine-specific protein detection workflow, and the test results can be issued on one report sheet, so that the disease can be judged more accurately and scientific decisions can be made.

19.3 Urinalysis Technology and Market Outlook

19.3.1 Application of AI Technology in Urine Formed Element Detection

With the rapid development of hardware computing power and Graphics Processing Unit (GPU) computing, AI technology has made a breakthrough. It plays an important role in laboratory medicine, especially in the automatic identification of cell morphology. The new generation of AI technology presents the characteristics of deep learning, autonomous learning and man-machine collaboration. Through continuous training of massive image databases and autonomous deep learning, the automatic identification ability of intelligent equipment for urine formed element has been continuously improved, and the burden of manual review has been gradually reduced.

Deep learning artificial intelligence technology develops rapidly, and there are many new deep learning algorithm models. At present, the most widely used is multi-layer neural network, because of its more neurons, the recognition effect is much better than single-layer and two-layer networks. Contemporary giants such as Google, Microsoft, and Facebook have all participated in the research and design war of deep learning framework. From widely used Caffe to TensorFlow, from supervised training learning to unsupervised training learning, the application of deep learning artificial intelligence in morphology is becoming more accurate and effective.

Unsupervised learning is also applied to the self-learning mechanism. Deep learning algorithms can self-learn cell features by outputting a large number of classified and labeled cell pictures. But other algorithms only learn features that people require them to learn. Just like a person with self-learning ability and a cramming person, it is self-evident who is better.

In addition, some manufacturers also use the amplification learning method. Firstly, deep learning adopts the mode of self-learning features, and then we introduce the amplification learning feature technology. In this way, the cell features learned by the algorithm are more accurate and comprehensive, and the classification compatibility is better. The advantage of overfitting recognition technology is that even when unlearned cells or impurities appear, there is no misclassification, which makes the recognition system more stable.

The development of Internet technology and the analysis and processing ability of big data have accelerated the improvement in the recognition algorithm and the recognition effect. Through the summary, analysis and training of a large number of clinicopathological sample image data, it is believed that AI technology can make a further breakthrough in the detection of urine formed elements.

19.3.2 Future Trends of Urine Exosomes

Exosomes are extracellular vesicles (EVs) secreted by cells. Its size is 30 nm–150 nm, like a saucer, has a bilayer structure, contains rich inclusions (including nucleic acids, proteins and lipids), and involves in molecular transmission from cell to cell. It is widely distributed in various body fluids, such as urine, saliva, blood, amniotic fluid, and cerebrospinal fluid and pathological ascites. Compared with other body fluids, urine has the advantages of simple and safe sampling, large volume and non-invasive. Therefore, the study of urine exosomes is of great significance for the early diagnosis, treatment, monitoring targets, and the study of disease mechanism of urinary system diseases. The following describes the relevant studies of urine exosomes in renal and bladder cancer.

The kidney is a urine producing organ. Urine exosome proteomics has found the expression of various proteins in kidney cells, and also identified proteins in bladder transitional epithelium, indicating that exosomes produced by kidney tumors can directly enter the urine [1]. Therefore, urine exosomes can be used as a new method to detect renal cancer.

Bladder is the direct organ that stores urine, and the changes related to bladder cancer (BCa) may be detected more quickly in urine than in blood. Some researchers have analyzed that exosomes secreted by bladder cancer cells contain a variety of proteins, and these proteins can also be detected in the urine of bladder cancer patients, so by labeling these proteins, bladder cancer can be effectively diagnosed. Smalley et al. [2] detected 307 proteins in urine exosomes from BCa patients and healthy controls by mass spectrometry, and identified 8 proteins highly expressed in urine exosomes from BCa patients and 1 protein highly expressed in urine exosomes from healthy people. Perez et al. [3]analyzed urine exosomal RNA from BCa patients and confirmed that RNA in urine exosomes is a stable molecular marker, among which mucin glycosylase 1 and human longevity guarantee gene 2 can be used as diagnostic indicators for BCa patients. By studying the expression profile of urinary exosomes in patients with bladder transitional cell carcinoma, it was found that the expression of 7 miRNA was significantly higher than that of healthy controls, and it has reference significance for the staging and grading of bladder transitional cell carcinoma [4].

Liquid biopsies are a hot track right now. The main biomarkers are circulating tumor DNA (ctDNA), circulating tumor cell (CTC), exosome, miRNA, and so on. Proteomic analysis and genomics-related studies based on LC-MS/MS and next-generation sequencing (NGS) technology have screened out a large number of candidate molecular markers related to kidney disease. In the future, it will have broad prospects in early diagnosis of tumors, definition of tumor typing, detection of pathological development, monitoring of drug resistance, and judgment of prognosis.

Declaration Jun Jiang, Chuanjun Su, Kun Wang and Yongqing Zhou are employees of URIT Medical Electronic Co., Ltd., Guilin, Guangxi, China.

References

1. Pisitkun T, Shen R F, Knepper MA. Identification and proteomic profiling of exosomes in human urine[J]. Proc Natl Acad Sci USA , 2004, 101: 13368-13373
2. Chen CL, Lai YF, Tang P, et al. Comparative and targeted proteomic analyses of urinary microparticles from bladder cancer and hernia patients [J]. J Proteome Res, 2012, 11(12): 5611-5629.
3. Butz H, Nofech-Mozes R, Ding Q, et al. Exosomal microRNAs are diagnostic biomarkers and can mediate cell-cell communication in renal cell carcinoma[J]. Eur Urol Focus, 2016, 2: 210-218
4. Armstrong DA, Green BB, Seigne JD, et al. MicroRNA molecular profiling from matched tumor and bio-fluids in bladder cancer[J]. Mol Cancer, 2015, 14: 194.

Stool and Intestinal Microbiota Examination

20

Tingting Wang, Xianglong Li, and Qinghua Liao

20.1 Introduction

Stool examination detects the changes in appearance, morphology, particles, and biochemistry of the human fecal samples, in order to study the human gene information, pathogenic microorganisms, commensal microorganisms, and other relevant information carried in the feces. The examination plays significant roles in helping the diagnosis of gastrointestinal dysfunction, and gastrointestinal ulcers, obstruction, bleeding, tumor, etc. Additionally, inflammation and lesions of the adjacent organs (i.e., liver and gallbladder), as well as parasitic diseases can also be diagnosed via stool examination. Its advantage includes ease to obtain specimens, non-invasive, and wide application potential of a variety of diseases. Stool examination is applicable to hospitalized patients and all patients suspected of digestive diseases, and is also frequently used for chronic disease screening in physical examination.

Recent studies have shown that detection of genetic information from the human digestive tract epidermal cells, which are partially shed in feces, provides particular reference significance for the early screening of colorectal tumors. In recent years, therefore, fecal DNA testing has shown a good market scale and application prospect in early cancer screening. A series of companies in China have developed colorectal cancer (CRC) early screening products based on fecal DNA testing. Target genes include mutations of KARS and APC genes, methylation of SDC2, BMP3 and NDRG4 genes, etc. The Chinese Guidelines for Colorectal Cancer

T. Wang (✉)
Hangzhou Hailu Medical Technology Co., Ltd., Hangzhou, China

X. Li
Hunan Hailu Biotechnology Co., Ltd., Changsha, China

Q. Liao
Sciendox Biotechnology Co., Ltd., Xiamen, China

H. Song, L. Dai (eds.), *In Vitro Diagnostic Industry in China*,
https://doi.org/10.1007/978-981-99-3110-1_20

Screening and Early Diagnosis and Treatment (2020, Beijing), published in the Chinese Journal of Cancer on January 15, 2021, clearly recommended multitarget fecal immunochemical testing (FIT)-DNA combined detection technology as one of the important means of early screening for colorectal cancer.

In addition, investigation of the bacterial DNA and metabolites in feces can also be used to assess the health status of human intestinal microecosystem. Intestinal microbiota accounts for more than 90% of the human symbiotic microorganisms, and together with the organs of the human digestive tract, constitutes the human intestinal microecosystem. They significantly affect host metabolism, immunity, and health. Intestinal microbiota degrades food components that human cells cannot digest, thus constructing a host-microbiota co-metabolic network. A healthy micro-ecosystem in balance also helps maintain the host immune response, resists against pathogens, and regulates the function of the whole human body directly or indirectly. Dysbiosis of the intestinal microbiota is demonstrated to be associated with various diseases. Feces contain a large number of microbial cells and metabolic substances from the gut microbiota; thus, they can be used as a "window" to assess the health status of the human gut microecosystem.

20.2 Routine Stool Examination and Stool Analyzer

20.2.1 Content of Routine Stool Examination

The routine examination of stool includes appearance and morphology, fecal chemistry, and immunology biomarkers.

Appearance description is judged by visual observation, which includes stool color (light yellow, green and jam color, etc.), shape (flat ribbon, spherical, etc.), hardness (soft, hard, watery, conjee-like, etc.). Commonly, stool samples can be classified into seven groups according to "the Bristol Stool Scale," which was first published in 1997 in the Scandinavian Journal of Gastroenterology by Heaton and Lewis of the University of Bristol, UK. In detail, types 1 and 2 (hard) indicate constipation; types 3 and 4 are ideal stool shapes, especially type 4 is the easiest shape to defecate; types 5 to 7 (loose) indicate probable diarrhea (normal for newborns is type 6). As the character of stool is related to the time it stays in the large intestine, it can be used to speculate the time it takes for food to pass through the large intestine, and to judge the host digestive ability and intestinal health. In addition, mucous stool (with pus, bloody, etc.), various intestinal parasitic worms (hookworms, roundworms, pinworms, tapeworm, etc.), can also be detected by visual observation.

The morphological examination refers to the observation of the morphological characteristics of fecal components, include cells (red cells, eosinophils, epithelial cells, macrophages, etc.), parasite eggs and protozoa, food residues, crystals, bacteria, etc. Presently, wet smear under microscope is generally used for the morphological examination. Traditionally, the operator drops an appropriate amount of normal saline on the slide and smear fecal sample on it with a sterile bamboo skewer. The smear should be of appropriate thickness, so that handwriting on the slide can still be seen. The slides are then placed under a microscope for observation. Recently, morphological examination is often performed on stool analyzer with integrated morphology detection module, image transmission system, and high automation degree.

Chemical and immunological tests detect the chemical and immunological properties of specific substance in the feces. Common fecal immunological tests with clinical significance include occult blood test, transferrin test, rotavirus disease antigen test, adenovirus antigen test, and *Helicobacter pylori* antigen test. Since 2000, FIT (Fecal Immuno-Test) or called iFOBT has been used detect hemoglobin as an indicator of occult blood, which is different from the earliest chemical fecal occult blood test (gFOBT, or called GuaiacFecal-Occult Blood Test). The most salient significance of fecal occult blood test is to predict and reduce the mortality of colorectal cancer. According to incomplete data, fecal occult blood test can reduce the mortality of colorectal cancer by 10–30%. With its advantages as non-invasive, easy to use, and low-cost, clinical guidelines strongly recommend it as a first-line screening program. Fecal immunology test can also be used to detect intestinal pathogenic viruses, bacteria, and parasites.

With the popularization of automated stool analyzers, the convenience, efficiency, and accuracy of routine stool detection have made great progress in recent years.

20.2.2 The Multi-Function Stool Analyzer

"Multi-function stool analyzer," or called "Feces analysis system," is commonly used for routine examination of stool samples in research and clinical laboratories. An integrated stool analyzer generally includes four functional modules: specimen processing, morphological detection, immunological detection, and waste disposal. In recent years, stool analyzers often incorporate another specimen image recognition and processing system. Compared with hand processing, the efficiency of feces analysis is significantly improved, and results are more reliable and reproducible attributed to the standardized operation. The waste disposal device makes it environment friendly.

The specimen processing module is to process solid and semi-solid feces into application solution to meet the needs of morphological and immunological testing. The specimen processing module generally includes sample injection system, liquid adding system, mixing system, and filtration system. According to the specific model of the instrument and the actual operation requirements, the injection system can be classified as disk type or strip type; The mixing system can be classified as rotating mixing, mechanical mixing, bubble mixing, etc.; The filtration system can be classified as full filtration separation method, the lateral filtration method, the bottom filtration method, the suction filtration method. Some instruments use direct smear strategy without filtration. Some devices also have the ability to photograph and record the specimen's appearance.

The morphology detection module consists of an automatic or semi-automatic microscope, a flow counting cell fixed to the microscope or a disposable counting plate, as well as the liquid sample delivery system. Microscopes are mated with lenses with different magnifications and image transmission systems; The flow counting cell has a single channel or multiple channels; The single-use counting board can be a single pool or made of multiple pools. Fecal analyzer equipped with automatic microscope can automatically complete the image acquisition and storage, and the operator can screen and edit photos at any time. For the analyzers equipped with a semi-automatic microscope system, image acquisition and analysis are completed manually.

The immunological detection module generally uses colloidal gold method to qualitatively analyze certain objects in fecal samples. Three-waste disposal module refers to the control of waste water, gas, other waste liquid, so as to avoid environment contamination. The data processing module generally includes basic information setting, patient information collection, report processing, data import and backup, and even report processing.

20.2.3 Major Manufacturers and the Market Forecasting

Development of automatic stool analyzers is still in its infancy. In February 2013, the first "multifunctional fecal analysis workstation" in China was approved by National Medical Products Administration, China. On this early generation analyzer, stool specimens treatment, microscopic examination of the morphology, and immunology test were integrated on a single device for the first time. It adopted the filtration separation specimen processing technology, used automatic microscope to get images, and developed the first immunology examination module with four reagent channels and 20 detection sites. In the recent 5 years, many domestic enterprises have made great efforts to improve the instrument performance. Development of stool analyzer in China has experienced three stages: stool specimen processing instrument, semi-automatic analyzer, and "quasi" fully automated multifunctional analyzer. At present, equipment of these three stages coexists in the market, and undoubtedly, the automated multi-function analyzer has a broader market prospect. By the end of 2021, the automatic stool producer KeyuBio Co., Ltd. has been listed on the New Third Board, AVE Technology Co., Ltd. has been successfully listed on the Shanghai Stock Exchange science and Technology Innovation Board. Orienter Co., Ltd. submitted the application for listing on the GEM in June 2021, but it was suspended in August the same year. Up to now, the manufacturers with high market share in the domestic market include Sciendox Co., Ltd., KeyuBio Co., Ltd., Orienter Co., Ltd., Hailu Co., Ltd., etc. (Table 20.1).

Automatic stool analyzers are one of the few "domestic brand only" segments in the in vitro diagnostics industry in China. The overall penetration rate is still low relative to the number of medical institutions in China, and the market is not fully stimulated. According to "the Development History of Stool Automatic Analyzer and National Product Status in 2015" released by China in Vitro Diagnostic Network (CAIVD) in 2016, there are about 1500 sets of automatic stool analyzers in the China domestic market, distributed in tertiary hospitals and secondary hospitals in

Table 20.1 manufacturers with high market share in the domestic market

Manufacturer	Products	Details
Sciendox Biotechnology Co., ltd., Xiamen, China	Multi-function stool analyzer 2000R/6000R	In 2009, They invented the "total filtration separation method for specimen processing" and got invention patent authorization from China, the United States, Japan and the European Union. Using this technology, their firstly developed "specimen liquefaction processing instrument" and "multifunctional fecal analysis workstation" in the China market. After 10 years of improvement and technical accumulation, the company possesses leading techniques in the field of liquefication and analysis of stool sample. They published the first version of "Fecal Morphology Atlas (Volume 1)" in China
Hunan Hailu Biotechnology Co., Ltd., Changsha, China	HALO-F280 automatic stool analyzer	The company presided the project of "research on the metabolism mechanism of key food nutrition components based on intestinal microbiome and probiotics" in the 13th five-year plan National key Research and development fund. The HALO-F280 analyzer is equipped with a fully enclosed system, the specimen box is designed with the head to ensure effective mixing. The detection speed is 40–120 samples per hour, and the counting pool is automatically perfused. The automatic stool analyzer has been patented and supported by the innovation Fund of the Ministry of science and technology
Sichuan Orienter Biotechnology Co., Ltd., Chengdu, China	FA160 automatic stool analyzer	The FA160 analyzer can perform tests including fecal characteristics and constituents, fecal occult blood, transferrin, rotavirus, adenovirus, *helicobacter pylori* and calprotectin. The main technical parameters are as follows: Detection speed is 60 samples/hour; sample tube filter 60–10 mesh; the suction needle was upside-down and quantitatively aspirated (0.8 mL). Low magnification (10×, 12 preset views), high magnification (40×, 18 preset views)
AVE Technology Co., Ltd., Changsha, Hunan	AVE-562 automatic stool analyzer	Comprehensive detection speed >90 samples/h, recovery of tangible components >80%; the sample delivery device is track-type sample delivery, with a capacity of 40 specimens in the waiting area; using disposable counting board, counting board storage capacity of 200. Equipped with multi-level automatic focusing, hierarchical photography and data collection modules, the recognition and classification is completed by manual auxiliary
Jinan Lanjie BioTech Co., Ltd., Jinan, China	Stool analysis workstation LJ-5000	The stool analyzer has won a number of national intellectual property invention patents. The whole inspection process including automatic processing, mixing, suspension, filtration and perfusion is completed in a sealed environment, avoiding specimen contamination and directly improving work efficiency and the operating environment of the hospital laboratory

(continued)

Table 20.1 (continued)

Manufacturer	Products	Details
KeyuBio Co., Ltd., Zhuhai, China	KU-F10/20 automatic stool analyzer	The detection techniques include: Microscope image; immunity test module; chemical test module. The main technical parameters are as follows: Orbital injection, 50 specimen sites; 5 test bins; holding 100–200 reagent cards; carry out 1–10 projects at the same time. Two or three channel microscopic examination count. Equipped with quality control module
Jiangxi Tecom Technology Co., Ltd., Nanchang, China	TEX760z automatic stool analyzer	The TEX760z analyzer can perform quantitative sample dilution, with high speed and effective mixing, do not destroy all kinds of ingredients in the sample. It is equipped with automatic built-in original imported microscope examination system, with image analysis, transmission, storage function modules. Automatic interpretation of the results can be completed according to the color. The instrument automatically selects the dipstick card. The waiting area can hold 50 samples at one time. The waste liquid produced by the instrument can be discharged automatically and treated in a centralized manner
Xiangyang Courager Medical Device Co., Ltd., Xiangyang, China	Automatic stool analyzer KRJ/FJ2-1 T 16 DC	In 2014, the automatic stool analyzer independently developed by the company was introduced on the national "12th Five-Year Plan" textbooks for general higher education. It is the only stool automation instrument that does not need to filter specimens and is equipped with external eyepieces
Chongqing Tianhai Medical Device Co., Ltd., Chongqing, China	DBFJ-1000 automatic stool analyzer	1 Multi-index automatic detection of upper and lower gastrointestinal bleeding by fecal appearance, cell morphology, fecal occult blood and other indicators; 2 The stool sampler is directly put on the machine without pretreatment, and the test process is completely hermetic to avoid environment contamination
Lituo Biotech Co., Ltd., Zhuhai, China	LTS-E100 stool analysis workstation	Microscopic examination was performed with specially designed glass slides to simulate manual production. Two steps including automatic loading and shirking help complete the detection process. With a continuous circulation injection, up to 5 emergency specimens can be added at any time; LIS network help automatically generate color graphic reports

various provinces and cities. However, a large part of them is not in frequent use. There may be the following reasons for this phenomenon: (1) as the focus of stool detection at home and abroad is different, foreign big brands have little interest in developing automatic stool instrument, the reference data that domestic manufacturers can rely on is insufficient; (2) as there is no unified and effective standard for sample collection and pretreatment, considerable technical difficulty exists in product design; (3) The routine charge of stool analysis is low, which limits the enthusiasm of the clinical laboratories to carry out stool analysis.

In spite of the negative factors, stool analysis is still one of the most widely used basic test items in medical institutions and laboratories at all levels in China. Stool examination covers the vast majority of clinical path examination items and is an important diagnostic basis for doctors to make clinical diagnosis. Therefore, with the continuous optimization of the product technology, it is believed that automatic stool analyzer will be more popular in the future in medical institutions at all levels. Especially since the beginning of 2020, types and transmission modes of new infectious diseases such as coronavirus disease 2019 (COVID-19) have become increasingly complex, which has brought great challenges to public health. Viruses in patients' feces can be transmitted by aerosols, posing a risk of spread. Therefore, it is of great significance for clinical laboratories to equip fully enclosed, automatic and zero-contact automatic stool analyzer. According to public information, by the end of 2020, the number of stool analyzers installed by Sichuan Orienter in China was about 1500 (data from its prospectus), and the number of other manufacturers is also increasing year by year. Compared to a few years ago, the market acceptance has grown tremendously, and a sustainable growth will be seen in the future.

20.3 Early Screening for CRC Based on Stool Testing

20.3.1 CRC Early Screening Technology and Products

Colorectal cancer (CRC) is a common malignant tumor that seriously endangers human health. Its incidence ranks the third and mortality ranks the fifth among all kinds of tumors in China. Early screening and diagnosis are crucial to the survival of patients. Colonoscopy is currently the gold standard for early detection of CRC and precancerous lesions. However, due to its traumatic nature and requirements for medical conditions, patient compliance is limited. In the past 20 years, the overall survival rate of CRC patients in China has improved to some extent, which may be related to the improvement of access to primary health care services, the development of screening and early diagnosis technology, and the improvement of surgery and medicine. However, there is still a considerable gap between China's CRC survival rate and that of the United States and other developed countries. Screening is an effective method to strengthen the early diagnosis of colorectal cancer, which can be used for primary and secondary prevention. In recent years, stool analysis has become one of the key research directions in CRC screening because it can be sampled at home, and is non-invasive, convenient and fast.

At present, early screening methods for CRC via stool examination mainly include fecal immunochemical testing (FIT) and fecal DNA testing. The Chinese Guidelines for Colorectal Cancer Screening and Early Diagnosis and Treatment (2020, Beijing), published in the Chinese Journal of Cancer on January 15, 2021, clearly recommended multi-target FIT -DNA combined approach as one of the important means of CRC early screening. Other technical means (imaging, biopsy, etc.) are needed to confirm the diagnosis of cancer positive patients by early screening.

Technical principle of the FIT method is the detection of fecal occult blood using an immune antigen response. According to the results of a meta-analysis published in Annals of Internal Medicine, FIT has a high overall diagnostic accuracy for CRC [1]. The diagnostic performance of FIT mainly depends on the cutoff value of positive test results. The researchers analyzed 19 trials involving more than 113,000 subjects and provided data from eight different datasets in the United States. In addition to the sensitivity and specificity, positive and negative likelihood ratios (LRS) were calculated to assess the ability of these tests to "include" or "exclude" the diagnosis of CRC, respectively. The cutoff point was set as a value >5 for positive LR and 0.2 for negative LR. The results showed that FIT had a sensitivity of 79% and a specificity of 94% for the diagnosis of CRC. Pooled data from these trials showed a positive LR of 13.10 and a negative LR of 0.23. Increasing the number of FIT samples did not affect the sensitivity, specificity, positive LR, or negative LR of the pooled FIT for CRC. The performance of different FIT producers evaluated in the study showed no significant difference. However, the researchers acknowledge that these results need to be interpreted with caution because most studies did not conduct head-to-head comparisons. In June 2021, Molecular Diagnostic Group of Laboratory Medicine Society of Chinese Medical Association published the article named "Chinese Expert Consensus on Experimental Diagnostic Techniques for Early colorectal Cancer and precancerous Lesions" in the Chinese Journal of Laboratory Medicine, which further affirmed the important role of quantitative FIT technology in early CRC screening. They also recommended that screening population and age should be defined as "people aged 40 to 74 years without special risk."

Fecal DNA testing works by detecting mutations in DNA fragments in the stool sample. As abnormal cells carrying the tumor mutation signal will shed into the feces, researchers can effectively detect the mutant genes by extracting and interpretation of the DNA information from the stool sample. In detail, KRAS mutation is an important early event in the development of CRC. Hypermethylation of tumor suppressor gene promoters is another important mechanism of tumorigenesis. Previous studies have confirmed that hypermethylation of tumor suppressors BMP3 and NDRG4 is also an important biological feature in the early stage of CRC. Combined detection of such multiple genes is more sensitive than any single mutation. In 2014, a large sample size prospective study in the United States showed that combination of FIT and multi-target DNA markers (KRAS mutation, BMP3 methylation and NDRG4 methylation) was more sensitive in detecting CRC and advanced adenoma than FIT alone, with a sensitivity of 92.3% for CRC. The sensitivity and specificity of advanced adenoma reached 42.4 and 86.6%, respectively [2].

Products based on FIT and/or DNA targets are now commercially available and are booming in China, with a number of products successfully marketed (Table 20.2). Colosafe® Human SDC2 gene methylation detection Kit (fluorescent PCR method) is the first commercial companion diagnostic product for colorectal cancer using stool DNA, which is approved by the National Medical Products Administration (NMPA) in China. It is developed by Creative Biosciences (Guangzhou) Co., Ltd. It

Table 20.2 CRC screening products by fecal DNA test in the Chinese market

The product name	The company name	Technology description	Application scenario	Approval by NMPA (up to the end of 2021)
Coloclear®	New Horizon Health Technology (Hangzhou) Co., Ltd.	Human KRAS gene mutation, BMP3/NDRG4 gene methylation and stool occulted blood combined detection kit (PCR fluorescent probe method and colloidal gold method)	Sampling at home/ physical examination/ hospitals	NMPAClass III Medical device License (20203400845)
Colosafe®	Creative Biosciences (Guangzhou) Co., Ltd	Human SDC2 gene methylation detection kit (fluorescent PCR method)		NMPAClass III Medical device License (20183400506)
Changqingsong®	Amoy Diagnostics Co., Ltd. (AmoyDx, Xiamen)	SDC2 gene methylation detection kit (fluorescent PCR method)		NMPAClass III Medical device License (20213400007)
ColoWell®	Shanghai RealBio Technology Co., Ltd	SDC2 and SFRP2 gene promoter methylation combined detection kit (fluorescent PCR method)		None
HuaChangkang®	Envelope Health of BGI (Shenzhen) Co., LTD	Multi-gene methylation test		None
ColoComf®	Wuhan Ammunition Life-tech Co.,Ltd	SDC2 and TFPI2 gene methylation combined detection kit (fluorescent PCR method)		None
REColon®	GeneBioHealth (Shenzhen) Co.,ltd	miR-92a qualitative detection kit (fluorescent RT-PCR method)		None

was included in the special approval channel for innovative medical devices by NMPA in March 2017, and was officially approved and listed as a Class III medical device On November 20, 2018. In March 2020, Colosafe® was approved by the European Union (CE) for marketing. The registration data show that the kit is used as a basis for clinicians to recommend a colonoscopy, and is not used as a basis for early diagnosis or definitive diagnosis of cancer. According to the clinical trial technology review report published by the NMPA, the Colosafe® Human SDC2 gene methylation detection Kit (CSZ1800035) reached the Kappa value of 0.85 in 1213 test samples (374 CRC cases and 839 non-CRC cases). This value above 0.75 indicated good consistency between the product and the gold standard (colonoscopy + pathology). In May 2021, Creative Biosciences hosted the "5.29 Gut Safety Day" activity. On the same day, they disclosed a comprehensive combined dataset including a variety of prospect researches on the effectiveness of the Colosafe® kit. They reported that up to March 2021, A total of 78,773 prospective screening cases were completed in three hospitals including the Sixth Affiliated Hospital of Sun Yat-sen University, the First Affiliated Hospital of Nanchang University, and Dongguan People's Hospital. Among all cases, 4913 were positive for Colosafe® test (positive rate 6.24%), among which 1964 cases underwent colonoscopy reexamination (colonoscopy compliance 39.98%). A total of 413 cases of CRC, 469 cases of adenoma, and 427 cases of other polyps were identified, with a positive predictive value (PPV) of 66.6% (21% for CRC).

In November 2020, the Coloclear® human KRAS gene mutation, BMP3/NDRG4 gene methylation and stool occulted blood combined detection kit (PCR fluorescent probe method and colloidal gold method) developed by New Horizon Health Technology (Hangzhou) Co., Ltd. was approved to be marketed by NMPA. The product's intended use description states that it is "suitable for screening people aged 40-74 years at high risk of CRC," that it cannot replace colonoscopy, cannot be used for tumor screening in the general population, and should not be used as the sole basis for clinical diagnosis. In September 2020, the company publicly released data of the first prospective large-scale multicenter registered clinical trial of Cancer Early Screening in China (Clear-C) related to Coloclear® in the 2020 Annual Meeting of Chinese Society of Clinical Oncology (CSCO). According to its public information, the "Clear-C" registered clinical trial was jointly carried out by the Second Affiliated Hospital of Zhejiang University School of Medicine as the lead research unit and 8 ClassIII Grade A hospitals. It was officially launched in September 2018. Nearly 6000 cases were enrolled, and 4758 cases were actually included in the statistical analysis. The sensitivity of Coloclear® was 91.94% for CRC screening and 63.5% for advanced adenoma detection.

In addition to the above two CRC molecular detection products approved by NMPA up to the end of 2021, a number of domestic companies are also developing similar products and have obtained a series of achievements. For example, in 2019, Shanghai RealBio Technology Co., Ltd. published the data of their SDC2 and SFRP2 gene promoter methylation combined detection approach in the Chinese Journal of Digestive Endoscopy. They announced that this specific PCR method was applied to 500 patients (132 cases of CRC, 38 cases of advanced adenoma). The sensitivity of combined detection of SDC2 and SFRP2 genes was 97.73% (129/132) in CRC group, which was significantly higher than detection of SDC2 only [70.45% (93/132), P = 0.000], SFRP2 only [81.82% (108/132), P = 0.000] or FIT [69.70% (92/132), P = 0.000]. The sensitivity of combined detection of SDC2 and SFRP2 in adenoma group was 57.89% (22/38), which was significantly higher than detection of SDC2 only [15.79% (6/38), P = 0.000] or FIT detection [21.05% (8/38), P = 0.021]. This study was completed together with Changhai Hospital Affiliated to the Naval Military Medical University, the Tenth People's Hospital Affiliated to Tongji University, and the seventh Medical Center, General Hospital of the People's Liberation Army. Their commercial product, ColoWell®, is currently being declared to the NMPA.

The listed company BGI also released its self-developed CRC early screening product "HuaChangkang®" in March 2019, and published the results of retrospective clinical trials. In November 2021, BGI, in cooperation with Shaxian District Health Bureau and Shaxian District General Hospital of Sanming, Fujian Province, launched the "People's Livelihood Project of Shaxian District CRC Early Screening Testing," which planned to organize free tests for people of 40–60 years old in community health centers. By the end of 2021, 5000 people of appropriate age were screened. No data from the project has been released publicly yet. HuaChangkang® obtained CE certification in May 2021 and is currently applying to NMPA.

20.3.2 Market Segmentation and Prospect of CRC Early Screening

Occurrence and development of CRC mostly follow the "adenoma-carcinoma" principle, and generally take 5–10 years to progress from precancerous lesions to carcinoma, which provides an important time window for early diagnosis and clinical intervention. In addition, the prognosis of CRC is closely related to the diagnostic stage. According to domestic and foreign data, the 5-year relative survival rate of stage I CRC is 90%, while that of stage IV CRC with distant metastasis is only 14%. Therefore, early diagnosis is essential to improve the survival rate. However, the awareness of CRC screening is far from enough. In order to improve public health and disease prevention, China's medium - and long-term Plan for the Prevention and Treatment of Chronic Diseases (2017–2025) was released in January 2017, which stated that by the years 2020 and 2025, the early diagnosis rate of key cancer types in high-risk areas should be increased to 55 and 60%, respectively. The Healthy China Action Plan for Cancer Prevention and Treatment (2019–2022), released in 2019, further mentioned that the government would promote development of early cancer screening, diagnosis and treatment, construction of regional cancer medical centers, and the simultaneous listing of new drugs from overseas.

However, at present, the marketing data of CRC testing products in the Chinese market is still small. Analysts believe that the future likelihood of the CRC early screening market in China will be influenced by the following key factors: (1) price of the product. At present, Huachangkang®'s price on the official website is 799 CNY, while price of Colosafe® and Coloclear® on the market is 1108 CNY and 1726 CNY, respectively. The price of such products is higher than that of ordinary colonoscopy. For most patients, stool DNA test is still a relatively expensive expenditure. (2) Effectiveness of the product. Although stool DNA test can give high sensitivity and specificity results, some people with negative result will still be advised to do colonoscopy, especially the ones classified into high-risk groups; this reduces the value of stool DNA test. Therefore, if future large-scale clinical studies can help further improve the sensitivity and specificity, it is believed that it will be more attractive to consumers. (3) Recognition by the medical profession and the general public. With the improvement in economic conditions, the general awareness of routine physical examination and cancer screening will also have a significant positive impact on the market development prospects; (4) The possibility of including stool screening in public medical insurance and commercial insurance. At present, fecal DNA testing is still a high economic burden for individuals or families in China. However, starting from 2021, some provincial-level public medical insurance has begun to gradually include cancer early screening, which is believed to be a development trend in the future. By comparing the sales of similar products in developed countries, it can be concluded that the possibility of including stool screening in public medical insurance, the standardization and risk control of the process, and the subsequent compensation problems if it is included in commercial insurance will determine the possibility of China's CRC early screening market to a certain extent.

On February 18, 2021, New Horizon Health Technology (Hangzhou) Co., Ltd. was officially listed on the Hong Kong Stock Exchange with an offering price of HK $26.66, raising more than HK $2 billion in total and achieving a market capitalization of HK $30 billion. According to the first-half yearly performance report of the company in 2021, its total revenue, gross profit, and gross margin have achieved significant growth. Total income of Coloclear® was 14.2 million CNY. But with a 137% year-on-year increase in its sales team size, there is still plenty of room for improvement in sales per capita. In addition, Huachangkang® of Envelope Health BGI has won the bidding of Wuhan Health Commission's collection project in May 2021 with a unit price of 210 CNY, and the estimated size is 100,000 cases/year. In July 2021, it reached a strategic cooperation with the First People's Hospital of Changsha County, Hunan under the auspices of the National Health Commission, planning to screen 450,000 people aged 45–74 years in Changsha County within 3 years. It is believed that under the promotion of relevant policies, the CRC early screening industry will have broad prospects in the future.

20.4 Microbiota Examination

20.4.1 Microbiota Examination Technology and Applications

Ever since the beginning of 2020, the widespread spread of COVID-19 around the world has once again reminded people that today's world is still faced with major infectious disease outbreaks, drug-resistant "superbugs," and other threats from microorganisms. Among them, human symbiotic microorganisms play most close roles with public health. Nowadays, microbiome studies gradually become the research focus, and consumers of related health intervention products have become a growth market in the health industry.

Human intestinal microbiota is characterized by high diversity and complex functions. There are 1000 to 1150 species of bacteria in the human gut, mainly located in the lower gastrointestinal tract; the total number of the bacteria is about 10 times the total number of human cells. The adult gut microbiota encodes about three million genes, about 150 times the number encoded in the human genome. The differences in gut microbiota between different individuals can reach 80–90% [3]. The food ingredients (such as dietary fiber) that cannot be absorbed by the upper gastrointestinal tract are metabolized by the microorganisms in the colon, producing a large amount of active materials (including short chain fatty acids, bile acid, amino acid, vitamin, tryptamine, etc.), participating in the enterohepatic circulation, and mediating metabolism, These metabolites further enter the blood circulation through the intestinal barrier and participate in the regulation of human gene expression and the maintenance of normal immune function.

Because of its complexity, scientists are using the emerging multi-omics technology to examine and evaluate the composition and functions of the gut microbiota, and feces are the simplest sample type for collection. Quantitative fluorescent PCR (qPCR) and metagenomic sequencing (mNGS) are the most commonly used methods to detect microbial composition. Biochemical assays, gas and liquid chromatography, and mass spectrometry have also been used to measure microbial metabolites and assess their metabolic functions. The structural and functional imbalance of intestinal microecosystem is believed to be closely related to the occurrence and development of a series of human diseases. A large number of basic and clinical studies have focused on revealing microbial molecular biomarkers in the development of various diseases. Researchers are also trying to establish disease and health monitoring models using such biomarkers. The ultimate goal of microbiota examination is to provide targets and recommendations for health intervention and disease treatment, like special medical food, probiotics/prebiotics, special dietary interventions, and fecal microbiota transplantation (FMT).

In 2018, Professor Liping Zhao and his team at Shanghai Jiao Tong University published a research paper in Science, reporting a dietary intervention targeting gut microbiota among people with type 2 diabetes [4]. A total of 43 patients were enrolled in this study. Group U (16 patients) was given a self-created diet intervention following the 2013 edition of the Chinese Diabetes Society Patient Education and Dietary Guidelines, while group W (27 patients) followed a diet rich in diverse dietary fiber (dietary fiber intake of approximately 40 g per day). Both groups had equal daily intakes of total energy and nutrient components. The only medicine treatment for both groups is acarbose. After 3 months of intervention, the glycosylated hemoglobin level of 89% of the patients in the W group had fallen below 7%, and only 50% of the patients in the U group had achieved this level. In addition, patients in group W lost more weight and improved their blood lipids more significantly. Microbiota examination-based metagenomic sequencing showed that at the end of the intervention, the gut microbiota of two groups differed significantly in the species and gene richness and composition. In detail, bacteria genes enriched in W group involved the ones in the pathways of resistant starch and inulin degradation, butyrate producing, etc. Also, the concentrations of acetic acid and butyrate in fecal samples increased only in the W group after dietary treatment. As representatives of short chain fatty acids (SCFAs), butyrate and acetic acid are indicated to help increase two glucagon-like peptides (known as sugar controlling molecules) in the gut and also have anti-inflammatory properties. This study further identified 15 functional strains, including a strain of *Faecalibacterium prausnitzii*, which may be closely related to the metabolic response of high dietary fiber and contribute to the remission of type 2 diabetes and the improvement in metabolic functions. This study shows that microbiota examination using fecal samples can help identify the key strains playing important roles during the diet intervention of metabolic syndrome, and clarify the mechanism inside. The findings would also help develop potential probiotics/prebiotics, and establish a clinical scheme for the prevention and treatment of diabetes by regulating the microbiota, which will benefit the majority of patients with metabolic syndromes.

In 2019, a research group led by Professor Jun Yu of the Chinese University of Hong Kong published a review article in the journal Nature reviews Gastroenterology & Hepatology. The article pointed out that some important markers of the gut microbiota are closely related to the occurrence and development of CRC and precancerous adenoma. Yu's group has found that the combination of molecular markers composed of four kinds of bacteria can be used to distinguish CRC patients from healthy people, and its effect is even better than FIT detection. Furthermore, they found that *Fusobacterium nucleatum* concentration is an ideal indicator for predicting chemotherapy resistance and poor prognosis of CRC patients, which is even better than TNM stage classification. In the future, it may even be possible to determine which chemotherapy drugs to choose based on the concentration of *Fusobacterium nucleatum* in surgically resectable specimens [5]. In March 2020, Professor Yu Jun and Professor Jingyuan Fang from the Department of Gastroenterology of Shanghai Renji Hospital received a public interview with the new media "Digestive Community," saying that it is promising to combine host small RNA or methylation markers with fecal bacterial markers in the future to build a new diagnostic tool. A combination of diagnostic markers has been successfully screened with a sensitivity and specificity of more than 92%. In 2021, Lixin Zhu's research group from the Institute of Gastroenterology, The Sixth Affiliated Hospital of Sun Yat-sen University published a study in Nature Communications, proposing an early screening method for CRC based on fecal microbial markers, and providing the screening targets and study results of colorectal adenoma (CRA). A total of 775 subjects including healthy controls, colorectal adenoma (CRA) and CRC patients were enrolled and fecal microbial sequencing was carried out. A cross-validated random forest model was constructed based on molecular markers of 11 microbial species, with a detection sensitivity of 0.82 in healthy and CRA populations. At the same time, the molecular markers identified in this study can significantly distinguish other diseases, such as inflammatory bowel disease, nonalcoholic fatty liver disease, metabolic syndrome, etc., indicating that this CRA microbiota marker has high disease specificity and has the potential to be transformed into accurate early screening products for CRC [6].

Until the end of 2021, the above potential diagnostic tools have not been successfully marketed as commercially available products. However, we expect that in the future, stool microbiota testing can become a powerful supplement to FIT and human DNA testing, jointly establish markers for early non-invasive diagnosis or early warning of adenoma carcinogenesis, and promote the further optimization of CRC early screening technology and product performance.

In addition to bacterial species targets, specific metabolites of the microbiota, such as SCFAs and bile acids, can also be used as objects for stool microbiota examination. From 2018 to 2021, supported by the Natural Science Foundation of Zhejiang Province, Dr. Xin Wang, chief scientist of Hangzhou Hailu Medical Technology Co., LTD., Researcher of Zhejiang Academy of Agricultural Sciences, and Ning Dai, Professor of Run Run Shaw Hospital of Zhejiang Province, led the largest dietary intervention study on diarrhea-type irritable bowel syndrome (IBS-D) in China [7]. A total of 108 adult Chinese IBS-D patients were randomly given Low FODMAPs Diet (LFD) or clinical empirical traditional Chinese dietary advice (TDA). After 3 weeks of intervention, fecal SCFAs were measured in both groups. Patients in the LFD group showed earlier improvement in stool frequency. With the improvement in symptoms, LFD also showed significantly lower metabolic activity of sugar fermentators such as *bifidobacterium* and *Bacteroides*, and the production of some metabolites that may stimulate excessive intestinal peristalsis were inhibited. Researchers have also found that patients can be classified into "protein fermentation pattern" and "carbohydrate fermentation pattern" based on their SCFA levels. The latter has a better response to LFD intervention programs. This study suggests that according to the fecal microbiota metabolites levels, individual dietary metabolic types can be accurately classified, and precise nutritional intervention programs suitable for people with high carbohydrate metabolism and high protein metabolism, respectively, can be formulated to help IBS-D patients better benefit from the intervention.

Fecal microbiota transplantation (FMT) is a therapeutic method in which functional microbiota from the feces of healthy people is transplanted into the gastrointestinal tract of patients. The purpose of FMT is to help patients rebuild a new intestinal microecosystem and help with the treatment of intestinal and extra-intestinal diseases. FMT has been widely used in the treatment of diseases including diarrhea caused by *Clostridium difficile* infection, inflammatory bowel disease, intractable constipation, metabolic disease, intestinal immune deficiency, intestinal allergy, and is considered as a breakthrough medical progress in recent years. The safety of FMT is a primary consideration in clinical decision making. The Asia Pacific Society of Gastroenterology (APAGE) and the Asia Pacific Society of Digestive Endoscopy (APSDE) summarized the most clinical concerns in the field of FMT and published the consensus of clinical experts on FMT in the Asia-Pacific region on Gut. Chinese experts, including Xiujuan Huang from the Chinese University of Hong Kong, Yongjian Zhou from Guangzhou First People's Hospital, and Faming Zhang from the Second Affiliated Hospital of Nanjing Medical

University, participated in the writing of the consensus [8]. It is clearly mentioned in the consensus that the different clinical outcomes of FMT are tightly related to the differences in intestinal microbial composition and functions between the donor and the recipient. Therefore, stool microbiota testing may be one of the necessary methods for donor screening and recipient matching. Specifically, through 16S rRNA gene sequencing or metagenomic sequencing, the intestinal microbiota structure and function of fecal donors and patients were evaluated, respectively, and the donor was matched according to the specific indications and species and metabolic indicators. Furthermore, according to the microbiota assessment before and after treatment, the course of treatment should be reasonably designed and strictly controlled. In August 2021, Health and Wellness Commission of Shanghai released "Notice on the publication of Surveillance specification for technology and process management of Fecal microbiota transplantation (2021 edition)" (http://wsjkw.sh.gov.cn/yzgl3/20210830/26e28dcc06b045cc8684674277d66f9e.html), It is clearly mentioned that departments that can independently develop FMT treatment should have the ability to detect gut microbiota structure and metabolism capabilities, *Clostridium difficile* (CDI) levels, drug-resistant bacteria amounts, COVID-19, and human monogenic genes using molecular biological techniques. It is also clearly proposed that stool test is one of the necessary means of donor screening, and qualified donors must meet the following conditions: normal stool routine examination; negative in occult blood test; negative in CDI, *Campylobacteria*, *Salmonella*, *Shigella*, *E. coli* producing shiga toxin, worm eggs, vesicles, parasites, *Yersinia enterocolitica*, pathogenic *Vibrio* (*Vibrio parahaemolyticus*, *Vibrio cholerae*), *Aeromonas*, amoeba, spores, norovirus, rotavirus and novel coronavirus (COVID-19); negative in multidrug resistance genes (ultra-broad spectrum β-lactamase, carbapenemase and vancomycin resistance); negative in *Helicobacter pylori* antigen (in stool). In addition, the quality control criteria for donor bacterial solutions also include "each preparation of bacterial solutions should be randomly sampled for pathogenic bacteria checking, cell counting, and 16s rRNA gene sequencing/metagenomic sequencing." The formal presentation of this document further illustrates the necessary and important significance of stool microbiota examination in the clinical application using intestinal microbiota as a target.

20.4.2 Market Segmentation and Prospect of Microbiota Examination

Advances in microbiota detection technology not only promote the progress of scientific research but also bring the possibility of personalized intestinal healthcare for the majority of consumers. At present, many biotechnology companies in China and abroad are committed to application of breakthroughs in various clinical research fields to consumer products, and provide personalized dietary interventions and recommendations on disease diagnosis and treatment (Table 20.3).

It must be admitted that, on the one hand, researches related to intestinal microbiota based on multi-omics techniques have been flourishing and have made

Table 20.3 Companies providing services on microbiota examination and personalized dietary interventions

Company	Products
BGI Nutrition Technology (Shenzhen) Co. Ltd	Use NGS technology to analyze the composition and metabolic characteristics of intestinal microbiota, which is used to assess the nutritional metabolism status, and to provide customers with personalized health management plans. It also includes a sales platform for nutritional products, food ingredients and probiotics
Shanghai Biotecan Pharmaceuticals Co. Ltd	Use NGS technology to analyze the diversity of intestinal microbiota in the subjects, indicating the risk of various diseases, and providing follow-up health management programs. Meanwhile, intestinal microecological therapy based on probiotics, prebiotics, nutritional support and FMT is provided. It is applicable to subhealthy people without immune deficiency diseases, diabetes patients, enteritis patients, constipation patients, obese people, etc.
Beijing Coyote Biotechnology Co., ltd.	To provide quantitative detection of seven core functional bacteria in the intestinal microbiota of children, and to assess the risk of constipation, diarrhea, allergy, eczema and other diseases
Hangzhou Hailu Medical Technology Co., Ltd.	Use the unique in vitro simulated fermentation technology to assess the metabolic characteristics of intestinal microbiota, including intestinal gas production, SCFFA index and bile acid index. The metabolic potential of subjects for specific foods and prebiotics is evaluated, and the corresponding precise health management plan is provided
Thalys Medical Group Co., Ltd.	In collaboration with genetic analysis co., ltd., a Norwegian high-tech molecular diagnostics company, the company is developing intestinal microbiotal testing protocols for irritable bowel syndrome (IBS) and inflammatory enteritis (IBD), mainly using multiplex probe technology

breakthroughs in various clinical research fields. The rise of microbiome-related industries seems to be brewing a revolution in the medical and health industry. On the other hand, the fecal microbiota examination products for the public in China are still in the initial stage, and the products mainly focus on consumer-level testing, that is, assessing the imbalance of the microbial structure and giving personalized nutritional recommendations. For example, Shanghai Biotecan, BGI Nutrition, and other similar companies mainly use high-throughput sequencing technology to detect the composition of the microbiota. Combined with other clinical indicators, they give the microbiota diversity score, chronic disease risk index, and nutritional balance index. Hangzhou Hailu Medical Technology Co., Ltd. provides intestinal microecological metabolic index and prebiotic metabolic ability test to comprehensively evaluated the nutritional metabolic capability. The test is achieved by an in vitro fermentation platform established together with Zhejiang Academy of Agricultural Sciences. At the same time, there are also some companies trying to develop live biotherapeutic products (LBP) on the basis of microbiota testing. For example, Bacteroides fragilis SK08 initially developed by Guangzhou Zhiyi Biotech was approved in the phase I clinical trial by NMPA in November 2019 as living biological drugs. Phase II clinical trials were launched in May 2021. Although some data and achievements have been accumulated, at present, domestic companies are still mainly focused on the assessment of the overall health status and nutrition utilization of the human body, and its applicability and conclusions are still difficult to meet the standard of clinical in vitro diagnosis. The market size is heavily dependent on probiotics, health food, and other industries.

New Media like Arterial Network and Probe Capital have written articles analyzing the characteristics and future development trend of the microbiome industry. They believe that the difficulties of commercialization of microbiota examination are mainly in the following aspects:

First, the uncertainty of basic research findings. Most of the studies related to microbiome use the method of multi-omics association, and the research results are mainly about the correlation between the changes of microbiota and the occurrence and development of diseases. There is no clear causal relationship, and the mechanism of many host-microbiota interactions is still unclear. The microecological imbalance found in many studies is not specific enough to be associated with a certain type of disease. The significant deficiencies reflected in the examination include: it is difficult to find indicator markers clearly related to diseases, insufficient data evidence, and difficulties to create products that meet the requirements of clinical diagnosis and treatment with high sensitivity and specificity. Great challenges exist in all the three main industrial application fields: microbiota examination, FMT and LBP.

Second, the policy details are not perfect. In China, there is no clear regulation on FMT and live bacteria drugs, and the attitude of the NMPA towards intestinal microbial therapy is not clear enough. The use of FMT is currently not regulated. It is a medical technique, not a drug, and does not require official approval for clinical trials. Each hospital carries out its own treatment, and there is no enough unified standard for the evaluation of treatment effect yet.

Third, lack of data management norms. The main data acquisition channels for microbiome sequencing and metabolomics testing are in the scientific research field, with only a small amount of data coming from clinicians and individual consumers. However, at present, the target population of commercial microbiota testing is consumer-level testing users, and the data quality is different from that of scientific research data, which brings certain difficulties to the establishment of database and data processing process. At present, there is a lack of clinical and consumer microbial data standards, which need to be promoted at the policy level. In addition to testing, domestic companies will face greater risks of policy uncertainty in the layout of the therapy field;

Fourth, the market cognition is not mature enough. The lack of corresponding microbial market education, the relatively low level of technological development, the low level of microbial treatment or drug research and development in China, and the high dependence of the microbial industry on government and social funds all bring challenges to the development of the industry. The professional understanding of microbial therapy in domestic capital needs to be improved, and it is difficult to start without breakthrough researches and industry development in developed countries. At present, the industry's research and data accumulation on intestinal microbes are insufficient, which cannot support the drug development and treatment corresponding to the strain-level function, and also weaken the appeal of microbiota examination products to a certain extent.

Therefore, for the future development of the industry, it depends on continuous breakthroughs in basic research, encouragement from the government and capital to improve product development, collection to the market in clinical diagnosis, public health, precision nutrition, and other aspects. On the other hand, accumulating enough clinical application data will help the microbiota examination technology be more applied in the field of disease screening and concomitant diagnosis in China, such as the screening of early CRC and the concomitant diagnosis of inflammatory bowel diseases. The mainstream market is in the future still needs further exploration and observation.

Declaration Tingting Wang is an employee of Hangzhou Hailu Medical Technology Co., Ltd., Hangzhou, China.

Xianglong Li is an employee of Hunan Hailu Biotechnology Co., Ltd., Changsha, China.

Qinghua Liao is an employee of Sciendox Biotechnology Co., Ltd., Xiamen, China.

References

1. Lee Jeffrey K, Liles Elizabeth G, Stephen B, et al. Accuracy of fecal immunochemical tests for colorectal cancer: systematic review and meta-analysis. Ann Int Med. 2014;160:171.
2. Imperiale Thomas F, Ransohoff David F, Itzkowitz Steven H, et al. Multitarget stool DNA testing for colorectal- cancer screening. N Eng J Med. 2014;371:187–8.
3. Jason L-P, Anup M, Gholamali R, et al. Strains, functions, and dynamics in the expanded Human Microbiome Project. Nature. 2017;550:61–6.
4. Li-ping Z, Feng Z, Xiao-ying D, et al. Gut bacteria selectively promoted by dietary fibers alleviate type 2 diabetes. Science. 2018;359:1151–6.
5. Wong Sunny H, Jun Y. Gut microbiota in colorectal cancer: mechanisms of action and clinical applications. Nat Rev Gastroenterol Hepatol. 2019;16:690–704.
6. Yuan-qi W, Na J, Rui-xin Z, et al. Identification of microbial markers across populations in early detection of colorectal cancer. Nat Commun. 2021;12:3063.
7. Ya-wen Z, Li-Jun F, Xin W, et al. Low fermentable oligosaccharides, disaccharides, monosaccharides,and polyols diet compared with traditional dietary advice for diarrhea-predominant irritable bowel syndrome: a parallel-group, randomized controlled trial with analysis of clinical and microbiological factors associated with patient outcomes. Am J Clin Nutr. 2021;113:1531–45.
8. Siew-C NG, Kamm Michael A, Yun-Kit Y, et al. Scientific frontiers in faecal microbiota transplantation: joint document of Asia-Pacific Association of Gastroenterology (APAGE) and Asia Pacific Society for Digestive Endoscopy (APSDE). Gut. 2020;69:83–91.

Semen

21

Yufeng Cui, Bin Hu, Chenyue Dou, Yanyan Kang, Yongliang Ni, and Qifeng Nie

21.1 Overview of Test

Semen consists of sperm and seminal plasma. Sperm, differentiated and derived from testicular spermatogenic cells, matures in the epididymis, and is ejaculated through the ductus deferens. By the time of ejaculation, semen is generated by the highly concentrated sperm suspension in the bilateral epididymis mixed and diluted with the secretions of the epididymis. About 90% come from secretions from the accessory organs, mainly from the prostate and seminal vesicles, and the remaining small amount from the bulbourethral glands and epididymis [1].

Semen test assesses sperm concentration, motility, viability, morphology, and DNA fragmentation, as well as seminal plasma biochemical, immunological, microbiological items, and sperm function.

Clinically, semen test (1) assesses male reproductive function and provides a basis for diagnosing infertility and observing curative effects; (2) aids the diagnosis of male reproductive system-related diseases; (3) tracks curative effects after vasectomy; (4) contributes to family planning and scientific research; (5) screens high-quality sperm for artificial insemination and sperm bank; (6) and serves forensic identification [2].

Y. Cui (✉) · B. Hu · C. Dou · Y. Kang
Shanghai Beion Medical Technology Co., LTD, Shanghai, China
e-mail: cyf@beion.com.cn

Y. Ni · Q. Nie
Dirui Industrial Co., Ltd. Changchun, Jilin, China

H. Song, L. Dai (eds.), *In Vitro Diagnostic Industry in China*,
https://doi.org/10.1007/978-981-99-3110-1_21

21.2 Status Quo of Domestic Product and Technology

No dramatic advance has been made in upgrading the technology of sperm quality analysis since 2019, except the further integration of machine learning algorithms that aid the dominating one-piece equipment and split-type instrument, which has streamlined the performance and improved the accuracy of image processing and recognition algorithms.

The World Health Organization (WHO) Laboratory Manual for the Examination and Processing of Human Semen (fifth edition) was well landed in the newly released sperm quality analyzer in 2019. Further standardized equipment operating procedures issued by manufacturers enhanced awareness of operators in medical institutions and textbook-level processing of specimens before testing all avail the improvement of semen analysis standardization and quality control.

The new product comes with more simplified operation. Some analyzer manufacturers have facilitated the usage by integrating pH value detection function. However, some enabled sperm dynamics, morphology, viability, and DNA damage analysis all at once. Now computers can draw conclusions on the kinetic results and morphological classification of sperm by dissecting sperm images taken by a microscopic imaging system. From this, clinicians can further correct the test results by observing the sperm images to secure the reliability.

Image analysis involves two recognition algorithms in most cases: one classifies sperm morphology in virtue of the traditional morphological and geometric shape data. The other extracts features of sperm shape with advanced machine learning or deep learning, then sorts it out using classic machine learning classification algorithm.

Regarding technology R&D, the artificial intelligence (AI) algorithm for sperm dynamics and morphological images is still in the test stage. The established AI image recognition plays a limited role in improving the accuracy of results, and is lagged far behind by the high accuracy requirements of clinical reports. So that AI assumes an auxiliary role only, and the test results are subject to professional opinions.

COMET assay, sperm chromatin dispersion test (SCD), TUNEL, and AO fluorescent staining method all can test DNA damage in sperm. And the detection method of AO fluorescence staining combined with flow cytometry, namely sperm chromatin structure assay (SCSA), is faster, more accurate, and intuitive in terms of sperm DNA fragmentation index (DFI) detection. The flow cytometry can detect tens of thousands of sperm stained by AO fluorescence within a few seconds, and the test results are objective, and secures reliable and highly repeatable outcomes. Because of such excellent performance, it has been widely used in clinical practice. In addition to detecting DNA damage in sperm, SCSA also shines on marking the percentage of immature sperm in the tested sample, enhancing the applicability [3].

Semi-automatic microplate reader and automatic biochemical analyzer are widely used for seminal plasma biochemical detection. Higher requirement for manual operations by semi-automatic microplate reader, however, leads to quite varying results due to the technical personnel's operating familiarity and operating habits. In this regard, the automatic biochemical instrument stands out for less manual intervention and better repeatability. Domestic institutions now go for their own analyzers according to their specific needs. Because of lower costs, hospitals in districts and counties prefer semi-automatic microplate readers. However, medical institutions such as reproductive centers, genetic rooms, and large tertiary hospitals give preference to automatic biochemical analyzers for their large amounts of specimens and high-quality requirements.

21.3 Domestic Influential Brands and Manufacturers

21.3.1 Influential Companies and Products in Semen Analysis Industry

21.3.1.1 S-Series Sperm Quality Analyzer of Shanghai Beion Pharmaceutical Technology Co., Ltd.

Shanghai Beion, a high-tech enterprise specializing in the R&D, manufacturing and marketing of in vitro diagnostic (IVD) instruments and reagents with an integrated industry chain, provides reproductive, genetic, cellular, pathological, biochemical, immunological, molecular and microbiological precision analytical instruments, diagnostic reagents (chips) and services in the field of IVD, is the first to apply AI in microscopic products, and is committed to creating high-end IVD products with independent hard-core technology brands and enabling import substitution and upgrading.

BEION S series mainly covers BEION S3, BEION S3–3, BEION S4, BEION S5, BEION S6, and sperm quality module software in medical image software V4.90.

BEION S series, all-in-one design, are designed with built-in XYZO fully electronically controlled biological microscope, computer system and touch screen display, temperature control system, power supply system, sperm counting pool, and sperm quality analysis management system software.

Main technical indicators of BEION S series sperm quality analyzer:

1. Automatic microscope control: automatic focusing and scanning collects sperm dynamic video and morphological images.
2. Constant temperature control: keep semen samples at 37 °C for detection and analysis.
3. Sperm dynamics analysis

   Under conditions of light field and phase contrast, the coincidence rate of sperm identification ≧95%, the coincidence rate of sperm motility classification ≧90%, the coincidence rate of sperm concentration ≧90%, and the misidentification rate of impurities ≦10%, the analysis time of a single specimen ≦ 60 s.
4. Morphological analysis

   The coincidence rate of the total number of sperm ≧90%, the coincidence rate of normal shape sperm ≧60%, and the coincidence rate of abnormal head sperm ≧80%, the analysis time of a single specimen ≤2 min.

Normal and abnormal classification: normal morphology sperm, abnormal morphology sperm, abnormal head sperm, cervical and midcourse abnormal sperm, main segment abnormal sperm, excessive residual cytoplasm, pear-shaped sperm, large-headed sperm, small-headed sperm, conical-headed sperm, round sperm, amorphous sperm with vacuolar head, small or large acrosome, posterior vacuolar sperm, double-headed sperm, acutely curved sperm, asymmetric inserted sperm, midsection thin sperm, thick or irregular sperm in the middle, spermatozoa with acute angle curved tail, spermatozoa with curly tail, spermatozoa with multiple tails, spermatozoa with short tail.

5. DNA damage analysis

   Automatic identification and counting of sperm, sperm with DNA fragments, and sperm without DNA fragments secures a coincidence rate of $\geq$80% and takes less than or equal to 90 s for analyzing a single specimen.

6. Quality control

   Automatically save quality control results, draws monthly quality control chart curves, and prints them out.

   The quality control video recording of sperm dynamics and viability supported enables loading and analyzing the quality control video recorded by a third party;

   Automatically generate X_{bar} chart, S chart, personnel difference quality control chart (Bland-Altman chart; Youden chart);

7. Case data management and reporting system

   The large-scale backstage database management system adds and modifies reports and inspection items according to specific needs, and supports customized reports.

   The report items are all open and editable. In addition to fixed items, semen physical characteristics, sperm microscope kinetic analysis, morphological analysis, DNA damage analysis, sperm function experiments, chemical analysis, and immunological analysis are all included.

21.3.1.2 SAS-II Sperm Quality Analyzer of Saisi Medical Technology (Beijing) Co., Ltd.

Saisi Medical Technology (Beijing) Co., Ltd., renamed from Beijing Yuchuang Hengyuan Technology Co., Ltd. and established in 2013, is a medical device production company taking medical image processing, pattern and AI recognition, automatic control as its core edges and integrating R&D, production and sales.

SAS-II sperm quality analyzer, comprising microscopic image scanning module, computer system, counting pool module, sperm quality analyzer software (version: V2.3), supports grayscale version analysis and phase contrast version analysis, and automatically detects and analyzes the total number of sperm, concentration/concentration, speed classification, total sperm motility, average curve speed, average linear speed, average path speed, side swing amplitude, whipping frequency, average angle, number of fast straight lines, fast straight line concentration, fast linear vitality, linearity, oscillation, forwardness, average size, average circumference, detection time, etc. More than that, the fourth and fifth editions of the WHO

Laboratory Manual for the Examination and Processing of Human Semen can be switched at will.

Main performance indicators: the acquisition and analysis time < 1.5 s, the maximum number of static samples collected per image reaches 500 (for calculating sperm concentration only) at least, with an error ≤ ±0.2%; the linear velocity of the dynamic sample measured by the sperm quality analyzer is not less than 500 m/s; the number of images collected for each field of view is 2 to 120; the error of the capture accuracy of the sperm count is ≤ ± 5%; the CV value of sperm concentration and motility measurement results ≤5%; the coincidence rate of sperm morphology and number analysis ≥94%; the coincidence rate of normal morphology sperm analysis ≥98%; the coincidence rate of abnormal morphology sperm analysis ≥94%; the analyzer recognizes sperm chromatin The coincidence rate of the number ≥ 93%.

21.3.1.3 Sperm Quality Analysis System of Jiangsu Ruiqi Life Science Instrument Co., Ltd.

Jiangsu Ruiqi Life Science Instrument Co., Ltd. mainly runs medical equipment and life science instruments.

Its sperm quality analysis system series of CFT-9201, CFT-9202, CFT-9203 and workbench table type structure designed according to the WHO5 standard is used for sperm quality analysis and enables sperm concentration and motility analysis, sperm morphology analysis, DNA fragmentation analysis, and quality control. All are equipped with sperm concentration and motility analysis software, sperm morphology analysis software, DNA fragmentation analysis software, automatic drawing software for monthly concentration monitoring table, automatic drawing software for monthly monitoring table for morphology, automatic drawing software for concentration indoor quality control X_{bar} chart, and morphology indoor quality control X_{bar} chart automatic drawing software, video recording software, and LIS connection software.

21.3.1.4 SSA-II Sperm Automatic Detection and Analysis System of Beijing Suijia Software Co., Ltd.

Founded in 2012, Beijing Suijia Software Co., Ltd., an innovative computer software development enterprise, specializes in the development and sales of medical software, Class I and II medical devices, as well as the medical and professional software development.

The SSA-II sperm automatic detection and analysis system conforms to the fifth edition of the WHO standard, is equipped with functions including sperm concentration and motility analysis (phase difference technology, contrast analysis), automatic morphological analysis, and quality control module, and supports LIS system connection, POE technology, GDI+ Interface technology, touch technology, wireless printing and automatic backup technology. With built-in national patented hardware system: phase contrast microscope + high frame rate Fireware B/GigE interface camera + Apple IMAC integrated computer, the system enables Tablet PC presentations such as Microsoft Surface, quality control, man-machine comparative analysis, and automatically counts the average and standard deviation between multiple researchers and computer detection values; moreover, it automatically identifies and divides sperm into acrosome, head, and midsection and enables color filling or edge filling; calculates sperm's length, width, area, circumference, acrosome ratio, ellipticity and other 11 sperm morphological data, as well as DFI; counts weekly, monthly, quarterly, annual case detection and daily average; sorts out the normal and abnormal averages and standard deviations of various semen indicators of all detected cases, and customizes the standard values of semen indicators.

21.3.1.5 LensHooke Sperm Quality Analysis Detector of Bonray Biotech Co., Ltd.

Bonray Biotech Co., Ltd. specializes in developing high-precision and user-friendly in vitro diagnostic equipment to help improve global medical care.

The LensHooke Sperm Quality Analyzer, a handheld automatic sperm quality analyzer, detects pH value, concentration, morphology and motility, is equipped with automatic focusing system and compatible with large electronic display to present images; furthermore, it issues medical-grade test reports and shares test reports through a local area network; supports quality control tests of pH value and concentration under 3 different concentration benchmarks, bar-code scanning; and takes about 2–5 min for each detection.

21.3.2 Manufacturers and Products of Seminal Plasma Biochemical Testing

Seminal plasma biochemistry detects fructose, zinc, neutral α-glucosidase, elastase and lactate dehydrogenase in seminal plasma. In this regard, BRED and Sinothinker stand out.

21.3.2.1 Reproductive Medicine Biochemical Analyzer of Shenzhen BRED Biotechnology Co., Ltd.

Shenzhen BRED Biotechnology Co., Ltd., a high-tech enterprise integrating R&D, production, and sales, provides automated testing platforms and supporting products for infertility diagnosis and assisted reproductive treatment.

Reproductive medicine biochemical analyzers cover CHEMWELLBRED reproductive medicine automatic biochemical analyzer (sm001) and reproductive medicine semi-automatic biochemical analyzer (sm002), and is equipped with the automatic detection function of WHO recommended methodology. The equipment realizes the accurate sample addition of high viscosity seminal plasma samples, and caters to the automatic detection requirements of some special reproductive testing items. sm001, with biochemical and ELISA detection functions, meets the requirements of quality control and standardization given a stable seminal plasma compound quality control material, and can detect other types of specimens except seminal plasma, as well as various other biochemical immune items.

21.3.2.2 Reproductive Medicine Biochemical Analyzer of Shenzhen Sinothinker Technology Co., Ltd.

Shenzhen Sinothinker Technology Co., Ltd., committed to the R&D, production and sales of medical testing products, has developed semi-automatic biochemical immune analyzer for reproductive medicine, automatic biochemical analyzer for reproductive medicine, automatic drying and washing machine, microplate reader, automatic blood analyzer, biochemical analyzer, blood coagulation analyzer, and other testing and analysis instruments.

Reproductive medicine biochemical analyzer models, of SK6000 reproductive medicine automatic biochemical analyzer and SK3002 reproductive medicine semi-automatic biochemical immunoassay analyzer, are specially designed for semen biochemical and immune quantitative analysis. Their test results are qualified by the fifth edition of the World Health Organization, with the carrying pollution rate $\leq 0.1\%$, absorbance repeatability $\leq 1.0\%$, and the function of sample-addition halfway.

21.4 Market Capacity

21.4.1 Sperm Analyzer Market Analysis

By the end of 2020, about 100,000 sets of sperm analyzers circulated in the domestic medical and health field, with a worth of about 2 billion yuan.

Year of 2014 reported 63.36 million yuan in the market size of sperm analyzers in the domestic medical and health field. That number has grown into 125 million yuan in 2019, with a 5-year compound growth rate of 25%.

Domestic sperm analyzer brands classified according to domestic imports are domestic brands such as Shanghai Beion, Beijing Saisi, Beijing Suijia, Beijing Weili, and Nanjing Ruiqi, and imported brands include Israel SQA, Spanish SCA, and American Hamilton. Domestic sperm analyzer market accounts for more than 85% of the market of sperm analyzers produced in China, and domestic brands are gradually replacing imported brands, revealed the statistics.

The infertility rate of couples of childbearing age in China is close to 13% and continues to increase. Male reproduction and health are now jostling for increasing attention of the public. The market demand for sperm analyzers in the domestic medical and health field will further expand, which will accordingly raise a higher threshold for the quality and function for domestic sperm analyzers, as the pandemic is gradually under control, the national "three-child" policy is unveiled to encourage fertility, and the general trend of "domestic substitutes imported" medical devices prevails.

21.4.2 Seminal Plasma Biochemical Market Analysis

Seminal plasma biochemistry detects fructose, zinc, neutral α-glucosidase, elastase, and lactate dehydrogenase in seminal plasma. So far, semi-automatic biochemical analyzers for reproductive medicine and semi-automatic biochemical immune analyzers for reproductive medicine are mainly used for biochemical detection of seminal plasma.

Domestic seminal plasma biochemical immunoassay analyzers such as Shenzhen BRED, Shenzhen Sinothink, and Nanjing Xindi are dominating the market. The said brand manufacturers provide seminal plasma biochemical detection reagents (boxes).

The current domestic market for seminal plasma biochemical analysis is about 500 million yuan, found the statistics. As the number of infertile couples continues to increase, Chinese people are paying more attention to male reproduction and health. Meanwhile, the national "three-child" policy to encourage fertility further stimulates the growth of the male sperm fertility test market. The seminal plasma biochemical analysis market will sustain growth.

21.4.3 Portable Sperm Analyzer Market Analysis

Portable sperm analyzers mainly POCT sperm analyze, simplify, and speed up the detection. It supports the immediate analysis at the sampling site, saves the trouble for complex processing procedures in laboratory testing, and enables semen sample collection at home. Till now, The LensHooke Sperm Quality Analyzer has acquired its registration certificate for the portable sperm analyzer in the domestic market, a huge blue ocean left to be fully developed.

A series of issues such as the accuracy of portable sperm analyzer detection and whether the test results are clinically recognized as the basis for diagnosis and treatment still demand further efforts. Compared with mature POCT-based medical testing projects, the POCT sperm analyzer is still in its infancy. That is, the portable sperm analyzer just gets started.

21.5 Future Development Expectations and Orientation of Semen Analysis

From the initial stage of manual inspection and semi-automatic analysis, to the rapid development of fully automated analysis, semen analysis has stepped into a new era of full laboratory automation and informatization. The next hot spot and leap in the development of laboratory medicine may be artificial intelligence.

With continuous updating and development of deep learning and image recognition algorithms, it's more and more common to use computers to learn people's thinking ability and experience to assist people to handle daily work. Smart healthcare is to land more artificial intelligence technologies to diagnose and treat clinical diseases. Wielding deep learning and image recognition technology to the medical field to identify and analyze medical images and processing a large number of medical pictures in virtue of high-performance computers make a significant research orientation of medical big data and constitute an important branch of expediting the construction of a smart medical system.

Declaration Yufeng Cui, Bin Hu, Chenyue Dou and Yanyan Kang are employees of Shanghai Beion Medical Technology Co., Ltd.

Yongliang Ni and Qifeng Nie are employees of Dirui Industrial Co., Ltd.

References

1. World Health Organization. The WHO laboratory manual for the examination of human semen and sperm–cervical mucus interaction. Geneva: WHO; 1980.
2. World Health Organization. WHO laboratory manual for the examination and processing of human semen. 5th ed. Geneva: WHO; 2010.
3. World Health Organization. WHO laboratory manual for the examination and processing of human semen. Sixth ed; 2021.

Vaginal Secretions

22

Yongliang Ni, Qifeng Nie, Shang Gao, and Zhengxu Kang

22.1 Summary

Leucorrhea, namely the vaginal secretions, appears in the form of mucus secreted by labia majora and labia minora, greater vestibular gland, cervical gland, endometrium, and fallopian tubes, exudates from vaginal mucosa, exfoliated epidermic cells of uterus and vagina, a small amount of white blood cells and non-pathogenic vaginal bacillus, and so forth. Normal vaginal secretions are acidic, with a pH of 4.0–4.5.

A routine item in gynecological examination, vaginal secretion inspection is mainly used for the diagnosis of female reproductive system inflammation, tumor, etc., serving as an important basis for clinical diagnosis of vaginal diseases. The specific detection items of vaginal secretions may vary slightly in different hospitals, but mainly cover physical inspection, dry chemical inspection, sediment analysis, etc.

Among them, the physical inspection mainly involves appearance and pH. Appearance detection, to be specific, is to judge the color, character, mucus, smell, and quantity of the sample. In the late 1980s, people discovered the unique microbial metabolites in the vagina and successively developed a series of new diagnostic techniques and methods, which, through medical practice, have been proved to be superior to traditional manual methods in terms of operational performance, sensitivity and specificity and suitable for batch operation and popularization in clinical practice. So far, the technology has come closer to maturity at home, with various single, multiple or combined bacterial vaginosis (BV)products having been produced by dozens of domestic enterprises applying the enzyme-based

Y. Ni · Q. Nie · S. Gao (✉) · Z. Kang
Dirui Industrial Co., Ltd., Changchun, Jilin, China
e-mail: gaoshang1@dirui.com.cn

H. Song, L. Dai (eds.), *In Vitro Diagnostic Industry in China*,
https://doi.org/10.1007/978-981-99-3110-1_22

chemical reaction technology. The detection items mainly include hydrogen peroxide, white blood cell esterase, neuraminidase lactic acid, proline aminopeptidase, and oxidase (Table 22.1).

The analysis of sediments in vaginal secretions mainly relies on manual microscopic examination, with the detection items mainly including white blood cells, clue cells, trichomonad, fungi, epithelial cells, and bacillus. For interpretation of the results, the criteria for determination of vaginal cleanliness can be based for diagnosis (Tables 22.2 and 22.3). Among them, grades I to II are normal; grades III to IV

Table 22.1 Chemistry detection items and clinical significance

Indicator	Clinical significance
pH value	An important indicator reflecting vaginal microecological balance
Hydrogen peroxide (H_2O_2)	Used to evaluate the level of lactic acid bacillus and determine whether the vaginal microecological environment loses its balance
Leucocyte esterase (LE)	An inflammatory reaction marker that reflects the number of white blood cells in vaginal secretions
Lactic acid (LA)	Used to evaluate the number of lactic acid bacillus, the dominant bacteria in the vaginal microecosystem
Neuraminidase (SNa)	Secreted by Gardnerella and some other anaerobic bacteria, it is an indicator of pathogenic bacteria, and a positive result indicates bacterial vaginosis
β-Glucuronidase (GUS)	An enzyme synthesized and secreted by aerobic bacteria. A positive result indicates aerobic vaginitis
Coagulase (CG)	An enzyme produced by staphylococcus. A positive result indicates abnormal vaginal microenvironment
Proline aminopeptidase (PIP)	A positive result indicates fungal vaginitis or vaginitis with anaerobic infection
N-acetylglucosaminidase (NAG)	A specific enzyme secreted by fungi and trichomonad. Combined with pH, it can suggest fungal vaginitis (pH $\leq$ 4.6) and trichomonas vaginitis (pH $\geq$ 4.8)
Oxidase (OX)	Suggesting infection with gonococcus

Table 22.2 Analysis of sediments in vaginal secretions and interpretation of results

Cleanliness	Bacillus	Miscellaneous bacteria	Epithelial cell	White blood cell
Grade I	++++	None or a little	Full vision field	0–5/HP
Grade II	++	+	1/2 vision field	5–15/HP
Grade III	+	++	A little	15–30/HP
Grade IV	–	++++	None or a little	>30/HP

Table 22.3 Clinical significance of sediment detection items

Indicator	Clinical significance
White blood cell	An inflammatory reaction marker that can reflect the cleanliness of secretions
Epithelial cell	A normal cell in reproductive tract secretions, which can reflect the cleanliness of secretions
Clue cell	It is a squamous epithelial cell exfoliated from the vagina accompanied by a large number of Gardnerella bacillus and anaerobic bacteria. The presence of a mass of clue cells (≥20%) in the secretions indicates Gardnerella infection, hence an important indicator for the diagnosis of bacterial vaginitis
Trichomonad	A positive result may indicate trichomonas vaginitis
Coccus and bacillus	The number of cocci and bacilli can reflect the secretion cleanliness and microecological status
Fungus	A positive result may indicate fungal vaginitis

are abnormal, indicating that it may be vaginitis. Combined with the case for whether pathogenic bacteria, fungi, trichomonad, etc. are found, bacterial vaginosis, fungal vaginitis, trichomonas vaginitis, and so forth can thus be diagnosed. In case of female reproductive system diseases, the type and quantity of sediments in vaginal secretions will change. On that account, the morphological examination of the sediments is of great value for the diagnosis of female reproductive system inflammation and the observation of diagnosis effects, and they can also be used for the diagnosis of sexually transmitted diseases and reproductive tract tumors, as well as the monitoring of estrogen levels.

Microscopic examination and chemistry enzymatic detection are two common examination methods in clinical practice, with each holding both advantages and disadvantages: The former is simple and intuitive for sediment examination, while the latter is fast and convenient. The combination of the two can improve the sensitivity and specificity of the detection and enhance the diagnostic rate of vaginitis (Table 22.4). However, in practice, attention is often paid to routine examination of vaginal secretions, while the joint detection is ignored. The results lead to the missed diagnosis and incomplete treatment of fungal or trichomonas vaginitis, as well as mixed infection with bacterial vaginosis, thereby causing repeated illness and increasing the burden of patients. Therefore, the combination of sediment and chemistry enzymatic detection is of great significance for the clinical diagnosis of bacterial vaginosis, fungal vaginitis, trichomonas vaginitis, senile vaginitis, and other gynecological diseases.

Table 22.4 Guidance for joint interpretation of chemistry detection and sediment detection of vaginal secretions

No.	pH	H_2O_2	LA	LB	SNa	PIP	NAG	0X	GUS	Epithelial cell	Clue cell	Trichomonad	White blood cell	Red blood cell	Fungus	Bacillus	Miscellaneous bacteria	Prompt of joint interpretation results
1		+		+									15–30 or > 30	Yes				Indicating vaginal inflammation
2		+	+															Indicating decrease in lactic acid bacillus and abnormal vaginal environment
3					+/±	+/±					Yes						Medium or large amount	Indicating bacterial vaginosis
4		+								Little or none						Little or none		Indicating that vaginal flora is out of balance and that vaginal environment is in morbid state or sub-healthy state.
5	<4.6						+/±								Yes			Indicating fungal vaginitis
6	>4.8						+/±					Yes						Indicating trichomonas vaginitis
7		+		+					+				15–30 or > 30					Indicating aerobic vaginitis
8	<4.6				+		+/±				Yes				Yes			Indicating bacterial vaginosis + fungal vaginitis

No.	pH	H_2O_2	LA	LB	SNa	PIP	NAG	0X	GUS	Epithelial cell	Clue cell	Trichomonad	White blood cell	Red blood cell	Fungus	Bacillus	Miscellaneous bacteria	Prompt of joint interpretation results
9	>4.8				+		+/±				Yes	Yes						Indicating bacterial vaginosis + trichomonas vaginitis
10		+		+				+	+				15–30 or > 30				Medium or large amount	Indicating aerobic vaginitis + possible gonococcal vaginitis. Gram stain is thus recommended to observing whether there is gram-negative diplococcus

22.2 Status Quo and Development of Vaginal Secretion Inspection Technology

22.2.1 Technical Status

Despite the highly automated detection in clinical chemistry, immunology, hematology, etc., most hospitals still rely on manual microscopy for routine detection of vaginal secretions. Along with the gradual increase in the amount of clinical specimens, the limitation of manual microscopy has become increasingly prominent in the inspection work, with its main problems shown as follows: (1) the steps are cumbersome and the overall time consumed is long; (2) in the process of specimen pre-treatment and detection, human error has a great impact on aspects such as smear uniformity and smear reading ability of different personnel; (3) specimen exposure, resulting in biological contamination and cross-infection between specimens; (4) high experience requirements and strong subjectivity; (5) artificial dyeing, for which operators are long exposed to dangerous chemical reagents. Besides, it may also pollute the laboratory environment; (6) dye sediment, which can easily lead to complicated background of microscopic examination and interfere with observation as a result.

In view of the above problems, medical device manufacturers at home have launched semi-automatic and automatic instruments for vaginal secretion detection by visiting hospitals, interviewing experts, and combining with clinical needs.

22.2.2 Technological Development

The development of detection technology will surely lead to the development and application of detection instruments. Presented below is an introduction to the development of its inspection technology through the development course of the instruments transitioning from semi-automation to full automation.

1. Development of semi-automatic chemistry instruments: The semi-automatic joint inspection analyzer adopts the principle of photoelectric colorimetry to automatically interpret the joint inspection card. Specimen preparation, sample dripping, preheating, joint inspection card placement, and report integration all require manual operation. Representative instruments and their manufacturers include Auto woMO joint inspection analyzer of Autobio and bPR-2011A of Bioperfectus.
2. Development of the automatic chemistry instrument: The automatic dry chemical analyzer, embracing the principle of photoelectric colorimetry, realizes automatic sample injection, automatic incubation, automatic quantitative interpretation of results, batch processing, and improvement in the detection

speed. However, the specimen preparation and the integration of microscopic examination results and chemistry results still require manual operation. Despite the increased degree of automation of the instrument, too much manual participation still does not completely solve the problems facing the clinical laboratory.

3. Development of the automatic all-in-one machine: Against the backdrop of technological development, in order to achieve the joint detection of morphology and chemistry, the former applies flow image technology or natural sedimentation microscopic photography technology combined with photoelectric colorimetry technology to achieve the integrated detection of gynecological vaginal secretions, along with which the intelligent all-in-one machine for vaginal secretions also emerges. The machine supports automatic sample injection, preheating, result interpretation, and report generation of the instrument. Especially, the GMD-S600 automatic gynecological secretion analytical system represented by DIRUI realizes the automatic sample preparation, sample injection, preheating, staining, and result interpretation. Standardized sample preparation, result detection, and result interpretation ensure, therefore, the quality control of the whole detection results.

22.2.3 Market Capacity

Gynecological diseases are common clinical illnesses contracted by women, with a serious impact on women's physical and mental health and quality of life. In recent years, the incidence of gynecological diseases in China has remained high. According to the research results, the detection rate of gynecological diseases among Chinese women is as high as 68.3% [1], and the overall incidence of mixed vaginitis in various regions of China has fluctuated between 7.33 and 56.80% in the past decade. In 2015, the incidence of cervical cancer among Chinese women was 16.56/100,000. The gynecological diseases, with vaginal inflammation and gynecological tumors included, have caused great harm to women's health, given which the diagnosis and treatment of related diseases have become one of the important subjects in clinical research. Therefore, the market potential of gynecological secretion detection instruments and supporting reagents is great.

Along with the continuous improvement and optimization of the detection technology of reproductive tract detectors, automatic gynecological secretion detection products have emerged and been launched on the market. With continuous improvement in clinical application effect, those products have moved to gradually replace the semi-automatic and manual microscopic examinations, which have become an irresistible trend. According to the public data presented by Insight and Info, the market size of domestic gynecological secretion analyzers is about 3.544 billion, and that of supporting detection reagents is about 3.15 billion annually. With the growing awareness of health screening among Chinese women, the market acceptance of automatic gynecological secretion detection products has increased, the academic promotion of those products in the corresponding market by relevant enterprises has deepened, and the clinical demand for gynecological secretion detection has scaled new heights. On that account, the market scale of gynecological secretion detection instruments and supporting reagents is expected to maintain its rapid growth.

22.3 Hot Products of some Domestic Representative Manufacturers

The products mentioned above are just representatives of many excellent products of domestic IVD enterprises (Table 22.5). The representative of semi-automatic chemistry instruments is SHTARS, and that of the automatic all-in-one machine is DIRUI. These representative enterprises are committed to the development and innovation of new technologies and products, leading to the transition of vaginal secretion detection from manual operation and semi-automatic instruments to automatic artificial intelligence. By doing so, they not only address the increasing demand for specimen amount but also tackle the standardization of the whole process of specimen detection, thereby improving the sensitivity and specificity of detection results and providing more powerful basis for accurate diagnosis of vaginal secretion diseases and guidance on medication.

Table 22.5 Hot products of some representative manufacturers at home

Manufacturer	Name and model of main products	Product features
DIRUI	GD-S120 vaginal secretion analyzer, GMD-S600 vaginal infections analyzer	1. Full-process automatic and intelligent detection. 2. Sample pretreatment module improving the biosafety. 3. Complete quality control system. 4. Planar laminar flow cell technology + high-speed camera shooting technology + artificial intelligence recognition.
Bioperfectus	BPR2014A vaginitis automatic detection workstation, SS-AMIA3 automatic biological microscope, etc.	1. Dark room detection in a closed incubation environment to reduce the interference with chemical reactions. 2. Alarm detection set during the operation of the instrument. 3. Automatic identification of gram stain smears and generation of a standard vaginal microecology evaluation report.
Autobio	AutowoMo automatic reproductive tract secretion workstation, AutowoMo W500, AutowoMo500S automatic reproductive tract secretion analyzer	1. Chemistry enzymatic detection and micromorphology method. 2. Wet sheet dyeing technology + high-definition automatic microscopy system + morphological intelligent AI interpretation.

Table 22.5 (continued)

Manufacturer	Name and model of main products	Product features
SHTARS	Unit-700 vaginal microflora analyzer, Comet-800 multi-functional high-magnification microscopy analytical system, etc.	1. HSL color interpretation system. 2. Artificial intelligence DYF patented AI image recognition technology. 3. Multifunctional high-magnification microscopy analytical system supporting bright field, dark field, phase contrast field and camera conversion.
THME	BD-500 leucorrhea detection analyzer, BD-800 leucorrhea detection analyzer	1. One-time classic slide count, without hole blockage and cross contamination. 2. Automatic inspection and analysis, high degree of automation. 3. AI microscopic recognition system.
LITUO	LTS-V400 vaginitis detector, LTS-V800 vaginal secretion analyzer	1. Automatic microscopic examination realized by using accurate automatic interpretation technology of microscope images and disposable slide technology. 2. Unique slide technology + simulated artificial microscopy technology + big data identification technology.
REETOO	F600 vaginal secretion analyzer, F2000 vaginal secretion analyzer (high throughput)	1. AI DeepCell engine able to recognize cells with high accuracy. 2. Integrated chip, clip type mount. 3. Ten-million-pixel high-resolution CCD imaging. 4. Multi-layer dynamic focus scanning.
AVE	AVE-320 vaginal secretions analyzer, AVE-321 vaginal secretions analyzer	1. Automatic pretreatment technology. 2. Sediment enrichment technology. 3. Sediment dyeing technology. 4. Intelligent identification technology.
UZER	GY61 basement automatic vaginal microecology evaluation system, GY66 vaginal secretion comprehensive analyzer	1. Level dyeing and staining; 2. Automatic intelligent microscopic examination.

22.4 Industry Development Trend

According to the data provided by the World Health Organization, the global prevalence of gynecological diseases among women is as high as 93% [2]; the number of deaths from gynecological diseases reaches up to nine million every year; 20 women die of gynecological diseases every minute; what's worse, it is still increasing annually at a rate of 8%. It is especially so for vaginitis. Statistics show that the infection rate of vaginitis only among women over 55 years old has reached a peak of 42%. According to Xu H L et al., the routine and BV triple detection results of 3300 gynecological outpatients' vaginal secretions, combined with clinical symptoms, showed that bacterial vaginosis accounted for 32.6%, which was significantly higher than fungal vaginitis (12.2%) and trichomonal vaginitis (3.6%). The results were consistent with those reported by Zhu H et al. With the increasing incidence rate year by year and the growing demand for specimens, microscopic examination has encountered bottlenecks. For that matter, the development of technology and the emergence of automation equipment are not accidental, but necessary. However, the current penetration rate of automation equipment is less than 10%. The reasons for this are mainly as follows: (1) some doctors are used to viewing real images in microscopic examinations and do not believe in the result interpretation by instruments; (2) there are doubts about the agreement percent of the instruments; (3) how to interpret chemistry in conjunction with sediments; (4) how to combine the results of instrument detection with the expert consensus on clinical application of vaginal microecology evaluation; (5) how to reach a consensus on the standardization of automatic vaginal secretion detection methods and that of report items; (6) how to further improve the identification ability of AI equipment... All these are the problems that instrument manufacturers need to solve. However, the emergence of any new technology and new product requires a process of recognition and a stage of acceptance.

Maurizio Ferrari, chairman of the International Federation of Clinical Chemistry (IFCC), pointed out in a report titled How to Image the Future of Laboratory Medicine: "In the future, the development of laboratory medicine will rely on electronic computers and information technology, ranging from the creation and innovation of electronic highways to the interpretation of AI inspection results, especially the application of new technologies such as automatic cell recognition, which can play an important role in the development and construction of laboratory medicine in the future." The intelligence of laboratory medicine indicates that AI is taken as the platform. At present, automatic interpretation and review in the inspection fields such as clinical chemistry, immunology, hematology and so forth have been established, and the detection of gynecological vaginal secretions will also move towards an era of automation and intelligence. The treated specimen is injected into a specific analytical assay plate, and the sediment in the specimen is digitally photographed and intelligently identified through a digital imaging system, enabling the screening and detection of common elements such as cells, mold, and trichomoniasis.

Declaration Yongliang Ni, Qifeng Nie, Shang Gao, and Zhengxu Kang are employees of Dirui Industrial Co., Ltd.

References

1. Xing D, Wang D, Tian Q. Analysis on gynecological diseases screening quality in He'nan province in 2013[J]. Maternal Child Health Care China. 2015;30(34):5941–5944
2. Wang L, Zhao X, Wang H, et al. Census results analysis among 628 married women in gynecological disease[J]. Xinjiang Med J. 2016;11(15):1208–1210.

Hematology Analyzers and Reagents 23

Guangna Ma, Gengwen Chen, Jialin Lin, Lingyu Bai,
Biao Wu, Yong Tang, Yang Yang, and Kang Yu

23.1 Development, Production, and Market Size of Hematology Analyzers and Reagents

23.1.1 Blood Cell Detection Techniques and Methods

23.1.1.1 Blood Cell Detection Techniques

A hematology analyzer mainly detects formed elements in blood, including red blood cells (RBCs), platelets, white blood cells (WBCs), and hemoglobin in RBCs. Such detection can be accomplished with three main categories of techniques: electrical impedance, light scattering, and colorimetry, each including several subcategories. Here is a brief overview of them.

Electrical Impedance

It is based on the Coulter Principle, that is, when non-conducting particles pass through an aperture, concurrent with an electric current, the pulse amplitude changes, in a way that is directly proportional to the volume of the particles traversing the aperture. The aperture is typically made of ruby (hence the name ruby aperture), ranging from 50 to 100 μm in size.

When more than one particle passes through the aperture at the same time or in close proximity, the resultant pulse amplitude is distorted, making it vital to manage the single-particle passage. This requires blood samples to be substantially diluted first, since blood cells, especially RBCs, are present in very high concentrations in

G. Ma (✉) · G. Chen · J. Lin · L. Bai · B. Wu
Shenzhen Mindray Bio-Medical Electronics Co., Ltd., Shenzhen, Guangdong, China
e-mail: maguangna@mindray.com

Y. Tang · Y. Yang · K. Yu
Maccura Biotechnology Co. Ltd, Chengdu, Sichuan, China

H. Song, L. Dai (eds.), *In Vitro Diagnostic Industry in China*,
https://doi.org/10.1007/978-981-99-3110-1_23

the blood. Thus, two specific technical routes are created, which are classic impedance and sheath flow impedance.

Classic impedance: Apply a constant voltage to the test sample, so that it flows slowly through the ruby aperture. Since the cells in the sample pass through the aperture in a random, irregular path, a dilution ratio of up to 1:20,000 is required to minimize the interference of overlapping particles. Classic impedance can detect RBCs in vast numbers and volumes; but, when applied to platelets in tiny numbers and sizes, it has a limited statistical magnitude, low repeatability and accuracy, and is susceptible to pulse interference.

Sheath flow impedance: According to the principle of flow focusing, the width of sample flow is controlled at a level comparable to the cell diameter, allowing the cells to pass through the ruby aperture one by one in a straight line with no interference between them and thus ensuring a high quality of pulse signals. With a dilution ratio between 1:300 and 1:500, a large statistical magnitude, and superior performance, sheath flow impedance can dynamically detect system background and automatically identify interferents. It is, however, significantly more complicated and expensive than classic impedance in that it requires creating a flow-focusing system.

Following RBC lysis, the remaining WBCs in the sample may be counted by impedance and classified as lymphocytes, intermediate cells, and neutrophils based on their size. Due to the low concentration of WBCs (about one-thousandth that of RBCs), they can be measured by classic impedance using a small dilution ratio.

Light Scattering

It is based on the Mie scattering theory, which describes a proportional relationship between the internal complexity of particles and their scattered light intensity. It was first used to detect WBCs, classifying them into lymphocytes, monocytes, neutrophils, eosinophils, and basophils.

The excitation light is usually a monochromatic laser and a very narrow and uniform energy distribution spot is obtained by beam shaping and irradiated on an optical flow cell. The flow cell, a transparent rectangular device built on the flow-focusing technology, enables the cells in the blood sample to pass through one by one and be irradiated by the light spot in the detection area to generate scattered light. The scattered light is received by a photoelectric device and converted into electrical signals. PD or PMT can be used depending on the signal intensity.

Light scattering may leverage two or more information dimensions to improve recognition accuracy. The dimensions are described as follows:

Volume: It is often measured using the forward scattered light signal of roughly 1° (or, alternatively, the light absorption signal of 0°), or using electrical impedance by adding a tiny aperture to the front of the optical flow cell.

Complexity: It is often measured using side scatter signals which allow for a wide variety of angular ranges, such as a medium angle of about 10° to 20°, a medium-to-high angle of about 40°, or a side angle of 90°. Depolarized light signals have also been used to reflect differences in cellular contents.

Fluorescence information: Specific labeling dye is added, which enters the cell and binds to specific targets. Following laser excitation, the dye releases fluorescence at specific wavelengths that differ from the excitation wavelength. The fluorescence information is then detected by a photomultiplier tube with high sensitivity through optical filter selection.

Colorimetry

Colorimetry is based on the Beer–Lambert law, that is, the concentration of the target substance is directly proportional to the light absorption at a specific wavelength. It is used to measure hemoglobin. First, a specific hemolytic agent is used to lyse RBCs, release hemoglobin, and form complexes. After light irradiation at a specific wavelength, a photoelectric sensor is used to detect the light attenuation from absorption. Complexes formed by different hemolytic agents have slightly different maximum absorption spectra, usually between 500 and 550 nm.

23.1.1.2 Blood Cell Detection Methods

The clinical detection of blood cells is closely related to how they are processed by reagents. After the blood cells are processed by the supporting reagents, the above detection techniques (such as sheath flow impedance and laser light scattering) can be used for cell counting and differential detection of WBCs. The blood cells can be detected by the chemical method, chemical staining method, and fluorescence staining method. The chemical method is mainly used in 3-part and 5-part differential hematology analyzers; the chemical staining method is mainly used in blood cell morphology detection, such as blood smear analysis, and some manufacturers have used chemical staining reagents in 5-part differential hematology analyzers; while the fluorescence staining method is mainly used in high-end 5-part differential hematology analyzers and blood cell analysis modules on the automation line.

Chemical Method

It allows the blood cells to be processed with chemical reagents and then counted and differentially detected using relevant technologies. The method primarily employs two kinds of reagents: surfactant-containing special reagents and diluents that maintain cell morphology and provide the appropriate ionic environment. The surfactant-containing special reagents play different roles in detecting different parameters: For example, when detecting HGB, they lyse RBCs to expose hemoglobin; when performing cell counting and differential detection of WBCs, they differentiate cells and change the density or size of cells, providing the material basis for detection and classification. The diluents can provide an appropriate cell suspension environment, maintain cell morphology, and ensure the stability and reliability of the detection process. Due to its ease of implementation at the technical level, this method has been adopted by Mindray, Dymind, URIT, Landwind, and other Chinese manufacturers in the hemolytic agents for their 3-part differential hematology analyzers, such as Mindray's latest BC-20 and BC-30S and its earlier products BC-2800 and BC-3000Plus. The chemical method has also been used in the reagents for Dymind's DH31, DH36, URIT's URIT-2900, URIT-3000Plus, etc. Despite the stringent detection standards and difficult technical development process for its use in 5-part differential hematology analyzers, the chemical method has been used in the products of many manufacturers, such as URIT's URIT-5510, URIT-5380 series, Mindray's BC-5000 series, Dymind's DF55, Zybio's Z5, and Z3 series, for cell counting and differential detection. The 3-part differential hematology analyzers generally use only one special chemical reagent for hemolysis, while 5-part ones may use one to three chemical reagents to achieve accurate 5-part differential detection.

Chemical Staining Method

Chemical dyes used in chemical staining can specifically stain different cell structures, and display different optical characteristics after staining and deposition. After blood cells are treated by hemolysis with chemical dyes and special reagents, the size of cells and the density of cell structures are changed. With these differentiating factors between different cells, the detection system can apply appropriate techniques to classify and count blood cells. Among the 5-part differential hematology analyzers applying this method, the most typical ones are Mindray's mid-end BC-5390 and BC-5390CRP series. They used supporting reagents, in which the chemical dyes differentially classify different WBC subtypes by staining and hemolysis of blood cells. Then the detection system can use these differentiating factors for counting and classification. It is a technically mature method that has been used by most made-in-China 5-part differential hematology analyzers.

Fluorescent Staining Method

The primary difference between this method and the above two lies in its introduction of fluorescent staining reagents. A fluorescent staining reagent is a chemical substance that can target and bind to different cells or different components in the same cell, and when such substances are excited by light irradiation at different energy levels, they can also emit excitation light with energy of a corresponding wavelength, that is, fluorescence. The intensity and amount of fluorescence are calculated by a special device so as to achieve differential detection and counting of different cells. Different blood cells are distinguished from each other by size and structure (after WBCs are treated with surfactant-containing special reagents, neutrophils appear denser than lymphocytes in structure), by cellular component (RNA content differs between RBCs and reticulocytes (RETs)), or by the content of a certain cellular component (abnormal granulocytes contain more DNA than neutrophils). Fluorescent staining uses these differences and targeted binding of fluorescent dyes to achieve more accurate differential detection and counting. For example, special dyes can detect NRBCs indicative of myeloid hyperplasia, and the intensity of fluorescence signals helps to detect abnormal lymphocytes. Mindray's 6-series (BC-6000Plus and BC-6800Plus) and 7-series (BC-7500 CRP and BC-7500 CS) instruments have used fluorescence staining reagents. The addition of fluorescent dyes offers another approach to the accurate detection of WBCs and the counting and detection of some abnormal cells. Specifically, M-6FD dye can accurately detect abnormal cells such as eosinophils, abnormal lymphocytes, and immature granulocytes; RET channel dye and M-6FN dye can perform differential detection on RETs and nucleated red blood cells (NRBCs), respectively. Fluorescence staining improves the accuracy and efficiency of clinical detection. Despite its high technical threshold, an increasing number of Chinese manufacturers are using this method. In addition to Mindray's instruments mentioned above, it is also used by Maccura's 8-series (F 800/F 810/F 880) and Dirui's BF-7200 series hematology analyzers.

23.1.2 Development and Production Status of Hematology Analyzers and Reagents, and Main Hematology Analyzer Manufacturers

23.1.2.1 Development and Production Status of Hematology Analyzers and Reagents in China

Hematology analysis is one of the three major routine clinical tests. In the past, RBCs, WBCs, and platelets in the blood were counted manually by a microscope, followed by the classification of WBCs in the stained blood smear. This was a time-consuming and laborious process with limited test items and poor result accuracy and consistency. This was changed by the advent of hematology analyzers (also known as blood cell analyzers, complete blood count (CBC) analyzers, blood cell counters, hemocytometers, etc.) and the development of relevant technologies. They have now been widely used for clinical hematology analysis due to their ease of operation and high degree of automation, and become essential and fundamental automation instruments in the clinical laboratory. Chinese manufacturers can now produce hematology analyzers and reagents independently. The product portfolio encompasses 3-part and 5-part differential hematology analyzers, and other instruments along the hematology analysis line such as slide makers & stainers, morphological analyzers, specific protein analyzers, and glycosylated hemoglobin (HbA1c) analyzers. They have been widely used in hospitals as the core instruments.

At present, 5-part differential hematology analyzers and hematology analysis lines have been playing a key part in various hospitals in China, and 3-part differential hematology analyzers are primarily used in small private hospitals, private clinics, township/community health services, and other small medical and health institutions. The concentration ratio is high in terms of the R&D and manufacturing of hematology analyzers and reagents. There are presently over 20 manufacturers that can produce 5-part differential hematology analyzers and over 100 that can produce 3-part ones. However, there are just a select few with reliable core technology, innovative R&D capabilities, and mass-manufactured products. They include Mindray, Maccura, Dirui (Changchun), URIT (Guilin), and Dymind (Shenzhen).

The first decade of the twenty-first century witnessed the dominance of foreign brands in the field of hematology analysis in China, covering almost all market segments from secondary to tertiary hospitals. Mindray launched its first 5-part differential hematology analyzer in 2006 and BC-6800 in 2011. The latter features a 3D fluorescence staining platform, allowing for such detection functions as the 5-part differentiation of WBCs, RETs, and NRBCs. Since then, locally produced hematology analyzers have been commonly used in major tertiary hospitals. Following BC-6800, Mindray introduced more 6-series high-end hematology analyzers and 5-series and 7-series CBC + CRP and/or SAA integrated analyzers, as well as CAL 8000 series hematology analysis line; URIT developed 5-series 5-part differential hematology analyzers using four-angle laser scattering 5-part differential technology; Dymind obtained 5-part differential hematology analysis technology through the diffusion of cytochemical 5-part differential technology, and launched the D-series 5-part integrated analyzer that incorporated CRP analysis; JASDAQ from Jiashan County, Zhejiang Province independently developed 5-series 5-part differential hematology analyzers using nucleic acid fluorescence staining technology (the company was acquired by Maccura in 2015 and became the source of technology for Maccura's 5-part differential hematology analyzers).

At this stage, Chinese manufacturers had created a complete industrial chain for hematology analyzers and reagents, covering all upstream and downstream processes. They had made the shift from 3-part differential to 5-part differential hematology analyzers and to hematology analysis lines, gaining a significant market share in top tertiary level A hospitals. In 2020, the first year of the third decade of the twenty-first century, the production volume of hematology analyzers in China crossed the 60,000 mark, half of which were installed in the domestic market. This represented the great achievements Chinese manufacturers had made in the R&D and production of hematology analyzers and reagents.

23.1.2.2 Main Chinese Manufacturers, Their Products, and Detection Principles

Mindray

Shenzhen Mindray Bio-Medical Electronics Co., Ltd. (hereinafter referred to as "Mindray"), established in 1991, is a world-leading medical device supplier and China's largest IVD developer and manufacturer, covering eight different lines of business. Mindray launched the first quasi-3-part differential hematology analyzer in 1998 and the first 5-part differential hematology analyzer (BC-5500) in China in 2006, ushering in a new area of locally produced 5-part differential hematology analyzers; in 2011, Mindray spearheaded the Chinese industry again by launching the BC-6800 automated hematology analyzer that could measure RETs and NRBCs. The product relied on multi-dimensional analysis, which combined sheath flow impedance, laser light scattering, and fluorescence staining, for cell counting and classification and colorimetry for hemoglobin determination. In 2013, BC-6900 automated blood cell and body fluid analyzer was launched, which could count RBCs, WBCs, and nucleated cells in cerebrospinal fluid, pleural effusion, and peritoneal effusion, and further determine the counts and proportions of mononuclear and multi-nuclear cells. BC-6800/6900 created the technological groundwork for Mindray's high-end hematology analyzers. In 2014, Mindray launched CAL 8000, the first hematology analysis line independently developed in China. After several updates, this analysis line can now be designed to feature hematology analyzers, automated slide makers and stainers, automated specific protein analyzers, HbA1c analyzers, and automated digital cell morphology analyzers. New modules can be added later to accommodate the laboratory's evolving needs, making it possible to test up to 1000 blood cell samples per hour. In just over a decade, China's hematology analyzers have finally reached a high level that is on par with or even better than international peers.

To address the customers' real challenges and pain points, Mindray launched BC-5390CRP, a CBC + CRP integrated analyzer, in 2015. It could provide both CBC and CRP test results at a time with a much-improved testing workflow. Mindray's pace of progress has never stopped. In 2017, the company unveiled BC-6800 Plus, the world's fastest standalone hematology analyzer that could de-aggregate platelet clumps, provide the RBC scattergram, and process 200 CBC + DIFF samples per hour. It was a turning point as China started to overtake established powers in hematology analysis. Based on the needs of clinicians working in the front line as well as its previous 5-part differential + CRP integrated analyzer, in 2020, Mindray launched BC-7500 CRP series (the world's first 5-part differential + CRP integrated analyzer enabling automated loading and detection of trace peripheral blood while catering to the specific needs of Chinese customers) and CAL 7000 (the first hematology analysis line enabling automated loading and detection of trace peripheral blood). By allowing operation in batches, they eliminated the hassle of manual intervention for the 5-part differential analysis and CRP testing of trace peripheral blood samples, so laboratories could perform trace peripheral blood detection with significantly higher efficiency and a streamlined workflow. In 2021, Mindray released BC-7500 CS, a 5-part differential CBC + CRP integrated analyzer (CBC + CRP + SAA), which expanded the list of test items for hematology analyzers.

In September 2021, Mindray's MC-80 appeared on the market. As China's first automated digital cell morphology analyzer that can be connected with the hematology analysis line, it has ushered in a new area of automated microscopic examination in hematology analysis. Backed by such technologies as multilayer fusion, SOLID ROCK hyperstable antishake system, and edge and tail scanning, MC-80 has made three major breakthroughs. First, it delivers ultraclear images to reproduce the real view under the microscope. Second, it can automatically adjust the analysis mode to the blood cell detection results. Third, it analyzes up to 60 slides/hours, ensuring a fast TAT for blood cell samples. As a revolutionary analyzer among Chinese brands in automated digital cell morphology analysis, MC-80 has facilitated the widespread adoption of high-end medical devices in most medical institutions in China, taking automated peripheral blood cell morphology analysis to the next level. CAL 7000, a hematology analysis line connected with Mindray's 7-series high-end hematology analyzers to slide maker & stainer SC-120 and automated digital cell morphology analyzer MC-80, has provided additional solutions for medical institutions, thereby supporting the rapid advances in the hematology analysis field in China.

Maccura

Maccura Biotechnology Co., Ltd. (hereinafter referred to as Maccura) was founded in 1994, it has entered the field of hematology analysis as a manufacturer of whole-blood controls designed for 3-diff analyzers. With fast development, Maccura's hematology product line has covered analyzers, reagents, quality controls, and calibrators. The complete analysis system can meet the needs of all laboratory sizes, from small to large. Up to now, Maccura has successively launched multi-leveled hematology controls and calibrators of open system, and of hematology analyzers of F 5 and F 8 series. The controls and calibrators are designed for parameters of CBC, DIFF, RET, Fluorescent PLT, etc.

In 2017, Maccura introduced F 5 series automatic hematology analyzers to the market, including F 560 and F 580 models. Those models use flow cytometry and nucleic acid fluorescence staining technology to realize WBC classification by analyzing FSL (forward scattered light) signal, SSC (side scattered light) signal, and SFL (side fluorescence light) signal of cellular particles. Once the F 5 series was launched, the number of installed instruments has achieved a rapid growth, and the hematology analysis has become the third-largest part of Maccura's product line.

Subsequently, the F 8 series automatic hematology analyzers were introduced to the market in 2019, including F 800, F 810, and F 880 models. F 8 series adopts modular design to meet the requirement of free combination; Maccura also optimized the technology and added more channels on the basis of 5-series. In addition to CBC + DIFF channel, NRBC (nucleated red blood cells) and RET (reticulocytes) can also be detected. The special PLT-F and AWS channels are used to detect low-value platelets and abnormal white blood cells. F 8 series also has multiple detection modes, including whole-blood mode, low-value leukocyte mode, pre-dilution mode, and sample research mode, to further meet the detection needs of users for special samples. At the same time, the stability of analyzers and user experience have also been greatly improved. For instance, F 8 series supports RFID chip identification technology of dye reagents, those reagents are ready to use after being plugged in. Compared with previous generations of reagents, the RFID identification technology prevents misuse, also, the operation of the latest generation is more convenient and efficient.

In addition to single-module analyzers, Maccura has successively launched hematology assembly lines and workstations to connect multiple analyzers of different models. Users can choose different models according to their needs, and connect those models with track modules to achieve automatic detection. Different from the assembly line, the workstation can also connect the following models: the automatic glycosylated hemoglobin analyzer(G 01), the automatic specific protein analyzer (P 100), the automatic slide maker and stainer(AS 120), combined with the intelligent management software, to realize the total solution for laboratory hematology analysis with only one tube of whole-blood sample. The laboratory intelligent management software (Malab intelligent system) supports setting up re-detection rules. It will automatically review abnormal samples, and send them back for re-detection according to the rules. This system improves the efficiency and reduces the cost of re-detection of samples. The assembly line and the workstation can be connected with corner modules and cross-column modules according to the layout of the laboratory design, which optimizes floor space usage and detection efficiency. In the future, the workstation can also be connected with more efficiency oriented models such as morphological analyzers to further improve the level of laboratory automation.

Dymind

ShenZhen Dymind Biotechnology Co., Ltd. (hereinafter referred to as "Dymind"), established in 2013, boasts a hematology analysis line covering 3-part analyzers, 5-part analyzers, 3-part +5-part integrated analyzers, and CBC + CRP integrated analyzers. The 5-part differential hematology analyzer uses cytochemical staining and multi-angle laser light scattering in WBC differential detection. From 2015 to 2020, Dymind successively developed 5-part differential hematology analyzers DH53 and DH76, 3-part +5-part integrated analyzer DH73, and CBC + CRP integrated analyzers such as D5CRP, D7CRP, and DH76CRP. In 2019, Dymind released the DM79X integrated analyzer, which requires only one tube of blood to detect CBC, CRP, and serum amyloid A (SAA).

At present, community-based medical institutions make up the majority of Dymind's customer base in China. In the low-end market in the hematology analysis segment, Dymind has surpassed other brands at home and abroad, second only to Mindray.

Dirui

Dirui Industrial Co.,Ltd. (hereinafter referred to as "Dirui") was established in Changchun, China in 1992. Its hematology analysis products include 3-part differential, 5-part differential, and CBC + CRP integrated analyzers. It provides a vast selection of items to meet the diverse needs of medical institutions at all levels. As the company's flagship product, BF-6900 CRP automated hematology analyzer can detect CBC and CRP with only one tube of blood. The instrument uses cytochemical staining and flow cytometry to perform 5-part differentiation of WBCs, and latex-enhanced immunoturbidimetry to detect CRP. The detection results cover high-sensitivity and conventional CRP.

Dirui's BF-7200 automated hematology analysis system, built on the principle of nucleic acid fluorescence staining, was introduced in 2021. It could be connected online to build a modular hematology analysis line that caters to the demands of a wide variety of customer groups.

URIT

URIT Medical Electronic Co., Ltd. (hereinafter referred to as "URIT") developed the URIT-5500 automated 5-part differential hematology analyzer in 2009. It used multi-angle polarized scatter separation (MAPSS) for WBC classification. This is a technology that features prominently due to its ability to keep WBCs' internal structures as close to their natural form as possible without using any staining solution; it can also detect WBCs in just one channel, accurately displaying their total count and classification. This instrument can also semi-automatically detect RETs, thus providing a basis for experimentally evaluating the hematopoietic function of the bone marrow in clinical practice.

All of URIT's 5-part differential hematology analyzers, including the URIT-5500, URIT-5380, URIT-5250, and URIT-5180 series, are based on MAPSS technology. The BH-5380CRP series of "WBC 5-part differentiation + CRP + RET" integrated analyzer, was introduced in 2018, which could detect CBC and CRP with only one tube of blood. In 2019, URIT and Goldsite Diagnostics Inc. (Shenzhen) jointly launched the automated blood analysis line URIT-5510&Orbital Astep PLUS, which enabled rapid detection of CBC + CRP + SAA and accurate determination of infection types.

23.1.3 Size of China's Hematology Analysis Market

23.1.3.1 Size and Landscape of China's Hematology Analysis Market

Market size: Hematology analyzers and reagents have long been adopted in China to support common diagnostic test items in hospitals. Accordingly, Chinese manufacturers have long been able to independently produce hematology analyzers and reagents and reagents that provide comparable performance to those from global brands. In 2020, the domestic market size reached CNY4.2 billion (tax-exclusive ex-factory price), accounting for about 20% of the global market size. By 2024, the domestic market size is predicted to reach CNY5.8 billion (tax-exclusive ex-factory price), with a compound annual growth rate of about 8%.

Tier 1 manufacturers: Mindray is the only Tier 1 manufacturer of hematology analyzers and reagents in the Chinese market.

Mindray started developing and manufacturing hematology analyzers and reagents in 1998. With a significant number of technically proficient researchers on the staff, the company has the proprietary right to all the core technologies required in advanced hematology analysis. Its customers range from top tertiary level A hospitals to community health service centers, from large third-party chain laboratories to private clinics, and its products have played an active part in the reform of China's medical and health system and the performance evaluation of tertiary public hospitals. In 2020, Mindray's 6-series and 7-series hematology analyzers, as well as high-end instruments such as the hematology analysis line ranked first in the Chinese market in terms of the number of new installations. Its automated digital cell morphology analyzers have been marketed since 2021. Mindray remains the holder of the largest share of the low-end market.

Tier 2 manufacturers: Dymind, URIT, and Maccura are Tier 2 manufacturers in the Chinese market, whose annual sales have or will cross the "100,000,000 yuan mark."

Founded in 2013, Dymind has grown very rapidly with the 5-part differential CBC + CRP integrated analyzer as its flagship product. Dymind was the only Tier 2 manufacturer that had not yet made their advanced 5-part differential analysis technology available for mass production by the end of 2021. It had an installed capacity of 2000 to 3000 5-part differential hematology analyzers, serving mostly secondary or lower-level community medical and health institutions.

URIT launched its first automated 5-part differential hematology analyzer in 2009, developed a 5-part differential CRP integrated analyzer in 2018, and obtained the recordation certificate for the MP-8120 automated slide maker & stainer in 2020. Its customers are mainly secondary or lower-level community medical institutions and private hospitals, with an annual installed capacity of hematology analyzers (including 3-part differential hematology analyzers) second only to Mindray.

After Mindray, Maccura is the second company in China with its own high-end 5-part nucleic acid fluorescence staining technology and independent hematology analysis line. At the end of 2021, its AS 120 slide maker & stainer obtained the recordation certificate. Its products are mostly high end and are mostly found at tertiary hospitals.

Tier 3 manufacturers: Dirui, XPENARRAY, SonoScape, EDAN, and Zybio are Tier 3 manufacturers in the domestic market. XPENARRAY offers the 5-part differential CRP integrated analyzer as its key product, whereas the other four all have a comprehensive portfolio in which hematology analysis products account for less than 15% of their sales. The majority of their customers are public secondary or lower-level and private medical and health institutions.

23.2 Main Innovative Hematology Analyzers and Reagents in China

23.2.1 Main Innovative Hematology Analyzers

In the field of in vitro diagnostics (IVD), hematology analysis is the first segment where Chinese brands have a larger market share than foreign ones. In recent years, following the pace set by Mindray, Chinese hematology analyzer manufacturers have exhibited a surge in innovative products, including CBC + CRP integrated analyzers, hematology analyzers with automated peripheral blood loading, automated slide makers & stainers, automated digital cell morphology analyzers, and automated hematology analysis lines.

23.2.1.1 CBC + CRP Integrated Analyzers

Motivated by the increasing test volume and the technical maturity of whole blood CRP detection, Chinese hematology analyzer manufacturers have created a CBC+ CRP integrated analyzer that innovatively combines CBC and whole blood CRP tests previously running on two separate instruments. This allows the detection of both CBC and CRP items at the same time using only one sample. Reduced blood consumption, easier operation, and shorter TAT are just a few of its most notable advantages, which explain why it has been so extensively adopted and well received by laboratory operators since its debut. According to different blood cell analysis platforms, CBC + CRP integrated analyzers can be divided into fluorescence staining platform-based integrated analyzers (such as Mindray's BC-7500 CRP and

BC-7500 CS) and chemical staining platform-based ones (such as Mindray's BC-5390 CRP series, Dymind's D7-CRP, URIT's BH-5380CRP, and Dirui's BF-6900 CRP). According to different CRP test items, CBC + CRP integrated analyzers can be divided into CBC + CRP integrated analyzers (such as Mindray's BC-7500 CRP, BC-5390 CRP, Dymind's D7-CRP, URIT's BH-5380 CRP, and Dirui's BF-6900 CRP) and CBC + CRP + SAA integrated analyzers (such as Mindray's BC-7500 CS, Dymind's DM79X, and XPENARRAY's XPEN60/65).

23.2.1.2 Hematology Analyzers with Automated Peripheral Blood Loading

Certain clinical settings, such as children's hospitals and maternal and child health care hospitals, often need CBC samples from peripheral blood. In peripheral blood CBC tests, manual intervention is often required to complete barcode labeling, number entry, sample mixing, sample loading, and reexamination. This involves a complicated operating procedure, a low degree of automation, and a high risk of making mistakes, which necessitates automated batch detection of peripheral blood. In 2020, based on the principle of 3D fluorescence staining analysis, Mindray pioneered in developing BC-7500 series hematology analyzers for automated mixing and detection of peripheral blood, barcode management of peripheral blood samples, LIS two-way communication, and automated reexamination of abnormal samples. BC-7500 series hematology analyzers can not only automatically load peripheral blood in batch, but also enable simultaneous batch loading of venous blood and peripheral blood. Only a small amount of blood is required for batch loading of peripheral whole blood: 27.5 μL for CBC alone; 36.5 μL for CBC + CRP; and 40 μL for CBC + CRP + SAA.

23.2.1.3 Automated Slide Makers and Stainers

When abnormal CBC test results are found in blood samples, which triggers blood smear reexamination rules, blood smears should be prepared for microscopic reexamination. Artificial blood smear preparation requires tedious manual operating processes such as blood drop dripping, spreading, drying, staining, cleaning, and re-drying, which pose biosafety risks and lack automation and standardization. Blood smears were formerly made and stained using two separate devices; however, technological advancements have led to the widespread use of automated slide makers & stainers in hospitals. By the end of 2021, Mindray's SC-120 was the only Chinese automated slide maker & stainer extensively used in hospitals. Although SC-120 was released later than competing foreign brands, it has now incorporated more sophisticated and mature parts and achieved significant improvements to the manufacturing process, allowing it to overtake the foreign competitors in quality and stability. Besides venous blood, SC-120 also features automated slide making and staining for trace blood, i.e., only 25 μL of blood is required for one standard round of automated slide making and staining.

23.2.1.4 Automated Digital Cell Morphology Analyzers

When abnormal CBC test results are found in blood samples, which triggers blood smear reexamination rules, blood smears should be prepared for microscopic reexamination. Manual microscopic examination is time-consuming and labor-intensive; it not only requires morphological expertise but also lacks a uniform standard. With the advancement of technology, some automated digital cell morphology analyzers have emerged in China, such as BCM-2 from CELLDIFF (Beijing), CA-030S from CELL-IMAGE (Shanghai), and ME-150 from ICELL (Beijing). However, they are not widely used in hospitals and cannot be incorporated into an automation line together with hematology analyzers and automated slide makers & stainers. In 2021, Mindray introduced its in-house developed automated digital cell morphology analyzer MC-80. In response to the demands of Chinese customers, it has made daring breakthroughs and incorporated the most recent advances in materials science, digital imaging, and intelligent recognition technology into the manufacturing and production processes; it is now possible to connect MC-80 to the hematology analysis line. MC-80 has several merits in performance. First, it can analyze up to 60 slides/hour, twice as fast as that of foreign analyzers. Second, it delivers clearer and more authentic images: MC-80 performs 20-layer vertical scanning on each WBC to capture every detail of the cell and fuse them all into a clear and delicate image. This in turn truly reproduces the subtle structure of each cell and accurately captures their comprehensive pathological features. Such clarity and authenticity help to identify abnormal cells and timely diagnose various hematological diseases. Third, the analyzer can intelligently match the appropriate analysis mode based on CBC results, alarms, and reexamination rules. It also allows adjusting the analysis mode as needed any time, while supporting user customization and optimized review rules to ensure less manual intervention and improved detection quality.

23.2.1.5 Automated Hematology Analysis Line

The automated hematology analysis line connects together the automated hematology analyzer, automated slide maker and stainer, and automated digital cell morphology analyzer through tracks. In recent years, CRP, SAA, HbA1c, and other whole blood test items have also been integrated into the hematology analysis line, so that all whole blood test items can be completed with a single tube, as the market prefers. In the current Chinese market, Mindray and Maccura are among the very few OEMs that provide all the modules on the hematology analysis line to support all whole blood items with one tube". Mindray's CAL 8000 and CAL 7000 hematology analysis lines boast modules that can perform CBC, CRP, SAA, and HbA1c testing, automated slide making and staining, and automated cell morphological analysis; all the modules are in-house developed by Mindray, and the underlying information can be interconnected. Maccura's F 9000 X automated hematology workstation can also complete CBC, CRP, and HbA1c tests; all the analysis modules are in-house developed by Maccura.

23.2.2 Main Innovative Hematology Reagents in China

23.2.2.1 Platelet (PLT) Rapid and Accurate Detection Reagents

Platelet is one of the most important parameters in hematology analysis. Platelet clumping, low PLT counts, RBC fragment interferences are the main pain points to address to achieve rapid and accurate PLT detection. To further improve the detection accuracy of low PLT count, specialized manufacturers have conducted extensive research and developed their unique products.

Platelet clump de-aggregation reagent: Platelets are one of the most important indicators for clinical evaluation of bleeding and thrombosis risk. In clinical practice, anticoagulants may be replaced to recollect blood and retest platelets in response to serious concerns such as pseudothrombocytopenia induced by platelet clumping. If the issue remains after the replacement, several blood samples must be collected and detected by a laborious manual microscopic examination. In an effort to address the challenges associated with timely and accurate reporting of aggregated platelet samples in clinical laboratories, Mindray has investigated the mechanism of platelet aggregation and identified the key cell pathways for de-aggregation, such as the calcium ion channel and the tyrosine kinase pathway. By reformulating the platelet detection reagent using a number of novel essential de-aggregation chemicals, the platelet clumps are de-aggregated. The innovative reagent has been used in many hematology analyzers of Mindray and serves as the foundation of its first-of-its-kind platelet clump de-aggregation technology. International patent applications have been filed for this technology. It has been well received by both local and international specialists and has been recommended as best practice in national industry standards.

The optical platelet reagent detects low PLT counts and eliminates the interferences of RBC fragments: The platelet detection function of first-generation hematology analyzers is based on the impedance method, and its principle is to detect platelets according to the volume difference between platelets and other cells, but it is susceptible to the interference of cells with a similar volume. The second-generation platelet detection technology is based on the laser flow cytometry. The principle is to detect platelets by irradiating the reagent-treated platelets with a laser and then collecting forward scatter, side scatter, and side fluorescence signals generated after the sample passes through the flow cell. The key benefit is that it can accurately detect low PLT counts while eliminating the interferences of giant platelets and other factors. Platelet optical (PLT-O) detection is enabled by Mindray based on the laser flow cytometry and PLT-O reagent. In contrast to previous platelet detection reagents, the PLT-O reagent allows simultaneous specific staining of the nucleic acids in platelets and RETs, to detect low PLT counts, identify platelets with high forward scattered light and fluorescence intensities as immature platelet fractions (IPF), and clearly distinguish between platelets and RBC fragments to eliminate the interference. Typical products include Mindray's BC-6800, BC-6800Plus, BC-6000Plus, and BC-7500 series. Maccura's F810 and F880 have also employed similar technologies. In addition, Maccura's F880 has added a separate platelet detection channel and used a separate reagent for specific fluorescence staining of nucleic acids in platelets. The nucleic acid dyes do not stain RBC fragments, but only intracellular nucleic acids in platelets, thus greatly reducing the interference of RBC fragments in lateral fluorescence signals in platelet detection. It can prevent any platelet aggregation from affecting the staining of platelets by nucleic acid dyes so that fluorescence signals can be used to effectively detect platelets.

23.2.2.2 RET and NRBC Detection Reagents

RETs are immature RBCs produced in the bone marrow and released into the peripheral blood, and as they mature, the intracellular RNA content gradually decreases and finally disappears. The intracellular RNA content indicates the degree of maturation of RETs. RETs indicate pathologic exuberance of hematopoietic function of the bone marrow and are common in several proliferative anemias such as iron deficiency anemia, megaloblastic anemia, and hemorrhagic anemia. In particular, RETs increase most significantly when hemolytic anemia is present. NRBCs indicate erythroid hyperplasia and are diagnostic of both bone marrow hyperplasia and hemolytic anemia. Using both RET and NRBC reagents for detection is clinically significant for hematological disease diagnosis.

Mindray uses a novel cationic cyanine red fluorescent dye to label RNA in RETs. The dyeing promoter in the reagent effectively accelerates the staining effect, so that the fluorescent dye can quickly bind to RNA in RETs, and then distinguish mature erythrocytes from RETs based on the different fluorescence intensities. Furthermore, the spherical reagent component causes RBCs to be spherical in shape, boosting RBC and platelet discrimination in volume characteristics and significantly improving RBC and platelet classification accuracy in this channel. In a separate channel, mature RBCs are lysed by hemolytic agents, and nucleic acids in NRBCs and WBCs are stained with a basic cyanine fluorescent dye. Since NRBCs differ from WBCs in nucleic acid content and cellular structural characteristics, the staining intensity of reagent-treated NRBCs is lower than that of normal WBCs. This means NRBCs can be effectively classified and counted by detecting the fluorescence signals and forward scattered light signals of the cells.

Commercially available 5-part differential hematology analyzers for detecting RETs also include URIT's URIT-5510 series. Leveraging MAPSS for cell differentiation and counting, URIT-5510 performs pure physical analysis, providing three test parameters for RETs, without the need for staining. In addition, Maccura's F810 and F880 5-part differential hematology analyzers can also detect RETs.

23.2.2.3 Whole Blood CRP Detection Reagents

C-reactive protein (CRP) is a common acute phase reactive protein named after its ability to precipitate with capsular C polysaccharide of Streptococcus pneumonia. CRP is produced by hepatocytes in response to tissue injury, inflammation, or infection, and is increasingly used clinically as a monitoring indicator. CRP levels in peripheral blood are quite low in healthy people, with about 90% of the population having CRP < 3 mg/L and about 99% having CRP < 10 mg/L. Inflammation is indicated when CRP is >10 mg/L, with higher concentrations indicating more severe inflammation. CRP levels above 20 mg/L (> 2 mg/L in infants) suggest the risk of bacterial infection. Therefore, CRP can help to identify the types of bacterial or viral infections, as well as to evaluate antibiotic efficacy. High-sensitivity C-reactive protein (hs-CRP) may also aid in cardiovascular risk identification. Combined with traditional clinical diagnostic methods of acute coronary syndrome, hs-CRP can serve as an early warning indicator of coronary artery disease or recurrence of acute coronary syndrome. Serum amyloid A (SAA) is also an acute phase reactive protein and a sensitive indicator of infectious diseases, making it helpful for infection detection, disease evaluation, and outcome prediction. Inflammatory, infectious, and non-infectious disorders may cause a substantial increase in the concentration of SAA in blood within hours.

The current hematology analysis market is dominated by "CBC + CRP" integrated analyzers. As an example, Mindray's integrated analyzer with the biggest market share detects CRP and SAA using the latex-enhanced immunonephelometry principle. The reagent's antibody-labeled latex beads agglutinate with the sample analyte (CRP or SAA protein), increasing the turbidity of the solution. When incident light of a specific wavelength is directed horizontally toward an antigen-antibody reaction complex, refraction and diffraction cause the complex to scatter light, which is proportional to the specific protein concentration. Turbidimetric analysis of the sample can determine the specific protein concentration, which is further converted by the proportion of whole blood cell volume (BCV) in the sample (containing RBCs, WBCs, and platelets) to obtain the specific protein concentration in the serum, so that the whole blood test results are consistent with the serum test results.

23.3 Future Trends of Hematology Analyzers and Reagents

Multiple factors have contributed to the advancement of hematology analyzers and reagents. On the one hand, clinical diagnosis and treatment necessitate more accurate, rapid, and numerous parameters for blood analysis; on the other hand, advances in science and technology, especially electronic science and technology, computer technology, laser and other light sources, and biochemical and staining labeling technology, have laid the groundwork for the development of detection instruments. Furthermore, rising living standards and health awareness have led to a more comprehensive and in-depth understanding of and involvement in disease prediction, prevention, treatment, and monitoring. This has significantly increased the workload of clinical examinations. Generations of faster, more practical, and more intelligent devices are coming out to keep up with the advancements. Looking back and ahead, the hematology analyzers and reagents industry may see the following trends in the coming years:

23.3.1 Analysis of Many More Parameters

Currently, cell classification is becoming increasingly fine-grained, and the physical and chemical properties of cells are continuously uncovered and mined. Driven by computer technology and clinical research, hematology analyzers can provide clinicians with more and more parameters and data. These include the earliest red cell distribution width (RDW), which played a vital role in the diagnosis and treatment of various anemias, as well as the reticulocyte-related parameters such as reticulocyte count (RET#), reticulocyte percentage (RET%), mean reticulocyte hemoglobin content (MCHr), high fluorescence (HF), medium fluorescence (MF) and low fluorescence (LF) intensity reticulocyte percentage (HFR%, MFR%, LFR%), immature reticulocyte ratio (IRF%), and immature platelet ratio (IPF%). All these are important parameters in clinical disease diagnosis, differential diagnosis, treatment monitoring, prognosis, and follow-up. In addition to conventional hematology parameters, CRP and SAA, and even ESR can be directly reported by more and more integrated analyzers, satisfying the growing clinical need to incorporate CRP and SAA in CBC tests. In clinical practice, it is likely that more new parameters will be used if they help with disease diagnosis or make testing procedures more efficient.

23.3.2 Diverse Test Samples

With the advances in trace detection and signal processing, what can be detected by some newly introduced hematology analyzers is no longer limited to blood, but also includes cells in cerebrospinal fluid, pleural effusion, peritoneal effusion, synovial fluid, and other body fluids. The number of cells in these fluids, including RBCs, WBCs, nucleated cells, mononuclear cells, and multinuclear cells, can be rapidly and accurately detected. Besides, the line between blood cell and plasma test items is being blurred. With the maturity of immune response technology for whole blood samples, some conventional biochemical immune items are now incorporated into hematology analyzers, such as BC-5390 CRP, BC-7500 CS, and BC-760 CS. Not only can these analyzers quickly finish CBC tests, but they can also complete such items as CRP, SAA, and erythrocyte sedimentation rate (ESR). In the future, hematology analyzers will likely include procalcitonin (PCT) and many more parameters. In addition, assisted by monoclonal antibodies and immunofluorescence labeling techniques, blood cells can be immunophenotyped using antibodies against clusters of differentiation (CD) while counting cells, so as to obtain more accurate information and counting of cell subsets.

23.3.3 Highly Automated Instruments

The effort to automate hematology analyzers has never stopped. After more than a half-century of evolution from being manual, semi-automatic, to fully automatic, hematology analyzers are now capable of automated sampling, automated slide making and staining, and even automated cell morphology analysis. Multiple analyzers can be connected by tracks to the automation line. Now a single analyzer can test over 200 samples per hour. Using the autosampler, the analyzer automatically closes the tube to puncture and extract the sample, saving labor and improving operational safety. According to the system rules, connecting together the hematology analyzer, slide maker & stainer, and digital cell morphology analyzer together through tracks provides a centralized approach to conduct activities such as sample scheduling, distribution, retesting, slide making, staining, analysis, and HbA1c detection. This will lead to a significant increase in work efficiency, a reduction in operation mistakes and the workload for analysts, and much faster turn-around times (TAT) for sample testing, bringing an enhanced patient experience and savings on resources. Analysts can therefore focus more on result evaluation and quality improvement, allowing them to provide more valuable services in clinical practice. With the future diversification of test items, more products such as flow cytometers and blood-type analyzers can be added to the automation line.

23.3.4 Information- and Network-Based Development

As computing technology advances, hematology analyzers are becoming more and more "informatized." The built-in barcode scanner can perform automated tasks like scanning sample tube barcodes, reading test requests, and thus assigning samples in a flexible manner. High-end hematology analyzers feature built-in retest rules to enable automated selection of samples requiring retests, slide making, and staining, and the ability to obtain historical data of patients by communicating with the hospital information system (HIS). They can also perform trend analysis on the sample results or obtain results of other test items, so as to comprehensively analyze and evaluate the results of different items. By analyzing clinical diagnostic pathways, sample review requirements, and other data, intelligent information management and review systems may rapidly detect abnormal samples and subsequently process them in accordance with the set rules, such as retesting, slide making, and staining. The overall information-based solutions of the analyzers have enabled automated quality control, reagent information management, cross-hospital review, cross-department communication, and multi-dimensional training. The thriving mobile Internet and telemedicine markets have also paved the way for the information- and network-based growth of hematology analyzers and other instruments on the automation line in the long term.

23.3.5 Automated Cell Morphology Examination

Manual microscopic examination is the "gold standard" for hematology analysis, but only very limited examiners have the required expertise and skills. Moreover, due to the stringent TAT requirements for hematology analysis in clinical practice, laboratories are in dire need of automated morphology analyzers as an essential addition to manual microscopic analysis. Therefore, there is a rising need for automated digital cell morphology analyzers that are efficient, intelligent, information-based, and capable of delivering clear results. A hematology analyzer performs preliminary sample screening; an automated slide maker & stainer makes and stains blood smears for the abnormal samples selected based on the retest rules; then an automated digital cell morphology analyzer automatically analyzes and pre-classifies the stained blood smears; finally, an experienced analyst compares, analyzes, and reviews the pre-classification results of blood smears and the test results of the hematology analyzer, before sending a report. This approach results in a considerably shorter TAT, a higher analysis efficiency, and a lower false negative rate, avoiding missed detection of any blood disease samples. A typical example is MC-80 automated digital cell morphology analyzer from Mindray. To sum up, greater accomplishments can be anticipated in peripheral blood cell morphology in the future.

Declaration Guangna Ma, GengWen Chen, Jialin Lin, Linyu Bai and Biao Wu are employees of Shenzhen Mindray Bio-Medical Electronics Co., Ltd.

Yong Tang, Yang Yang and Kang Yu are employees of Maccura Biotechnology Co., Ltd.

Part VII

Microbiology and Companion Diagnostic

Instruments and Reagents for Microbial Culture Identification

24

Yehuan Zheng, Juan Fang, Xiaoli Cui, Xiangyu Wang, Mengmeng Lv, Guangyu Fu, Bingbing Zeng, Wei Xiong, and Yifeng Sun

24.1 General

With the continuous development of the national economy and the gradual improvement of people's living standards, people are becoming aware of the importance of health. The government has issued relevant policies and proposed requirements for promoting food safety and improving the level of medical services. The rapid diagnosis of pathogenic bacteria is particularly important for the treatment of patients. The spread of pathogenic microorganisms has driven the development of disease control and the reform of the public health system and promoted the iterative development of the microbiological testing techniques.

The microbiological testing can achieve the identification of pathogenic bacteria through the microbial cultivation, identification, and subsequent drug susceptibility test, etc., thus guiding the precision therapy of patients based on the drug susceptibility. The mild cases can be solved by the empirical treatment; however, for severe and critically infected patients, time is life; at this time, the rapid microbiological diagnosis, precision therapy, shortening the time to obtain the drug susceptibility results and give precision therapy, and improving the patient's cure rate are important clinical issues to be solved urgently.

Y. Zheng (✉) · J. Fang · X. Cui · G. Fu
Autobio Diagnostics Co., Ltd., Zhengzhou, Henan, China
e-mail: zhengyehuan@autobio.com.cn

X. Wang
The Second People's Hospital of Shenzhen, Shenzhen, Guangdong, China

M. Lv
The Sixth People's Hospital of Zhengzhou, Zhengzhou, Henan, China

B. Zeng · W. Xiong · Y. Sun
Zhuhai Encode Medical Engineering Co., Ltd., Zhuhai, Guangdong, China

H. Song, L. Dai (eds.), *In Vitro Diagnostic Industry in China*,
https://doi.org/10.1007/978-981-99-3110-1_24

In recent years, with the rapid development of science and technology, there are many updated techniques for microbiological testing, and their application and the relevant equipment R&D are continuously updating. Science and technology have driven the continuous, diversified development of microbiological testing techniques; domestic and foreign manufacturers of IVD reagents and instruments have shown a trend of diversification, and they developed innovative, advanced, and simple microbiological testing techniques and related products, and obtained the registration certificate at home and abroad to replace the traditional microbiological testing methods. Besides, due to the global epidemic of COVID-19 in 2020, the sales of conventional products of domestic and foreign representative manufacturers have been affected, but the development trend of the rapid IVD microbiological testing industry remains unchanged.

24.2 Registration of Related Instruments for Blood Culture and Drug Susceptibility Identification and Related Products in Recent 3 Years

24.2.1 Blood Culture

24.2.1.1 Registration of New Products in Recent 3 Years

Through searching on the NMPA platform, the registration of products related to the automatic microbiology blood culture systems from January 2019 to December 2021 is shown in Table 24.1.

24.2.1.2 Domestic Influential Brands and Products in the Recent 3 Years

1. Autobio Experimental Instrument (Zhengzhou) Co., Ltd.: BC120 automated blood culture system.
   (a) Basic principle: It adopts advanced noninvasive and visualization technology, combined with a unique optical testing system, to achieve the full automation of blood culture and testing.
   (b) Basic structure: It consists of a main machine and a control system; one set of control systems can realize the parallel connection of up to five main machines and the blood culture and testing of 600 bottles.
   (c) Type of reagents: seven types of supporting culture bottles: standard aerobic bottles, standard anaerobic bottles, standard bottles for children, resin aerobic bottles, resin anaerobic bottles, resin bottles for children, and mycobacterial culture bottles.
   (d) Features: It can be connected to Lis software and Autobio microbiology laboratory information system to realize the whole process management of sample information; besides, it can realize the parallel operation of five sets and expand to 600 bottles, to meet the uses of hospitals at all levels, and support the on-board culture of mycobacteria.

Table 24.1 Registration of products related to the automatic microbiology blood culture systems from January 2019 to December 2021

Serial No.	Manufacturer	Product	Management category	Model & specification	Approval date
1	Henan Maincare biological technology co., ltd.	Blood culture bottle (biochemical sensor)	Category II	20 bottles/box	March 12, 2019
2	Autobio experimental instrument (Zhengzhou) co., ltd.	Automated blood culture system	Category II	BC120	March 12, 2019
3	Hunan Mindray medical technology co., ltd.	Automated microbial cultivation system	Category II	Representative models: TDR-X060, TDR-X120, TDR-X240	April 19, 2019
4	Shandong Scenker biotechnology co., ltd.	Automated blood bacterial culture system	Category II	LABSTAR50, LABSTAR 60, LABSTAR 100, LABSTAR plus, LABSTAR EX	2019.10.29 October 29, 2019
5	Zosbio technology co., ltd.	Automated blood culture system	Category II	ZOS-BC60	2020.02.07 February 7, 2020
6	Zhuhai DL biotech. Co., ltd.	Anaerobic blood culture bottle (colorimetry)	Category II	II-1 20 bottles/box, 40 bottles/box	2020.07.22 July 22, 2020
7	Zhengzhou autobio diagnostics co., ltd.	Onboard blood culture bottles	Category II	20 tests/box	2021.03.01 March 1, 2021
8	Zhengzhou autobio diagnostics co., ltd.	Blood culture bottles	Category II	20 bottles/box, including aerobic culture bottles: Standard aerobic culture bottles, resin aerobic culture bottles, standard culture bottles for children, resin culture bottles for children; anaerobic blood culture bottles: Standard anaerobic culture bottles, resin anaerobic culture bottles	2021.03.01 March 1, 2021

(continued)

Table 24.1 (continued)

Serial No.	Manufacturer	Product	Management category	Model & specification	Approval date
9	Zhuhai DL biotech. Co., ltd.	Automated blood culture system	Category II	BT24, BT48, BT60, BT120, BT180, BT240	June 8, 2021
10	Zhuhai DL biotech. Co., ltd.	Automated blood culture system	Category II	DL-Bt32, DL-Bt64, DL-Bt80, DL-Bt112, DL-Bt224, DL-Bt336, DL-Bt240	July 8, 2021
11	Zhuhai Lituo biotechnology co., ltd.	Automated blood culture system	Category II	LTS-BMC60, LTS-BMC80, LTS-BMC90	July 29, 2021
12	Zhuhai DL biotech. Co., ltd.	Child blood culture bottle (colorimetry)	Category II	III-1 20 bottles/box, 40 bottles/box	August 24, 2021
13	Zhuhai DL biotech. Co., ltd.	Aerobic blood culture bottle (colorimetry)	Category II	I-1 20 bottles/box, 40 bottles/box	August 24, 2021
14	Zhejiang quark biotechnology co., ltd.	Aerobic culture bottles (fluorescence method)	Category II	Models: Standard aerobic culture bottles (for adults), resin aerobic culture bottles (for adults), resin aerobic culture bottles (for children); specifications: 20 bottles/box, 50 bottles/box, 100 bottles/box.	October 14, 2021
15	Zhejiang quark biotechnology co., ltd.	Anaerobic culture bottles (fluorescence method)	Category II	Models: Standard anaerobic culture bottles (for adults), resin anaerobic culture bottles (for adults); specifications: 20 bottles/box, 50 bottles/box, 100 bottles/box.	October 14, 2021
16	Jiangsu Zhongsheng medical diagnostic reagents co., ltd.	Aerobic culture bottles (colorimetry)	Category II	40 mL/bottle, 25 bottles/box, 50 bottles/box	October 15, 2021
17	Wuhan Diascie technology co., ltd.	Anaerobic culture bottles	Category II	80 mL × 50 bottles	November 25, 2021
18	Wuhan Diascie technology co., ltd.	Aerobic culture bottles	Category II	Standard aerobic bottles: 80 mL × 50 bottles; standard half-volume bottles: 40 mL × 50 bottles.	November 30, 2021

Table 24.1 (continued)

Serial No.	Manufacturer	Product	Management category	Model & specification	Approval date
19	Zhengzhou autobio diagnostics co., ltd.	Onboard blood culture bottles	Category II	Round bottles, 20 tests/ box. Aerobic culture bottles: Standard aerobic culture bottles, resin aerobic culture bottles, standard culture bottles for children, resin culture bottles for children; anaerobic blood culture bottles: Standard anaerobic culture bottles, resin anaerobic culture bottles	December 16, 2021

2. Zhuhai DL Biotech. Co., Ltd.: DL-Bt series of automated blood culture systems.
   (a) Basic principle: It adopts the measurement with photodetector and multi-mode mathematical operation analysis based on the principle of non-invasive testing, to obtain accurate testing results.
   (b) Instrument model: Depending on different onboard capacity, including DL-Bt32, DL-Bt64, DL-Bt80, DL-Bt112, DL-Bt224, DL-Bt336, DL-Bt240; BT24, BT48, BT60, BT120, BT180, BT240.
   (c) Type of reagents: including anaerobic bottles, aerobic bottles, and bottles for children.
   (d) Features: BT series are made of new materials and adopt integrated design, featured by small size, lightweight, more stable operation, low failure rate, and easy maintenance.
3. Hunan Mindray Medical Technology Co., Ltd.: TDR-X series of automated microbial cultivation systems.
   (a) Basic principle: It adopts the irreversible color developing technology and a variety of algorithm modes, to solve the problem of delayed submission and testing of samples.
   (b) Instrument model: representative models: TDR-X060, TDR-X120, TDR-X240.
   (c) Features: By adopting the patented solid direct heating technology and combing with the drawer-type partition sample injection, the temperature is kept constant; besides, it is equipped with the industry-leading negative pre-reporting function, which builds a communication bridge between the laboratory and the clinic.
4. Shandong Scenker Biotechnology Co., Ltd.: automated blood culture system.
   (a) Basic principle: It adopts continuous optical testing and color-developing methods to achieve the rapid testing of bacteria and fungi in the blood.

(b) Instrument model: LABSTAR series products, including five models, namely, LABSTAR 50, LABSTAR 60, LABSTAR 100, LABSTAR 120, and LABSTAR EX.
(c) Type of reagents: 25 mL/bottle, 40 mL/bottle; including antibiotic neutralization and enrichment culture bottles for adults, antibiotic neutralization and enrichment culture bottles for children, standard enrichment culture bottles, anaerobic antibiotic neutralization and enrichment culture bottles.
(d) Features: The series of products possess a variety of abnormal state data processing functions and automatic recovery functions to ensure accurate data; LABSTAR 50 series are for rotating and shaking culture; LABSTAR 100/LABSTAR 120 is for rocking and shaking culture, and depending on the needs of users, unique operation interfaces and software functions can be designed, and culture bottles with special nutritional conditions can be made. Different from the above three models, LABSTAR EX adopts a modular management mode and can be expanded to 64 units.

24.2.2 Microbial Sample Pretreatment

24.2.2.1 Recordation of New Products in Recent 3 Years

Through searching on the NMPA platform, the recordation of products related to the microbial sample pretreatment systems from January 2019 to December 2021 is shown in Table 24.2.

Domestic Influential Brands and Products in the Recent 3 Years

1. Autobio Experimental Instrument (Zhengzhou) Co., Ltd.
   (a) Instrument model: AutoStreak S1800 microbial sample pretreatment system independently developed by Autobio Experimental Instrument (Zhengzhou) Co., Ltd.
   (b) Features: It can complete the automatic liquefaction and inoculation streaking of sputum samples with one key, and is compatible with other liquid samples; it provides the quantitative inoculation and international patented streaking methods to improve the separation effect of pathogenic microorganisms; it is equipped with bio-safe cabinet-type negative pressure inner cavity, automatic sample opening and closing cover and efficient HEPA filter element, to achieve the periodic UV lamp disinfection and effective control over the biological safety risks; equipped with humanized interactive system, to monitor the consumables consumption and experimental progress in real time with dynamic large-screen display; its audible and visual alarm can be connected to the Lis software and Autobio microbiology laboratory information system to realize the whole process management of sample information.
2. Wuhan Diascie Technology Co., Ltd.
   (a) Instrument model: Microbial sample pretreatment systems PROBACT-40, PROBACT-70, PROBACT-90; automated transfer blood culture system AT-

Table 24.2 Recordation of products related to the microbial sample pretreatment systems from January 2019 to December 2021

Serial No.	Recordation entity	Product	Management category	Model and specification	Recordation date
1	Shandong Aotemeixin biotechnology co., ltd.	Microbial sample pretreatment system	Category I recordation	H.robot-1700i; H.robot-2700; H.robot-5700; H.robot-5700i	June 28, 2019
2	Shanghai Modury biotechnology co., ltd.	Microbial sample pretreatment system	Category I recordation	Blueyes calf, 1 set/ box	December 23, 2019
3	Zhengzhou Zopomed medical equipment co., ltd.	Microbial sample pretreatment system	Category I recordation	Models ZOPOMED-100, ZOPOMED-200, ZOPOMED-300, ZOPOMED-400, ZOPOMED-500 and ZOPOMED-600	December 24, 2019
4	Chongqing Kejie medical technology co., ltd.	Microbial sample intelligent pretreatment system	Category I recordation	KJMI6000/set, KJMI6300/set	April 15, 2020
5	Wuhan Diascie technology co., ltd.	Microbial sample pretreatment system	Category I recordation	PROBACT PLUS-90; PROBACT PLUS-70	April 17, 2020
6	Hunan Hailu biological technology co., ltd.	Microbial sample pretreatment system	Category I recordation	HALO-P100	July 13, 2020
7	Hunan Haili medical technology co., ltd.	Microbial sample pretreatment system	Category I recordation	HALO-P100	July 13, 2020
8	Jinan Babio biotechnology co., ltd.	Microbial sample pretreatment system	Category I recordation	ET-800+	September 23, 2020
9	Shanghai Modury biotechnology co., ltd.	Microbial sample pretreatment system	Category I recordation	Blueyes Buffalo, 1 set/box	October 20, 2020
10	Weihai Xianghe Yingchun medical technology co., ltd.	Microbial sample pretreatment intelligent device	Category I recordation	WY25–3/1850*840*1750	January 4, 2021

(continued)

Table 24.2 (continued)

Serial No.	Recordation entity	Product	Management category	Model and specification	Recordation date
11	Hunan Tianqi medical new technology co., ltd.	Microbial sample pretreatment system	Category I recordation	HJ-24	March 29, 2021
12	Shandong Ruixuyang biotechnology co., ltd.	Microbial sample pretreatment system	Category I recordation	RS-201	June 4, 2021
13	Autobio experimental instrument (Zhengzhou) co., ltd.	Microbial sample pretreatment system	Category I recordation	AutoStreak S1800	June 9, 2021
14	Well care Wuhan medical technology co., ltd.	Microbial sample pretreatment system	Category I recordation	FM-A	October 28, 2021
15	Langmai (Shandong) biotechnology co., ltd.	Microbial sample pretreatment system	Category I recordation	LAEK-3000; LARK-1800i	November 10, 2021

BACT SYSTEM, enhanced-type microbial sample pretreatment systems PROBACT-40 PLUS, PROBACT-70 PLUS, PROBACT-90 PLUS.

(b) Features: It has excellent sample pretreatment ability, including sputum digestion, feces enrichment, and swab homogenization; besides, sample streaking can be completed in the culture environment, so that the in vitro samples can be sent to the culture environment immediately; the culture medium device can provide two to three solid medium combinations simultaneously; provide normal, aerobic and anaerobic environments.

3. Jinan Babio Biotechnology Co., Ltd.
   (a) Instrument model: Microbial sample pretreatment systems ET-800, ET-800+, microbial sample treatment robot ET-2000.
   (b) Features: It has unique one-key operation technology and diverse and flexible streaking methods; in principle, the streaking method can be automatically selected by the system according to the sample type, or a special streaking method can be made depending on the user's requirements; it is equipped with a unique vision technology, which can monitor the processing progress of samples in real time and provide real-time feedback to the human-machine interface.
4. Langmai (Shandong) Biotechnology Co., Ltd.
   (a) Instrument model: LARK-1800, 1800i, and LARK-3200, 3200i series microbial sample pretreatment systems.

(b) Features: It is equipped with a built-in multi-joint 3D robotic arm, metal inoculating loop, sample homogenization processing position, different types of culture dishes, and high-speed streaking system. The advanced robotic technology is applied to the field of microbial sample processing, and the mechanical streaking is used to replace manual streaking, improving working efficiency.

24.2.3 Identification of Drug Susceptibility

24.2.3.1 Registration of New Products in Recent 3 Years

Through searching on the NMPA platform, the registration of products related to the drug susceptibility identification and analysis systems from January 2019 to December 2021 is shown in Table 24.3.

24.2.3.2 Domestic Influential Brands and Products

1. Autobio Experimental Instrument (Zhengzhou) Co., Ltd.
   (a) Instrument model: Automated drug susceptibility analyzer AutoMic i600 for microbiological assay.
   (b) Basic principle: The colorimetry/turbidimetry based on the biochemical reaction for the identification part; dilution combined with the redox method for the in vitro drug susceptibility testing.
   (c) Supporting reagents: Five susceptibility assay kits, namely Enterobacter susceptibility assay kit (colorimetry/turbidimetry), non-fermenting bacteria susceptibility assay kit (colorimetry/turbidimetry), Gram-positive bacteria susceptibility assay kit (colorimetry/turbidimetry), Streptococcus susceptibility assay kit (colorimetry/turbidimetry), fungi susceptibility assay kit (colorimetry/turbidimetry), can meet the needs for drug susceptibility testing of a majority of common clinical pathogenic bacteria. The kits are 120-well plates, covering a wide variety of antibiotics and a wide range of concentration gradients, and include newly marketed and to-be-marketed drugs such as ceftazidime/avibactam, ceftaroline, oritavancin, polymyxin B, tigecycline, to meet the diverse clinical needs.
   (d) Features: The multivariety plates are designed for random placement to achieve the two-way intelligent identification and matching of plates and specimens; the instrument can automatically complete the sample adding, incubation, and result interpretation; the 64-bit high-throughput incubation chamber can meet the testing needs of users at all levels; the colorimetry and turbidimetry are combined for simultaneous detection at 4 wavelengths and automatic interpretation of results without interruption.
2. Zhuhai DL Biotech. Co., Ltd.
   (a) Instrument model: mainly including three types of drug susceptibility test systems, namely bacterial identification and drug susceptibility analysis systems DL-96II, DL-96A, D2Mini.

Table 24.3 Registration of products related to the drug susceptibility identification and analysis systems from January 2019 to December 2020

Serial no.	Manufacturer	Product	Management category	Model and Specification	Approval date
1	Hunan Mindray medical technology co., ltd.	Bacillus detection kit	Category II	TDR BAC-64, TDR BAC-96, TDR BAC-128, TDR BAC-ID, TDR BAC-AST; 10 tests/kit	May 8, 2019
2	Hunan Mindray medical technology co., ltd.	Non-fermenting bacteria detection kit	Category II	TDR NF-64, TDR NF-96, TDR NF-128, TDR NF-ID, TDR NF-AST; 10 tests/kit	May 8, 2019
3	Hunan Mindray medical technology co., ltd.	Vibrionaceae detection kit	Category II	TDR VIB-64, TDR VIB-96, TDR VIB-128, TDR VIB-ID, TDR VIB-AST; 10 tests/kit	May 8, 2019
4	Hunan Mindray medical technology co., ltd.	Corynebacterium detection kit	Category II	TDR CB-64, TDR CB-96, TDR CB-128, TDR CB-ID, TDR CB-AST	May 8, 2019
5	Hunan Mindray medical technology co., ltd.	Staphylococcus detection kit	Category II	TDR STAPH-64, TDR STAPH-96, TDR STAPH-128, TDR STAPH-ID, TDR STAPH-AST	May 8, 2019
6	Hunan Mindray medical technology co., ltd.	Yeast-like fungi detection kit	Category II	TDR YEAST-64, TDR YEAST-96, TDR YEAST-128, TDR YEAST-ID, TDR YEAST-AST	May 8, 2019
7	Hunan Mindray medical technology co., ltd.	Neisseria/Haemophilus detection kit	Category II	TDR NH-64, TDR NH-96, TDR NH-128, TDR NH-ID, TDR NH-AST	May 8, 2019
8	Hunan Mindray medical technology co., ltd.	Streptococcaceae detection kit	Category II	TDR STR-64, TDR STR-96, TDR STR-128, TDR STR-ID, TDR STR-AST	May 8, 2019

Table 24.3 (continued)

Serial no.	Manufacturer	Product	Management category	Model and Specification	Approval date
9	Hunan Mindray medical technology co., ltd.	Enterobacteriaceae detection kit	Category II	TDR ONE-64, TDR ONE-96, TDR ONE-128, TDR ONE-ID, TDR ONE-AST	May 8, 2019
10	Shandong Scenker biotechnology co., ltd.	Bacterial identification and susceptibility assay kit (colorimetry/ turbidimetry)	Category II	XK-96A-C Enterobacteriaceae susceptibility assay kit, XK-96A-F non-fermenting bacteria susceptibility assay kit, XK-96A-P staphylococcus susceptibility assay kit, XK-96A-L streptococcus susceptibility assay kit, XK- 96B-C Enterobacteriaceae identification and susceptibility assay kit, XK-96B-F non-fermenting bacteria identification and susceptibility assay kit, XK-96B-P staphylococcus identification and susceptibility assay kit, XK-96B-L streptococcus identification and susceptibility assay kit	September 30, 2019
11	Shanghai Fosun pharmaceutical co., ltd.	Staphylococcus susceptibility test plate	Category II	MS2 specifications: 1 test/plate, 10 plates/box	November 7, 2019
12	Shanghai Fosun pharmaceutical co., ltd.	Non-fermenting bacteria susceptibility test plate	Category II	BIOFOSUN; specification: 1 test/ plate, 10 plates/box	November 13, 2019

(continued)

Table 24.3 (continued)

Serial no.	Manufacturer	Product	Management category	Model and Specification	Approval date
13	Fosun diagnostic technology (Changsha) co., ltd.	Automated microbial susceptibility analyzer	Category II	Droplet48	November 19, 2019
14	Fosun diagnostic technology (Changsha) co., ltd.	Fungus susceptibility assay kit (culture method), gram-negative bacteria susceptibility assay reagent (micro-broth dilution method), gram-positive bacteria susceptibility assay reagent (micro-broth dilution method)	Category II	Plate type/disc type, 10 tests/kit	November 19, 2019
15	Shanghai Fosun pharmaceutical co., ltd.	Gram-positive aerobic bacteria identification plate	Category II	BIOFOSUN; specifications: 2 tests/plate, 10 plates/box	April 8, 2020
16	Shanghai Fosun pharmaceutical co., ltd.	Gram-negative aerobic bacteria identification plate	Category II	BIOFOSUN; specifications: 2 tests/plate, 10 plates/box	April 10, 2020
17	Autobio experimental instrument (Zhengzhou) co., ltd.	Automated microbial identification and susceptibility analyzer	Category II	AutoMic-i600	July 16, 2020
18	Shanghai Fosun pharmaceutical co., ltd.	Enterobacter susceptibility test plate	Category II	MS2; specifications: 1 test/plate, 10 plates/box	September 8, 2020

Table 24.3 (continued)

Serial no.	Manufacturer	Product	Management category	Model and Specification	Approval date
19	Zhuhai DL biotech. Co., ltd.	Streptococcus/ enterococcus identification and susceptibility assay plate (colorimetry/ turbidimetry), staphylococcus identification and susceptibility assay plate (colorimetry/ turbidimetry), Enterobacter/ oxidase-negative gram-negative bacilli identification and susceptibility assay plate (colorimetry/ turbidimetry), non-fermenting bacteria/oxidase positive gram-negative bacilli identification and susceptibility assay plate (colorimetry/ turbidimetry)	Category II	10 tests/box DL-120STREP, DL-120STAPHE, DL-120E, DL-120NE	December 31, 2020
20	Zhengzhou autobio diagnostics co., ltd.	Enterobacter susceptibility assay kit (colorimetry/ turbidimetry)	Category II	10 tests/kit, 20 tests/kit, 50 tests/kit	March 1, 2021
21	Zhuhai DL biotech. Co., ltd.	Bacterial identification and drug susceptibility analysis system	Category II	DL-96A, D2Mini, D2Plus	March 3, 2021
22	Shanghai Fosun pharmaceutical co., ltd.	Microbial identification and susceptibility analysis system	Category II	BIOFOSUN-II	March 4, 2021
23	Zhengzhou autobio diagnostics co., ltd.	Gram-positive bacteria susceptibility assay kit (colorimetry/ turbidimetry), fungi susceptibility assay kit (colorimetry/ turbidimetry)	Category II	10 tests/kit, 20 tests/kit, 50 tests/kit	April 8, 2021

(continued)

Table 24.3 (continued)

Serial no.	Manufacturer	Product	Management category	Model and Specification	Approval date
24	Zhengzhou autobio diagnostics co., ltd.	Streptococcus susceptibility assay kit (colorimetry/ turbidimetry), non-fermenting bacteria susceptibility assay kit (colorimetry/ turbidimetry)	Category II	10 tests/kit, 20 tests/kit, 50 tests/kit	April 12, 2021
25	Zhuhai DL biotech. Co., ltd.	Yeast-like fungi identification and susceptibility assay plate (turbidimetry)	Category II	DL-96FUNGUS;10 tests/box	April 19, 2021
26	Zhuhai Baso biotechnology co., ltd.	Microbial and susceptibility analysis system	Category II	BSP-TB96	August 31, 2021
27	Shanghai Fosun Changzheng medical science co., ltd.	Automated microbial susceptibility analyzer	Category II	Droplet48	September 1, 2021

(b) Basic principle: Colorimetry/turbidimetry based on biochemical reaction for the identification part; turbidimetry for the drug susceptibility test part.

(c) Supporting reagents: Including 96-well plate and 120-well plate; reagents include Enterobacteriaceae, non-fermenting bacteria, Enterococcus/ Streptococcus, Staphylococcus, and fungi. All of them are composite identification and susceptibility plates.

(d) Features: DL-96A: It is automated equipment that meets the needs of domestic and foreign bacterial detection and drug susceptibility testing after upgrading on the basis of inheriting the advantages of DL-96II, to achieve the automatic interpretation. D2Mini: Lightweight interpretation module. The card reading speed is 2/3 shorter than that of the third-generation machine, which meets the needs of high-throughput testing.

3. Hunan Mindray Medical Technology Co., Ltd.
   (a) Instrument model: Including an automatic sampler TDR-J100, an automatic microbiological analysis system TDR-300B.
   (b) Basic principle: Biochemical method for the identification part; turbidimetry based on micro-broth dilution method.
   (c) Supporting reagents: Identification/drug susceptibility assay kits for Enterobacteriaceae, Staphylococcus, yeast-like fungi, Streptococcus, Neisseria/Haemophilus, non-fermenting bacteria, etc.

(d) Features: It can provide interpretation for 60 to 80 specimens per hour; provide a variety of statistical functions, including statistics of drug resistance rate, detection rate, enzyme production, and workload. Open result entry functions: entry and analysis of the test cards of different manufacturers. Combine with the drug susceptibility results obtained by K-B method.

4. Fosun Diagnostic Technology (Shanghai) Co., Ltd.
   (a) Instrument model: Automated microbial susceptibility analysis system Droplet48; susceptibility analysis system BIOFOSUN-II for microbial identification.
   (b) Basic principle: Droplet48: Fluorescence detection technology is used for drug susceptibility analysis.
   (c) Supporting reagents:

      BIOFOSUN-II supporting reagent: plate type; drug susceptibility test plates for Staphylococcus, Enterobacter, Enterococcus, non-fermenting bacteria; identification plates for Gram-positive aerobic bacteria and Gram-negative aerobic bacteria.

      Droplet48 supporting reagents: disc/plate types; plates for Candida, Cryptococcus, Aspergillus, Staphylococcus, Enterococcus, Streptococcus, Enterobacter, non-fermenting bacteria, Haemophilus influenzae.
   (d) Features: Droplet48 adopts unique fluorescence detection technology and combines it with the computer algorithm, which can quickly reflect the replication of pathogenic bacteria after drug action; the drug susceptibility test results can be obtained in as fast as 4 h. Only the bacterial suspension needs to be prepared manually; other processes such as bacterial liquid distribution, incubation, detection, removal of waste plates, and reporting can be automatically completed by the system.

24.3 Summary and Outlook

In the future, microbiological testing technology will present the following development trends: first, the testing efficiency of microbial content in the samples should be improved to reduce the time required for routine testing, and the testing of the count and type of microorganisms can be completed in a relatively short period of time. Second, the accuracy of the testing results should be ensured to improve the precision of the testing; finally, the automation of the testing technique should be realized to promote the development of intelligent microbiological testing technology.

As the microbial resistance increases, there is a growing need for rapid bacterial identification (ID) and antibiotic susceptibility testing (AST). The traditional culture-based method needs a long cycle. Physicians often have to treat patients empirically with antibiotics when necessary, which leads to inappropriate use of antibiotics, increases mortality and medical costs, and antibiotic resistance. In the future, the rapid bacterial identification (ID) and AST will be more promising solutions in miniaturization and automation development. With the advancement of policies and the increase in demand, in order to achieve better development of IVD industry, it is necessary to increase the support for product innovation, standardize the market environment of the industry, strengthen the corporate brand awareness and create a strong brand.

Declaration Yehuan Zheng, Juan Fang, Xiaoli Cui and Guangyu Fu are employees of Autobio Diagnostics Co., Ltd.

Bingbing Zeng, Wei Xiong and Yifeng Sun are employees of Zhuhai Encode Medical Engineering Co., Ltd.

25 Companion Diagnostics

Chengbo Fu, Yan Jiang, Yile Sun, and Yuqing Tang

25.1 Overview

Companion diagnostics (CDx), as a sub-field of in vitro diagnostics (IVD) industry, complements targeted therapy and is a necessary tool to achieve precision medicine. CDx mainly provides patients with the information of specific therapeutic efficacy and side effects by detecting the level of biomarkers such as genes and proteins related to the clinical responses of specific drugs, screening the most appropriate patients under treatment in the target population, and conducting targeted personalized medical treatment, so as to effectively improve the therapeutic efficiency of targeted agents and reduce unnecessary treatment costs.

CDx originated from the promotion and application of targeted agents. This industry first appeared in the 1980s and rose in the 1990s, with the commercial success of Herceptin® (generic name: trastuzumab, Roche) and Gleevec® (generic name: imatinib, Novartis). Thereafter, while quite some monoclonal antibodies and small molecule targeted agents manufacturers started to launch CDx products, the industry entered a rapid development period. Prior to 2010, the approved CDx products mainly adopted immunohistochemistry (IHC) and fluorescence in situ hybridization (FISH) technologies. After 2010, the combination of CDx and targeted agents based on polymerase chain reaction (PCR) technology was approved. On July 14, 2011, the U.S. Food and Drug Administration (FDA) officially issued *Guidance for Industry:* In Vitro *Companion Diagnostic Devices* on August 6, 2014. Since 2017, a large number of CDx and targeted agent combinations based on

C. Fu (✉) · Y. Jiang
Beijing Bohui Innovation Biotechnology Group Co., Ltd., Beijing, China
e-mail: fuchengbo@bohui-tech.com

Y. Sun · Y. Tang
Tellgen Corporation, Shanghai, China

H. Song, L. Dai (eds.), *In Vitro Diagnostic Industry in China*,
https://doi.org/10.1007/978-981-99-3110-1_25

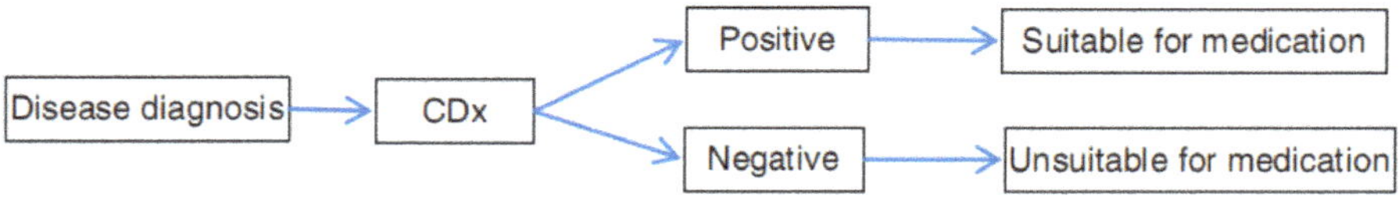

Fig. 25.1 Flow chart of CDx detection. CDx is a necessary detection for corresponding drug treatment.

next-generation sequencing (NGS) technology have been approved, marking a new era of CDx [1].

At present, there are more than 40 CDx products approved by FDA. See Fig. 25.1 for the CDx and detection process [1].

Clinically, CDx is mainly applied to the following two aspects [2]:

25.1.1 Treatment Selection

For the clinical application of new molecular targeted agents and other immunotherapeutic drugs, the patients should receive appropriate examinations to screen the patient population suitable or unsuitable for receiving (ineffective treatment or high side effects and risks) specific drug treatment, so as to formulate the corresponding personalized treatment scheme. This is the main application direction of CDx.

25.1.2 Efficacy Monitoring

The therapeutic effect on patients is judged by monitoring the efficacy of drugs and corresponding adjustments are made to the treatment scheme, so as to improve the safety and effectiveness of treatment.

According to indications, CDx can be divided into diagnostics for oncology, cardiovascular disease, central nervous system, inflammation, and virology. Among them, oncology is the hottest field in the CDx market. At present, a variety of CDx kits have been developed for the detection of various cancer biomarkers. Among the 35 CDx products approved by FDA before 2018, the products used for the diagnosis of breast cancer, non-small cell lung cancer (NSCLC), and colorectal cancer dominate, reaching 12, 8, and 6 products, respectively. At the same time, CDx is applied not only in the field of tumor treatment, but also in invasive systemic mast cell hyperplasia and thalassemia.

According to the technology platforms, the CDx market can be divided into immunodiagnosis (e.g., IHC) with proteins as the detection targets and molecular diagnosis (e.g., PCR, FISH, and NGS) with nucleic acids as the detection targets. In recent years, molecular diagnosis has gradually become the main detection platform; especially, because of its strong practicality, simple operation, low cost, and high clinical coincidence rate, the PCR technology has become the most commonly used methodology. In contrast, NGS has significant advantages for detecting unknown sequences, unknown mutations, and high-throughput multiple sites. Therefore, although NGS still has limitation in clinical application, it has a great development potential. Taking advantage of the technical features and advantages of NGS, the current research and development (R&D) efforts for CDx at home and abroad mainly focus on the direction of large-panel pan-cancers covering hundreds of genes.

According to the sample types, the CDx market can be divided into tumor tissue detection and liquid biopsy. Liquid biopsy refers to the detection method of extracting non-solid tissue samples from human body, which is a new non-invasive detection method. Liquid biopsy in a broad sense includes the collection and detection of blood, urine, saliva, cerebrospinal fluid, and other body fluids as well as feces. Compared with tissue detection, liquid biopsy has significant advantages such as convenient sampling, non-invasive or minimally invasive nature, and rapid, dynamic, and real-time monitoring. More importantly, many patients, whose tissue samples are difficult to obtain or have a small quantity and poor quality, can obtain targeted treatment opportunities through liquid biopsy.

At present, the mainstream liquid biopsy technology mainly uses circulating tumor cells (CTC) or cell-free DNA (cfDNA) for detection. Cell-free DNA (cfDNA) is the most easily obtained and most studied type of liquid biopsy samples. Circulating tumor DNA (ctDNA) is a kind of cfDNA that is released by tumor cells that may have specific mutations. CTC is also a common sample type in liquid biopsy. The isolation and identification of CTC can be used for prognosis, diagnosis, and drug-resistance monitoring.

Due to the technical advantages of liquid biopsy, in addition to its application in CDx, liquid biopsy is also suitable for tumor detection, especially for large-scale early screening of tumors and detection of minimal residual disease (MRD). In recent years, with the technological progress in NGS, the cost of detection has decreased significantly, which makes the application of liquid biopsy based on NGS platform in early screening of tumors possible. However, the cancer early screening industry is still in its fledgling stage, and the products can be roughly divided into two categories: one covers the early screening products for single cancers represented by liver cancer and colorectal cancer, such as domestic companies New Horizon Health and Berry Oncology; the other one contains early screening products for pan-cancers, including lung cancer, colorectal cancer, liver cancer, and breast cancer, such as domestic companies Burning Rock DX and GenePlus. The domestic early screening products for single cancers are now available, while the early screening products for pan-cancers are still in the stage of R&D and validation. See Table 25.1 for the mainstream markers associated with CDx products from domestic companies.

Cancer screening is an important field of public health, which helps improve the early diagnosis and treatment rate of cancer in target populations, and is the most effective way to reduce the burden of cancer treatment. In comparison, the single cancer screening and pan-cancer screening products face different populations and their application scenarios and commercialization models are different. For the

Table 25.1 Mainstream markers of CDx products from domestic companies

Company	Markers
Genetron health	NGS detection: ctDNA mutation + ctDNA methylation + protein markers
Berry oncology	NGS detection: Terminal sequence characteristics of cfDNA, nucleosome distribution, DNA fragmentation, and pentahydroxymethylation
Envelopo health	NGS detection: ctDNA mutation + methylation
New horizon health	Fecal DNA detection (PCR detection of gene mutation + methylation + fecal occult blood index)
Singlera	NGS detection: ctDNA methylation + AI
GenePlus	NGS detection: ctDNA mutation + methylation

Source: Data from the company's public information

population without high-risk factors of cancer, they are more suitable to use pan-cancer early screening products for preliminary screening. For the population with family history and high-risk factors of cancer, they are more suitable to select single cancer early screening products for fine screening. Therefore, single cancer early screening products have a stronger clinical attribute, while pan-cancer early screening products have a health management attribute. From the perspective of clinical ecology in China, the combination of the two is needed to achieve the goal of early screening of cancer in China. At present, both single cancer and pan-cancer early screening products focus on colorectal cancer, liver cancer, gastric cancer, lung cancer, breast cancer, and cervical cancer. These cancers basically belong to the cancer types (lung cancer, breast cancer, liver cancer, and colorectal cancer) with the highest incidence, or the cancer types (pancreatic cancer and ovarian cancer) lacking clinical screening means and with serious harm in China. Therefore, the clear clinical path value and the large-scale potential brought by the high incidence make these fields quite hot in the cancer early screening market.

25.2 Overview of CDx Industry

25.2.1 Domestic and Foreign Markets

The number of cancer patients is huge worldwide, and China is one of the countries with the largest number of cancer cases in the world. According to the data of the World Health Organization (WHO), it is predicted that the number of cancer patients in the world would be about 135 million in 2020. Those in Asia would account for 48.4% of the new cancer patients in the world. From 2014 to 2018, the Compound Annual Growth Rate (CAGR) of cancer patients in China was 9.7%; in 2018, about 4.28 million patients increased in China, accounting for about 24% of the world's total; about 2.87 million people died of cancer, accounting for 30% of the world's total; the numbers of new cases and deaths rank the first in the world. Among the new cancer cases in China in 2018, lung cancer, colorectal cancer, gastric cancer, liver cancer, and breast cancer accounted for the highest proportion, namely 18.1%, 12.2%, 10.6%, 9.2%, and 8.6%, respectively. The latest global cancer burden data in 2020 released by the International Agency for Research on Cancer (IARC) of the WHO shows that China has become the country with the largest number of new cancers in the world. In 2020, there were 19.29 million new cancers in the world, 4.57 million in China, while 9.96 million deaths in the world, and 3.5 million in China. The huge cancer population is giving birth to a huge cancer detection and treatment market.

According to the prediction of Markets and Markets, CDx would be the fastest growing sub-industry in the whole IVD industry in the future. In 2022, the global CDx market scale is expected to reach $6.51 billion, with a compound annual growth rate of 20.1% from 2017 to 2022, far higher than the compound growth rate of 5.5% in the IVD industry. In addition, the proportion of CDx in the whole IVD industry would also increase from 3.2% in 2016 to 7.8%.

According to relevant information released by China Industry Information Network and Smart Research Consulting, China accounted for only 4% of the global CDx market share in 2015. With the accelerated development of the CDx market in China, the market share of China is expected to reach 6.5% by 2021 due to factors such as the expansion of the number of new cancer cases, the continued improvement in medical standards, and the increased ability of patients to bear medical expenses. The business scale would reach RMB 10 billion by 2025. Figure 25.2 shows the market size and growth rate of CDx in China from 2012 to 2020.

In addition to its application in CDx, liquid biopsy based on NGS technology also shows the huge market space in China. It is estimated by Brilliance Consulting that by 2030, the potential market size of liquid biopsy in the three fields of cancer CDx, minimal residual disease monitoring, and early screening and detection of cancer in China will be $4.5 billion, $15 billion, and $29 billion, respectively, and the overall size will reach $48.5 billion, equivalent to about RMB 340 billion.

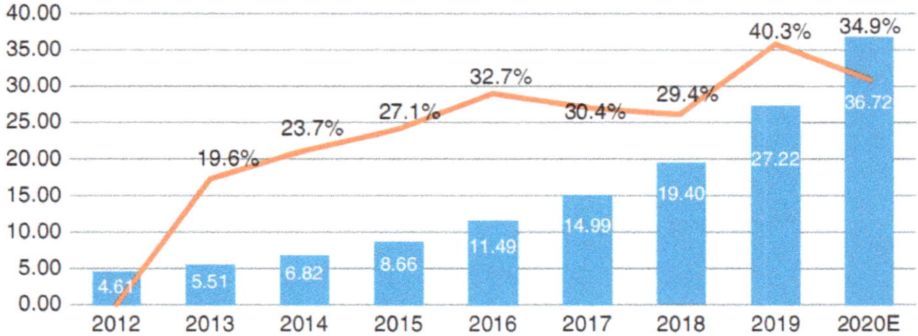

Fig. 25.2 The size and growth rate of the CDx market in China from 2012 to 2020. (Source: Visiongain)

Table 25.2 Current common biomarkers for CDx of cancers

Cancer	Markers for detection
Lung cancer	EGFR gene mutation, including deletion of exon 19; exon 21 mutation; abnormal expression of EGFR protein
	ALK gene fusion mutation and ALK protein expression
	ROS1 gene fusion mutation
Breast cancer	HER-2 gene amplification; HER-2 protein expression
Melanoma	BRAF gene mutation, including exon 15 V600E mutation
Hematological system tumor	Platelet-derived Growth Factor Receptors (PDGFR) gene mutation, including chromosomal rearrangement of chromosome 5q31 ~ 33
Nasopharyngeal carcinoma	Abnormal expression of EGFR protein

In terms of CDx, large international multinational companies have the most approved CDx products with different technical focuses. In recent years, FDA has approved several tissue-based NGS assays for tumor analysis and specific CDx requirements, including two large-panel pan-cancer liquid biopsy detection kit products.

The main types of common biomarkers for cancer CDx are shown in Table 25.2 [3].

CDx started late in China. In March 2015, the Ministry of Science and Technology held the first national "Precision Medicine Strategic Expert Conference." The conference plans to invest RMB 60 billion yuan in the field of precision medicine by 2030; in July 2015, the Individualized Medical Detection Technology Expert Committee of the Health and Family Planning Commission formulated *Technical Guidelines for Individualized Treatment and Detection of Tumors (Trial)* and *Technical Guidelines for Gene Detection of Drug Metabolizing Enzymes and Drug Action Targets (Trial)*, which advance the standardization and normalization requirements of drug and gene detection for precision medicine of tumors. In the "13th Five-Year Plan" released by the state in March 2016, precision medicine becomes a national strategy. On November 12, 2019, the National Medical Products Administration (NMPA) organized and formulated "*Guidelines for the Review of General Registration Technology for Performance Evaluation of Tumor-Related Mutation Gene Detection Reagents (High-Throughput Sequencing)*" and "*Guidelines for the Review of Registration Technology of CYP2C19 Drug Metabolic Enzyme Gene Polymorphism Detection Reagents*" (No. 83 in 2019), providing guidance for tumor mutation genes and CYP2C19 drug metabolism. From the perspective of the approved products, in January 2018, NMPA approved the super Amplification Refractory Mutation System (ARMS) Epidermal Growth Factor Receptor (EGFR) gene mutation detection kit of AmoyDx, which is the first ctDNA detection kit approved for marketing in China based on the CDx reagent standard. This is a milestone in the field of in vitro diagnosis in China, indicating that China has been in line with the international standard in CDx. Since the second half of 2018, NGS-based CDx kits have been approved successively. In July 2018, the "Human EGFR/ALK/BRAF/KRAS Gene Mutation Detection Kit" made by Burning Rock DX was successfully approved, and won the first certificate of tumor NGS in China. Soon later, Novogene, Geneseeq, and AmoyDx obtained the approval documents for tumor diagnosis products based on

NGS technology in the same year. Since then, CDx products on the NGS platform of BGI, GenePlus, and Genetron Health have been approved to market in 2019 and 2020, respectively. In terms of early screening of tumors, the "first certificate of early screening of cancer" was also approved by the regulatory authorities. On November 9, 2020, the NMPA approved the application for registration of innovative Class III medical device—ColoClear by Circle, a product of New Horizon Health—for "screening of high-risk colorectal cancer population aged 40–74." It shows that the domestic regulatory authorities have gradually recognized cancer early screening products, and the regulatory ideas are similar to those of developed countries such as Europe and the United States.

In recent years, in order to meet the growing demand of tumor patients for targeted therapy and immunotherapy, NMPA has accelerated the approval process for these new therapies. In order to achieve the safe application of targeted agents, it is necessary to carry out cancer genotyping before medication, which has given rise to the demand for CDx detection for a large number of related loci, thus greatly promoting the development of the CDx industry.

25.2.2 Industrial Chain

The upstream of the CDx industry is the supplier of equipment and consumable, mainly including gene sequencer, PCR amplification instrument, and nucleic acid extractor. The upstream industry of gene sequencer is dominated by imported products due to a high technical barrier. However, the technical threshold for nucleic acid extractor and PCR amplification instrument is relatively low, so these products are basically localized.

Consumables include enzyme, primer, and probe; due to the high difficulty in technology development and low industrialization maturity, the upstream raw material manufacturers are mainly foreign leading enterprises.

Domestic CDx and gene sequencing companies are mainly distributed in the midstream and downstream. The midstream industry supplies various diagnostic reagents. At present, domestic enterprises dominate the market. Through their own technical platforms and equipment, they have developed various diagnostic products to take a large market share. In this market segment, many outstanding companies have emerged. Take AmoyDx as an example: as the first manufacturer having launched EGFR detection reagent in China, it gets a high market share in the field of lung cancer, accounting for more than 60% of the hospital market. Currently, domestic CDx reagents develop single- or multi-gene detection kits that can cover main target loci, e.g., EGFR, KRAS, BRAF, EML4-ALK, PIK3CA, ROS1, NRAS, and Human Epidermal Growth Factor Receptor-2 (HER-2), and main targeted agents. These reagents are applicable for various types of samples, including tissue and blood ctDNA [4].The downstream industry of CDx covers users who purchase these reagents, including hospitals, independent clinical laboratories, blood stations, and health examination centers. Today, the domestic CDx purchasers are mainly the hospital pathologic departments. There are three detection service modes: patient-hospital, patient-hospital-service company (Independent Clinical

Laboratory (ICL) and diagnostic service company), and patient-service company. The first two are the most popular service modes, with hospital as the flow carriers. The flow proportion of the third mode will increase with the improvement in the market education.

25.2.3 Development Trend of CDx Industry

For diseases with known gene mutation principles and corresponding targeted agents, CDx detection is an indispensable step. From the demand side, supply side, policy side, and technology side, there are some key factors that promote the development of the CDx industry [5].

25.2.3.1 Demand Side

The number of tumor patients is gradually increasing, and the drug accessibility has improved

Cancer is the second leading cause of death in the world, which caused 9.6 million deaths in 2018. Among the new cases in the world in 2018, lung cancer, breast cancer, colorectal cancer, prostate cancer, and gastric cancer contributed the most, accounting for 11.6%, 11.6%, 10.2%, 7.1%, and 5.7%, respectively. The cost of cancer treatment has become a heavy burden on the global healthcare system [6, 7].

The world's largest number of new cancer patients is in Asia. In 2018, among the 18.1 million new cancer patients in the world, there were about 8.75 million new cancer patients in Asia, accounting for 48.4% of all, making Asia the continent with the largest number of new cancer patients worldwide. China is one of the countries with the most cancer cases in the world; and cancer is also one of the most deadly diseases in China. The total number of cancer patients in China will exceed 32 million in 2020. In the future, with the population aging and the improvement in the survival rate of cancer patients in China, the increasing number of cancer patients will increase the demand for CDx products in both aspects of stock and incremental market.

25.2.3.2 The Supply Side

Targeted agents and immunotherapy will become the main trend and continue to promote the demand for CDx products

The year 2005 was the first year that witnessed targeted agents entering China. With the approval of Gefitinib developed by AstraZeneca to enter the domestic market, China ushered in the era of targeted treatment for cancers. As the domestic pharmaceutical market began to set foot in targeted agents, icotinib, developed by Betta Pharmaceuticals, was approved in 2011 and became the first small molecule targeted anti-cancer drug with independent intellectual property rights in China. China's biomedical industry turned to molecular targeted agents in an all-round way. Since 2011, immunotherapy has begun to rise, which is expected to further promote the reform in the field of cancer treatment in the future. With the discovery of new pathogenic mechanisms and new gene loci, new targeted agents will be developed successively, so as to promote the continuous enrichment of CDx products and further expansion of the market.

In recent years, the diagnostic industry and pharmaceutical enterprises have more closely cooperated in the research and development and shared a common consensus and practice to keep pace with the development of diagnostic kits and drugs (synchronous research and development, clinical trials, and application for approval). On the one hand, this development model can provide effective CDx experiments for drug research and development, control drug development costs, obtain ideal clinical data, and ensure the safety and effectiveness of drugs; on the other hand, corresponding CDx reagents are developed based on the defined clinical application scenario, which can speed up the marketing of CDx products and improve business collaboration [8].

In addition, with the transformation of tumor treatment mode from malignant disease to chronic disease, one-shot detection will change to continuous detection during treatment, and the application frequency of CDx will increase.

25.2.3.3 Policy Side

The policy continuously promotes the development of CDx from the aspects of clinical standards and medical insurance payment

As a national strategy, precision medicine has been strongly supported by the government. Relevant departments have issued many policies and regulations to actively promote the development and clinical application of related products and instruments. The National Health Commission has successively issued two important documents—*Administrative Measures for the Clinical Application of Anti-tumor Drugs (Trial)* and *Guidelines for the Clinical Application of New Anti-tumor Drugs (2020)*—to strengthen the supervision and management of the clinical application of anti-tumor drugs. It is clearly stipulated in the documents that doctors should reasonably select anti-tumor drugs according to the pathological diagnosis results of tissue or cytology, or the special molecular pathological diagnosis results. In principle, doctors shall not prescribe anti-tumor drugs for treatment before the pathological diagnosis result is issued; according to the diagnosis and treatment specifications, clinical diagnosis and treatment guidelines, and clinical pathways or drug instructions issued by the National Health Commission, the targeted agents that are required to undergo gene target detection need to detect gene target before use, and can only be prescribed after it is confirmed that these agents are suitable for the patients.

In addition, in terms of medical insurance payment, the country has also made some systematic adjustments. Before the targeted agents were included in the medical insurance drug catalogue list, most patients could not afford the huge drug expenditure due to the high drug price. Therefore, the penetration rate of targeted agents in China had been at a low level, and CDx, as the pioneer procedure of targeted agents, was also affected by the drug market, resulting in a low penetration rate. In 2011, targeted agents were covered by medical insurance with significant price reduction; since 2017, the National Healthcare Security Administration started another three rounds of medical insurance negotiations to reduce prices, and the prices of most mainstream targeted agents decreased significantly. From 2017 to 2019, the average price decline of tumor targeted agents reached 59%, greatly reducing the economic pressure upon cancer patients, and the demand for targeted agents rose. More importantly, in order to avoid the waste of medical insurance funds, the medical insurance policy requires that targeted agents must pass target detection before being covered by medical insurance. Therefore, the expansion of the targeted agent market driven by medical insurance will also increase the penetration rate of its related diagnostic products. On the other hand, the national policy explicitly includes cancer gene detection in medical insurance, which is conducive to standardizing the hospital diagnosis and treatment path of CDx. In December 2018, the Beijing Municipal Medical Insurance Bureau issued the *Notice on Regulating the Price Adjustment of Pathology and Other Medical Services*, which stipulates that DNA sequencing of tumor tissues shall be included in medical insurance Class B service list and priced to RMB 3800. Since June 15, 2019, the comprehensive reform through linkage between medical services and medical supplies in Beijing has been officially implemented, and the city has implemented a new medical insurance policy for pathological examinations, which means that tumor gene detection is officially covered by the medical insurance [9].

25.2.3.4 Technology Side

The technology progress in large-panel pan-cancer products and liquid biopsy brings broader application prospects

At present, the penetration rate of CDx in China is less than 50%. With the technical innovation of large panels and NGS products, and the development speed of CDx products, clinical use scenarios and costs will be significantly improved, the penetration rate will be increased, and the market is expected to further expand.

At present, the hospital CDx is still dominated by single gene detection. For patients, it is more practical to detect all possible mutation types of a single cancer (multi-gene detection) at one time. Nowadays, the PCR technology is relatively mature and some recently marketed multi-gene detection products can meet the needs of tumor drug detection targets. With further innovation of NGS technology, it can be expected that large-panel pan-cancer products will be launched at home and abroad to promote further improvement in CDx penetration.

In addition, liquid biopsy based on NGS technology is expected to accelerate the reform of the CDx market. Liquid biopsy has the unique advantages of being non-invasive, convenient, and rapid. For patients who cannot obtain tissue biopsy on admission and in terms of continuous medication, liquid biopsy can play to its technical advantages, expand clinical application scenarios, continuously track patient conditions, and play a more active role in precision medicine. Up to now, liquid biopsy technology has four main development stages, namely, the scientific exploration period before the 1990s, the technological development period in the 1990s, the industrial development period in the twenty-first century and beyond (2000–2010), and the industrial explosion period (2011 to date). At present, liquid biopsy has been used clinically in reproductive health checkup, genetic disease diagnosis, and early cancer screening. The main technological development

Table 25.3 Research direction and commercialization progress of major domestic early screening enterprises

Application of early screening	Domestic Companies (Representative)	Technical validation → Retrospective study → Prospective study → Commercialization	
Pan-cancers	Burning Rock DX	"PREDICT" is expected to enroll 14,000 subjects; the study is expected to be completed in 2023	
Liver cancer	Genetron Health	IVD registration for application in 2,000 people started in the second half of 2021	"Mutation Capsule": launched in the form
	Berry Oncology	"" Liver Screening" launched in the form of LDT in August 2020 and the study is expected to be completed in 2023	August 2020: LDT
Colorectal cancer	New Horizon Health	Approved for early screening of cancer in November 2020	
	Creative Biosciences	Approved for auxiliary diagnosis in November 2018	
	AmoyDx	Approved for listing in January 2021	

directions in the future include tissue traceability technology for different components, very early cancer discovery technology, technology to detect tumor heterogeneity by liquid biopsy, and technology to infer the stage and size of tumor from the amount of ctDNA and allele frequency and other information. In addition, comprehensive multidimensional component analysis combined with machine learning algorithm is the development trend of cancer liquid biopsy technology. Therefore, the progress in NGS technology platform and artificial intelligence (AI) algorithm will certainly open a wide space for the application of liquid biopsy in more clinical fields [10]. The research direction and commercialization progress of major domestic early screening enterprises are shown in Table 25.3.

25.3 Main Technical Platforms and Related Clinical Applications of CDx

The main technology platforms for CDx detection can be divided into immune method, such as IHC based on protein, and molecular diagnostic method based on nucleic acid, including PCR, FISH, and NGS high-throughput gene sequencing. Among them, the molecular diagnostic method is the most common [6].

At present, the main molecular diagnostic technologies in the world can be divided into nucleic acid detection and biochip. Nucleic acid detection includes PCR, FISH, and gene sequencing. Biochip technology can be divided into gene chip technology and protein chip technology. Nucleic acid detection technology is mainly used in CDx.

25.3.1 IHC

Immunohistochemistry (IHC) is based on the basic principle of immunology—antigen/antibody reaction, that is, the principle of the specific combination of antigen and antibody. It uses chemical reaction to color the antibody-labeled chromogenic agents (including fluorescein, enzyme, metal ions, and isotopes) to determine the antigens (polypeptides or proteins) in tissues and cells, so as to conduct localization, qualitative, and relative quantitative studies.

25.3.2 Fish

Fluorescence in situ hybridization (FISH for short) is an important non-radioactive in situ hybridization technology. It uses nucleic acid probes directly or indirectly labeled with fluorescein to hybridize with target nucleic acid sequences to be detected in the samples, so as to conduct qualitative, quantitative, or relative location analysis of DNA.

FISH has many advantages, such as safety and speed, good probe stability, long-term preservation, simple and intuitive multicolor labeling, and analysis of metaphase chromosomes and interphase cells. As a visual molecular cytogenetic technology, FISH is currently widely used in the detection of chromosome aberrations, such as aneuploidy, chromosome recombination, and the detection of viral gene expression. At present, FISH has been extensively applied in genetic disease diagnosis, virus infection analysis, prenatal diagnosis, tumor genetics, genome research, and many other fields. However, FISH technology is currently only applicable to detect the fusion or amplification of single gene fragments, and requires more professional interpretation technology, so it has certain limitations in clinical use.

25.3.3 PCR

Polymerase chain reaction (PCR) is a molecular biological technology used to amplify specific nucleic acid fragments in vitro. Born in 1992, the second generation of PCR technology, namely real-time PCR (RT-PCR), has the advantages of low contamination risk with closed tube detection, small sample size, and being simple and cost-effective, and is the first choice for clinical gene detection. Fluorescence PCR instrument can hold 96 or 384 samples at one time, and the detection throughput is higher than FISH and IHC. In addition to high-throughput sequencing, fluorescent PCR is also the method to detect most DNA mutation types.

However, the weakness of fluorescence PCR is also obvious. Due to the limitation of principle, this method can only detect mutations at known loci and cannot cover all bases of the gene. As a result, some rare mutations may be ignored to obtain false negative results, leading to misjudgment.

Digital PCR (dPCR), which appeared at the end of the twentieth century, is an absolute quantitative technology for nucleic acid molecules. Compared with conventional qPCR, dPCR can directly count the number of DNA molecules and absolutely quantify the initial sample. This method disperses a large number of diluted nucleic acid molecules into the reactor formed by micropores or micro-droplets of the chip, and the number of nucleic acid templates in each reactor is less than or equal to one. In this way, after PCR cycle, the reactor with nucleic acid molecular template will give out fluorescence signal; otherwise, there is no signal. According to the relative proportion and reactor volume, the nucleic acid concentration of the original solution can be inferred, so that the target molecules with very low copy number can be detected directly and quantitatively, independent of any calibrator or external reference. This method is particularly suitable for applications that cannot be well distinguished with Ct value, e.g., copy number variation, low-frequency mutation detection, relative gene expression research (e.g., allele imbalance expression), validation of second-generation sequencing results, gene expression analysis, etc.

25.3.4 High-Throughput Next-Generation Sequencing (NGS)

High-throughput sequencing technology, also known as "next-generation sequencing technology," can sequence hundreds of thousands to millions of DNA molecules in parallel at one time with short reading length through sequencing by synthesis. At present, FDA has approved six NGS-based CDx products.

NGS can obtain all the information of the whole genome from a small number of samples, so it is applicable to the detection of point mutation, fusion gene, gene amplification, and other mutation types, providing better technical support and selection for tumor susceptibility gene detection, CDx, personalized drug use, etc. However, there are still bottlenecks such as high cost (about RMB 1000–10,000 for a sample) and long time (varying in different platforms, generally at least 1 week). In practical use, the technical requirements for the laboratory technician are also relatively high and the popularity is relatively low compared with other technical platforms. In addition, high-throughput sequencing often generates huge amounts of data, which often exceeds the need for detecting a limited number of site mutations in clinical practice. Therefore, targeted amplification or hybrid capture will be used in clinical application to enrich the DNA fragments of interest, followed by high-throughput sequencing, so as to form different gene sequencing panels. In the future, with the R&D and marketing of various large-panel pan-cancer products, the acceleration of automation, and progress in industrialization, NGS detection will be faster and more cost-effective. Therefore, NGS will be the key development direction of CDx in the future.

25.3.5 Comparison of Application Prospects of PCR and NGS in the Field of CDx

In the clinical application, as far as the existing targets of targeted therapy are concerned, PCR detection can basically meet the clinical needs. For most cancers, there are no more than ten targets of targeted agents on the market. Taking lung cancer with the most abundant targeted agents as an example, the existing PCR diagnostic products can meet the rapid detection needs of the core driver genes in the first-line treatment of lung cancer, including the new-generation multi-gene detection kit (trade name: Aihuijian) launched by AmoyDx. This kit can simultaneously detect the core driver genes of lung cancer, such as EGFR, ALK, ROS1, KRAS, BRAF, HER-2, rearranged during transfection (RET), Mesenchymal to Epithelial Transition factor (MET), NRAS, and PIK3CA, covering all the core gene targets of targeted agents that have been marketed or will be marketed in the coming three to 5 years (Fig. 25.3). Therefore, PCR will be sufficient to meet the detection needs of targeted treatment of lung cancer for each gene in the coming several years. However, the large-panel NGS can detect the tumor mutation burden (TMB) used to guide immunotherapy, which is an irreplaceable technology of PCR and other methods.

Similarly, for other specific cancers, it is not necessary to detect as many gene loci as possible. The genes with detection value should meet two conditions: one is the mutant gene in the cancer; the other one is the ability to predict the effect of targeted agents. For gene detection, the corresponding gene detection items should be selected according to the actual needs of targeted agents to be evaluated. At present, the marketed targeted agents act on relatively fixed target genes. When sequencing covers enough target genes, increasing the number of genes may not provide more guidance for targeted agents. It is of little significance to detect genes with few mutations in a certain cancer or genes without targeted agents at present. For example, BRCA is mutated a lot in breast cancer and ovarian cancer, and rarely in lung cancer. For another example, SMARCA4 is often mutated in lung cancer. Because there is no targeted agent, even if the mutation is detected, it has no value in predicting the drug efficacy. At present, most targeted agents need to detect no more than ten genes. Correspondingly, the 11 NGS-based detection kits that have been approved in China can cover less than 10 targets, and tumor types are limited to

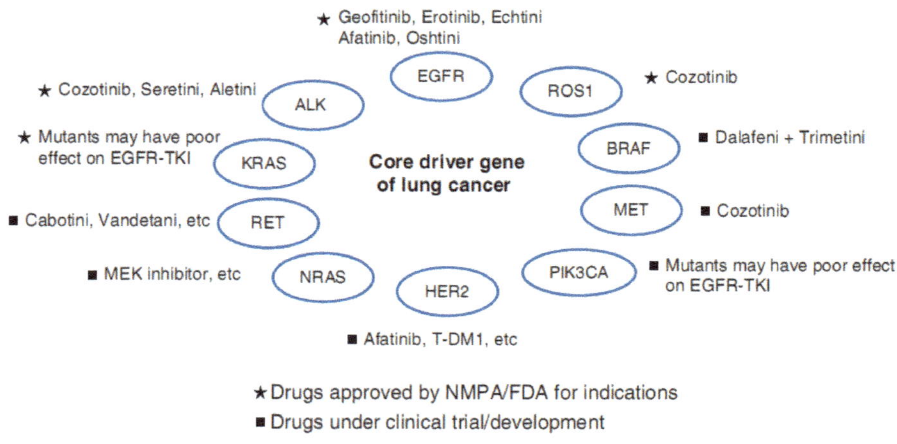

Fig. 25.3 Detection kit for AmoyDx lung cancer multigene (fluorescence PCR). Clinical value of detection of first-line core driver genes in lung cancer

NSCLC and colorectal cancer. The technical characteristics of NGS determine that its advantages are mainly reflected in the field of medium and large panels, which is also the main direction of research and development for domestic NGS companies. At present, all gene detection companies can provide large-panel NGS detection kits that cover hundreds of genes, as well as the approved and existing tumor markers, including TMB for PD-1/Programmed Death-Ligand 1 (PD-L1) monoclonal antibody immunotherapy. For targeted agents detecting less than ten genes, PCR has significant advantages over NGS, such as simple operation, high accuracy, short reporting time, and high cost performance, and hence it becomes the best choice for most hospitals and patients. At present, PCR still plays the main role in clinical practice in China with NGS as supplement. In terms of cost and feasibility, the reasonable combination of various technical routes is still the most economical and effective plan.

From the perspective of clinical application, PCR is suitable to detect the known gene loci and those with high sensitivity, while NGS is more advantageous in finding unknown genes; qPCR is more suitable for clinical gene diagnosis of tumor tissue samples, while NGS is more advantageous in blood ctDNA detection. According to the *Expert Consensus on the Application of Liquid Biopsy in Clinical Tumor Diagnosis and Treatment and Medical Laboratory Practice* jointly formulated by the Laboratory Medicine Branch of the Chinese Medical Association and the National Health Commission in 2019, ARMS-PCR is recommended when known and single-targeted treatment-sensitive or drug-resistant mutations are detected; and NGS method is recommended for known and multiple parallel clinical treatment targets, or when unknown genes are discovered and clinical value and relevant mechanisms are explored.

From the angle of combined use of targeted agents, the application of PCR and NGS is related to the type of targets and the targeted agents recommended. The two dimensions of clinical needs for CDx are target and treatment plan. Among the current first-line targeted agents developed, PCR technology is used for CDx of EGFR, BRAF, and other targets, while NTRK, RET, and other targets coexist with PCR and NGS. At present, the CDx of second-line/third-line targeted agents is only applicable to EGFR and ALK targets. PCR technology is used for EGFR mutation, while NGS has not been effectively applied. To sum up, looking at the above four technical platforms for CDx, NGS, IHC, FISH, and PCR, as the most widely used traditional CDx technologies, are technically different from each other. Taking ALK gene fusion detection as an example, FISH has obvious advantages in clinical agreement rate, so it is the standard method recommended by the guidelines for detecting ALK gene fusion. It can detect all fusion types but cannot distinguish them and its detection cost is high. Comparatively, although the cost of IHC detection is low, the clinical agreement rate is low because of its subjective judgment and lack of uniform positive standard. RT-PCR is very practical, simple to operate, and low in cost, and has a higher clinical agreement rate compared with IHC, and especially with the introduction of new technologies such as dPCR, there will be more opportunities for clinical application. However, PCR has its disadvantages: detection of known mutations only and failure to detect unknown mutations or fusion types. Even so, PCR is

Table 25.4 Performance comparison of common technical platforms for CDx

Method	Cost	Operation complexity	Time	Throughput	Mutation	Application
qPCR	★	★	★	★★	Point mutation Gene expression Gene amplification Gene fusion	Most widely used currently for single or combined detections of multiple targets(EGFR, ROS, ALK)for lung cancer, colorectal cancer, etc.
FISH	★★	★★	★★	★	Gene amplification	
					Gene rearrangement	*HER-2, ALK*
NGS	★★★★★	★★★★★	★★★★★	★★★★★	All types of mutation	*BRCA 1/2*
IHC	★	★★	★★	★	Protein expression	*PD-L1*
					Mutation	

still the mainstream CDx detection technology. Comparatively, NGS has significant advantages in detecting unknown sequences, unknown mutations, and high-throughput multiple loci, but its operation and data analysis are difficult, and its detection cost is relatively high. Although NGS has great development potential, its current application still has some limitations. See Table 25.4 for the performance comparison of common technology platforms for CDx.

25.4 Major Domestic CDx Enterprises

Thanks to the strong support of the country since 2014, the rapid development of technology, and the increasing market demand for targeted agents, the domestic CDx has entered the fast lane of sustainable development. In January 2018, NMPA approved the "Super ARMS EGFR gene mutation detection kit" of AmoyDx, which is the first ctDNA detection kit in China that has been approved to market according to the CDx reagent standard in the form of liquid biopsy. On July 23, 2018, the "human EGFR/ALK/BRAF/KRAS gene mutation detection kit" of Burning Rock DX was successfully approved, and won the first certificate of tumor NGS in China. Soon later, Novogene, Geneseeq, and AmoyDx obtained the production approval documents of CDx products based on NGS technology on August 13, September 30, and November 20, 2018, respectively. The first three approved CDx products are targeted at gene mutations on EGFR, ALK, and ROS1, and their main indications are NSCLC. The targeted agents that can be used together with them include gefitinib, icotinib hydrochloride, osimertinib mesylate, and crizotinib. What is more on above three products, the approved CDx product—human 10 gene mutation detection kit (sequencing by reversible termination)—of AmoyDx not only includes the detection of ten genes, but also includes colorectal cancer in the detection range for the first time. It can be used with cetuximab injection, and became the first pan-cancer NGS detection product in China.

According to the approval list, as of December 2021, the PCR method is still the development mainstream of CDx products.

From 2014 to 2021, more than 100 tumor gene detection kit products based on molecular diagnostic technology were approved in China. Since 2018 when AmoyDx's Super ARMS® EGFR gene mutation ctDNA detection kit as the first product in the form of liquid biopsy was approved according to CDx reagent standard for marketing, NMPA has approved more than 110 CDx products, most of which are PCR products, and 11 are NGS products. Among the domestic CDx products approved, AmoyDx, SINOMD, YZY Medical, GP Medical, SUREXAM, and ACCB Biotech contributed more than 50% of total, leading the industry. See Table 25.5 for the methods and manufacturers of CDx products approved in the field of tumor detection; see Table 25.6 for major gene targets detected and relative kit manufacturers based on PCR method, and Table 25.7 for those CDx products based on NGS method.

Table 25.5 Method and manufacturers of CDx products approved for tumor detection (as of December 31, 2021)

SN	Company	FISH	NGS	PCR	Gene chip	IHC	Sanger sequencing	Other methods	Total
1	AmoyDx	1	2	17					20
2	LBP	7				1			8
3	SUREXAM	4						4	8
4	GP medical	5		2					7
5	SINOMD	1		3			3		7
6	YZY medical			7					7
7	ACCB biotech			6					6
8	Tellgen			4					4
9	MicroDiag biomedicine			4					4
10	RIGHTONGENE			3			1		4
11	Wuhan HealthCare	4							4
12	Daan gene	1					2		3
13	SHENRI BIO			3					3
14	Genetron health		1	2					3
15	Haijili biotechnology			2					2
16	RIQIGEN			2					2
17	HEAS biotech			2					2
18	BGI GBI			2					2
19	Mole bioscience			2					2
20	Sinochips				2				2
21	Gene tech		1	1					2
22	Biotron technology			1					1
23	HELIXGEN (Guangzhou)			1					1
24	BGI		1						1
25	GenePlus technology		1						1
26	Novogene		1						1
27	Burning rock DX		1						1
28	XIAMEN SPACEGEN		1						1
29	Geneseeq		1						1
30	Hybiome biomedical							1	1
31	Zeesan biotech			1					1
32	Suzhou DMD biomed	1							1
33	Geneis		1						1
34	Zhenrui biotech		1						1

Table 25.5 (continued)

SN	Company	FISH	NGS	PCR	Gene chip	IHC	Sanger sequencing	Other methods	Total
35	GenomePrecision			1					1
36	HaploX		1						1
	Total	24	13	66	2	1	6	5	117

Note: Data from NMPA website and relevant public information

Table 25.6 Major gene targets detected and reagent kit manufacturers: approved CDx products based on PCR method (as of December 31, 2021)

Gene locus	Product name	Manufacturer
HER-2	*HER-2* gene amplification detection kit (fluorescence in situ hybridization)	GP medical
	HER-2/neu gene amplification detection kit (fluorescence in situ hybridization)	Daan gene
	HER-2 gene amplification detection kit (fluorescence in situ hybridization)	Suzhou DMD biomed
	HER-2 gene amplification detection kit (fluorescence in situ hybridization)	SINOMD
	Human HER-2 gene amplification detection kit (fluorescence in situ hybridization)	AmoyDx
	HER-2 gene amplification detection kit (fluorescence in situ *hybridization)*	SUREXAM
	HER-2/neu (17q12)/TOP2A (17q21)/csp17 multicolor detection kit for breast cancer (fluorescence in situ hybridization)	LBP
	HER-2 detection kit for breast cancer (immunohistochemical method)	LBP

(continued)

Table 25.6 (continued)

Gene locus	Product name	Manufacturer
EGFR	Human EGFR mutant gene detection kit (multiplex fluorescent PCR method)	AmoyDx
	EGFR gene amplification detection kit (fluorescence in situ hybridization)	GP medical
	EGFR gene amplification detection kit (fluorescence in situ hybridization)	SUREXAM
	EGFR gene detection kit (fluorescence in situ hybridization)	LBP
	EGFR gene mutation detection kit (fluorescent PCR method)	GP medical
	Human EGFR/ALK/ROS1 gene mutation detection kit (fluorescent PCR)	AmoyDx
	Human EGFR gene 22 mutation detection kit (fluorescent PCR method)	AmoyDx
	Human EGFR gene mutation detection kit (fluorescent PCR method)	ACCB biotech
	EGFR gene mutation detection kit (fluorescent PCR method)	MicroDiag biomedicine
	Human EGFR gene mutation detection kit (fluorescent PCR method)	RIQIGEN
	Human EGFR gene mutation detection kit (fluorescent PCR method)	Haijili biotechnology
	Human EGFR gene mutation detection kit (PCR fluorescence method)	Tellgen corporation
	Human EGFR gene mutation detection kit (fluorescent PCR method)	SHENRI BIO
	EGFR gene mutation detection kit (fluorescent PCR capillary electrophoresis)	SINOMD
	Human EGFR gene mutation detection kit (PCR fluorescence probing)	RIGHTONGENE
	Human EGFR gene mutation detection kit (PCR fluorescence probing)	YZY medical
	Human EGFR gene 20 mutation detection kit (PCR fluorescence probing)	BGI GBI
	EGFR gene mutation detection kit (PCR fluorescence probing)	HEAS biotech
	Human EGFR gene mutation detection kit (Taqman ARMS method)	MicroDiag biomedicine
	Human EGFR gene mutation detection kit (flow cytometry)	SUREXAM

Table 25.6 (continued)

Gene locus	Product name	Manufacturer
ALK	Human EML4-ALK fusion gene detection kit (fluorescent PCR method)	AmoyDx
	Human ALK gene fusion and ROS1 gene fusion detection kit (fluorescent PCR method)	AmoyDx
	Human EGFR/ALK/ROS1 gene mutation detection kit (fluorescent PCR)	AmoyDx
	Human EML4-ALK fusion gene detection kit (fluorescent PCR method)	AmoyDx
	Human EML5-ALK fusion gene detection kit (fluorescent PCR method)	ACCB biotech
	ALK gene rearrangement detection kit (fluorescence in situ hybridization)	SUREXAM
	Human ALK fusion gene detection kit (fluorescence in situ hybridization)	Wuhan HealthCare
	Human EML4-ALK fusion gene detection kit (PCR fluorescence probing)	YZY medical

(continued)

Table 25.6 (continued)

Gene locus	Product name	Manufacturer
KRAS	Human KRAS gene mutation detection kit (fluorescent PCR method)	ACCB biotech
	Human KRAS gene 7 mutation detection kit (fluorescent PCR method)	Tellgen corporation
	Human KRAS gene mutation detection kit (Taqman ARMS method)	MicroDiag biomedicine
	Human KRAS gene mutation detection kit (PCR fluorescence probing)	YZY medical
	Human KRAS gene codon 12/13 mutation detection kit (pyrosequencing)	Gene tech
	Human KRAS gene 7 mutation detection kit (fluorescent PCR method)	AmoyDx
	KRAS gene mutation detection kit (sequencing method)	Daan gene
	Human KRAS gene mutation detection kit (fluorescent PCR method)	SHENRI BIO
	KRAS gene mutation detection kit (PCR fluorescence probing)	HEAS biotech
	Human KRAS gene mutation detection kit (fluorescent PCR method)	AmoyDx
	Human KRAS gene mutation detection kit (PCR fluorescence probing)	YZY medical
	Human KRAS gene mutation detection kit (fluorescent PCR method)	ACCB biotech
	Human KRAS gene mutation detection kit (fluorescent PCR method)	ACCB biotech
	Human KRAS gene V600E mutation detection kit (fluorescent PCR method)	AmoyDx
	Human KRAS gene mutation detection kit (fluorescent PCR method)	YZY medical
	Human KRAS gene V600E mutation detection kit (PCR fluorescence probing)	YZY medical
	Human KRAS gene mutation detection kit (fluorescent PCR method)	ACCB biotech
IDH1	Human IDH1 gene mutation detection kit (PCR fluorescence probing)	Genetron health
	Human IDH1 gene mutation detection kit (fluorescent PCR capillary electrophoresis sequencing)	GenomePrecision
Polygene detection	Human KRAS/NRAS/PIK3CA/BRAF gene mutation detection kit (fluorescent PCR method)	AmoyDx
	Human KRAS/NRAS gene mutation detection kit (fluorescent PCR method)	AmoyDx
	Human KRAS/NRAS/BRAF gene mutation detection kit (fluorescent PCR method)	AmoyDx
	Human KRAS/NRAS/PIK3CA/BRAF gene mutation detection kit (fluorescent PCR method)	AmoyDx
	Human KRAS gene mutation detection kit (fluorescent PCR method)	AmoyDx

Note: Data from NMPA website and relevant public information

Table 25.7 Approved CDx products based on NGS method (as of December 31, 2021)

Manufacturer	Approved date	Method	Locus	Indications and diagnostic drugs
Burning rock DX	2018.07.18	Sequencing by reversible termination	EGFR, ALK, BRAF, KRAS	Gefitinib, Icotinib, Crizotinib, Osimertinib
Novogene	2018.08.13	Semiconductor sequencing	EGFR, KRAS, BRAF, PIK3CA, ALK, ROS1	Gefitinib, Osimertinib, Crizotinib
Geneseeq	2018.09.30	Sequencing by reversible termination	EGFR, ALK, ROS1, BRAF, KRAS	Gefitinib, Icotinib, Crizotinib, Osimertinib
AmoyDx	2018.11.16	Sequencing by reversible termination	EGFR, ALK, ROS1, RET, KRAS, NRAS, PIK3CA, BRAF, MET, HER-2	Gefitinib, Osimertinib, Crizotinib, Cetuximab
BGI	2019.08.26	Combined probe anchoring polymerization sequencing	EGFR, KRAS, ALK	Gefitinib, Icotinib, Crizotinib
GenePlus	2019.12.31	Combined probe anchoring polymerization sequencing	EGFR, KRAS, ALK	Gefitinib, Icotinib hydrochloride, Osimertinib mesylate, Crizotinib
Genetron health	2020.01.22	Sequencing by reversible termination	EGFR, KRAS, BRAF, HER-2, PIK3CA, ALK, ROS1, MET	Gefitinib, Icotinib, Osimertinib, Crizotinib
XIAMEN SPACEGEN	2020.01.22	Semiconductor sequencing	EGFR, KRAS, BRAF, HER-2, ALK, ROS1	Gefitinib, Icotinib hydrochloride, Crizotinib
Zhenrui biotech	2021.02.24	Sequencing by reversible termination	KARS, NRAS, BRAF, PIK3CA	CRC cetuximab
Geneis	2021.07.14	Sequencing by reversible termination	EGFR, KRAS, BRAF, PIK3CA, ALK, ROS1	Gefitinib, Icotinib hydrochloride, Osimertinib mesylate, Crizotinib
HaploX	2021.10.20	Combined probe anchoring polymerization sequencing	EGFR, ALK	Gefitinib, Icotinib hydrochloride, Osimertinib mesylate, Crizotinib

Note: Data from NMPA website

Declaration Chengbo Fu and Yan Jiang are employees of Beijing Bohui Innovation Biotechnology Group Co., Ltd.

Yile Sun and Yuqing Tang are employees of Tellgen Corporation, Shanghai, China.

References

1. Nucleic Acid Based Tests. https://www.fda.gov/medical-devices/in-vitro-diagnostics/nucleic -acid-based-tests.
2. List of Cleared or Approved Companion Diagnostic Devices (In Vitro and Imaging Tools). https://www.fda.gov/medical-devices/in-vitro-diagnostics/list-cleared-or-approved-companion-diagnostic-devices-in-vitro-and-imaging-tools.
3. Jan Trøst Jørgensen. The current landscape of the FDA approved companion diagnostics. Transl Oncol. 2021;14:101063. https://doi.org/10.1016/j.tranon.2021.101063.
4. Agarwal A, Ressler D, Snyder G. The current and future state of companion diagnostics. Pharmgenomics Pers Med. 2015;8:99–110. https://doi.org/10.2147/PGPM.S49493. eCollection 2015.
5. Guidance for Industry: In Vitro Companion Diagnostic Devices. https://www.fda.gov/media/81309/download.
6. Jørgensen JT, Hersom M. Companion diagnostics-a tool to improve pharmacotherapy. Ann Transl Med. 2016;4(24):482. https://doi.org/10.21037/atm.2016.12.26.
7. Valla V, Alzabin S, Koukoura A, Lewis A, Nielsen AA, Vassiliadis E. Companion diagnostics: State of the art and new regulations. Biomark Insights. 2021;16:11772719211047763. https://doi.org/10.1177/11772719211047763.
8. Milne C-P, Bryan C, Garafalo S, McKiernan M. Complementary versus companion diagnostics: apples and oranges? Biomark Med. 2015;9(1):25–34. https://doi.org/10.2217/bmm.14.84.
9. Roscoe DM, Hu Y-F, Philip R. Companion diagnostics: a regulatory perspective from the last 5 years of molecular companion diagnostic approvals. Expert Rev Mol Diagn. 2015;15(7):869–80. https://doi.org/10.1586/14737159.2015.1045490.
10. Principles for Codevelopment of an In Vitro Companion Diagnostic Device with a Therapeutic Product. https://www.fda.gov/media/99030/download.

Part VIII

Mass Spectrometry

26 Matrix-Assisted Laser Desorption Ionization Time-of-Flight Mass Spectrometry

Zengli Yang, Keya Cai, Gaoling Zhao, Meili Liu, and Zhimin Lin

26.1 Introduction

Mass spectrometry (MS) is a kind of technology that ionizes material particles (atoms and molecules) into charged ions, separates them according to the location space, time sequence, etc. by appropriately stable or changing electromagnetic fields, and detects their strength for qualitative and quantitative analysis. Since the twentieth century, especially after the 1980s, with the rapid development of new ion sources (such as *Matrix-Assisted Laser Desorption Ionization* [MALDI], *Electron Spray Ionization* [ESI]) and ion optics theory, after decades of technical iteration and theoretical innovation, mass spectrometry has already become an indispensable new measurement technology in the field of modern chemical analysis and biological analysis. It is widely used in chemical engineering, life science, food safety, environmental monitoring, medical and health, and other fields. Compared with traditional detection methods, it has the advantages of rapid analysis, high throughput, high sensitivity, high specificity, simultaneous detection of multiple indicators, low cost, and so on.

The appearance of new ion source-MALDI breaks the application limitation of mass spectrometry in life science, and MALDI makes it possible to detect biomacromolecules at the level of pmol even fmol, with molecular weight of several hundreds of thousand Daltons (Da). As a new mass spectrometry detection technology, MALDI-TOF-MS (*Matrix-Assisted Laser Desorption Ionization Time-of-Flight Mass Spectrometry*) has been applied to chemical engineering, life science, and other scientific research.

Z. Yang (✉) · K. Cai · G. Zhao · M. Liu
Autobio Diagnostics Co., Ltd., Zhengzhou, Henan, China
e-mail: yangzengli@autobio.com.cn

Z. Lin
Zybio Inc., Chongqing, China

H. Song, L. Dai (eds.), *In Vitro Diagnostic Industry in China*,
https://doi.org/10.1007/978-981-99-3110-1_26

In 2013, the U.S. Food and Drug Administration (FDA) first approved the use of MALDI-TOF-MS to identify pathogenic microorganisms, which marked that MALDI-TOF-MS began to be officially used in the clinical field. Studies have shown that MALDI-TOF-MS can achieve the identification results of microbial colonies within a few minutes and the identification accuracy rate is up to 98%, which is obviously superior to traditional microbial identification methods such as morphology, physiology, and biochemistry, and has received extensive attention and research from international clinical experts. In recent years, MALDI-TOF-MS, in addition to being used for microbial identification, has been expanded in the application of biomarker analysis and single nucleotide polymorphism (SNP) analysis.

26.2 Technical Principles and Working Mode of MALDI-TOF-MS

26.2.1 Technical Principle

MALDI-TOF is mainly composed of a matrix-assisted laser desorption ionization ion source (MALDI) and a time-of-flight mass analyzer (TOF). MALDI is a soft ionization technology that is applicable to the determination of mixtures and biological macromolecules. Its principle is to irradiate the co-crystalline film formed by sample and matrix with laser, the matrix absorbs energy from the laser and transfers it to biomolecules, and the process of ionization transfers protons to biomolecules or gets protons from biomolecules, which ionizes biomolecules. The principle of TOF is that ions accelerate under the action of electric field to obtain the same kinetic energy. The flying speed of ions with different mass charge ratio (m/z) is different. The flying speed of ions with small mass charge ratio is faster than that of ions with large mass charge ratio. After flying through the field-free flight tube, the ions arrive at the detector in turn. The ion mass charge ratio can be converted by recording the time when the ions arrive at the detector.

26.2.2 Working Mode

At present, the main types of MALDI-TOF-MS on the market are linear mode and reflection mode.

26.2.2.1 Linear Mode

In the linear mode, the ions fly in a straight line. The main factors that affect the resolution of MALDI-TOF-MS in this mode are the kinetic energy dispersion and spatial dispersion of the initial ions. The technologies adopted to solve the above problems include dual field acceleration technology and delayed extraction technology. The kinetic energy dispersion is the main factor affecting the resolution, and the ion delay extraction technology can better overcome the initial kinetic energy dispersion and improve the resolution. For the same m/z ions, before the pulse arrives, the ions fly freely according to their own kinetic energy. After a certain time delay, the ions with higher energy move more toward the detector than the ions with lower energy, and the ions with lower energy are farther away from the detector. After the extraction pulse is applied, the ions with higher initial energy will obtain less energy because they are close to the outlet, while the ions with lower initial energy will obtain more energy on the contrary. Adjusting the appropriate delay and pulse voltage can greatly compensate for the initial energy dispersion, so that the ions can reach the detector at the same time, thus improving the resolution.

The identification of microorganisms by MALDI-TOF-MS is based on the comparison between the ribosomal protein fingerprint of the microorganism to be tested and the standard protein fingerprint in the database. Although the ribosomal protein size of different microorganisms is different, the molecular weight is basically concentrated in 2000 Da ~ 20,000 Da, and the requirements for the resolution of the instrument are generally about 1000. The resolution, sensitivity, and other performance parameters of the linear mode can fully meet their identification requirements.

26.2.2.2 Reflection Mode

For the pulsed ion source, the delayed extraction technology can eliminate the impact of kinetic energy dispersion on the resolution, but there are still some limitations, including the mass discrimination effect, which is difficult to apply in the detection of continuous ion flow sources. For this reason, B.A. Mamyrin proposed reflective time-of-flight mass spectrometry in 1973. A reflective electrostatic field was placed in the field-free flight zone to improve the problem of ion energy focusing, which to some extent solved the problem of insufficient desorption capacity in linear mode. In the reflection mode, the ionized sample molecules obtain energy under the action of the acceleration voltage and fly into the field-free flight tube. When they fly to the end of the tube, the charged ions enter the reflection field. The ions with high kinetic energy will rush into the deeper reflection area, while the ions with low kinetic energy will be pushed back by the reflection field earlier. Thus, the ions with low kinetic energy can leave the reflection area in less time to make up for the longer flight time in the field-free area. Thus, the mass resolution is greatly improved. In addition, the flight distance of ions in the reflection mode is longer than that in the linear mode, which can further improve the mass resolution.

26.3 Development History, Research and Development (R&D), and Production Status

26.3.1 International MALDI-TOF-MS Development

In 1912, British physicist Joseph John Thomson developed a simple mass spectrometer and discovered the neon isotope, which laid the foundation for the development of mass spectrometry. In 1919, Francis William Aston improved the initial mass spectrometer and developed the first high-precision mass spectrometer. In 1946, W. Stephens first put forward the idea of TOF. Two years later, Cameron and Eggers designed and developed the experimental prototype of the world's TOF-MS. The TOF-MS technology has officially entered practice from the theoretical stage. In 1988, Hillenkamp and Karas, scientists from the University of Münster, Germany, first proposed MALDI. Later, Kenichi Tanaka found that the technology could be used for the analysis of biological macromolecules and published a paper. In 2002, Kenichi Tanaka won the Nobel Prize in Chemistry for his discovery.

26.3.2 Development of MALDI-TOF-MS Technology in China

The research of MALDI-TOF-MS in China started late. In the mid-1980s, the Jiou Group of the Department of Scientific Instrument Engineering of Xiamen University was one of the first units to develop TOF-MS in China. It mainly studied the mass spectrometer of linear and reflective structures, but it was not until 1990 that the first spectrum was obtained on an oscilloscope. In 1987, Zheng Lansun set about establishing a pulsed laser ion source time-of-flight mass spectrometer in the Department of Chemistry of Xiamen University. The ions were obtained by ionizing solid samples with a Nd: Yttrium Aluminum Garnet (YAG) pulsed laser. In 1990, the time-of-flight mass spectrum of aluminum standard samples was obtained for the first time. In the early 1990s, Xu Zhenlin Group of the Department of Precision Instruments of Tianjin University and H. Wollnik's team worked together to develop a high-resolution mass spectrometer. After entering the twenty-first century, although many mass spectrometry manufacturers have emerged in China and made a lot of attempts in terms of the structure and principle of analytical instruments, there is still a certain gap between the overall performance and foreign products, and China's time-of-flight mass spectrometry is still in its infancy and maturity. In 2018, Autobio launched a fully automatic microbial mass spectrometry detection system independently researched, developed, produced, and registered for commercial use in China, and has initially achieved large-scale sales, which has also been sold to many countries abroad, marking that China's MALDI-TOF-MS is gradually being recognized by international peers, and the overall competitiveness of China's mass spectrometry equipment has been greatly improved.

26.3.3 R&D and Production Status

At present, the application in the field of clinical microbiological diagnosis is the main driving force behind the rapid development of MALDI-TOF-MS technology. From the market of MALDI-TOF-MS in China, the market share of imported brands (Bruker, Shimadzu, bioMérieux, etc.) dropped from more than 95% in 2017 to about 65% in 2021. The development of MALDI-TOF-MS in China will enter a "blowout period," relying on the rapid development of national science, technology, and economy. A large number of mass spectrometry R&D and production enterprises have sprung up (see Part V of this section for details). The rapid development of mass spectrometry in China shows that some enterprises have achieved breakthroughs in the key technologies of MALDI-TOF-MS and broken the technological monopoly of imported brands. However, it is reported that some key components of MALDI-TOF-MS still have "choke" technology, such as laser, molecular pump, detector, and other core components, which are restricted by upstream enterprises and still need to be solved.

26.4 Market

China's MALDI-TOF-MS mass spectrometry market was mainly monopolized by imported brands before 2015. By the end of 2021, the installed capacity of microbial mass spectrometers in China has reached about 1500 units, of which Chinese brand mass spectrometers account for about 35%, and the installed capacity is growing rapidly. According to the official statistics of the Statistical Information Center of the National Health and Family Planning Commission at the end of March 2020, there are 2996 tertiary hospitals, 10,404 secondary hospitals, 3384 CDCs (China Center for Disease Control and Prevention), and 3052 maternal and child health care institutions in the country. Referring to the penetration rate of time-of-flight mass spectrometry instruments in foreign clinical microbiology laboratories, it is estimated that in the next 5 years, the number of MALDI-TOF-MS instruments purchased by the Chinese medical system will be about 4000–5000 units, and the Chinese market capacity of instruments and consumables is conservatively estimated to be 7 billion RMB. In the future, with the continuous advancement of China's scientific and technological level, the application direction of mass spectrometers will continue to expand, and the market demand will also continue to increase. From the overall distribution of mass spectrometry brands, bioMérieux and Bruker are still dominant, but with the continuous improvement in competitiveness of domestic brands, the market competition will be more intense in the future.

26.5 Major Production Enterprises in China

According to the official statistics of the National Medical Products Administration (NMPA), as of December 2021, a total of 12 Chinese manufacturers have obtained time-of-flight mass spectrometer medical device registration certificates. See Table 26.1 for details.

26.5.1 Autobio

Autobio started to develop time-of-flight mass spectrometry earlier. After 4 years of research and development, it officially launched the Automated Mass Spectrometry Microbial Identification System Autof ms1000 (hereinafter referred to as Autof

Table 26.1 Time-of-flight mass spectrometry with NMPA registration certificate

Product name	Model specifications	Manufacturer	Approval date
Time-of-flight mass spectrometry system	Clin-Tof-II	Bioyong technologies Inc.	2016/11/1
Time-of-flight mass spectrometry detection system	DR MassARRAY	Guangzhou Darui biotechnology co., ltd.	2018/9/30
Time-of-flight mass spectrometer for microbial identification	microTyper MS	Jiangsu Skyray instrument co., ltd.	2019/6/10
Mass spectrometry detector	M-discover 100, M-discover 100 excellence	Zhuhai Meihua medical technology co., ltd.	2020/2/24
Fully automated microbial mass spectrometry detection system	Autof ms1000, autof ms2000, autof ms600, autof ms800, autof ms1600, autof ms2600	Autobio diagnostics co., ltd.	2020/9/11
Fully automated microbial mass spectrometry detection system	CMI-1600	Guangzhou Hexin instrument co., ltd.	2020/5/27
Matrix-assisted laser desorption ionization time-of-flight mass spectrometer	MS-S800, MS-S820	Medicalsystem biotechnology co., ltd.	2020/5/12
Time-of-flight mass spectrometry detection system	SDxMassARRAY	Jiangsu Simcere medical device co., ltd.	2020/7/14
Fully automated microbial mass spectrometry detection system	EXS1000, EXS2000, EXS2600	Zybio Inc.	2020/8/4
Microbial rapid identification mass spectrometry	Smart MS	Zhuhai DL biotech. Co., ltd.	2020/11/5
Time-of-flight mass spectrometry detection system	DP-TOF	Zhejiang Digena diagnostic technology co., ltd.	2020/12/28
Time-of-flight mass spectrometer	Type I	Rongzhi biotechnology (Qingdao) co., ltd.	2021/6/11

Data source: National Medical Products Administration

ms1000) in September 2017. In April 2018, it received the NMPA certification, mainly used for detection of bacteria, yeast-like fungi, filamentous fungi, and mycobacteria. The database contains 5000 species of microbial protein fingerprints of more than 17,000 strains, ranking in the forefront of the global industry, and the global sales volume has exceeded 500 units, covering many application fields such as medical treatment, disease control, food and medicine, and marine scientific research institutions. In 2020, the sales volume of instruments exceeded the two major imported brands for the first time, and won the trust and recognition of a large number of top-level hospital customers.

Following the Autof ms1000, Autobio successively launched Autof ms2000, Autof ms600, Autof ms800, Autof ms1600, and Autof ms2600 in 2020 to meet the diversified selection needs of users. In the same year, Autobio launched the full-automatic sample adding system AutoMimo 1200, which is equipped with mass spectrometry, greatly liberating laboratory manpower and providing users with an integrated mass spectrometry solution.

26.5.2 Bioyong

Bioyong Technologies Inc. (hereinafter referred to as Bioyong) was founded in 2003. It is the first enterprise focusing on the research and development of clinical mass spectrometry. The time-of-flight mass spectrometry (Clin-Tof-II) produced by Bioyong received the medical device certification from National Medical Products Administration (NMPA) in June 2016. As the first clinical mass spectrometry enterprise in China to obtain an NMPA certification, Clin-Tof-II can achieve rapid, simple, low-cost, and high-throughput detection of microorganisms while ensuring high accuracy and sensitivity. It can be widely used in clinical diagnosis, biological safety, food quality control, environmental safety, and other fields. The database covers more than 7900 strains of 370 genera and 2200 species. In 2017, Bioyong developed a series of new products, detection items, and scientific research services based on the Clin-Tof-II nucleic acid application platform. Due to the high sensitivity and good stability of nucleic acid mass spectrometry detection, it provides a new idea and method for clinical genetic detection.

26.5.3 Zybio

Zybio Inc. (hereinafter referred to as Zybio) is a high-tech enterprise specialized in R&D, manufacture, sales, and technical services of in vitro diagnostic (IVD) reagents and equipment. The company's main product covers clinical chemistry, immunoassay, molecular diagnosis, Point of Care Testing (POCT), hematology, microbiology, pathological and other diagnostic products, and the upstream raw materials.

On May 19, 2020, Zybio officially acquired Xiamen Mass Spectrometry Instrument Co., Ltd. (referred to as Xiamen Mass Spectrometry). On the basis of the original research of Xiamen Mass Spectrometry, the new EXS3000 launched by Zybio obtained the NMPA certification on August 4, 2020. The EXS3000 database contains a local database (2000 species) and a cloud database, with more than 4000 species.

26.5.4 Meihua

Zhuhai Meihua Medical Technology Co., Ltd. (hereinafter referred to as Meihua) is a high-tech enterprise that specializes in R&D, production, sales, and service of clinical IVD instruments and supporting reagents.

The MALDI-TOF-MS mass spectrometry rapid identification system launched by Meihua in 2018 covers nearly 1000 species of bacteria, yeasts, molds, mycobacteria, and other strains, and can be widely used in clinical diagnosis, food and animal (import and export) inspection and quarantine, food processing safety and quality control, environmental microbiology detection, and other fields. On February 24, 2020, Meihua mass spectrometer M-Discover 100 and M-Discover 100 Excellence obtained the NMPA certificate.

26.5.5 IntelliBio

Rongzhi Biotechnology (Qingdao) Co., Ltd. (hereinafter referred to as IntelliBio) is a state-level high-tech company founded by Dr. Zhou Xiaoguang, a senior mass spectrometry R&D expert, specializing in the R&D, production, and sales of life science analytical instruments, consumables, and solutions.

The MALDI-TOF-MS Quan series of IntelliBio can be used in microbial identification, glycosylated hemoglobin, nucleic acid typing, mass spectrometry imaging, and other fields. Among them, Quan TOF I obtained the NMPA certificate on June 11, 2021. The database contains more than 4500 species of microorganisms belonging to 500 genera.

26.5.6 Medicalsystem

Medicalsystem Biotechnology Co., Ltd. (Ningbo) (hereinafter referred to as Medicalsystem) was founded in June 2018. Major industries of Medicalsystem are in vitro diagnostic reagents, instruments, and independent third-party medical diagnostic services.

The MALDI TOF MS-S800 and MALDI TOF MS-S820 of Medicalsystem obtained NMPA certificates on May 12, 2020. The instruments are composed of Mass Spectrometers and identification software (name: MT Master; version number: V1.0), mainly used to identify bacteria and fungi, covering more than 1000 species.

26.5.7 DL

Zhuhai DL Biotech Co., Ltd. (hereinafter referred to as DL) is a Chinese high-tech enterprise specialized in microbial medical instruments and in vitro diagnostic reagents, including Fully automated Microbial Identification/Antibacterial Susceptibility Test (ID/AST) System and Microbial Rapid Identification Mass Spectrometry.

Auto Microbial Rapid Identification Mass Spectrometer System Smart MS uses MALDI-TOF-MS technology to identify clinically isolated bacteria and fungi. The Smart MS database contains peptide mass fingerprinting (PMF) data of more than 180 genera.

26.5.8 Hexin

Guangzhou Hexin Instrument Co., Ltd. (hereinafter referred to as Hexin) was founded in 2004. It is a key high-tech enterprise of China Torch Program integrating mass spectrometer R&D, production, sales, and technical services. It mainly provides customers with mass spectrometers and related technical services.

The automatic microbial mass spectrometry detection system CMI-1600 is a mass spectrometry detection system independently developed by Hexin. The database originated from the research accumulation of China Center for Disease Control and Prevention (CDC) for many years and with quality assurance. It contains more than 3500 species and 68,000 strains of bacteria spectrum, which can meet the detection needs of multiple application fields.

26.5.9 EWAI

Beijing East & West Analytical Instruments, Inc. (hereinafter referred to as EWAI) was founded in 1988. The company's products involve hundreds of Gas Chromatography (GC), Gas Chromatography Mass Spectrometry (GC-MS), High Performance Liquid Chromatography (HPLC), Atomic Absorption Spectroscopy (AAS), Automatic Flight System (AFS), X-Ray Fluorescence Spectrometer (XRF), and related supporting products.

Ebio Reader™ 3700 M is a multifunctional biological information reader developed by EWAI based on MALDI-TOF platform, which can be used for both clinical medical detection and non-clinical fields such as food safety, illegal additives, disease control and prevention, industrial microorganisms, and so on; the database is under construction.

26.5.10 Skyray

The microTyper MS high-throughput microbial rapid identification system is the first commercialized MALDI-TOF-MS in China with completely independent intellectual property rights jointly developed by Jiangsu Skyray Instrument Co., Ltd. (hereinafter referred to as Skyray Instrument) and its holding subsidiary Xiamen Mass Spectrometry. The product is produced and sold by Skyray Instrument Fujian Branch, and was approved by the Fujian Provincial Drug Administration to obtain the NMPA registration certificate on June 10, 2019. The instrument has a supporting database of more than 2300 bacterial species, which can be used for the identification of bacteria and fungi.

In May 2020, Skyray transferred the "MALDI-TOF" business, personnel, and related assets as well as all the "MALDI-TOF" related assets owned by Xiamen Mass Spectrometry to Zybio, with a transaction price of ¥76.16 million. Since then, Skyray Instrument cannot continue to develop and produce MALDI-TOF, but it can continue to sell.

26.5.11 Darui Biotech

Guangzhou Darui Biotechnology Co., Ltd. (hereinafter referred to as Darui Biotech) was founded in 2003 and is a subsidiary of Daan Gene Co., Ltd. It is a biomedical high-tech enterprise integrating in vitro diagnostic products, medical testing, and innovation incubation.

The time-of-flight mass spectrometry detection system DR MassARRAY is an automated medium-throughput gene detection system specially designed for hospitals and clinical detection centers. The system obtained the NMPA registration certificate of Guangdong Food and Drug Administration on September 30, 2018. It is mainly an in vitro diagnostic equipment that detects SNPs on the DNA of living organisms.

26.5.12 Digena

Zhejiang Digena Diagnostic Technology Co., Ltd. (hereinafter referred to as Digena) was founded on July 2, 2018. It is a company that serves the field of life and health with innovative diagnostic technology.

The Dipu (DP)-TOF time-of-flight mass spectrometry detection system is the first approved general-purpose time-of-flight nucleic acid mass spectrometry detection system in China. The system obtained the NMPA registration certificate on December 28, 2020. The product is based on MALDI-TOF-MS technology, which can be used for the detection of known nucleotides in samples derived from living organisms (such as blood, body fluids, and tissues) in combination with supporting reagents. The scope of application covers various fields of biology, such as infectious disease prevention and control, genetic disease detection (birth defect prevention and control), pharmacogenomics (precision medication), cancer analysis of solid tumors and liquid biopsy (tumor prevention and control), health management (functional medicine), and clinical translational medicine research.

26.5.13 Simcere

Jiangsu Simcere Medical Device Co., Ltd. (hereinafter referred to as Simcere) is a precision medical solution provider under Simcere Holdings, a leading pharmaceutical group in China. In February 2017, Simcere Diagnostics was founded on the platform of the "State Key Laboratory of Translational Medicine and Innovative Drug Development" of the Ministry of Science and Technology of the People's Republic of China. By integrating a variety of leading molecular detection platforms and bioinformatics analysis capabilities, Simcere Diagnostics provides medical workers and medical institutions with a decision-making basis for precision medicine in the fields of tumors, autoimmune diseases, infections, and pharmacogenomics. It also provides direct-to-consumer medical testing services.

In March 2018, Simcere and America Agena officially signed a strategic partnership agreement based on MassARRAY nucleic acid mass spectrometry technology platform. On July 14, 2020, the Simcere time-of-flight mass spectrometry detection system SDx MassARRAY obtained the NMPA certificate, which is mainly an in vitro diagnostic equipment for detecting SNPs on the DNA of living organisms.

Declaration Zengli Yang, Keya Cai, Gaoling Zhao and Meili Liu are employees of Autobio Diagnostics Co., Ltd.

Zhimin Lin is an employee of Zybio Inc.

Tandem Mass Spectrometry

27

Quan Ji, Zhimin Lin, Sixing Chen, and Zengli Yang

The tandem mass spectrometry, in which two or more mass spectrometers are integrated, is a combination of two-step mass analyzers in time or space. The spatial tandem mass spectrometry is made up of two or more mass analyzers, including common triple quadrupole tandem mass spectrometry (QQQ), quadrupole linear ion trap mass spectrometry (Q-TRAP), and quadrupole time-of-flight tandem mass spectrometry (Q-TOF).

The triple quadrupole mass spectrometry is characterized by an excellent quantitative capability, as well as high sensitivity and robust qualitative capability. In addition to the general full-scan functionality, it also supports such modes as multiple-reaction monitoring (MRM), precursor ion scanning and product ion scanning, and neutral loss scanning, making it a useful tool for the research on the structures of characteristic groups. The liquid chromatography-triple quadrupole tandem mass spectrometry, in which liquid chromatography is coupled to tandem mass spectrometry (LC-MS/MS), features a higher sensitivity and a more powerful quantitative capability. Currently, LC-MS/MS has been widely applied in the industries of pharmaceuticals, medicine, health, environmental protection, food, etc.

27.1 Technical History

A mass spectrometer with two or more mass analyzers coupled together is called a tandem mass spectrometer. In the early 1980s, on the basis of the conventional mass spectrometry procedures, a new technology of tandem mass spectrometry emerged.

Q. Ji (✉) · Z. Lin · S. Chen
Zybio Inc., Chongqing, China
e-mail: jiquan@zy-ivd.com

Z. Yang
Autobio Diagnostics Co., Ltd., Zhengzhou, Henan, China

H. Song, L. Dai (eds.), *In Vitro Diagnostic Industry in China*,
https://doi.org/10.1007/978-981-99-3110-1_27

The development of the magnetic sector mass spectrometry and hybrid quadrupole tandem mass spectrometry advanced the double-stage mass spectrometry (MS/MS) technique to the triple-stage mass spectrometry (MS/MS/MS), for which scanning modes were greatly expanded. Due to a variety of mass analyzers, there are diversified tandem mass spectrometry techniques. The common ones include triple quadrupole tandem mass spectrometry (QQQ), quadrupole ion trap mass spectrometry (Q-TRAP), quadrupole time-of-flight tandem mass spectrometry (Q-TOF), hybrid quadrupole and magnetic mass spectrometry (QQB), and multiple sector magnetic mass spectrometry (BBB). The triple quadrupole mass spectrometry had its origin in 1981 when Rick Yost published an article on selective ion fragmentation, which triggered a new era of triple quadrupole analytical techniques [1]. In the article, the author described the principles of the triple quadrupole mass analyzer and the advantages of its practical applications for the first time.

27.2 Principle Description

In 1952, Wolfgang Paul (Professor of Physics at the University of Bonn, Germany) et al. [2] put forward and experimentally validated the idea of filtering ions using the radio-frequency quadrupole electric field, leading to the birth of quadrupole mass analyzers available today, based on which triple quadrupole mass spectrometry was developed. In a triple quadrupole mass spectrometer, upon the ionization of the analyte by the ion source, the analyte is transferred into the quadrupole, and the applied electric potential on the quadrupole creates a quadrupole electric field, under which the ions deflects, and only the ions satisfying certain conditions can pass through the quadrupole, while other ions hit the electrode. The quadrupole analyzer consists of four precisely machined hyperbolic electrodes. The Radio Frequency (RF) voltages with the same amplitude and a phase difference of 180° are applied to the two pairs of horizontal and vertical electrodes, respectively. A cross section of the electrode system is shown in Fig. 27.1.

Where r_0 denotes the radius of the in-circle of the four electrodes, U is the DC voltage component in the RF power supply, V is the AC voltage component in the RF power supply, $\omega = 2\pi f$ represents the angular frequency of the AC voltage, f is the AC voltage frequency, and t is the time. As the potential indicated in Fig. 27.1 is applied to the corresponding pole, the field space enclosed by the quadrupole electrodes will generate an electric field distribution as follows:

$$\Phi(x,y,t) = (U - V\cos\omega t)\frac{(x^2 - y^2)}{r_0^2} \tag{27.1}$$

The motion of ions in the quadrupole field constitutes the basis for ion binding and mass analysis by the quadrupole, for which solution can be performed based on Newton's Second Law. The stability of the motion of ions may be described with the solution of the Mathieu Equation, from which the formulas for the two important parameters a and q [3] can be obtained:

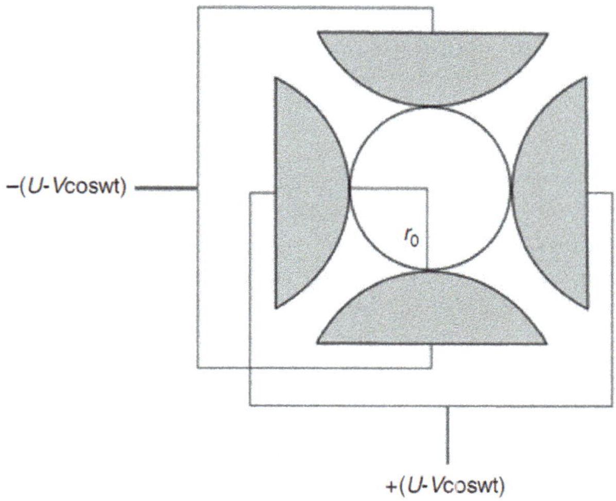

Fig. 27.1 Schematic diagram of cross section of the quadrupole analyzer

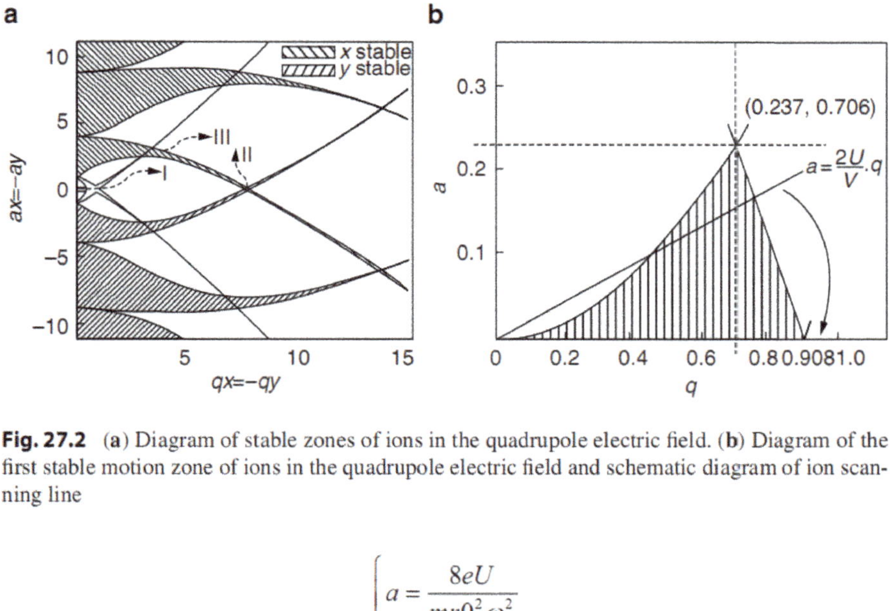

Fig. 27.2 (**a**) Diagram of stable zones of ions in the quadrupole electric field. (**b**) Diagram of the first stable motion zone of ions in the quadrupole electric field and schematic diagram of ion scanning line

$$\begin{cases} a = \dfrac{8eU}{mr0^{2}\omega^{2}} \\ \hline q = \dfrac{4eV}{mr_{0}^{2}\omega^{2}} \end{cases} \tag{27.2}$$

The stable motion zones of ions in the quadrupole electric field are plotted from a and q, as shown in Fig. 27.2:

As shown in Fig. 27.2a, ions show multiple stable motion zones, and it is necessary to ensure the stability in the x and y directions simultaneously, such as zones I, II, and III, to enable ions to pass through the quadrupole smoothly. Theoretically, all x–y stable motion zones can be used as the working zones for quadrupole mass spectrometry.

Currently, all the commonly used quadrupole mass analyzers operate in the first stable motion zone, as shown in Fig. 27.2b. The ranges of a and q within the first stable motion zone are $0 < a < 0.237$ and $0 < q < 0.908$, respectively. If (a, q) falls within the first stable motion zone, the corresponding ion can pass through the quadrupole electrode system; otherwise, the radius of motion of ions in the x or y direction will become increasingly larger until it finally escapes from the field space. The principles of the quadrupole as a mass analyzer is to continuously alter the DC and AC voltages so that only the ions of a certain mass-to-charge ratio can reach the detector at a certain moment, and these ion signals are recorded separately to obtain the mass spectra of the ions of various mass-to-charge ratios.

The above is the working principle of the single quadrupole mass spectrometry, which features simple structure, low cost, easy maintenance, and high quantification capability, as well as obvious drawbacks. The major drawbacks include low resolution, poor specificity, interference from adjacent m/z ions, and difficulty in qualitative analysis, all of which, however, have been well resolved due to the emerging tandem mass spectrometry. Tandem mass spectrometry induces molecular ion cleavage by second mass spectrometry, which is conducive to the research on the relationship between precursor ions and fragments. It provides the structural information of molecular ions, and quantifies the sample by multiple-reaction monitoring (MRM) to significantly improve the specificity. In the triple quadrupole mass spectrometry system, the collision cell at the early stage is also made up of quadrupoles. Therefore, it is referred to as a triple quadrupole mass spectrometer.

27.3 Development Trend of Triple Quadrupole Mass Spectrometry

The triple quadrupole technology has developed for over 40 years and its working principles have been well established. With the continuous advancement of science and technology, the growing demand for applications, and the constant investments from mass spectrometry system manufacturers, continuous development and progress of the triple quadrupole technology has been promoted. The technical upgrades mainly focus on more efficient and stable ion sources, and higher ion transmission efficiency, resolution, and fragmentation and detection efficiency. Furthermore, user friendly, intelligence, and portability also become the development trends.

27.3.1 Atmospheric Pressure Interface

The atmospheric pressure interface is a key component of a mass spectrometer and plays two significant roles in a mass spectrometry system: one is to limit the inlet airflow and the other is to transmit ions from the atmospheric pressure zone to the low vacuum zone. As a mass analyzer generally operates under high vacuum, in order to maintain the vacuum inside the mass spectrometer, an atmospheric pressure interface such as a capillary or an orifice is commonly used to restrict the airflow.

However, while limiting the flow, the atmospheric pressure interface also limits the effective ion collection area due to its size, and thus only a small part of ions can enter into the atmospheric pressure interface. Furthermore, once ions enter into the flow limiting device, the Coulomb force between ions diffuses the ions outward and thereby results in secondary losses. When ions enter into the low vacuum zone via the atmospheric pressure interface, the ion beam further diverges due to the ultrasonic expansion arising from the high air pressure difference. Ultimately, the ion transmission efficiency is typically less than 0.2%. Therefore, the development of the atmospheric pressure interface technology is mainly concentrated on the improvement of the ion collection efficiency.

27.3.2 Ion Transmission

The ion transmission zone is mainly located between the atmospheric pressure interface and the mass analyzer, with the function of efficiently transmitting the ions introduced via the atmospheric pressure interface to the mass analyzer so as to complete the processes of further ionization, removal of neutral molecules, and vacuum transition of charged droplets. As both airflow and electric field have a large impact on the ion motion state within this zone, the ion motion is highly complex, and it is also one of the zones with the most serious ion loss. Therefore, major mass spectrometry system manufacturers have been introducing various devices and technologies to improve the performance of their instruments with respect to this zone, for example, ion funnel and RF multipoles.

The ion funnel technology has its origin on the stacked-ring ion guide (SRIG), and consists of a series of pellet metal electrodes arranged at intervals. RF and DC voltages are applied to the metal electrodes, with the RF voltage for ion binding and the DC voltage to produce a gradient field for ion transmission. Ion funnels are ideally suitable for operation in the vacuum zone of tens to hundreds of Pa, and are therefore generally arranged after the capillary for the first-step ion transmission. In some mass spectrometry systems, in order to improve the capability to filter neutral molecules and ion transmission efficiency, multiple ion funnels are connected in off-axis tandem, such as the off-axis dual ion funnels employed by Agilent.

The RF-only multipole ion guide is the most widely used ion transmission device in the mass spectrometry system, which features simple structure, high ion transmission efficiency, easy driving, etc. These multipoles mainly include quadrupole, hexapole, octopole, and dodecapole. The quadrupole ion guide has the strongest ion-binding capability and the highest transmission efficiency, while the dodecapole ion guide provides the broadest mass transmission range and is more suitable for operation under a slightly higher air pressure. For the purpose of improving the ion transmission efficiency, capability to filter neutral molecules, mass transmission range, and operating pressure, the multipole ion guide has a variety of variants with respect to the structure, such as segmented quadrupole, square quadrupole, and curved multipole.

27.3.3 Collision Cell

The collision cell is positioned between two quadrupole mass analyzers. As the collision cell in the early days was also designed with a quadrupole structure, the mass spectrometry system formed by three quadrupoles was called triple quadrupole mass spectrometry. The collision cell serves as a place for the precursor ions to produce fragment ions and is one of the key components of the triple quadrupole mass spectrometer. At present, the collision cells from major mass spectrometer manufacturers are designed with multi-electrode rods or rings, most of which are multipoles, such as quadrupole, hexapole, and octopole, with a wider mass transmission range for higher-order multipoles compared to the quadrupole. The development trend of the collision cell technology is mainly centered on the improvement of collision-induced dissociation efficiency, enhancing the capability to remove the interference from neutral molecules, and solving MRM crosstalk.

The collision dissociation efficiency is related to the collision energy, the neutral molecule size, as well as the operating air pressure of the collision cell. The ion fragmentation efficiency can be improved by increasing the collision energy or the operating air pressure. It is an effective approach to increase the collision energy by applying a linear accelerating electric field to the collision cell, for example, the linear high-pressure collision cell technology introduced by Agilent, which can improve the fragmentation efficiency by increasing the air pressure inside the collision cell and accelerating the ions axially. Moreover, to better filter out neutral molecules, linear collision cells have been gradually replaced by curved (90- or 180-degree) ones. In a curved collision cell, the charged ions move along the curved path, while the neutral molecules remain in linear motion and are filtered out. MRM crosstalk refers to a condition that the MRM product ions from the next channel enter into the collision cell before the MRM product ions from the previous channel have completely passed through the collision cell. In the event that the product ions for the previous MRM have the same mass-to-charge ratio as the product ions for the next MRM, the signal of the product ions from the previous channel will have an effect on the signal of the next channel, leading to a false positive result. An effective way to resolve MRM crosstalk is to shorten the time for ions to pass through the collision cell, and a typical solution is to apply a DC gradient electric field between the inlet and outlet.

27.4 Advantages and Disadvantages of LC-MS/MS

The LC-MS/MS technique has distinct advantages, especially in the detection of small molecules at low concentrations. It is extensively used in developed countries such as Europe and the United States. The technical advantages of the triple quadrupole mass spectrometry primarily include high sensitivity and specificity, low sample consumption, and multiple tests on the same blood sample. The distribution of the most important performance indices is shown in Fig. 27.3.

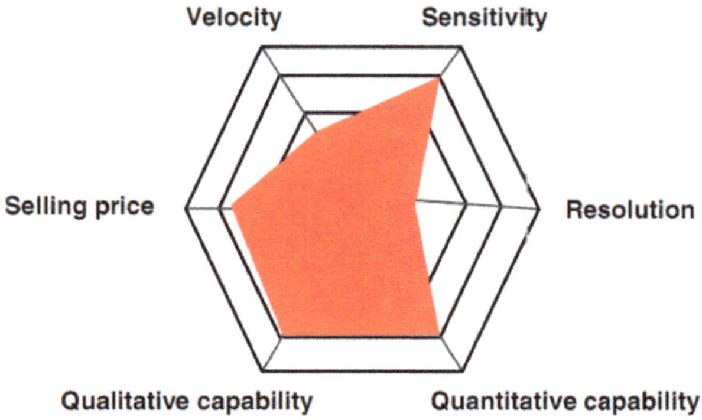

Fig. 27.3 Distribution of characteristics of triple quadrupole mass spectrometry

27.4.1 High Sensitivity and Specificity

Currently, the LC-MS/MS instruments are provided with the sensitivity of ppt and ppb grades, for which they play an irreplaceable role in clinical testing. LC-MS/MS is a procedure to effectively separate substances using a chromatographic system, and then analyze the composition or structure of the substances by using the mass spectrometry to determine the ion strength based on the mass-to-charge ratio (*m/z*) difference. The triple quadrupole mass spectrometer delivers a wide range of ion scanning capabilities, with multiple scan modes besides the general full-scan mode. For example, for a precursor ion scan, Q1 is used to determine the precursor ion and Q3 to determine some specific fragment ion, thereby enabling the monitoring of a specific molecule in a highly complex mixture. For a neutral loss scan, the combination of Q1 and Q3 analyzers maximizes the sensitivity. In addition, there are reaction monitoring scan (SRM) mode and multiple-reaction monitoring scan (MRM) mode to avoid the impact of structural analogs.

27.4.2 Low Sample Consumption

An accurate analysis of a sample at the microliter or microgram level can be carried out.

27.4.3 Multiple Tests on One Blood Sample

The simultaneous evaluation of various indices is often involved in any screening operation, while conventional immunological procedures generally evaluate only one index in a single analysis, for which there are limitations on the throughput and costs of testing. LC-MS/MS has a simultaneous multi-component analysis capability to reduce the costs of a single test. Therefore, LC-MS/MS is expected to serve as a powerful tool for screening tests.

However, the detection technique with LC-MS/MS also has significant drawbacks, which limit its extensive clinical use, especially in less developed regions. The drawbacks of this technique mainly include high instrumentation costs, difficulty in personnel training, difficulty in standardization of clinical tests, complexity of pre-treatment, and limited related policies and industry standards.

27.4.4 High Cost of Instrument and Initial Investment

LC-MS/MS devices are high in cost, mostly imported from abroad, and require supporting accessories (nitrogen generator, Uninterruptible Power Supply (UPS), and sample pre-treatment supporting devices), as well as a laboratory with appropriate temperature and humidity. Furthermore, their daily maintenance costs are also high. Therefore, there is still a long way to go before LC-MS/MS is fully generalized and widely applied. Though the mass spectrometry platform features a demanding working environment and substantial one-time input, in the long run the costs of reagents for an individual sample .will be significantly lower than that of conventional immunoassay methods.

27.4.5 High Technical Expertise and Lack of Talents

The use of a mass spectrometer requires a complicated procedure such as sample pre-treatment, which places much more demand on the laboratory technicians compared to the existing conventional equipment. Apart from the need for talents with both clinical and mass spectrometry testing knowledge, there are also urgent needs for trained personnel in equipment maintenance and laboratory management. Moreover, large amount of data are generated by mass spectrometry, which makes the quantitative analysis more complicated.

27.4.6 Difficult Standardization of Clinical Testing

Currently, the majority of clinical testing using LC-MS/MS are laboratory developed test (LDT) without proper quality controls, making it difficult to trace the test results to reference substances. There are different brand manufacturers for the mass spectrometers for clinical use, even different models under the same brand. For different instruments, samples, and substances to be tested, it is often necessary to establish different pre-treatment and detection methods, for which it is difficult to standardize the detection using LC-MS/MS.

27.4.7 Complicated Pre-Treatment and Low Automation Level

The composition of clinical specimens is often very complicated. The high sensitivity of the mass spectrometer instruments requires pre-treatment of samples to remove the interfering components. Different sample pre-treatment methods are required to be optimized based on different sample types and analytes with different physicochemical properties. For the complicated sample pre-treatment requirements, manual operations are always required, making it difficult to conduct automated clinical testing. Compared to biochemistry/immunoassay methods, there are difficulties with LC-MS/MS technique for random insertion of any urgent samples, and the reporting period is longer (at least one working day), making it impossible to satisfy the requirements of any test with small sample size and rapid reporting of results.

27.4.8 Shortage of Criteria and Guidelines

At present, there are few standards, guidelines, experts' consensus, or other normative documents available for the application of the LC-MS/MS technique in clinical testing. Furthermore, the application of clinical laboratory testing equipment often requires relevant certificates with national recognition, while the equipment at many manufacturers does not have such certificates yet. Meanwhile, there is a lack of regulations on test admission and pricing, and LC-MS/MS test is not currently in the directory of insured drugs, which has restricted its development.

Fig. 27.4 Market size of global mass spectrometry and LC-MS/MS clinical applications

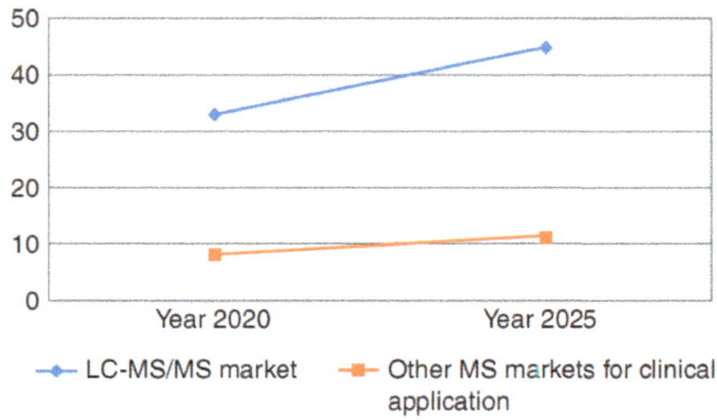

27.5 LC-MS/MS Market Conditions

27.5.1 International LC-MS/MS Market

27.5.1.1 International LC-MS/MS Market Continues to Grow

As estimated by "MarketsandMarkets," the global mass spectrometry market will reach $4.1 billion in 2020 (Fig. 27.4), of which LC-MS/MS tests account for approximately 80%, which is $3.3 billion. End-users include institutions such as medical institutions, pharmaceutical companies, and life science institutes, where LC-MS/MS tests by pharmaceutical companies in North America have accounted for the largest market share, while new screening and vitamin tests in China are the applications with the largest share.

The mass spectrometry market is expected to reach $5.6 billion by 2025, with an average annual growth rate of 6.5%, and the share of LC-MS/MS is expected to remain at about 80%, or about $4.5 billion.

27.5.1.2 Factors Driving Industry Growth

Factors driving the industry growth mainly include investment in new drug development and increased application in developing countries.

1. Investment in new drug R&D

   Over the past 20 years, investment in pharmaceutical R&D has been increasing. Pharmaceutical enterprises and life-science-related institutions have always been highly sought after by the capital industry, and it is estimated that 18.9% of all investment project funds were invested in pharmaceutical R&D in Europe in 2018. However, mass spectrometry has taken an important place in pharmaceutical R&D, from early drug development to later drug evaluation and then to clinical trials, all of which require accurate detection of drug concentrations. Therefore, with the continuous investment in drug development, it is expected to stimulate the growth of the mass spectrometry market.
2. Increased applications in developing countries.

   The increase in mass spectrometry applications in developing countries, especially in China and India, represents a significant driving factor for the future growth of the global mass spectrometry industry, providing a huge demand for mass spectrometry applications. Currently, the application of mass spectrometry in these two countries is still not well developed and the application field is also limited. In the future, with the continuous expansion of new drug R&D and clinical application of mass spectrometry in developing countries, the scale of mass spectrometry industry is expected to expand rapidly and drive the promotion and application of mass spectrometry technology worldwide.

27.5.2 Chinese LC-MS/MS Market

27.5.2.1 The Chinese LC-MS/MS Market Is Still in the Start-Up Period with Relatively Slow Growth of Market Size

The global mass spectrometry market has a development history of over 100 years. Comparatively speaking, China had a relatively late start in the development of mass spectrometry technology and a relatively shortage of talent pool, and it was only until after 2000 that it started to develop mass spectrometry technology progressively. In 2006, Beijing East & West Analytical Instruments, Inc. launched a quadrupole gas-mass spectrometer GC-MS-3100, which was the first commercial mass spectrometry product in China. Presently, only one company in China has launched its self-developed commercial LC-MS/MS instruments, and most of the companies selected foreign manufacturers as "Original Equipment Manufacturer (OEM)," or sold their own testing products on the platforms of international manufacturers.

Since there is a certain gap between the medical market in China and that in developed countries such as Europe and the United States, the clinical application market of mass spectrometry in China is still in the start-up period, and mass spectrometry has not been widely applied in the medical industry, and the industry scale is growing relatively slowly.

The market size of mass spectrometry in the medical industry in China amounted to about RMB 2 billion in 2017, and grew to RMB 2.5 billion in 2019, and the market for LC-MS/MS applications was RMB 2 billion, with a compound annual growth rate of 11.8% (as shown in Fig. 27.5). The major types of mass spectrometers commonly used in the biopharmaceutical field are LC-MS/MS, gas chromatography mass spectrometry (GC-MS), Q-TOF-MS/Orbitrap, and matrix-assisted laser desorption ionization (MALDI)-TOF, with LC-MS/MS being the major model for clinical detection. The LC-MS/MS application market was RMB 1.6 billion in 2017, accounting for about 80% of the market for all mass spectrometry applications, which grew to RMB 2 billion in 2019, still accounting for about 80%.

27.5.2.2 The Market Development Space Is Enormous with Good Prospect for LC-MS/MS Clinical Application

LC-MS/MS has been applied in several clinical testing fields due to its performance characteristics. However, different from foreign countries, the main application

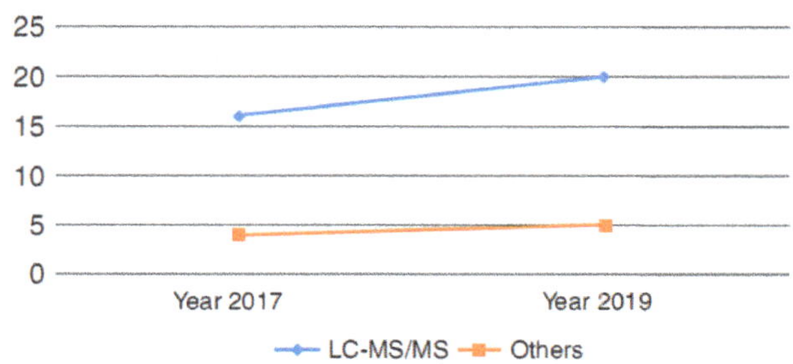

Fig. 27.5 Market size of LC-MS/MS clinical applications in China (Unit: RMB 100 million). (Data source: Terminal access, collated by Zybio)

areas in China are newborn screening and vitamin detection, with other scenarios still to be developed, including drug concentration detection, hormone detection, etc.

Neonatal Screening

LC-MS/MS is mainly applied to screen newborns for inherited metabolic disease (IMD), a type of disease resulting from the accumulation of genetic metabolites or deficiencies of important physiological substances caused by defects in the genetic metabolic pathway, causing corresponding clinical symptoms. It involves metabolic abnormalities of several substances such as amino acids, organic acids, fatty acids, steroids, and vitamins, and may result in damage to several systems. In 1991, Millington et al. [4] utilized MS/MS techniques for the first time to detect multiple amino acids and acylcarnitine in dried blood filter sheets for newborn screening. A series of subsequent laboratory efforts also verified the advancement and rationality of this approach. In 2002, Xuefan Gu et al. introduced LC-MS/MS to China, thereby enabling increasingly widespread application of LC-MS/MS in the detection of genetic metabolic diseases.

The mass spectrometry enables multiple tests on one blood sample, and the more the tests the lower the average cost. In traditional neonatal screening for genetic metabolic diseases, immunological methodology is mostly employed that only one disease can be detected at a time. The mass spectrometry technique enables the simultaneous analysis of nearly 100 metabolites and the detection of over 40 genetic metabolic diseases in a few minutes, thereby greatly improving the screening efficiency, making it an important tool for IMD screening, and has been widely applied for IMD screening and its clinical detection outside of China. The American College of Medical Genetics (ACMG) has included 54 genetic disorders into the newborn screening program, including 29 primary and 25 secondary disorders, and LC-MS/MS is widely applied for screening. In China, genetic metabolic diseases are eligible for subsidies include neonatal phenylketonuria (PKU), congenital hypothyroidism (CH), and, in some southern regions, congenital adrenocortical hyperplasia (CAH), and glucose-6-phosphate dehydrogenase deficiency (G-6-PD). The remaining over 40 tests are out-of-pocket and are optional based on family history of genetic disorders.

Currently, a number of hospitals and medical service institutions nationwide have launched programs for genetic metabolic disease testing by tandem mass spectrometry, and these institutions are mainly centralized in maternal and child health hospitals in the Yangtze River Delta, Pearl River Delta, Beijing, and Tianjin. Xinhua Hospital, Zhejiang Children's Hospital, and Guangdong Maternal and Child Health Hospital are the first medical institutions to adopt this technology. The current model adopted in most places is to have additional items of own choice based on family genetic history on top of the government subsidized items, involving more than 40 items in total, at a combined cost of up to RMB 500–1500 per person. Given the fact that most families are not knowledgeable about family medical history, a simple traditional screening for three to four diseases may be preferred in the short term. However, the cost-effectiveness benefits are expected to become increasingly apparent in the future as more newborn screening programs become available.

Taking into account the continued impact of the newly adopted multiple-child policy, the number of future annual births is expected to be above 15 million. The average national newborn screening rate was 39% in 2007 and over 50% in 2010, and is expected to reach 70% in the next 5 years. Based on the mass spectrometry detection rate of 40% and a per capita cost of RMB 300, the market space is estimated to be about RMB 1.8 billion. In the future, with the increase in mass spectrometry penetration, the prospect of the market is promising.

Vitamin Testing

Vitamins are important active substances for maintaining the health of the human body, which participate in the normal metabolic and cellular regulation processes of living organisms and are necessary for human growth and development. Insufficient or lack of vitamin intake may result in a relatively large impact on human health. Therefore, the vitamin levels in the human body have attracted extensive attention from nutritionists and clinicians, and accurate test results can assist them in accurately assessing the nutritional status, impaired absorption, or toxicity levels of vitamins in the human body. Different vitamins feature different molecular structures, chemical properties, as well as physiological concentrations with thousand-fold differences, making accurate detection of vitamins a challenge from sample handling to assay methods. The article "Application of Liquid Chromatography-Tandem Mass Spectrometry in Vitamin Detection," published in *Chinese Journal of Laboratory Medicine*, recommends using LC-MS/MS to achieve accurate detection of vitamin levels.

Currently, Vitamin D testing has the largest market in China. As a fat-soluble vitamin, vitamin D is involved in several physiological processes in the human body and has been significantly associated with the incidence of not only orthopedic diseases, but also autoimmune system, infectious diseases, cancer, and cardiovascular diseases. According to statistics, there are 1 billion people worldwide with vitamin D deficiency (serum concentration less than 20 μg/L), and the introduction of a high-throughput and high-accuracy LC-MS/MS testing technology to assess vitamin D levels presents excellent market value and application prospects. In practical operations, Vitamin D testing is mainly performed on perinatal women, newborns, and middle-aged and elderly people.

Depending on the level of hospital and methodology, a traditional vitamin D test may cost RMB 100–200. According to estimates by China International Capital Corporation limited (CICC), assuming that the cost of vitamin D testing is RMB 150 per person, and the testing rates for perinatal women, newborns, and the elderly over 60 years old are 40%, 40%, and 5%, respectively, the mass spectrometry market of vitamin D is over RMB 7.6 billion.

Therapeutic Drug Monitoring

Therapeutic drug monitoring (TDM) refers to the observation of drug efficacy in the process of clinical drug therapy; meanwhile, the administration of drug regimen is adjusted by measuring the concentration of total drug components in blood, urine, and saliva, in conjunction with clinical characteristics and pharmacokinetics and pharmacodynamics, so as to improve the efficacy and reduce the probability of toxic side effects.

Drugs theoretically requiring TDM are mainly: (1) drugs with low therapeutic index, limited safety range, and strong toxic reactions; (2) drugs with large individual differences in pharmacokinetics; (3) drugs with non-linear kinetic characteristics; (4) drugs that are consumed for a long time and the efficacy of which cannot be easily and quickly judged, etc. In China, the development of TDM is still at an early stage, with existing clinical guidelines available for reference, such as the 128 psychotropic drugs specified in the Arbeitsgemeinschaft für Neuropsychopharmakologie und Pharmakopsy- chiatrie *(AGNP) Consensus Guidelines for Psychiatric Therapeutic Drug Monitoring: 2011* in 2011 and the 15 drugs identified in the *Expert Consensus on Therapeutic Drug Monitoring in Children* of the Chinese Medical Association Branch Clinical Pharmacology Group in 2015.

The *Expert Consensus on Specifications for Therapeutic Drug Monitoring (2019 Edition)* has listed the analytical techniques for determining drug concentrations (primarily blood drug concentrations) in biological samples, which mainly include technical methods such as spectroscopic analysis, chromatographic analysis, liquid chromatography-mass spectrometry, and immunological detection, with liquid chromatography-mass spectrometry and high-performance liquid chromatography recommended for drug monitoring in terms of specificity. According to estimates, the market for psychiatric mass spectrometry in China is about RMB 540 million, and the market for immunosuppressive drugs for organ transplantation is about RMB three million, with a total market of about RMB 600 million along with other minor drug classes.

Steroid Hormones

Presently, chemiluminescence serves as the main method used for steroid hormone detection; however, the wide variety of steroid hormones in the human body with similar structures is prone to cross-interference. For example, the structures of estradiol and testosterone are extremely close to each other, and the amount of estradiol in the female body is several times higher than that of testosterone. Even if only a small percentage of estradiol and testosterone assay reagents cross-react, this could result in serious errors in the results of the immunoassay for testosterone in women. Second, steroid hormone testing has placed higher demands on the performance of the testing instruments. In most of the normal human body fluid samples, steroid hormone levels are extremely low, generally at the ng/mL level, and plasma 21-deoxycortisol even to the pg/mL level. Therefore, steroid hormone testing requires high sensitivity and specificity of the methodology.

This year, LC-MS/MS testing for steroid hormones has become a main choice for medical testing laboratories. Besides the high sensitivity, LC-MS/MS test samples are subject to pre-treatment before testing, which usually removes proteins, including hormone-binding proteins, and additionally removes impurity interferences; consequently, the specificity is significantly improved. In an article published in the *Chinese Journal of Laboratory Medicine* in 2019, "Liquid

Chromatography-Mass Spectrometry for Steroid Hormone Testing: Methodological Changes for Precision Diagnosis," it is reported that LC-MS/MS is leading the methodological changes in clinical steroid hormone testing.

In addition to instrumentation costs, pre-treatment represents another major challenge for steroid hormone mass spectrometry. Due to the relatively low concentration in vivo, the pre-treatment requires the removal of as many impurities as possible while retaining and concentrating the substance to be tested. For clinical test, the accessibility of the pre-treatment method is also very important. The commonly applied pre-treatment methods for clinical use include protein precipitation, liquid–liquid extraction, and solid-phase extraction, of which solid-phase extraction methods can use commercial extraction plates and are relatively easy and safe to operate.

According to Frost & Sullivan estimates, the market size of chemiluminescence detection of steroid hormones in China amounted to RMB 5 billion in 2019, and if LC-MS/MS can take over 50% of the market in the future, the market space can reach RMB 2.5 billion.

27.5.3 Future Trends

27.5.3.1 The Clinical Application Market for LC-MS/MS in China Has a Significant Upward Potential

According to a grassroots industry research, clinical mass spectrometry testing in the United States accounts for about 15% of the total medical testing market, and the size of the US clinical mass spectrometry market is about USD 9 billion. In benchmarking with the market share of clinical mass spectrometry in the United States, the market size of medical testing terminal in China is about RMB 200 billion, and the potential market of clinical mass spectrometry is about RMB 30 billion. According to a grassroots research, most of the mass spectrometry in Independent Clinical Laboratories (ICLs) in China are only at the level of RMB ten million, among which the relatively large ones are Guangzhou Kingmed and Beijing Harmony Health with the total not exceeding RMB 300 million. We estimate that the total size of mass spectrometry market in China is no more than RMB 2 billion, accounting for no more than 1% of the total medical testing market, which is still

Table 27.1 Comparison of liquid chromatography tandem mass spectrometry markets in China and the United States

	China	United States
Total market size	RMB 2 billion	USD 9 billion
Percentage of total testing market	<1%	15%
Number of test items	About 100 items	About 500 items
Instrument holdings and increment	250 sets, with an annual increase of 100 sets	3000 sets, with an annual increase of 700 sets
Number of mass spectrometers in each first-line hospital	<10 sets	40–60 sets

Note: All figures in the table are for 2017

Data source: Broker Research Report, network, collated by Zybio much less than the 15% in the United States. The comparison of the mass spectrometry market between China and the United States is shown in Table 27.1.

27.5.3.2 Central Hospitals Are Gradually Attaching Importance to Mass Spectrometry, Accelerating the Entry of LC-MS/MS into Hospitals

Due to the relatively high sensitivity of LC-MS/MS, and the obvious advantage of detecting low concentrations of substances, many central hospitals in China have established their own LC-MS/MS testing platforms, such as Peking Union Medical College Hospital, Beijing Fuwai Hospital, Beijing Anding Hospital, Shanghai Zhongshan Hospital, Shanghai Xuhui Central Hospital, and Sichuan Huaxi Hospital. In 2018, the Shanghai Municipal Health Care Commission released the *Assessment Criteria for Grade III General Hospitals in Shanghai* (2018 Edition), which included LC-MS/MS and time-of-flight mass spectrometry in the assessment criteria for First-class Hospital at Grade 3. It can be seen that in China, LC-MS/MS testing is being gradually recognized in leading hospitals and its use is expected to continue to expand.

27.5.4 The Emergence of the LC-MS/MS Testing Market Is Pending the Maturation of the ICL Testing Market

27.5.4.1 Reasons for the Limitation in the Development of the Mass Spectrometry Industry in China

The development of mass spectrometry industry in China is limited by two important factors: (1) large investment in the instrument in early stage; and (2) complicated instrument operation and high requirements for operators. For leading hospitals, though they have the financial strength to purchase instruments, the complicated operation consumes a lot of labor costs. In addition, leading hospitals in China tend to use automated instruments to improve efficiency due to the large number of patients admitted and the high workload. And, LC-MS/MS places a relatively high financial pressure and sample pressure on Grade I and II hospitals.

27.5.4.2 Established Independent Clinical Laboratory Can Contribute to the Rise of the LC-MS/MS Testing Market

Due to the high operator requirements and initial investment in LC-MS/MS, testing institutions are required to train dedicated personnel and then rely on a large number of samples to recover costs. It is possible for third parties to purchase a large number of high-priced high-end testing equipment only after the formation of the scale effect of testing; it will also bring a large number of testing samples.

In addition, as LC-MS/MS enables "multiple tests on one blood sample," the cost of individual testing is lower when more samples are tested; therefore, when ICL is in a large scale, the use of LC-MS/MS is more likely to reduce operating costs. In the United States, the ICL is relatively well developed, accounting for approximately 34% of the overall laboratory testing market. The mature ICL market has provided the soil for the development of the LC-MS/MS testing industry.

27.5.4.3 The ICL Market in China Is Developing and Progressively Maturing

Currently, the overall ICL industry in China is characterized as "small, scattered, and vulnerable." As of the end of 2020, there were 48,919 testing institutions in China, of which 6414 have an annual revenue of over RMB ten million, accounting for only 13.11% of the entire industry, and 47,173 small and micro testing organizations with less than 100 employees, accounting for 96.43% of the total number of organizations (Data Source: Broker Research Report). On the other hand, the ICL in China is also at a high growth stage. By the end of 2020, the number of total testing institutions in China increased by 11.16% compared to 2019.

The related laws and policies in China are being gradually improved, which is expected to promote the rapid development of the industry. On June 1, 2021, the newly revised *Regulations for the Supervision and Administration of Medical Devices* in China came into force. In accordance with Article 53 of the Regulations, for in vitro diagnostic reagents that are not yet available in China with the same variety of products on the market, the specific management of eligible medical measures shall be developed by the drug regulatory department under the State Council jointly with the competent health department under the State Council. The new Regulations for the first time legislatively and explicitly conferred the legal status of Laboratory Developed Test (LDT) in the in vitro diagnostic industry. Second, with the reform in medical insurance payment methods in China, the laboratory departments are likely to become a cost growth sector in hospitals, which will certainly lead to a large number of samples sent out for testing, and can also vigorously promote the development of ICL industry.

27.5.5 The Industry Is Gradually Standardized to Boost the Market Development

Previously, the mass spectrometry industry in China had been lacking in related industry norms, and the industry development was chaotic without certain standards, and the sample pre-treatment, internal standard selection, and methodological validation were different among manufacturers.

In recent years, the industry has progressively introduced a number of consensus guidelines and industry standards to regulate industry behaviors. For example, *Recommendations for Clinical Application of Liquid Chromatography-Mass Spectrometry, Development and Validation of Clinical Assays for Liquid Chromatography-Tandem Mass Spectrometry, Expert Consensus on Standardization of 25-Hydroxyvitamin D Detection by Liquid Chromatography-Tandem Mass Spectrometry, Current Status of Free Hormone Detection, and Clinical Application of Liquid Chromatography-Tandem Mass Spectrometry*. These documents have progressively established various standards for the mass spectrometry industry, including multiple methods for the test method development, project traceability, and data validation.

Declaration Quan Ji, Zhimin Lin and Sixing Chen are employees of Zybio Inc. Zengli Yang is an employee of Autobio Diagnostics Co., Ltd.

Part IX

Pathological Diagnosis

28 Overview of Pathological Diagnosis

Xiaojun Zhou

28.1 History of Pathological Diagnosis

Pathology as a medical discipline, on the one hand, studies the etiology and occurrence mechanism of diseases and provides an important theoretical basis for human beings to understand and master the laws of the occurrence and development of diseases, and for the prevention and treatment of diseases. From its inception, pathology has assumed an important mission in the practice of clinical medicine, that is, to diagnose various diseases together with clinicians. Therefore, pathology is also an important clinical discipline. The earliest ancient scholars connected the changes in human organs with clinical signs by observing the changes in human organs with the naked eye. After the advent of cytopathology, pathologists provided clinical diagnosis of diseases from changes in cell and tissue structure. In the 1870s, German pathologists first advocated surgical biopsy as an important means of disease diagnosis [1]. Since then, with the continuous promotion of this work around the world, on the basis of continuous summarization of experience, surgical pathology has gradually developed.

Traditional surgical pathology mainly provides clinical diagnosis of diseases based on biopsy (referred to as biopsy) and surgical resection specimens. These specimens were routinely embedded in paraffin, sectioned, stained with hematoxylin-eosin (HE; with some special staining and histochemical staining if necessary), and observed under light microscope to make pathological diagnosis. In recent decades, with the advancement in biological technology, the application of various new technologies and new methods such as electron microscopy, immunohistochemistry, in situ hybridization, single-gene or multi-gene sequencing, and other molecular biology technologies has been made in pathological diagnosis. At the same time, due to the development of clinical medicine and imaging technology, not only various

X. Zhou (✉)
Medical School of Nanjing University, Nanjing, Jiangsu, China

H. Song, L. Dai (eds.), *In Vitro Diagnostic Industry in China*,
https://doi.org/10.1007/978-981-99-3110-1_28

specialties of the surgical system send various tissue samples to the pathology department for pathological diagnosis, but also various specialties of the internal medicine system, dermatology, and radiology. Other departments also send tissue or cytology specimens to the pathology department for examination; pathologists not only provide pathological diagnosis based on biopsy or surgical specimen examination, but also conduct pathological diagnosis through the examination of various exfoliated cells, fine needle aspiration, and even body fluids and other specimens. Therefore, the scope of current pathological diagnosis work has been greatly expanded, involving all clinical departments of the hospital, and has become an indispensable and important part of the medical work of hospitals at all levels. Since the source of pathological examination is not just from the surgical system, it has also been suggested to change the name of surgical pathology to diagnostic pathology [2].

28.2 The Role and Importance of Diagnostic Pathology

28.2.1 Determining the Diagnosis of the Disease

With the development of clinical inspection technology and imaging medicine, there are many diseases that can be initially diagnosed after clinical examination, and some diseases mainly based on functional or metabolic disorders do not need pathological examination. For diseases with organic lesions, pathological diagnosis is still the most correct, reliable, and final diagnosis [3]. No matter how much the various clinical examination techniques (imaging, molecular biology, etc.) are advanced, the final diagnosis of many diseases still requires pathological examination. For example, for any palpable mass or space-occupying lesions detected by imaging, or for various ulcers, local stiffness, and masses seen in endoscopy, the diagnosis can only be established by biopsy pathological examination, which helps make the right judgment. In the diagnosis of various tumor diseases, only the pathological diagnosis is the most reliable diagnosis.

28.2.2 Providing a Basis for Clinical Selection of Treatment Options

First of all, correct pathological diagnosis, especially through morphological analysis, immunohistochemistry, molecular pathology, and other techniques, provides further evidence for the etiology or possible pathogens of the disease, which is very important for timely, effective, and reasonable targeted treatment. Secondly, due to the different sensitivities of different pathological types of tumors to chemotherapy and radiotherapy, different tumor-targeted drugs are also suitable for different tumors. Therefore, the pathological staging of the tumor as well as the results of various hormone receptors and targeted genes, etc. are essential factors to consider in selecting the appropriate chemotherapy, radiotherapy, and targeted therapy.

28.2.3 Providing Information on Prognostic Factors

The prognosis of different diseases can be very different, and even the same disease may have different prognosis in different individuals. Many parameters of pathomorphology can be used as important indicators for judging the prognosis of the disease. For example, in case of breast cancer, its histological type, degree of infiltration, presence or absence of metastasis, degree of differentiation of cancer cells, expression of sex hormone receptors, expression of oncogene proteins such as C-erbB-2, number and subgroups of inflammatory cells in the interstitium [4, 5] can provide a reference for the correct clinical judgment of prognosis.

28.2.4 Understanding the Development of the Disease and Judging the Curative Effect

Any kind of disease has its own development features, and there is also a progressive evolution relationship between different diseases. Through the pathological examination of multiple biopsies, the dynamic changes in the disease can be understood, which can provide important information for correctly judging the prognosis of the disease, so that the patient can receive reasonable treatment; in addition, the pathological examination results can also objectively and truly reflect various treatments, regimen, or efficacy of different drugs. Although the changes in various serological indicators and the changes in imaging results can be used as an important basis for evaluating the curative effect, for many diseases with organic lesions, the pathological changes are still the most objective and the most direct efficacy evaluation index.

28.3 Types of Pathological Diagnosis

28.3.1 Cytological Diagnosis

Cytological diagnosis, also known as cytology examination, is an important part of diagnosing pathology. Diagnosis of certain diseases is mainly based on the observation of the morphology and properties of cells that fall off, scrape, and puncture from the diseased part of the human body. Cytological examination is currently mainly used in the diagnosis of tumors, and can also be used in the examination and diagnosis of certain diseases, such as the diagnosis of inflammatory diseases of various internal organs and the judgment of hormone levels.

28.3.2 Histological Diagnosis

Histology diagnosis is the most important part of pathological diagnosis and is the final diagnosis in most cases. Histological diagnosis relies on the naked eye and light microscope observation of biopsy tissue or surgical specimen, and diagnoses various diseases by analyzing and identifying the morphology of diseased tissue and cells. Specimens for pathological examination are routinely fixed with formaldehyde (formalin), embedded in paraffin, sectioned, and stained with hematoxylin-eosin (HE) for histological observation [6]. Diagnosis can be obtained, but difficult cases should be assisted by techniques such as immunohistochemistry, special staining, electron microscopy, or molecular biology.

28.3.3 Intraoperative Pathological Diagnosis

Intraoperation pathology diagnosis includes frozen section, rapid paraffin section, and intraoperative cytology diagnosis, among which frozen section is the most used. At present, frozen section technology or rapid paraffin section technology is commonly used at home and abroad to solve the problem of diagnosis in surgery. The requirement of accuracy and speed is one of the most important and difficult tasks that pathologists do in their practice. The main role of pathological diagnosis in surgery is to decide the surgical plan, and its specific role includes the following aspects [7–11]: (1) Determine the nature of the lesion, whether it is an inflammatory lesion or a tumor; whether it is a benign tumor or a malignant tumor. This is crucial for clinicians to decide on surgical options during surgery, whether radical surgery, amputation, or partial excision is required. (2) To understand the infiltration and spread of malignant tumor, such as whether the edge is involved, whether there is disease in the surrounding tissue, or whether there is metastasis in the surrounding and distant lymph nodes of the tumor, so as to determine the scope of surgery. (3) Determine whether the sample taken contains enough tissue to make a diagnosis.

28.3.4 Pathological Autopsy

Pathological autopsy examination (autopsy for short) has played an important role in the development of clinical medicine or pathology. Autopsy can be divided into medicolegal autopsy and clinical autopsy. The former is at the request of a legal institution, performed by a forensic doctor or a pathologist to clarify deaths related to medical corrections, accidents, murders, etc. The latter is an autopsy performed at the request of the clinician and with the consent of the relatives of the deceased or at the request of the relatives, to improve the level of medical care. The function of pathological autopsy is to improve the level of clinical diagnosis and the quality of treatment first. Even if the pathological diagnosis is obtained by biopsy or surgical specimen examination before the patient's death, autopsy can still provide a more comprehensive and accurate pathological diagnosis. At the same time, autopsy also provides detailed information on the patient's disease evolution process, pathogenesis, clinicopathological links, and the role of treatment. So far, summarizing the experience and lessons of diagnosis and treatment through autopsy results is still the most important means to improve the medical level. Pathological autopsy is an indispensable means for training clinical and pathological professionals [12]. Through good training in autopsy, pathology professionals can more systematically improve the theoretical level and practical diagnosis ability of pathology. In addition, autopsy also provides important specimens and data for clinical education and medical research. It not only ensures the quality of medical education, but also promotes the development of pathology and medical epidemiology, human anatomy, histo-embryology, and other disciplines.

28.4 Development Trend of Pathology Diagnosis Industry and Discipline

Pathological diagnosis belongs to the in vitro diagnosis of diseases. The progress of pathological diagnosis technology in each period is closely related to the development of related instruments and equipment and its reagent consumables. It is the innovative development of instruments, equipment, and reagent consumables related to pathological diagnosis technology that has promoted the progress of pathological diagnosis [13, 14].

At present, the conventional pathological technical equipment mainly includes microtome series, microscope series, and automatic tissue dehydration and embedding instrument series. Although they have been continuously updated over the years, the basic principle and structure have not fundamentally changed. In the past, almost all of these equipment were imported. In recent years, domestic products have been significantly improved, and new instruments and equipment such as rapid dehydration treatment have been developed. With further improvement in the quality and efficiency of conventional pathological instruments and equipment developed in China, more and more pathological products will occupy the domestic market in the future. At the same time, it is expected that pathological instruments and equipment with a higher degree of automation and systematization will come out and promote the standardization of pathological technology and automation.

Immunohistochemical diagnosis technology was widely used in China in the 1990s. In recent years, it has developed rapidly and has become a necessary pathological diagnosis technology for almost every pathology department in China [15]. There is a steady stream of new monoclonal and polyclonal antibodies that are developed and marketed every year. Currently, there are 100–200 kinds of antibodies used in daily detection, and thousands of antibodies can be selected for application. In the past, the manual operation of immunohistochemistry has greatly promoted the standardization of immunohistochemistry technology with the popularization and application of immunohistochemistry automated stainers in recent years. At present, the domestic market of immunohistochemical reagents and equipment is mainly dominated by imported products, though domestic enterprises have a variety of antibodies and immunohistochemical automatic stainers with independent intellectual property rights. Most of the immunohistochemical reagents used for diagnosis are not registered, and the staining results depend on the subjective judgment of pathologists. However, immunohistochemical reagents related to targeted drug therapy must be reviewed and registered by relevant national departments. In the future, more specific and sensitive antibodies will continue to be launched. With the development of artificial intelligence, the results of immunohistochemistry will gradually be interpreted by machines, not only qualitatively but also quantitatively.

Molecular pathology detection technologies include in situ hybridization, fluorescent probe nucleic acid amplification detection (real-time polymerase chain reaction [PCR]), microarray detection, and single-gene and multi-gene gene sequencing, which are rapidly developed for pathological diagnosis and targeted therapy. Different molecular pathology detection technologies require different special precision equipment and specific reagents, and the application requirements of multiple varieties and large quantities have rapidly promoted the in vitro diagnosis industry related to disease diagnosis, which has become the most active high-tech industry today [16]. Domestic-related enterprises have made rapid progress in the past 10 years. Some relatively low-end equipment such as PCR instruments and in situ hybridization instruments can be provided, but the high-end instruments leading the times such as second-generation sequencers and digital PCR instruments are still unique patented products of international companies, including molecules currently routinely used in domestic pathology departments. Pathological detection reagents are basically produced by domestic manufacturers, and most of them have passed the examination and registration of relevant national departments (except for some high-throughput sequencing reagents). A few new companion diagnostic detection reagents also need to be provided by foreign manufacturers. In the future, it is up to domestic enterprises to further integrate their strengths and enter the ranks of international advanced industries in the research and development of high-end, precision, automated equipment, and innovative reagents.

As one of the important diagnostic departments of hospitals in my country, the pathology department of a hospital in China has undergone the following major changes with the development of the discipline in the past decade or two [17, 18]: (1) the number of biopsy and cytology examinations has increased several times; (2) the clinical specialties are highly refined, and objectively requires the subspecialization of pathology to adapt; and (3) new technologies and new equipment are constantly emerging and highly specialized, requiring the pathology department to be equipped with a variety of technical platforms. Facing the changes in the pathology market in the future, the pathology departments of large domestic hospitals should appropriately increase personnel, adjust the professional structure of personnel, continuously increase equipment platforms, and select characteristic development areas, which can fully adapt to the progress and development of contemporary pathological diagnosis, but relatively small hospitals (county-level hospitals). The pathology department of the hospital is limited by personnel and equipment, the development is limited, and even survival is very difficult. Obviously, in the face of the general trend of the reform of national tiered medical care and medical insurance fees in the future, the establishment and integration of regional pathology centers or the establishment of third-party laboratories with the help of social forces to support the pathological diagnosis business of small- and medium-sized hospitals will become an inevitable choice for the development of pathological diagnosis in China in the future. In recent years, central ministries and local governments have successively issued "Several Opinions of the State Council on Promoting the Development of the Health Service Industry" (Document of State Council [2013] No. 40), "Guiding Opinions of the General Office of the State Council on Promoting the Construction of a Hierarchical Diagnosis and Treatment System" (Document of State Council [2015] No. 70), "National Health and Family Planning Commission on Printing and Distributing Basic Standards and Management Regulations for Pathological Diagnosis Centers," "Basic Standards for Pathological Diagnosis Centers (Trial)," "Management Regulations for Pathological Diagnosis Centers (Trial)," and other guiding documents to further promote the domestic pathological diagnosis industry to usher in a new stage of integration and development.

Compared with clinical laboratory departments in hospitals, pathology departments in hospitals in China lag behind in laboratory institutionalization and quality control management. In the past, there was almost a lack of systematic and standardized quality control management. In recent years, under the leadership of national, provincial, and municipal pathological quality control institutions, the management institutions have been gradually improved from top to bottom, and a number of immunohistochemistry and molecular pathology domestic and even international inter-laboratory quality assessments and standardized experiments are carried out regularly every year. As regards laboratory quality certification, the nucleic acid amplification clinical laboratory (i.e., PCR laboratory) built in the pathology department has basically obtained the evaluation and certification of clinical testing centers at all levels. Many third-party pathology laboratories and hospital pathology departments in China have carried out pathological quality control construction with reference to the norms formulated by College of American Pathologists (CAP) or ISO15189 in the United States, and many departments have passed the certification of CAP or ISO15189 pathology laboratories. With the strengthening of the national medical quality construction, under the active promotion of the pathological quality control institutions at the national, provincial, and municipal levels, China will gradually improve the pathological diagnosis quality control system in the future. My country's pathological diagnosis industry provides a strong guarantee for the healthy and rapid development of the industry.

References

1. Angel. Other: Rudolf Virchow: Doctor, Statesman, Anthropologist. Erwin H. Ac 100 kerknecht. American Anthropologist, 2010,56(5):933-934.
2. Parslow Tristram G, Volkan AN, Krasinskas Alyssa M, et al. Impacts of new concepts and technologies on the practice of diagnostic pathology: an Emory University perspective. Arch Pathol Lab Med. 2017;141(3):325.
3. Academician Liu Tonghua talks about pathological diagnosis. Encyclopedia. 2020;25:40.
4. Tuncel F, Satici F, Bozkurt F, et al. Clinicopathological features of breast cancer cases and their relationship with immunohistochemical findings. Ann Med Res. 2020;27(6):1715.

5. Maheshwari P, Rajesh Kumar KS, Hazarika D, Naik R. A correlation of pathological characteristics and immuno histo chemistry (IHC) based biomarker expression in triple negative breast carcinomas. J Clin Cell Immunol. 2021;12(6):631.
6. Wu LN, Zhang LN, Weng SX, et al. Effect of different thyroid decalcification on HE staining, immunohistochemistry and nucleic acid quality. Chin J Pathol. 2020;49(1):80.
7. Onieva-González FG, Galeano-Díaz F, Matito-Díaz MJ, López-Guerra D, Fernández-Pérez J, Blanco-Fernández G. Inflammatory pseudotumor of the liver. Importance of intraoperative pathology. Cir Cir (English Edition). 2015;83(2):151.
8. Sosuke M, Kentaro Y, Haruo M, Tomoyuki T, Tomoko T, Yoshiaki O, Kazuo N, Toshifumi O, Takehiro T. Assessment of the concordance rate between intraoperative pathological diagnosis and the final pathological diagnosis of spinal cord tumors. Acta Med Okayama. 2021;75(4):455.
9. Liping W, Bing L, Debby R. Five-year review of intraoperative pathology consultation in a single institution. Proc (Bayl Univ Med Cent). 2021;34(6):649.
10. Montesinos Manuel R, Fernanda MM, Alejandro I. Value of the intraoperative pathology in thyroid surgery. Comparison with preoperative aspiration puncture and deferred pathology. Medicina. 2021;81(4):611.
11. John D, Boughey Judy C, Hoskin Tanya L, et al. Locoregional management of the axilla in mastectomy patients with one or two positive sentinel nodes: the role of intraoperative pathology. Clin Breast Cancer. 2021;21(5):458.
12. Westphal SE, Apitzsch JC, Penzkofer T, et al. Contrast-enhanced postmortem computed tomography in clinical pathology: enhanced value of 20 clinical autopsies. Hum Pathol. 2014;45(9):1813.
13. Talat Z, Asma S. Adoption of digital pathology in developing countries: from benefits to challenges. JCPSP. 2021;31(9):1120.
14. Tonghua L. Opportunities and challenges for the development of diagnostic pathology in China. Chin J Pathol. 2005;34(8):466–7.
15. Jie C, Jie Z, Linming H. Attach importance to quality control and standardization of immunohistochemistry. Chin J Pathol. 2005;34(2):65–6.
16. Anon. Ten years of methods. Nat Methods. 2014;11(10):1000–1.
17. Jie C. Keep up with the pace of the times and do a good job in pathological work in the new era. Chin J Pathol. 2018;47(1):1.
18. Jianming Y, Ning L. Development status, opportunities and challenges of pathological diagnosis of tumor tissue. Chi J Pathol. 2020;49(11):1097–101.

Conventional Pathology 29

Xiaolu Wang and Xiaojun Zhou

29.1 Concepts and Applications

Conventional pathology is the behind-the-scenes work performed by pathologists on living tissue removed from patients to help clinicians diagnose disease and determine treatment plans. Pathologists provide pathological consultation services for various organ systems and medical subspecialties of the human body for doctors and patients.

Conventional pathology is the basis of pathology, and the diagnostic indications include various benign and malignant lesions, and even microscopic examination of non-biological and inorganic substances such as kidney stones can be performed. Is the tissue obtained by puncturing the mediastinal lymph nodes small cell carcinoma or granulomatous inflammation? Is it non-small cell carcinoma or lymphoma? These diseases cannot be diagnosed by imaging examination alone, but conventional pathology can be done, and clinicians can be informed in time to adjust the treatment plan according to the pathological diagnosis, and even prevent patients from receiving unnecessary overtreatment or surgery.

During the operation, the surgeon needs an intraoperative pathological biopsy to check the resection range of tumor infiltration, the pathologist needs to conduct intraoperative consultation to identify the benign and malignant lesions, and even needs to examine the surrounding lymph nodes to determine the subsequent clinical decision. After surgery, accurate pathological diagnosis is related to clinical staging and determines the prognosis of patients. Conventional pathology is also used in the follow-up of the treatment process to determine whether the tumor has recurred or recovered.

X. Wang (✉)
Central Capital of Yichang, Yichang, Hubei, China

X. Zhou
Medical School of Nanjing University, Nanjing, Jiangsu, China

H. Song, L. Dai (eds.), *In Vitro Diagnostic Industry in China*,
https://doi.org/10.1007/978-981-99-3110-1_29

29.2 Technical Status of Conventional Pathology

Technical work in conventional pathology has been under pressure to do more with less money, less people, and less time. Sectioning is a complex process involving many steps, including tissue fixation, dehydration, clearing, embedding, paraffin block preparation, sectioning, staining, and mounting. The emergence of automatic instruments such as automatic paraffin microtome and automatic dyeing and sealing all-in-one machine has solved the manual operation of some links, but currently there is no single instrument that can complete the entire experimental operation.

With the rapid development of the pathology examination market, conventional pathology also faces a series of problems, mainly the lack of skilled and well-trained pathologists and pathology technicians. In addition, the high cost of pathology examinations, lack of compensation policies, and high initial investment expenses will also hinder the growth of the conventional pathology examination market.

29.3 Conventional Pathology-Related Products and Market Situation

Commonly used reagents for conventional pathology include formaldehyde, ethanol, and routine staining solutions (hematoxylin, eosin). The prices are low, the overall market space is small, and most suppliers are comprehensive manufacturers. On the contrary, there are many commonly used equipment, including tissue dehydrator, tissue embedding machine, cryostat, paraffin microtome, etc. There are many types and models of equipment, see Table 29.1 for details.

29.3.1 Conventional Pathological Equipment Has a High Threshold and Many Varieties

The traditional manual operation has many disadvantages, such as complicated operation, high technical requirements, lengthy time, and low output rate. Therefore,

Table 29.1 Corresponding equipment and representative manufacturers in each link of histopathological preparation

Production process	Required equipment	Representative manufacturers
Fixed, dehydrated, transparent	Tissue dehydrator	Leica, Sakura, Dakewe
Waxing, embedding	Tissue embedding machine	Sakura, Hengsong
Slice, patch	Paraffin microtome, frozen microtome, bleaching and drying machine, slicer, etc.	Leica, Sakura, Hengsong, Dakewe
Dyeing	Fully automatic dyeing machine	Leica, Sakura, Dakewe
Cover slip	Automatic coverslipping machine	Leica, Sakura

automation equipment is the common direction of users and enterprises. The current status of conventional pathological equipment is a wide variety and poor substitution. There are as many as dozens of various equipment required for the simple production process. In addition, some equipment is weak in substitution, and specific instruments can only do specific links. Automation equipment covers a variety of disciplines such as medicine, biology, chemistry, physics, and electronics combined with engineering. The intersection of multiple disciplines determines that this type of product has better technicality and has a higher entry threshold.

29.3.2 Domestic Substitution Is in Progress

At present, the domestic conventional pathology equipment market is dominated by multinational companies such as Leica and Thermo Fisher. The product lines of foreign brands are relatively complete, which can cover the whole process of pathology production and occupy more than 60% of the overall market. After the new medical reform in 2009, the State Council has invested a total of 850 billion yuan in medical reform, which will bring development opportunities for national enterprises. With the investment of capital, domestic enterprises represented by Dakewe are constantly rising. The fully automatic tissue dehydrator and fully automatic intelligent dyeing and sealing system developed by Dakewe have been on the international stage and sold at home and abroad. On the whole, the market capacity of conventional pathological diagnosis has not changed much, and the fully automatic integrated operation platform will be the direction for enterprises to move forward.

Cytopathology

30

Xuedong Fu and Yinghao Yu

30.1 Overview of Cytopathology

30.1.1 Cytopathology Concepts and Classification

Cytopathology is mainly to observe the morphology of cells under the microscope, and to study the occurrence of diseases according to the abnormal conditions of cells, so as to provide the basis for the diagnosis and prevention of diseases.

30.1.1.1 Exfoliative Cytology

Exfoliative cytology refers to the diagnosis of cells that are naturally exfoliated by the body. The purpose of diagnosing cancer and precancerous lesions is achieved by collecting exfoliated cell samples from the body for smears and observing their cytological morphology. At present, it is mainly used in cervical exfoliative cytology. The main application scenarios of exfoliative cytology are shown in Table 30.1.

30.1.1.2 Fine-Needle Aspiration Cytology

Fine-needle aspiration cytology (FNAC) refers to the use of fine needle aspiration to absorb cells and other components in the lesion to make a smear, and observe the morphological changes and interstitial changes of tumor and non-tumor cells. Because of its simplicity, safety, rapidity, good sensitivity, high diagnosis rate, strong reliability, and almost non-invasiveness to patients, it has become one of the important diagnostic methods for clinical diseases [1–3]. At present, fine needle

X. Fu (✉)
Fuzhou Maixin Biotech. Co., Ltd, Fuzhou, Fujian, China
e-mail: fxd@maxim.com.cn

Y. Yu
No. 900 Hospital of Joint Logistics Support Force, Fuzhou, Fujian, China

H. Song, L. Dai (eds.), *In Vitro Diagnostic Industry in China*,
https://doi.org/10.1007/978-981-99-3110-1_30

Table 30.1 Main application scenarios of exfoliative cytology

Target organ	Operation method	Main purpose
Cervix, vagina, vulva, endometrium	Specimens are obtained by brushing or scraping, and the smears are immediately fixed with ethanol	Precancerous lesions, early cancer diagnosis and differential diagnosis, identification of infectious agents
Ascites and flushing fluids	Liquid specimens are collected in fixative	Diagnosis of residual or recurrent ovarian, fallopian tube, endometrial, or cervical cancer
Respiratory tract	Bronchial lavage and bronchoalveolar lavage	Differential diagnosis of precancerous lesions, lung cancer and infection, identification of infectious agents, chemical and immunological analysis of chronic bronchial and lung lesions
Oral vestibule and adjacent organs	Brush directly on the smear	Differential diagnosis of precancerous lesions and cancer
Urinary tract	Urine and bladder washes	Differential diagnosis of carcinoma in situ and related lesions, therapeutic testing, DNA analysis by flow cytometry or image analysis

aspiration cytology is widely used in thyroid-diagnosing pathology. In addition, it also has applications in breast, lymph nodes, head and neck masses, pericardial effusion, pleural effusion, cerebrospinal fluid, and vitreous fluid.

30.1.2 The Application and Value of Cytopathology in Clinical Diagnosis

30.1.2.1 Carry Out Census of Population or Areas with High Cancer Incidence

Regular screening of certain cancers can detect tumors that patients cannot perceive, including some precancerous lesions or early malignant tumors, buy time for patients' treatment, and improve their prognosis. For example, cervical cancer screening is to identify patients with potential precancerous lesions through early cytopathological screening, thereby greatly reducing their mortality.

30.1.2.2 Diagnose Early Malignant Tumors and Provide Basis for Early Treatment

As a non-invasive or minimally invasive technique, cytology can be used as a physical examination item to enable patients to detect early-stage cancer that they do not perceive, and to provide the basis for early treatment.

30.1.2.3 Postoperative Follow-Up of Malignant Tumor

As one of the most convenient methods for patients to regularly review after treatment for malignant tumors.

30.1.2.4 Indication of Benign Lesions

It suggests inflammatory infection and other benign lesions. For example, cervical liquid-based cytology may indicate whether the patient is infected with inflammation or trichomoniasis.

30.1.2.5 When It Is Difficult to Obtain Histopathological Specimens, Cytopathology Can Achieve the Purpose of Morphological Diagnosis

For example, in cases in the lung, mediastinum, or abdominal cavity that are not suitable for surgery, most of the percutaneous cytology can identify the nature and basic tissue type of the tumor, and provide a morphological diagnosis basis for radiotherapy and chemotherapy.

30.2 Cytopathology-Related Manufacturers

30.2.1 Major Manufacturers and Their Representative Products

30.2.1.1 Representative Manufacturers of Liquid-Based Cytology

Liquid-based cytology products are mainly composed of liquid-based cell preparation instrument and its supporting reagent consumables such as Pasteur staining solution and staining tank. From the production method, it can be divided into: membrane type, sedimentation type, centrifugal throwing type. Membrane and sedimentation liquid-based cell preparation methods are widely used in public tertiary hospitals because of their better effect and high accuracy; Tripartite medical inspection institutions are widely used. The common liquid-based cytology manufacturers and their representative products currently on the market are shown in Table 30.2.

It is worth mentioning that many third-party testing institutions are also developing their own liquid-based brands, such as "Jinxianrui" under King Med; "Jindian" under Dian. It can be seen that third-party testing institutions are actively deploying upstream industrial chains to enrich their entire industrial lines.

30.2.1.2 Representative Manufacturers of Immunocytochemical p16/Ki-67 Double Staining Detection

As the application of cervical cancer screening in cytology becomes more and more important, many auxiliary detection technologies for cervical cancer diagnosis have been derived. Among them, immunocytochemical p16/Ki-67 double staining detection technology has developed rapidly [4]. In less than 5 years of development, more than 30 manufacturers have produced related products, among which the more prominent manufacturers are Roche, Maixin, Zhongshan, Yaneng, Detong, and the representative manufacturers and details are shown in Table 30.3. This field will also become the driving force for cervical cancer screening to move toward a new era of "precision and individualization."

Table 30.2 List of representative products of liquid-based cytology

Manufacturer	Production method	Instrument model	Degree of automation	Production throughput
BD	Subsidence	BD PrepStain	Fully automatic production dyeing	48 slices
Hologic	Membrane	ThinPrep 5000	Fully automatic production dyeing	20 slices
IBP	Subsidence	LBP-2264	Fully automatic production dyeing	64 slices
TIB	Subsidence	TIB-AutoPrep4806	Fully automatic production	48 slices
Maccura	Subsidence	PC 2000	Fully automatic production dyeing	20 slices
Lituo	Subsidence	LTS-3000B	Fully automatic production dyeing	24 slices
Healthsky	Subsidence	ALP-4800A	Fully automatic production dyeing	48 slices

Note: As each manufacturer has multiple products of the same type, this table only reflects the product with the largest throughput

Table 30.3 List of related manufacturers of immunocytochemical p16/Ki-67 double staining technology

Manufacturer	Product name	Product filing time	Sensitivity	Specificity
Roche	CINtecPLUS	2019.1.22	94.4%	78.7%
Maixin	p16/Ki-67 detection kit	2018.3.1	90.9%	71.7%
Zhongshan	p16/Ki-67 detection kit	2018.8.28	–	–
Yaneng	p16/Ki-67 detection kit	2021.3.22	–	–
Detong	p16/Ki-67 detection kit	2019.11.6	86.7%	68.5%

Note: Sensitivity and specificity are the cases of detection ≥CIN2; marked "–" means no big data analysis

30.3 Analysis of Current Market Application

30.3.1 Market Capacity

Cytopathology is widely used in pathological diagnosis, among which the most prominent is the diagnostic application of cervical precancer screening. Cervical cancer is currently the only cancer that can be prevented and controlled through vaccination and regular screening. It has been listed by the World Health Organization (WHO) as "the first cancer that can be eliminated" [5], and its significance in screening can be imagined. Taking cervical cancer screening in my country as an example, according to the statistics of the seventh national census, the number of women aged 21–65 in my country is about 458 million. Assuming that cervical cancer screening is carried out every 3 years, about 122 million people are screened for cervical cancer every year in the country according to an estimate of 80%. The price of a single cytology test ranges from 150 to 200 yuan. Assuming that the price of a single cytology test is 160 yuan, the terminal market capacity of cervical cancer screening in my country is about 19.52 billion yuan. With the continuous and in-depth development of precision medicine, more and more auxiliary methods are used in cervical cancer screening, and the market potential is unpredictable.

30.3.2 Product Application

Currently, cervical liquid-based cytology is widely used in the field of cytopathological diagnosis [6]. In the cervical liquid-based cytology test, the domestic and imported products are in a state of mutual radiance. Some large tertiary hospitals mainly use imported Thinprep or BD liquid-based cell preparation and staining systems. At the same time, domestic cytology preparation products with excellent effects are also used in tertiary hospitals, and their product effects are gradually approaching international first-class brands, such as IBP liquid-based cell preparation staining system.

In addition to the traditional Pap smear and liquid-based preparation methods, various emerging technologies have also begun to be used in cytopathological diagnosis in recent years, such as immunocytochemical staining technology and DNA ploidy technology. At present, major tertiary hospitals have successively carried out immunocytochemical p16/Ki-67 double staining detection technology for cervical cancer diagnosis. This technology has higher sensitivity than cytology, and can help cytology doctors make diagnosis of difficult cases. In western regions or small and medium-sized hospitals where cytology doctors are relatively scarce, DNA ploidy technology occupies the market due to its advantages of not requiring doctors to read pictures and automatically issuing reports by machines, but because it has no clear charges and clinical significance, so it cannot be carried out on a large scale. The application of artificial intelligence (AI) in cytopathological diagnosis has been a hot spot in recent years [7], and the use of AI-assisted image reading technology can enable cytology doctors to focus on "diagnosis" rather than "search." At present, many large tertiary hospitals and third-party testing institutions have introduced AI intelligent image reading technology. In many provinces and regions, "Cervical Computer Aided Diagnosis" has been added to the charging code. For example, the charging code for "Cervical Computer Aided Diagnosis" in Fujian is: 270800002, the charge price is 230 yuan. However, the development of this technology is also limited due to the constraints of high cost and the power and responsibility of issuing reports.

30.3.3 Market Development Trend

The application of immunocytochemistry in cytopathological diagnosis will become more and more extensive. One is the p16/Ki-67 double staining detection technology in cervical cytopathological diagnosis; AI artificial intelligence is in hot development, and will also become the direction of development in the field of cytopathological diagnosis.

30.4 Summary and Outlook

Since Professor Yang Dawang established the first batch of cytology laboratories in China in the early 1950s, cytopathology has made great progress in China, but there is still a certain gap with developed countries. Cytopathology can make great contributions to early tumor screening due to its advantages of minimally invasive, safe, reliable, and reproducible sample acquisition. At present, the most successful early tumor screening is cervical liquid-based cytology screening, but in other non-gynecological cytology screening and diagnosis such as thyroid puncture, pleural ascites, and lymph node aspiration, further exploration and more accurate screening and diagnosis are needed. At present, for the application of cytopathological diagnosis technology, many new technologies have appeared in the market, such as immunocytochemistry technology and AI artificial intelligence assisted reading technology. More and more technical participation means that cytopathology will develop toward a more accurate and convenient diagnosis. The tumor risk can be diagnosed earlier with early intervention and early treatment, so that some tumor patients will no longer have the situation of "late stage as soon as it is detected."

Declaration Xuedong Fu is an employee of Fuzhou Maixin Biotech. Co., Ltd.

References

1. Thierauf J, Hoffmann TK, Bommer M, Veit JA, Lindemann J. [Value of fine needle aspiration cytology and core needle biopsy in the head and neck region.]. Laryngorhinootologie. 2015;94(5):311–6.
2. Musayev J. The diagnostic value of fine needle aspiration cytology in minor salivary gland lesions. Oral Surg Oral Med Oral Pathol Oral Radiol. 2015;119(3):e135.
3. Haider SA, Memon S, Laghari MS, et al. Efficacy of fine needle aspiration and cytology in solitary thyroid nodule. J Pharm Res Int. 2021;33(17):1–6.
4. Toliman PJ, Phillips S, de Jong S, et al. Evaluation of p16/Ki-67 dual-stain cytology performed on self-collected vaginal and clinician-collected cervical specimens for the detection of cervical pre-cancer. Clin Microbiol Infect. 2020;26(6):748–52.
5. Lin S, Gao K, Gu S, et al. Worldwide trends in cervical cancer incidence and mortality, with predictions for the next 15 years. Cancer. 2021;127(21):4030–9.
6. Gad M, Jean-Claude D, Theogene R, et al. Protocol for the study of cervical cancer screening technologies in HIV-infected women living in Rwanda. BMJ Open. 2018;8(8):e020432.
7. Yousif M, van Diest PJ, Laurinavicius A, et al. Artificial intelligence applied to breast pathology. Virchows Arch. 2022;480(1):191–209.

Immunohistochemistry 31

Qinghai Yang, Qixin Lin, and Yun Shi

31.1 Immunohistochemical-Related Products and Development Status

Immunohistochemical technology has been developed in China for more than 20 years. And it has become an indispensable part of pathologists' daily work with the continuous enrichment and improvement of technical methods, the increase of new technologies and the gradual automation of staining process. Although the majority of our immunohistochemical-related reagents and automated staining systems rely on imports, immunohistochemical industry in China developed rapidly in recent years. As the growing of market demand and products domestication awareness is increasing, many domestic enterprises seize the opportunity to vigorously carry out independent innovation, constantly develop immunohistochemical reagents and automated staining systems with independent intellectual property rights. For example, Fuzhou Maxim successfully developed CD10, CD20, and CK8 diagnostic antibodies in 2012, breaking the monopoly of foreign companies. In 2016, China's first independently full-automatic immunohistochemical staining system (Titan) was successfully developed and launched by Fuzhou Maxim. In 2019, Celnovte Bio developed its own core technology "Microstucker" secondary antibody polymer, and Hangzhou Biolynx's AS310 Automatic Immunohistochemical Staining System was officially released. Enterprises of China broke the monopoly of foreign enterprises with high-quality products and good services and gradually became competitive.

Q. Yang · Q. Lin · Y. Shi (✉)
Fuzhou Maixin Biotech. Co., Ltd, Fuzhou, Fujian, China
e-mail: shiyun@maxim.com.cn

H. Song, L. Dai (eds.), *In Vitro Diagnostic Industry in China*,
https://doi.org/10.1007/978-981-99-3110-1_31

31.1.1 Antibody

There are hundreds of immunohistochemical antibodies used in the daily work of the pathology department, which are also known as primary antibodies, playing an important role in the diagnosis and treatment of human diseases. With the deepen understanding of diseases, the types of antibodies are gradually increasing. Immunohistochemical antibodies can be divided into monoclonal antibodies and polyclonal antibodies according to their preparation methods. Monoclonal antibodies include mouse monoclonal antibodies and rabbit monoclonal antibodies. They are widely favored by users because of high specificity, and account for the vast majority of antibodies used in pathology. Mouse monoclonal antibody technology has been developed for more than 40 years since 1975, and it has been mastered by most immunohistochemical enterprises with R&D capabilities. However, only a few enterprises master the technology to prepare rabbit monoclonal antibodies due to the development patent limitation of rabbit myeloma cell line, such as Abcam's production of "EP" series rabbit monoclonal antibodies and Spring Bioscience's production of series antibodies with a clone name beginning with "SP."

There are three types of enterprises that can produce and sell immunohistochemical antibodies to pathology department in China: (1) Multinational enterprises, such as Roche, Leica, and Dako. These companies own antibody development, preparation, and production capacity. (2) Most small immunohistochemical enterprises in China, which don't have antibody development and preparation capacity. They buy concentrated antibodies as raw materials to repackage or process them into ready to use antibodies. (3) A few domestic enterprises, such as Fuzhou Maxim Biotech. Co., Ltd, have antibody development, preparation and production capacity, and able to produce immunohistochemical monoclonal antibodies of diagnostic level in vitro.

31.1.2 Detection Amplification System

The antigen-antibody binding is weak and invisible in immunohistochemical staining. Usually, a staining system that can specifically bind to the primary antibody and amplify the antigen-antibody binding signal is used. This combined system is called detection amplification system. The earliest detection amplification system used direct method to label fluorescent dye or visible color source at the end of antibody, but the staining signal was weak. Indirect detection amplification system (Biotin detection system) has emerged with the continuous progress of technology. But it is gradually deprecated because endogenous biotin is easy to cause false positive results. The main representatives are ABC detection system, Maxim's SP detection system and Dako's LSAB detection system. The polymer method detection system is the main immunohistochemical detection amplification system at present. The secondary antibodies and enzymes are linked to the polymer to form a chelate. And the chelate combines with the primary antibody, effectively solves the false positive problem of biotin method, and makes the immunohistochemical technology more specific, more sensitive, and simpler, such as EnVision detection system of Dako, MaxVision detection system of Maxim, and Novalinker detection system of Leica.

31.1.3 Full-Automatic Immunohistochemical Staining System

Automatic immunohistochemical staining system has become an inevitable trend in the development of pathological technology. Its appearance is an important progress and innovation in the field of histopathology technology. In the past decade, automatic immunohistochemical staining systems have sprung up like mushrooms. After the automation of immunohistochemistry, the staining process can be automatically controlled by the computer, and technicians can be freed from a large number of experiments, reducing the possibility of human operation errors, thus improving the consistency, reproducibility and reliability of staining, and promoting the standardization of immunohistochemistry technology.

There are many types and models of immunohistochemical automation systems at home and abroad. Only representative products widely used in the market are introduced here. See Table 31.1 for specific parameters.

Table 31.1 Summary of representative immunohistochemical automation products

Manufacturer	Model	Placement	Design principle	Antigen repair mode	Maximum antigen repair temperature	Slice capacity/ batch	Reagent capacity
Ventana	BenchMark GX	Floor type	Liquid cap membrane	On line	100 °C	20	25
	BenchMark XT	Floor type	Liquid cap membrane	On line	100 °C	30	35
	BenchMark Ultra	Floor type	Liquid cap membrane	On line	100 °C	30	35
Leica	Bond-Max	Desk type	Capillary siphon	On line	100 °C	30	36
	Bond-III	Floor type	Capillary siphon	On line	100 °C	30	36
DAKO	Link48	Desk type	General system	Off line	–	48	42
	Omnis	Floor type	Capillary siphon	On line	100 °C	30 + 30	60
Lumatas	Titan	Floor type	General system	On line	102 °C	72	70
	Titan S	Floor type	General system	On line	102 °C	36	42
BioGenex	Elite/Infinity/ Ultra	Floor type	Capillary siphon	On line	100 °C	40	40
PathCom	SS1	Desk type	Solid cover plate	On line	103 °C	36	40
LabVision	360/480/720	Desk type	General system	Off line	–	36/48/84	40/49/40

31.2 Development Status of Immunohistochemistry

31.2.1 Immunohistochemical Application: Companion Diagnostics

Immunohistochemistry provides objective evidence for pathological diagnosis and differential diagnosis. Identifying specific bacteria, viruses, and other microorganisms through immunohistochemical technology can improve the accuracy of pathological diagnosis of infectious diseases. For neoplastic disease, immunohistochemistry also provides objective diagnostic evidence to assist pathological diagnosis through various ways. These are the general impressions of immunohistochemical application by pathological workers. Since 2000, with the emergence of targeted drugs and the rapid development of immunotherapy. Some specific immunohistochemical tests, together with fluorescence in situ hybridization, fluorescence polymerase chain reaction (PCR), high-throughput sequencing, and other molecular tests, have been given a new mission which is called companion diagnostics (CDx). It can provide patients with individualized diagnosis and treatment plan. As of December 29, 2021, FDA has approved 49 companion diagnostics products. The products related to immunohistochemistry are mainly including: (1) Companion diagnostics with human epidermal growth factor receptor-2 (HER2) as the target gene. (2) Companion diagnostics with epidermal growth factor receptor (EGFR) as the target gene. (3) Companion diagnostics with anaplastic lymphoma kinase (ALK) as the target gene. (4) Companion diagnostics with the detection of stem cell factor receptor (c-KIT) protein. (5) Companion diagnostics with the detection of programmed cell death 1/programmed cell death-ligand 1 (PD-1/PD-L1) protein. See Table 31.2 for FDA approved immunohistochemical-related companion diagnostics, manufacturers, corresponding targeted drugs and indications. The development of companion diagnostics industry is in full swing abroad, and the domestic medical device industry is also in a thriving state. Only from 2019 to 2021, the National Drug Administration (NMPA) approved and marketed three PD-L1 companion diagnostics kits and one PD-L1 antibody: PD-L1 test kit (immunohistochemical method) PD-L1 IHC 22C3 pharmDx, PD-L1 antibody reagent (immunohistochemical method) Monoclonal Mouse Anti-Human PD-L1 Clone 22C3, PD-L1 test kit (immunohistochemical method) PD-L1 IHC 28-8 pharmDx and Anti PD-L1 antibody detection reagent (immunohistochemical method) VENTANA PD-L1 (SP263) Assay. PD-L1 (clone 22C3) was used to detect PD-L1 protein in non-small cell lung cancer tissues and assist in identifying patients who can be treated with pembrolizumab. The survival period of patients with non-squamous NSCLC may be prolonged after using nivolumab if their PD-L1 expression level were $\geq 1\%$ detected by PD-L1 (clone 28-8). PD-L1 (clone SP263) is used to detect PD-L1 protein in urothelial carcinoma and assists in identifying patients who is failure of platinum chemotherapy but can use tirelizumab, including patients who have locally advanced or metastatic urothelial carcinoma that progressed in 12 months with neoadjuvant or adjuvant chemotherapy [1]. In addition, CD117 is used

Table 31.2 FDA certified immunohistochemical related products

Target protein	Companion diagnostics products	Manufacturer	Targeted drug	Indication
HER2	PATHWAY antiHer2/neu (4B5)	Ventana	Trastuzumab	Breast cancer
	Rabbit monoclonal primary antibody			
	Bond oracle HER2 IHC system	LEICA	Trastuzumab	Breast cancer
	HercepTest	DAKO	Trastuzumab, pertuzumab, ado-trastuzumab emtansine	Breast cancer
			Trastuzumab	Gastric cancer, gastroesophageal carcinoma
EGFR	Dako EGFR pharmDx Kit	DAKO	Cetuximab, Panitumumab	Colorectal cancer
ALK	VENTANA ALK (D5F3) CDx assay	Ventana	Ceritinib, crizotinib, alectinib	NSCLC
c-KIT	Dako c-KIT pharmDx	DAKO	Imatinib	Gastrointestinal stromal tumor
PD-L1	VENTANA PD-L1 (SP142) Assay	Ventana	Atezolizumab	Urothelial carcinoma, triple-negative breast cancer, NSCLC
	PD-L1 IHC 28-8 pharmDx	DAKO	Nivolumab and ipilimumab	NSCLC
	PD-L1 IHC 22C3 pharmDx	DAKO	Pembrolizumab	NSCLC, adenocarcinoma of stomach or gastroesophageal junction, cervical carcinoma, urothelial carcinoma, head and neck squamous cell carcinoma (HNSCC), esophageal squamous cell carcinoma, triple-negative breast cancer

for the identification of gastrointestinal stromal tumors and determining the targeted use of Glivec. ER and PR are used for predicting the therapeutic effect of tamoxifen in breast cancer patients. ALK (clone D5F3) staining results guide the use of cozotinib in non-small cell lung cancer patients. HER-2 staining results of breast cancers can guide the use of trastuzumab, etc.

31.2.2 Application Status of Immunohistochemical Automation

At present, there are 29 manufacturers of immunohistochemical staining instruments with 42 types all around the world, and 18 domestic manufacturers with 23 types. Although there are multitudinous manufacturers of immunohistochemical staining instruments, the industry is almost monopolized by a few foreign enterprises. Most of them adopt the business model of "free instruments and monopolize reagents". Manufacturers sell or lease the instruments to customers at a very low price but limit the reagents used in the instruments by technical means, and finally obtain highly profits by selling special reagents for the instruments.

The current situation of domestic industry is similar, foreign brands monopolize more than 80% market share. Only a few domestic immunohistochemical instruments researched and developed on our own. The automatic immunohistochemical staining instrument Titan series of Fuzhou Maxim is a truly self-developed product. Most domestic immunohistochemical staining instruments are imitations of Leica Bond series. The main reasons for the above industry status including: (1) Core technology is still in the hands of a few large foreign-funded enterprises. (2) Foreign funded enterprises have more mature technology to deal with factors that affect the staining quality, such as dewaxing effect, antigen repair effect, reagent coverage effect, reagent dropping accuracy, temperature control system, and cleaning effect (3) The R&D cycle is long, which generally takes more than 5 years, and it requires a long-term stable core R&D team. (4) The R&D funds are huge, usually cost tens of millions of dollars, while domestic enterprises often have limited capital. (5) Immunohistochemical automation manufacturers usually have many years' experience in R&D of immunohistochemical reagents, while domestic enterprises often do not master the core technology.

31.3 Analysis of Domestic Immunohistochemical Market

According to the data from intelligent research consulting, the demand for immunohistochemical reagents in China increased from 924 million CNY in 2012 to 1.8 billion CNY in 2018, and exceeded 2 billion CNY in 2020 with a growth rate of 10–20%, which is about 10% higher than the global demand. However, the demand has not been met due to limited technology and lack of pathologists, and there is still a strong growth momentum because the following five aspects.

31.3.1 The Incidence of Cancer Is Increasing

According to the latest data from International Agency for Cancer Research (IARC) of the World Health Organization, China has more than 4.5 million new cancer cases and 3 million cancer deaths in 2020, ranking first in the world [2]. Multiple factors, such as population aging and poor lifestyle, have led to an increasing incidence of cancer. It is estimated that the total number of cancer cases will reach 5.1 million in 2025. The number of patients admitted to tumor hospitals has continued to increase, flowing the increase demand for relevant diagnosis.

31.3.2 Increase of Differential Diagnosis Items

With the discovery of antibodies' new uses and the emergence of increasing new antibodies, the application of immunohistochemistry in tumor diagnosis and differential diagnosis, classification, prognosis judgment will be more accurate. New markers are not substitutes for old one, and the number of diagnostic items for the same cancer will increase with its increase, driving the industry to further expand.

31.3.3 Development of Targeted Drugs and Companion Diagnostics

Companion diagnostics can provide information about the patient's response to specific therapeutic drugs. The common immunohistochemical companion diagnostics items include HER2, ER/PR, CD20, and PD-L1. Taking PD-1/L1 as an example, it is estimated that the potential drug users will reach 4.5 million according to new cancer cases of China in 2020. Assuming that the price of immunohistochemical test for companion diagnostics is 150 CNY, the potential market for PD-1/L1 will be nearly 700 million CNY. The demand will continue to increase with the constantly marketing of new targeted drugs.

31.3.4 Popularization of Automation Will Increase the Whole Market Scale of Immunohistochemistry in Terms of Reagent Usage

Automation has promoted the rapid development of this industry in recent years. The automated staining system can complete a larger number of immunohistochemical detection without increasing personnel. At present, there are 2217 grade-A tertiary hospital and 8833 general hospital of level II in China. Assume that the grade-A tertiary hospital and tumor hospital are equipped with five automatic machines on average, and the annual output of a single machine is about one million CNY. Other tertiary hospitals are equipped with 2 machines on average with an annual output of 500,000 CNY, and general hospital of level II are equipped with 1 machine on average with an annual output of 200,000 CNY. It can be estimated that the potential market of reagents brought by domestic automatic dyeing machines is more than 11 billion CNY, which is 4 times larger than the current market scale.

31.3.5 Rising of Domestic Enterprises with Large Market Replacement Space

At present, foreign enterprises account for about 65% and domestic enterprises account for about 35% in the domestic immunohistochemical market. The import mainly occupied the equipment and its bound secondary antibody market as the R&D of automation equipment started late in China. Domestic enterprises occupied the open primary antibody market mainly by virtue of price advantage. With the marketing and entering terminal of domestic automation equipment, domestic brands are expected to share the market occupied by foreign enterprises, and further realize import substitution on the basis of rapid expansion of the market.

31.4 Summary and Prospect

There is still a gap between the research and production of immunohistochemistry (reagents and instruments) at home and abroad. Further improvement of technology is the major premise for the development of immunodiagnosis in the future. More kinds, more specific, and more sensitive diagnostic and companion diagnostics immunohistochemical reagents and more convenient, more reliable, and more intelligent automatic immunohistochemical staining instruments will increase the application of immunohistochemistry. The standardized and scientific management of immunohistochemical products by the state and the self-management of pathology department will further increase the application, and promote the development of immunohistochemistry in vitro diagnosis in China.

Declaration Qinghai Yang, Qixin Lin and Yun Shi are employees of Fuzhou Maixin Biotech. Co., Ltd.

References

1. Ilie M, Khambata-Ford S, Copie-Bergman C, Huang L, Juco J, Hofman V, Hofman P. Use of the 22C3 anti-PD-L1 antibody to determine PD-L1 expression in multiple automated immunohistochemistry platforms. PLoS One. 2017;12(8):e0183023. https://doi.org/10.1371/journal.pone.0183023.
2. Latest global cancer data: cancer burden rises to 19.3 million new cases and 10.0 million cancer deaths in 2020 questions and answers (Q&A). iarc.who.int/faq/latest-global-cancer-data-2020-qa/. Accessed 16 Dec 2020.

32 Molecular Pathology

Chun Meng

32.1 Polymerase Chain Reaction (PCR)

32.1.1 Principle and Classification of PCR

PCR is the abbreviation of polymerase chain reaction, the basic process is taking fundamental chain as template and specific primer as starting point of extension under the catalysis of DNA polymerase, then the sub-strand DNA complementary to the fundamental chain is replicated in vitro through denaturation, annealing, extension, and other steps. Its specificity depends on the oligonucleotide primers which are complementary to both ends of the target sequence.

The basic principle of PCR has not changed, but many kinds of PCR technologies have been derived with the substantial improvement of DNA polymerase and reagent performance, as well as the continuous innovation of instruments and plastic reaction tubes, such as Inverse PCR (IPCR), Anchored PCR (APCR), Asymmetric PCR, Reverse Transcription PCR (RT-PCR), NEST-PCR, Multiplex PCR, fluorescence quantitative real-time PCR, etc. [1].

32.1.2 Development and Comparison of PCR Technology

In the 1980s, the first generation of traditional PCR technology appeared and it used agarose electrophoresis to analyze PCR products, but there were some shortcomings such as cumbersome operation, only applicable to qualitative research, and

C. Meng (✉)
Fuzhou University, Fuzhou, Fujian, China
e-mail: mengchun@fzu.edu.cn

H. Song, L. Dai (eds.), *In Vitro Diagnostic Industry in China*,
https://doi.org/10.1007/978-981-99-3110-1_32

high risk of cross contamination. In order to avoid the defects of traditional PCR and conduct quantitative analysis of target gene, the second-generation PCR named fluorescent quantitative real-time PCR was created in 1992. Fluorescent quantitative PCR (qPCR) is the mainstream technology at current. It uses specific fluorescent probes to conduct real-time monitoring of the target fragment's amplified fluorescent signal in the exponential phase. At the same time, it realizes absolute gene expression and relative quantitative detection, overcoming the defects of previous endpoint PCR quantification.

The quantitative PCR is only relative because relying on the Ct value is still the biggest technical bottleneck of quantitative PCR at present. Moreover, the sensitivity and accuracy of the detection are limited under the condition of low copy target molecules and slight difference in template concentration. Under this circumstance, the "third generation PCR" came into being, such as QX100 micro-drop digital PCR system of Bio-Rad (Table 32.1).

32.1.3 Analysis of PCR Industry Chain

The PCR industry chain can be divided into upstream biochemical raw materials, midstream PCR instruments and equipment, and downstream medical institutions and third-party testing centers.

1. Upstream

   The upstream of PCR industry chain is mainly biochemical raw materials, including enzymes, primers, etc. The manufacturers are mainly foreign tycoon, including Roche, Meridian Life Science, Solulink, and Surmodics. Due to the high difficulty in technological development and low industrialization maturity, domestic enterprises mainly focus on agency business, such as Shanghai Bioleaf.
2. Midstream

   The midstream of PCR industry chain are PCR instruments and equipment. Domestic PCR instrument participants mainly include DAAN Gene, Targeting One, Sansure Biotech, Rain Sure Biotech, and Tellgen. And foreign PCR instrument participants mainly include Roche, Qiagen, Thermo Fisher Scientific. Domestic PCR reagent participants mainly include Amoydx, Sansure Biotech, DAAN Gene, BGI, Hybri Biotech.
3. Downstream

   The downstream of PCR industry chain are mainly medical institutions and third-party testing centers. Medical institutions mainly refer to pathology department and clinical laboratory department of hospital. PCR instruments and reagents can be used for tumor detection in the pathology department and virus detection in the clinical laboratory. PCR products can also be used in third-party testing centers.

Table 32.1 Comparison of third-generation PCR technologies

Technical stage	Technical classification	Target	Advantage	Defect	Application	Representative companies
First generation	Ordinary PCR+ colloidal gold	SNP+ single nucleotide polymorphism, single locus	Rapid detection of nucleic acid	Poor accuracy and low sensitivity	Individualization drug gene detection	Xi'an Goldmag
Second generation	Fluorescence quantification PCR	Nucleic acid of pathogenic microorganism	High-precision and quantitative	–	Hepatitis virus, HPV, Coxsackie virus, *Mycobacterium tuberculosis*, etc. Genetic disease gene detection, Thalassemia, etc. Individualization drug gene detection	Sansure Biotech, DAAN Gene, SKHB, Liferiver Biotech, Lepu Gene, etc. (more than 30)
	Amplification refractory mutation system, ARMS	Oncogene mutation	High-precision (0.01–1.0%)	–	Single gene detection of tumor	Foreign: Qiangen (Germany), Roche (Switzerland), Biomerieux (France). Domestic: Amoydx
	High resolution melting, HRM	Two sites allele	High throughput, high sensitivity, good specificity, good repeatability and simple operation	–	Single gene detection of tumor	Foreign: Thermo Fisher, etc.
						Domestic: Suzhou MicroDiag Biomedicine, Wuxi Riqi Gene, etc.
Third generation	Multiplex PCR	Multi-site at the same time	Efficient, systematic, economical, simple, and convenient	Difficult to unify conditions	HPV detection	Foreign: Biofire Diagnostics (USA), Cepheid (USA)
						Domestic: Tellgen
	Digital PCR	Absolute nucleic acid quantification and detection of rare alleles	High precision, strong tolerance and high sensitivity	Expensive	Study of differential gene expression, companion diagnostics and real-time monitoring of tumor therapy, non-invasive prenatal screening	Foreign: Bio-Rad, Thermo Fisher, Stilla Technologies. Domestic: Pilot Gene, Targeting One

32.1.4 Main Enterprises and Market Pattern

32.1.4.1 Clinical Application of qPCR

qPCR is the most widely used technology for clinical molecular diagnosis at home and abroad, especially in infectious diseases (viral hepatitis, venereal diseases, and other bacteria/viruses) and tumor companion diagnostics. According to incomplete statistics, the State Food and Drug Administration had approved 806 PCR products as of December 31, 2020, and fluorescent quantitative PCR (qPCR) products accounted for 85.11%. In the field of companion diagnostics, 60% of NMPA approved products are based on qPCR technology. Besides, among 39 companion diagnostics products approved by FDA, the proportion based on qPCR technology also accounts for 38.46% (Fig. 32.1, Table 32.2).

The domestic PCR industry is highly competitive, and the leading effect in different subdivisions is significant. There are many approved PCR detection products in China, and the competition is fierce due to the relatively low threshold of second-generation PCR technology. Main enterprises include DAAN Gene, Amoydx, Hybri Biotech, Liferiver Biotech, Bioperfectus Technologies, Tellgen, SanSure Biotech. From the quantity of approved PCR detection kits, DAAN Gene has 38 kits based on qPCR technology that obtain NMPA's approval. From the perspective of different subdivided application fields (Table 32.3), the product lines of each enterprise have high overlap and fierce competition, especially in eugenics, STD, and HPV detection. However, Amoydx, Hybri Biotech, and Yaneng Biotech are absolutely leading in the field of companion diagnostics, HPV, and thalassemia detection by virtue of their first mover advantages, technology accumulation, and channel advantages. Hybri Biotech occupies 1/3 market share in the HPV detection field, and Amoydx is absolutely leading in PCR companion diagnostics (Table 32.4).

32.1.4.2 Clinical Application of Digital PCR (dPCR)

Digital PCR is still in its infancy in China. At present, only the HER2 gene amplification test kit (dPCR method) of Nanjing Quest genomics has been approved. It has great clinical application potential and advantages in tumor companion diagnostics,

Fig. 32.1 NMPA approved PCR products

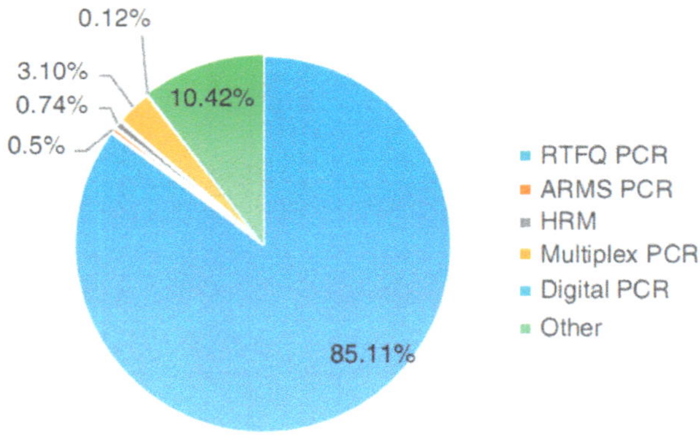

Table 32.2 Testing fields' statistics of second-generation PCR products approved by NMPA

Disease classification	Specific test kit	Approved quantity
Viral hepatitis	HBV	81
	HCV	33
	HEV	4
Venereal disease	HPV	108
	EB virus	12
	Chlamydia trachomatis, Gonococcus, *M. urealyticum*	53
	HIV/AIDS	22
Eugenics	Measles virus, Rubella virus	4
	Human cytomegalovirus	20
	Herpes simplex virus (HSV)	24
	Chromosome deletion, polyploidy	8
Other pathogenic bacteria and viruses	*Mycobacterium tuberculosis*	35
	Mycoplasma pneumoniae	15
	Influenza virus	38
	Enterovirus	43
	Respiratory syncytial virus	8
	Coxsackie virus	15
Tumor	Oncogene detection	75

early tumor screening, infectious disease detection, NIPT, pharmacogenomics, and other fields. According to Frost & Sullivan's data, the market size of China's dPCR industry has increased from 1.46 billion CNY in 2013 to 7.2 billion CNY in 2017 with CAGR = 29.2%. And the market size is expected to reach 26.66 billion CNY by 2022 (Fig. 32.2).

The favorable domestic policies and the demand for precision medical care have driven the rapid growth of dPCR, which has huge developmental potential in the future. The key drivers include: (1) Population growth and aging: The aging trend of China's population has led to the growth of tumor medicine market and the demand for in vitro detection. Digital PCR has obvious advantages in disease detection, such as tumor, infectious disease, and genetic disease. And the expansion of medical market will further promote the growth of digital PCR. (2) Favorable domestic policies: According to the 13th Five Year Special Plan for Scientific and Technological Innovation of Medical Devices issued by the General Office of the Ministry of Science and Technology of the People's Republic of China, it is required to focus on the development of POCT detection, new gene sequencer, random inspection full-automatic nucleic acid detection system, quantitative digital PCR, etc. (3) Demand for precision medicine and tumor treatment: The foundation of precision medicine lies in individualized medicine. It's highly required in the accuracy of pathogenic mutation detection and quantitative analysis. Therefore, the application of a new PCR technology is urgently needed, and Digital PCR has obvious advantages in this

Table 32.3 Comparison of detection fields covered by PCR test kits of major domestic molecular diagnostic enterprises

Manufacturer	Hepatitis	HPV	Thalassemia	STD	Eugenics	Respiratory infections	Deafness	Y chromosome deletion	Tumor
Hybri Biotech	√	√	√	√		√	√	√	
Yaneng	√	√	√				√	√	
DAAN	√	√		√	√	√			√
Bioperfectus		√		√		√			
Tellgen		√		√				√	√
Liferivwe	√	√		√	√				√
Sansure	√	√	√	√	√	√			
Amoydx									√

Table 32.4 Competition pattern of qPCR in different segmented application fields

Field	Leading enterprises	Market share	Remarks
HPV	Hybri Biotech	Hybri: about 26%, Yaneng: 17%, Qiagen:14%	First mover advantage: Hybri Biotech obtained approval of the first HPV detection kit in China in 2006.
Thalassemia	Yaneng	Yaneng: about 50%, Qiagen: about 20%, Others: 30%	Powerful government resources and earliest layout: Obtained α-Thalassemia and β-Thalassemia gene detection kit in 2008 and 2009 respectively.
Companion diagnostics	Amoydx	–	–
Viral hepatitis	DAAN	–	–
Genetic deafness	CapitalBioPro	CapitalBioPro: >50%, BGI Gene and Hybri: 10–20%	In 2019, CapitalBioPro R&D the first genetic detection kit for hereditary deafness in the world, undertook a large number of government detection projects, and has obvious advantages in government procurement.

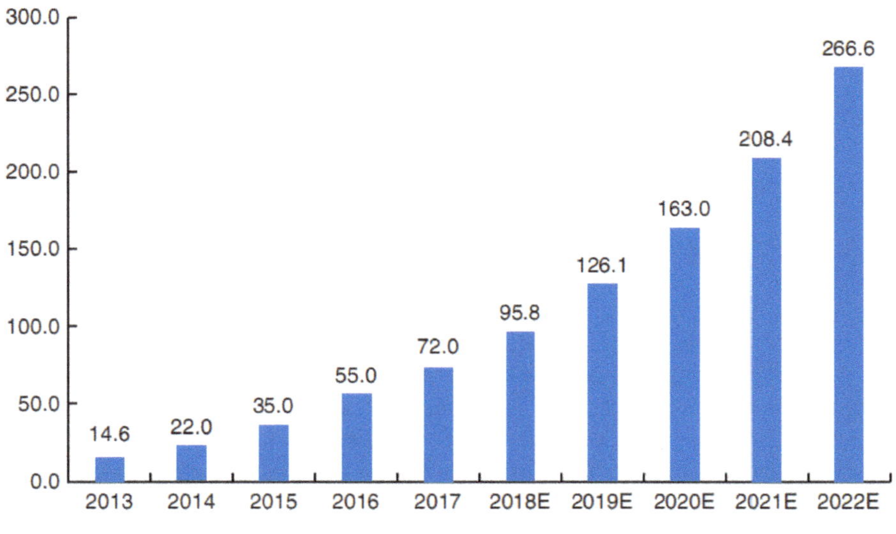

Fig. 32.2 Forecast of dPCR market scale (100 million CNY)

regard. (4) Rapid change of PCR technology: The sensitivity has been continuously improved from traditional ordinary PCR to the emerging digital PCR. The fluorescent quantitative PCR of second generation is the mainstream of PCR technology at present, and the digital PCR of third generation is the future directions with broad application prospects.

32.1.5 Analysis of PCR Industry Development Trend

32.1.5.1 The Sinking of PCR Laboratory Resources Is Expected to Drive the Release Volume of Various Diagnostic Instruments and Reagents

Due to the lack of detection capacity at the grassroots unit, the sinking of PCR laboratory resources is expected to drive the volume of various diagnostic instruments and reagents. PCR detection requires a special PCR laboratory to distinguish the operation processes of reagent preparation, sample processing, amplification and analysis, and to ensure the air cleanliness by controlling the airflow direction. The requirements for the area and operators are high. Therefore, the laboratories are concentrated in the grade-A tertiary hospitals and major third-party detection centers. According to the statistics by the middle of 2020, there are 2831 tertiary hospitals, 9901 secondary hospitals, 1102 specialized hospitals, and 3402 disease control institutions in China. It is conservatively assumed that before the introduction of policy, all tertiary hospitals have nucleic acid detection capabilities, 60% of specialized hospitals and disease control institutions, and 10% of secondary hospitals have the capabilities. A total of 10,700 medical institutions still need to complete the construction of nucleic acid detection capabilities this year. If a single laboratory is conservatively estimated to cost 1.34 million CNY, it will bring an incremental market space of 14.3 billion CNY, including 3.2 billion for nucleic acid extractor and 5.9 billion for fluorescent quantitative PCR instrument.

32.1.5.2 Domestic Substitution and Export Prospects Drive Industry Development

Foreign enterprises account for a large proportion in the domestic PCR instrument industry. Domestication of products is expected in the future, and the high-quality PCR reagents have export potential. The macroenvironment of the past 2 years has provided an opportunity for high-quality China-made instruments to be found and recognized by global customers. For example, BGI's comprehensive "Huo-Yan" laboratory has been built in batches around the world and become a multinational epidemic prevention and control outpost. The nucleic acid detection products of SanSure Biotech are exported to more than 140 countries and regions, including France, the Philippines, the United Arab Emirates, Turkey, Serbia, Bangladesh, Thailand, and the market share of some countries exceeds 80%. It's expected that domestic products will quickly catch up with foreign ones through depth contact with international customers, constantly improving products to meet international market needs and rapid iteration in the window period. Then fully opening up the space for domestication of medical apparatus and instruments, as well as the export road of domestic medium and high-end medical manufacturing.

32.1.5.3 Digital PCR Is Future Development Direction

Digital PCR is the third-generation PCR technology, its popularity is expected to continuously increase. The related technology and industrialization have developed rapidly since the advent of digital PCR. With the powerful national policies, China's digital PCR industry has maintained steady growth. At present, there is no high-end dPCR instrument in China. From the experience of foreign countries, dPCR is expected to become one of the main directions in the PCR field, leading the progress of PCR technology in the future. Domestic enterprises still need to make more progress in dPCR field.

32.1.5.4 Combined Application of Multiple Technologies in Molecular Diagnosis

At present, molecular diagnosis technology shows a trend of combining with biology, physics, and other disciplines. For example, fluorescent PCR technology is a combination of biology and physics, biochip is a combination of biology, physics, and computer science. New detection technologies such as sequencing technology, biochip technology, biosensor technology, surface plasmon resonance technology, microarray chip technology have emerged in the market. In the future, the molecular diagnosis industry will combine multiple technologies, it can not only detect in real time and quickly, but also detect multiple genes at the same time and achieve genotyping, greatly improving the level of disease diagnosis.

32.2 Gene Sequencing

Gene sequencing technology is also called DNA sequencing technology, which is aimed to obtain the base sequence of target DNA segment. The development of sequencing technology is mainly based on the two milestone concepts of "life is sequential" and "life is data." Sequence is the most basic and important data in genomics, and also the core part of big data era in the life science field.

32.2.1 The Development of Sequencing Technology

In 1977, Sanger invented the landmark terminal sequencing method, which is called the first-generation sequencing. Sanger method has become the mainstream of DNA sequencing for decades because of its simplicity, rapidity, and continuous improvement. However, it can no longer fully meet the needs of research with the development of science. The genome re-sequencing of model organism and the genome sequencing of non-model organism require lower cost, higher throughput, and faster sequencing technology. So, the next-generation sequencing came into being.

The core idea of the next-generation sequencing technology is sequencing by synthesis (SBS) or sequencing by alignment (SBL) which determines the sequence of DNA by capturing newly synthesized end labeling, and its prominent feature is high-throughput and automation. The next-generation sequencing technology not only greatly reduces the cost and improves the speed of sequencing, but also maintains high accuracy. Its limitation and bottleneck are high-throughput with short-read but long-read with low-throughput. Throughput determines the time and cost required for sequencing, while reading length determines the difficulty of reverting the real situation of genome. The third-generation sequencing technology that has solved this problem is a new milestone [2].

PacBio's SMRT and Oxford Nanopore Technologies' single molecule nanopore sequencing technology are the third-generation sequencing technology. Its biggest feature is single molecule sequencing which doesn't require PCR amplification to achieve high throughput and long-read. So the error of PCR amplification can be avoided and methylation DNA sequencing can be performed. However, there are still some shortcomings, such as high error rate, dependence on the activity of DNA polymerase, high cost, insufficient bioinformation analysis software, and less data accumulation [3, 4]. The comparison of different sequencing technologies is shown in Table 32.5.

32.2.2 Clinical Application of NGS

NGS technology is widely used in routine clinical practice, including non-invasive prenatal test (NIPT), preimplantation genetic diagnosis/preimplantation genetic screening (PGD/PGS), genetic diseases, tumors, and drug genomics. In June 2014, NMPA approved the first NGS diagnostic product for fetal chromosome aneuploidy detection. NIPT is the most mature field of NGS application at the moment in China. The advantage of NGS applied to PGD/PGS is that it can use a single platform to analyze monogenic disease and chromosome abnormalities. With the lower cost and the improvement of gene interpretation ability, the application of NGS in genetic diseases, especially rare diseases, has changed from genome to whole exome sequencing (WES) and whole genome sequencing (WGS). In 2016, a prospective study confirmed the clinical effectiveness of WES as a first-line molecular detection technology for the diagnosis and treatment of neonatal monogenic disease. Another study carried out in 2016, involving 1000 families in 54 countries, showed that WGS had a higher diagnostic rate of undiagnosed diseases than classical methods.

The tumor NGS detection used in hereditary tumor syndrome screening and somatic mutation analysis make the cancer prevention and treatment move forward to the prevention stage. The 2017 National Comprehensive Cancer Network Guide points out that NGS could be used to detect related gene mutations and genetic counseling, such as some high penetrance gene mutations related to hereditary breast cancer and ovarian carcinoma, Lynch syndrome and neurofibroma, and some middle and low penetrance genes. NGS is most widely used in the field of somatic mutation analysis. The NGS analysis of genetic variation and related driving and companion mutation in tumor initiation, development and metastasis stages are helpful to the classification, prognosis, targeted therapy, and drug resistance analysis of tumor patients. Several sequencing programs have been set up internationally to decipher cancer cell mutation patterns. The Cancer Genome Project has discovered nearly five million tumor somatic gene mutations and established the largest and most extensive cancer somatic mutation database in the world. A lot of preliminary work has laid a solid foundation for the follow-up clinical application of NGS.

Table 32.5 Comparison of the first, next, and third-generation sequencing technologies

Sequencing technology	Typical sequencing platform	Sequencing principle	Read	Throughput	Accuracy rate	Advantage	Defect
First generation	ABI/LIFE3730	Sanger dideoxy chain termination method, capillary electrophoresis	400–900 bp	0.2 Mb/run	>99%	Long-read, high accuracy	Low-throughput, high cost
	ABI/LIFE3500						
Next-generation	Illumina HiSeq	Sequencing by Synthesis, Bridge PCR, Reversible Terminator Chemistry	50–150 bp (×2)	750–1500 Gb/run	>99%	High-throughput, low cost	Short-read, complicated sample preparation
	SOLiD	Ligase sequencing	50–75 bp	50 Gb/run	>99%		
	MGI	High-density DNA Nanoball	28–100 bp	150–1440 Gb/run	>99%		
	Roche 454	Pyrosequencing	200–600 bp	0.45 Gb/run	>99%		
Third generation	PacBio SMRT	Sequencing by Synthesis/DNA Polymerase	1000–10,000 bp	0.5–0.9 Gb/run	<90%	Fast, long-read, simple sample preparation	Low accuracy, high cost
	Oxford Nanopore MinION	Nanopore exonuclease sequencing	135,000 bp	20 Gb/run	92–98%		

Tumor liquid biopsy and single cell sequencing are new directions of NGS application. The peripheral blood of tumor patients contains circulating tumor cell (CTC) or circulating tumor DNA (ctDNA), which is convenient to obtain and suitable for individualized diagnosis, prognosis, and recurrence risk assessment of tumors. Single cell NGS can reveal the differences between individual cells, providing refined guidance for tumor molecular typing and individualized treatment, which can help to accurately understand the internal heterogeneity and evolution of tumors.

32.2.3 Analysis of Gene Sequencing Industrial Chain

With the development of gene sequencing technology, the marketization of technology has attracted the attention of global capital. China has basically formed a complete industrial chain. The gene sequencing industry chain is divided into upstream equipment, reagents and consumables, midstream sequencing service, gene big data service, and downstream application (Table 32.6).

32.2.3.1 Upstream

The upstream manufacturers determine the market capacity, development prospects, and business model characteristics of the midstream service. The upstream detection instruments are mainly imported, and domestic equipment seeks to break through in many ways. Instruments and reagents form a complete set. Reagents and consumables are the core profit sources of upstream suppliers. In the long run, the integration and automation of equipment and supporting reagent consumables required for routine testing processes will become a trend. The upstream of gene sequencing industrial chain involves complex interdisciplinary and manufacturing and assembly of precision instruments. The headstream technology and patent portfolio build high barrier which promote the formation of a highly concentrated competition pattern in the upstream of the industry.

Instruments: Imported brands, mainly Illumina and Thermo have high market share and a certain monopoly position because first mover advantage. Domestic enterprises layout the R&D and production of gene sequencing equipment through acquisition, cooperative R&D, independent R&D. For example, BGI purchased Complete Genomics in 2013 and acquired the intellectual property rights of gene sequencing equipment. At present, MGI has become the leader of domestic gene sequencer R&D enterprises. NextSeq CN500, a gene sequencer jointly developed by Berry Genomics and Illumina, was marketed in 2015. In September 2020, QITAN Tech released the first independently developed fourth generation nanopore gene sequencer QNome-9604 in China, which could read more than 150 kbp. The pace of domestic substitution is accelerating.

Reagents and consumables: The localization degree is gradually increasing. The business models of testing kit mainly include IVD or LDT. It is required to register in NMPA in IVD mode, for example, Novo Gene's tumor six gene mutation detection kit based on semiconductor sequencing was approved in 2018. LDT is a

Table 32.6 Gene sequencing industrial chain

<table>
<tr><th colspan="2">Upstream (Device side)</th><th colspan="2">Midstream (Server)</th><th colspan="2">Downstream (Application side)</th></tr>
<tr><td rowspan="8">R&D and manufacture of sequencing equipment</td><td rowspan="8">Illumina, Thermo Fisher life, pacbio, Oxford Nanopore, BGI, HYK GENE, DAAN GENE, Berry Genomics</td><td rowspan="10">Gene sequencing service</td><td rowspan="10">BGI, HYK GENE, DAAN GENE, Berry Genomics, CapitalBio Corp, Novo Gene, BNR, ADICON, KingMed, GTH, WEGENE, TOPGEN</td><td rowspan="3">Scientific institution</td><td>Basic Biology Research</td></tr>
<tr><td>Basic Agronomy Research</td></tr>
<tr><td>Basic Medical Research</td></tr>
<tr><td rowspan="5">Hospital</td><td>Basic Medical Research</td></tr>
<tr><td>Non-invasive prenatal examination</td></tr>
<tr><td>Assisted reproduction testing</td></tr>
<tr><td>Tumor diagnosis and treatment</td></tr>
<tr><td>Genetic disease detection</td></tr>
<tr><td rowspan="6">Production of consumables and reagents</td><td rowspan="6">Illumina, Thermo Fisher life, pacbio, Oxford Nanopore, BGI, HYK GENE, DAAN GENE, Berry Genomics</td><td rowspan="2">Pharmaceutical enterprises</td><td>Basic Drug Research</td></tr>
<tr><td>Clinical drug testing</td></tr>
<tr><td rowspan="4">Data service</td><td rowspan="4">Illumina, Thermo Fisher life, DNAnexus, BGI, HYK GENE, UEC, QYNODE, GeneDock, Berry Genomics</td><td rowspan="4">Individual</td><td>Screening of disease susceptibility genes</td></tr>
<tr><td>Family test</td></tr>
<tr><td>Tumor diagnosis and treatment</td></tr>
<tr><td>Drug metabolism test</td></tr>
</table>

self-built project of the medical laboratory. Genetron heath, a cancer precision medical enterprise, focuses on LDT in its diagnosis and monitoring business.

32.2.3.2 Midstream

Sequencing service is the fastest growing part of the industrial chain and occupies the largest market. Data analysis is key to the development of gene sequencing industry. Enterprises that are ahead of layout data analysis platform are expected to win the first opportunity in the competition.

The midstream of global gene sequencing industrial chain has accelerated expansion. According to BCC data, the market share of gene sequencing services in global gene sequencing market is 51.4% in 2018 and 57.4% in 2023 (predicted). And the gene sequencing service market will occupy 51.5% and 62.1% of the overall market share of China's gene sequencing in 2017 and 2022 (predicted) respectively. The application in downstream of the industrial chain is constantly enriched to promote the expansion of the midstream market scale.

The business model of gene sequencing service enterprises is mainly to earn income by providing sample testing, processing, data analysis, and other charging items. The technical and financial barriers in the midstream are lower than those in the upstream equipment manufacturing, so many domestic enterprises cut into the gene sequencing industry from the midstream. As the number of sequencing service enterprises continues to increase, the intensified competition has driven the sequencing price down to a certain extent. Most enterprises have a high revenue from sample testing, which is highly dependent on equipment. The operating performance is greatly affected by the prime cost, because the upstream manufacturers have greater bargaining power. In addition, the original data from the sequencer can only obtain the variation information through genome comparison, data filtering and screening and other steps, providing reference for disease diagnosis and treatment. Data analysis is the key to the development of gene sequencing service industry and the differentiation point of enterprises' comprehensive technical strength.

Gene data analysis and interpretation are related to the application of downstream gene sequencing. In the future, the gene sequencing industry will move from product phase to data platform phase. Gene cloud platform service is required and inevitable trend of industry development. Sequencing service is seriously homogeneous. But sequencing data analysis mainly relies on bioinformatics, medical big data, cloud platform, and other technologies to form a gene database, thereby optimizing data analysis capabilities and improving efficiency and accuracy. Leading enterprises like Novo Gene, BGI, and Illumina have vertically extended to gene cloud platform services based on their original businesses.

32.2.3.3 Downstream

The application side determines market size of the midstream gene sequencing service segmentation. The scientific research market has the most mature development, the clinical market has the largest capacity, and the penetration and recognition of the consumer market have increased rapidly.

The scientific research gene detection market started early, with the most mature application, few detection institutions, large market share of leading companies, and technical and resource barriers. Its segmentation and market scale are not as broad as clinical, so most companies' business models tend to be integrated solutions, clinical and scientific research parallel. For example, Novo Gene is a leading scientific research company on gene sequencing, which has accumulated rich technology and customer resources, at the same time, it has actively deployed clinical applications to further open up growth space.

The main users of clinical market are medical institutions and patients, whose demand for disease treatment is relatively stable and has the most developmental potential. Reproductive health is one of the most mature clinical application fields at present. Its gene testing mainly includes premarital and prenatal testing, embryo transfer screening, non-invasive prenatal diagnosis (NIPT), neonatal monogenic inherited disease testing, etc. NIPT has the most mature development among them. BGI and Berry Genomics occupy more than 90% market share of NIPT. However, NIPT market penetration rate is about 10% at present, with huge potential to increase. The application of gene detection in tumor mainly includes tumor susceptibility prediction, early diagnosis and screening of tumors, personalized medication, and postoperative detection. The maturity of technology development is personalized medication > postoperative detection > early diagnosis and screening > tumor susceptibility prediction. Based on the large number of cancer patients and urgent demand in China, the development of tumor gene detection industry is expected.

The consumer gene detection market is dominated by the public, with a large scale of potential users. However, the public's awareness of gene testing and willingness to pay still need to be cultivated, and capital may be the key factor to promote public awareness and penetration. At present, the business model of consumer application enterprises is mainly to obtain users through preferential prices, card returns, low price trials, etc. It explores derivative business models with gene data as the core on the basis of data accumulation.

32.2.4 Summary and Prospect

NGS is one of the most important technological advances in biological science in past 30 years. At present, the domestic hardware of gene sequencing technology is simultaneously developing as that of foreign countries, but the software construction lags behind slightly. High throughput and long-read will be the development trend due to continuous improvement of NGS technology, and the detection target will be transferred from DNA to RNA. The current disadvantages, such as data processing, quality control, ethics, will be readily solved with the continuous decline of testing costs, optimization and upgrading of sequencing methods, intelligent data interpretation, and accumulation of clinical experience. And NSG will gradually become a routine clinical testing item.

References

1. Yu M, Cao Y, Ji Y. The principle and application of new PCR Technologies. IOP Conf Ser Earth Environ Sci. 2017;100:012065. https://doi.org/10.1088/1755-1315/100/1/012065.
2. Park ST, Kim J. Trends in next-generation sequencing and a new era for whole genome sequencing. Int Neurourol J. 2016;20(Suppl 2):S76–83. https://doi.org/10.5213/inj.1632742.371.
3. Eid J, et al. Real-time DNA sequencing from single polymerase molecules. Science. 2009;323(5910):133–8.
4. Guo Y. Review of the application and advantages and disadvantages of sequencing technology in gene diagnosis. Hereditas (Beijing). 2014;36(11):1121–30.

Part X

Development Report of IVD Reagent Raw Materials

Classification and Status of IVD Reagent Raw Materials

33

Guangyu Yang, Hongsen Jin, Shuai Han, Huisheng Zhang, and Peng Cui

In 2019 and 2020, the in vitro diagnostic (IVD) industry presented a trend of accelerated growth due to the impact of Coronavirus Disease-2019 (COVID-19). In 2019, the market size of the IVD industry increased by about 10–15%. In 2020, it achieved an accelerated growth of above 40%, driving the market size of core IVD reagent raw materials to grow from 6–7 billion to over 10 billion. It is estimated that the growth rate of IVD reagent raw materials in 2021 exceeded 20%. The market shares of Chinese IVD reagent raw materials manufacturers have continued to rise in various market segments, especially in the emergency supply of raw materials related to nucleic acid testing. The research and development (R&D) and large-scale manufacturing capabilities of domestic manufacturers have been verified. Seen from the overall market of IVD reagent raw materials, more than 80% of the products are provided by overseas brands. Over the next 3–5 years, supply chain assurance will still be the main trend of the IVD reagent raw materials market. In 2019 and 2020, the Ministry of Science and Technology, the State Council, and the China Securities Regulatory Commission all issued relevant policies to provide guidance for the development of the key IVD reagent raw materials industry. In 2019, there was a lack of financing in the IVD reagent raw materials industry. In 2020, five IVD reagent raw materials manufacturers successively submitted their initial public offering (IPO) applications, which planned to raise a total of 5.908

G. Yang (✉)
Shanghai Jiaotong University, Shanghai, China
e-mail: yang@hzymes.com

H. Jin · S. Han
Wuhan Hzymes Biotechnology Co., Ltd., Wuhan, Hubei, China

H. Zhang
Shenzhen University, Shenzhen, Guangdong, China

P. Cui
Fapon Biotech Inc., Shenzhen, Guangdong, China

H. Song, L. Dai (eds.), *In Vitro Diagnostic Industry in China*,
https://doi.org/10.1007/978-981-99-3110-1_33

billion. China's IVD reagent raw materials industry has taken a fast lane and received extensive attention from the capital market, but there are also restrictive factors. In this case, IVD reagent raw materials manufacturers need to look for breakthroughs in refined R&D, intra-industry collaboration, government–industry–university–research–employer–finance cooperation, and overseas market development.

Used to test blood, urine, body fluids, and other samples outside the human body, IVD reagents can provide a basis for disease diagnosis and health assessment. Their test results have a bearing on above 70% of medical decisions. In the background of the break of the COVID-19 pandemic in 2020, the polymerase chain reaction technology and the immune detection technology in the IVD field have played vital roles in the clinical diagnosis of severe acute respiratory syndrome coronavirus-2 (SARS-CoV-2), the screening of infected persons, and the epidemiological investigation.

The IVD reagent raw materials industry is divided into upstream, midstream, and downstream industries. Among them, the upstream industry involves core IVD reagent raw materials, mainly providing basic raw materials for midstream IVD reagent raw materials manufacturers, such as enzymes, coenzymes, substrates, antigen-antibodies, magnetic beads, and microspheres. It belongs to the field of basic materials. At present, this field is dominated by overseas brands, and the domestic IVD reagent raw materials industry is still in its infancy. The COVID-19 pandemic in 2020, however, has driven domestic raw materials manufacturers into a stage of rapid development.

According to the *Report on China's* In-vitro *Diagnosis Industry 2019* and the *Report on China's* In-vitro *Diagnosis Industry 2020*, the total size of China's IVD reagent market was about 80 billion in 2019, and reached around 115 billion in 2020, a growth of above 43% on the basis of 2019. On the basis of public data and survey questionnaire analysis, it is estimated that the market size of IVD reagent raw materials was 6–7 billion in 2019, and exceeded 10 billion yuan in 2020. Among them, antigen-antibodies accounted for nearly 50%; enzymes, coenzymes, and substrates accounted for nearly 30%; raw materials such as probe/primers accounted for about 10%; and magnetic beads, microspheres, and so forth accounted for about 10% (see Fig. 33.1 for details).

Depending on their application fields, IVD reagent raw materials can be classified into biochemical diagnosis raw materials, molecular diagnosis raw materials, immunodiagnosis raw materials, gene sequencing raw materials, and other raw materials (such as coagulation-related raw materials, biosensor enzyme raw materials, and mass spectrometry raw materials).

Biochemical diagnosis raw materials include enzymes, coenzymes, substrates, and antigen-antibodies. To be specific, the market sizes of enzymes, substrates, and coenzymes are estimated to be about 400–500 million, 100 million, and 100 million, respectively. At present, the major domestic suppliers of enzymes, coenzymes, and substrates used for biochemical diagnosis include Toyobo, Roche, Hzymes Biotech, Apis, and Dacheng Biotechnology. Overseas brands account for above 80% of the market size.

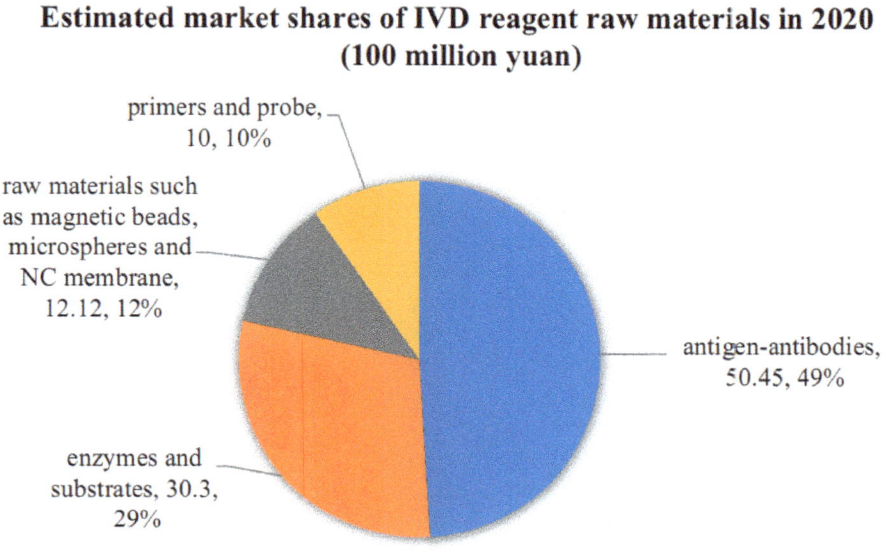

Fig. 33.1 Market shares of various products of IVD reagent raw materials

The market size of antigen-antibodies in the field of biochemical diagnosis is estimated to be about 100–200 million. The major suppliers include Roche, Dako, OYC, HyTest, and Fapon Biotech. Overseas brands account for above 80% of the market size in this field as well. The market size of latex microspheres used by the reagents for latex-enhanced immune turbidimetry is less than 100 million, and this field is dominated by overseas brands. The major suppliers in this field include ThermoFisher and Agilent. Some domestic biochemical reagent manufacturers can produce latex microspheres of certain particle sizes.

Biochemical diagnosis raw materials also involve the special form of original reagent production service (biochemical reagent Original Entrusted Manufacture (OEM)). The market size of enzyme-related reagents is about 400–500 million. The major suppliers include Toyobo, Sjodax, BCT Biotech, Hzymes Biotech, Holmes, and Juchuang Biotechnology. Immune reagents have a market size of 200–300 million, and are mainly supplied by DENKA SEIKEN and Sekisui Medical. Overseas brands account for above 70% of the overall OEM market size. Some biochemical reagent manufacturers, such as BSBE, EPNK, Zhicheng Biological Technology, and Xincheng Biological, also participate in the circulation of OEM reagents.

In the field of molecular diagnosis, the market size of pretreatment enzyme raw materials (proteinase K) is about 200 million, and the major suppliers are Merck, Roche, Hzymes Biotech, and Gproan. The market size of core enzyme raw materials is about 500–600 million. The market size of Polymerase Chain Reaction (PCR) and Reverse Transcription-Polymerase Chain Reaction (RT-PCR) premixes is about one billion, and the major suppliers include NEB, Takara, Vazyme, and Fapon Biotech. Overseas brands have seized above 70% of the market share. The market size of five deoxyribonucleotides including Deoxy-Ribonucleoside Triphosphate (dNTP) is about 100 million, and the major suppliers are Roche, C&W, and Huaren Pharmaceutical. The market size of Next-Generation Sequencing (NGS) platform raw materials is about 100–200 million, and overseas brands have seized above 90% of the market share. The market size of probe/primers for molecular diagnosis has grown rapidly due to COVID-19, reaching around one billion in 2020. The major suppliers include Sangon Biotech, Genscript, General Biol, Tsingke Biotechnology, and BiOligo.

In the field of immunodiagnosis, depending on the specific testing items involved, nearly 100 kinds of relevant antigens and corresponding antibodies are available as raw materials, and the market size is about 5 billion. The major suppliers include HyTest, Fapon Biotech, Genstars, KEY-BIO Biotech, CUSAg, MAIYUE, TRX Biotech, and Cnpair Biotech. The market size of immunodiagnostic enzyme raw materials and luminescent substrates is about 200–300 million. The major suppliers include Roche, MCT, and Hzymes Biotech. Overseas brands have seized above 80% of the market share.

The market size of coagulation-related raw materials in the field of in vitro diagnosis is about 100–200 million, and they are mainly provided by overseas brands.

The market size of biosensor enzyme raw materials is about 200–300 million. The major suppliers are all overseas brands, including Toyobo, Amano Enzyme, and Kikkoman.

Currently, the clinical and scientific research market of enzymes for mass spectrometry has a size of less than 100 million, but it is developing rapidly. The major suppliers are all overseas brands, including NEB.

Declaration Hongsen Jin and Shuai Han are employees of Wuhan Hzymes Biotechnology Co., Ltd.

Peng Cui is an employee of Fapon Biotech Inc.

34 Development Bottlenecks and Favorable Factors of IVD Reagent Raw Materials

Guangyu Yang, Hongsen Jin, Shuai Han, Huisheng Zhang, and Peng Cui

34.1 Development Bottlenecks of IVD Reagent Raw Materials

Core in vitro diagnostic (IVD) reagent raw materials constitute the basis for the research and development (R&D) and innovation of IVD reagents, and belong to the field of basic disciplines that require long-term investment. China's IVD reagent raw materials industry started relatively late. Enterprises specialized in the R&D and production of IVD reagent raw materials did not appear until around 2000. Compared with overseas brands of IVD reagent raw materials, domestic brands are lagged behind, no matter in terms of brand influence, innovative R&D capability, production process research, and quality control procedures. This gap is clearly reflected by the fact that overseas brands have seized above 80% of the market share of IVD reagent raw materials in China.

At present, the bottleneck problems restricting the development of core IVD reagent raw materials in China can be described from four aspects.

First, the domestic IVD reagent raw materials industry has its own shortcomings, and there is a gap between overseas and domestic brands in product performance. The process of localization substitution is not going smoothly.

G. Yang (✉)
Shanghai Jiaotong University, Shanghai, China
e-mail: yang@hzymes.com

H. Jin · S. Han
Wuhan Hzymes Biotechnology Co., Ltd., Wuhan, Hubei, China

H. Zhang
Shenzhen University, Shenzhen, Guangdong, China

P. Cui
Fapon Biotech Inc., Shenzhen, Guangdong, China

H. Song, L. Dai (eds.), *In Vitro Diagnostic Industry in China*,
https://doi.org/10.1007/978-981-99-3110-1_34

According to our survey, more than 50% of enterprises in the industry believe that the inability of products to meet customer demands is currently the biggest obstacle to the development of domestic raw materials. Specifically, domestic IVD reagent raw materials manufacturers are inadequate in terms of innovative R&D capability, large-scale production capacity, and quality control procedures.

Second, domestic IVD reagent raw materials manufacturers have small scale and weak policy and market influence.

Due to the wide variety, diverse professional fields, and long R&D cycle of IVD reagent raw materials, the scale of domestic IVD reagent raw materials manufacturers is generally small. According to our survey results, there were about 10 domestic manufacturers with a sales volume of above 100 million yuan in 2020, and more than 300 IVD reagent raw materials manufacturers participated in China Association of Clinical Laboratory Practice Expo (CACLP) and China IVD Supply Chain Expo (CISCE) in 2021. Quantitatively, all major overseas brands have at least 2000 kinds of products, while domestic IVD reagent raw materials manufacturers have only a little more than 1300 kinds at most, as detailed in Table 34.1.

Third, there is a lack of synergism between IVD reagent raw materials manufacturers and academic circles, and the transformation of scientific and technological achievements is not smooth.

On the one hand, academic circles face a lack of timely and accurate information about technical demands, and it is difficult to determine the direction of basic research. Besides the lack of industrialization and engineering management experience on the part of basic research teams, there is also a lack of research on processes supporting the transformation of R&D achievements into mass production. In the transformation of R&D achievements, there is also the scarcity of resources necessary for large-scale industrialization, and neither hardware nor software can meet the demands of industrial transformation.

On the other hand, business circles lack professional and forward-looking technical information sources. The forward-looking talents of basic disciplines are all in universities and research institutions, and are rarely available to enterprises. There is also a lack of high-end R&D talents that are essential for the R&D of innovative products, as high-end R&D talents are also concentrated in universities and scientific research institutes. In addition, there is also the inadequacy of high-end research equipment. This is because research on IVD reagent raw materials requires a large

Table 34.1 Comparison of domestic and overseas IVD reagent raw materials manufacturers in terms of number of products

Overseas manufacturers	Number of products	Domestic manufacturers	Number of products
Merck	>300,000	Fapon Biotech	>1300
ThermoFisher	>100,000	Vazyme	>500
NEB	>20,000	Yeasen	>500
Roche diagnostics	>10,000	Hzymes Biotech	>500
DSM	>5000		
Toyobo	>2000		

number of high-end research equipment in a wide range of fields, making it impossible for enterprises to make large-scale investment in the purchase of such equipment without forecasting the prospective earnings.

Fourth, the IVD reagent raw materials industry is scattered, and there is a lack of policy support at the local level.

China's IVD reagent raw materials manufacturers are distributed all over the country. In fact, they are scattered in various regions nationwide, except in the Yangtze River Delta, the Pearl River Delta, and the Beijing-Tianjin-Hebei region (where the distribution is relatively concentrated). The support policies formulated by local governments have a narrow coverage and little effect. IVD reagent raw materials manufacturers have to go through a long cycle from establishment to achievement of profitability. Due to the superposition of a variety of factors, the IVD reagent raw materials industry benefits little from local industrial policies.

34.2 Favorable Factors of IVD Reagent Raw Materials

The above four factors pose the main obstacles to the development of the IVD reagent raw materials industry. However, with the increase in the number and the improvement in the quality of core IVD reagent raw materials manufacturers in China, as well as the changes in domestic and foreign situations and the capital market's emphasis on the upstream raw materials industry, factors favorable for the development of the industry have begun to emerge.

First, midstream IVD reagent raw materials manufacturers are paying significantly more attention to the upstream raw materials industry.

Due to the impact of Coronavirus Disease-2019 (COVID-19) since 2020, many IVD reagent raw materials have been out-of-stock, prompting midstream IVD reagent raw materials manufacturers to take seriously the security of supply of upstream raw materials. During this period, more midstream IVD reagent raw materials manufacturers are open to the possibility of domestic upstream raw materials manufacturers serving as alternative suppliers, which creates more opportunities for domestic IVD reagent raw materials manufacturers. At the same time, midstream IVD reagent raw materials manufacturers, under the cost pressure of centralized bidding and procurement, are valuing the cooperation with upstream raw materials manufacturers, and even playing an active role in the layout of upstream raw material industries, thereby promoting the rapid development of raw material manufacturers.

Second, financial capitals are paying attention to the IVD reagent raw materials industry.

According to public statistics, in 2019, IVD reagent raw materials manufacturers have received the attention of only a few angel investment institutions. In 2020, IVD reagent raw materials manufacturers raised a total of more than 2.5 billion, involving areas such as antigen-antibodies, molecular diagnosis, magnetic beads, and microspheres. See Table 34.2 for details.

Table 34.2 Financing conditions of IVD reagent raw materials manufacturers in 2020

Enterprise name	Main product	Disclosure time	Round	Financing amount
AbMax Biotechnology	Antibodies	2020/3/18	Equity	Undisclosed
Yacoo	Biobuffer	2020/4/16	Equity	Undisclosed
Vazyme	Molecular enzyme	2020/5/8	C	550 million yuan
CW BIO	Molecular enzyme	2020/9/2	Equity	245 million yuan
Bioeast Biotech	Antibodies, enzymes, microspheres, etc.	2020/11/25	Angel investment	Tens of millions yuan
Vdo Biotech	Microspheres	2020/12/14	Equity	Undisclosed
ABclonal Technology	Antibodies, molecular enzymes	2020/12/18	C	600 million yuan
Fapon Biotech	Antigen-antibodies, molecular enzymes	2020/9	A+	About one billion yuan

Table 34.3 Summary of IPO filing by IVD reagent raw materials manufacturers in 2020 (as of October 2021)

Enterprise name	Sino Biological	ACRO Biosystems	Nanomicro Tech	Vazyme	Fapon Biotech
Application result	Passed	Passed	Passed	Passed	Pending approval by China Securities Regulatory Commission (CSRC)
Stock exchange	ChiNext Board of Shenzhen Stock Exchange	ChiNext Board of Shenzhen Stock Exchange	STAR Market of Shanghai stock exchange	STAR Market of Shanghai Stock Exchange	ChiNext Board of Shenzhen Stock Exchange
Time for deliberation	2021.3.4	2021.4.16	2021.4.21	2021.7.13	/
Number of shares issued	17 million shares	20 million shares	44 million shares	40.01 million shares	No more than 40.01 million shares
Amount raised	900 million	937 million	365 million	120 million	2.506 billion

In 2020, five IVD reagent raw materials manufacturers successively submitted their initial public offering (IPO) applications, planning to raise a total of 5.908 billion. The funds raised would mainly be used for R&D center construction, innovative product R&D, capacity expansion, and marketing investment. See Table 34.3 for details.

Third, the government attaches importance to the security of supply of key raw materials.

Since 2019, the State Council, the National Health Commission, and the China Securities Regulatory Commission have all issued relevant incentive policies, with particular emphasis on the security of the supply chain of key raw materials, providing directional guidance for the development of IVD reagent raw materials.

34.3 Development Suggestions for the IVD Reagent Raw Materials Industry

According to a survey on IVD reagent raw materials manufacturers, more than 50% of the respondents believed that the growth rate of the market size of the industry in 2021 would fall between 20% and 30%. However, according to the relevant statistics released in the prospectus of Vazyme, the market share of domestic IVD reagent raw materials is not expected to exceed 20% until 2024. Therefore, in the next 3–5 years, overseas brands will still be the major suppliers of IVD reagent raw materials in China. For domestic IVD reagent raw materials manufacturers, the joint efforts of all parties concerned are needed to break through the bottlenecks and realize leapfrog development.

First, R&D investment should be increased to advance toward refined quality standards. The R&D of IVD reagent raw materials is a long and ongoing process that requires continuous investment. Only by fully elevating product performance to an internationally advanced level can domestic brands be expected to compete with overseas brands on the domestic market. Especially, in terms of some refined quality standards, such as miscellaneous enzyme contamination, microbial load, and system suitability, the establishment of national standards on key IVD reagent raw materials should be promoted. Currently, there is a lack of relevant industries or national standards on IVD reagent raw materials, due to which the evaluation of product performance remains stagnant at the level of system adaptation at the application side. Regardless of enzyme activity determination, substrate purity analysis, and antibody titer determination, different enterprises have different methods and standards, which pose challenges to the evaluation of product quality. In this context, promoting the establishment of industrial or national standards will help to standardize and normalize the development of the industry, and avoid the phenomenon of "bad money driving out good money."

Second, the leading role of industry associations should be brought into full play to promote the coordinated development of the industry. The IVD reagent raw materials industry involves many fields and technical platforms, making it difficult for a single enterprise to achieve full coverage of product lines. In this case, industrial synergy and complementary advantages can be realized only through giving full play to the leading role of industry associations, uniting enterprises in the industry, and creating a favorable market competition atmosphere. Notably, in terms of the layout of product lines and the division of labor, guidance should be given to enterprises with different technological advantages, so as to rationally allocate R&D resources and avoid repeated construction.

Third, new "barrier-less" R&D institutions should be organized to improve the success rate of innovation and transformation.

A "six-in-one" synergistic system, i.e., government–industry–university–research–employer–finance, should be established in place relying on relevant industrial policies, and R&D institutions without the barriers of academic research or industrial enterprises should be developed. On the one hand, experts and scholars from universities and research institutions should be helped to understand the current situations of industrial development and market demands, and clarify the direction of basic research. On the other hand, industrial enterprises should be assisted in fully utilizing the high-end R&D talents and equipment of universities and research institutions, so as to accelerate the pace of innovation and R&D and improve the quality of raw materials. At the same time, the new product R&D demands of midstream manufacturers should be introduced to conduct joint application evaluation with downstream product users such as hospitals and Centers for Disease Controls (CDCs). Combined with the support of financial capitals, we can improve the success rate of innovation and transformation and catch up with the highest level of raw material R&D and production worldwide. At present, the establishment of the Institute of Key Raw Materials under the Shanghai Institute of Laboratory Medicine is an attempt to break the barriers between academic circles and industry, paving the way for the direct industrialization of academic research achievements. The in vitro diagnostic reagent raw material industry goes out. Currently, the main market shares of domestic IVD reagent raw materials are still based in China, and the size of the overseas market is several times that of the domestic market.

Fourth, as domestic IVD products go overseas, it is the responsibility of IVD reagent raw materials manufacturers to ensure the security of supply of IVD reagent raw materials in China. Meanwhile, with the improvement in the R&D level of IVD reagent raw materials manufacturers, joining the supply chain of overseas IVD reagent raw materials manufacturers has emerged as an important development direction. This has raised high requirements for the R&D, production, quality management, marketing, technical support, and other capabilities of IVD reagent raw materials manufacturers.

34.4 Conclusions

The IVD reagent raw materials industry is in an era of great change. There is not only the rapid growth and demonstration effect of leading enterprises, but also the rapid expansion of characteristic small and micro enterprises in market segments. Coupled with the attention of financial capitals, the IVD reagent raw materials industry has entered a stage of rapid development.

The development of the IVD reagent raw materials industry requires policy support and the guidance of industry associations, which create a favorable competitive atmosphere and promote industrial synergy. Driven by the rapid development of the IVD reagent raw materials industry and the intensification of competition among midstream manufacturers, collaboration with upstream raw materials manufacturers will be the future trend. The industrial layout and capacity building for overseas markets will be the next hotspot of competition for IVD reagent raw materials manufacturers. In view of the bottlenecks and difficulties currently faced by IVD reagent raw materials manufacturers, improving product quality, investing in innovative R&D, promoting refined quality standards, and strengthening industry–university–research–application–cooperation are key breakthrough directions. In conclusion, the development trend of the IVD reagent raw materials industry is promising, but there are still challenges to overcome. In this context, the joint efforts of the whole industry chain are needed to maintain the healthy and stable growth of the industry.

Declaration Hongsen Jin and Shuai Han are employees of Wuhan Hzymes Biotechnology Co., Ltd.

Peng Cui is an employee of Fapon Biotech Inc.

Part XI

Reference Standards and Controls for In Vitro Diagnostic Reagents

35 Development and Application Status of National Reference Materials for in Vitro Diagnostic Reagents

Jian Zhang, Junli Zu, and Gongcheng Liu

35.1 General

In vitro diagnosis refers to the activity of analyzing and testing samples (blood, body fluids, tissues, etc.) taken from a human body by means of chemical, physical, or biological analysis, so as to evaluate the physiological and pathological state of the human body. Corresponding instruments and reagents are required in the analysis and testing process of in vitro diagnosis, which then constitutes a measurement system. Due to the huge market demand, there are a huge number of in vitro diagnostic (IVD) manufacturers for the same measurand. Meanwhile, due to the differences in technological development, IVD reagents with different detection principles for the same measurand are developed. However, in clinical use scenarios, the laboratory results need to be as consistent as possible between different measurement systems to decrease the differences between different laboratory results and improve the comparability. Therefore, building a reference measurement system for IVD reagents is an effective method to achieve such purpose.

In 1998, the European Union approved the Directive 98/79/EC on In Vitro Diagnostic Medical Devices (hereinafter referred to as the EU Directive). The EU Directive stipulates that available reference measurement procedures and/or available high-order reference materials must be used to ensure the traceability of the assigned values of calibrators for IVD reagents. Thereafter, the International Organization for Standardization (ISO) has successively issued ISO17511 and

J. Zhang (✉)
Shanghai Bioyuan Biotech Co., Ltd., Shanghai, China
e-mail: zhangjian@bioyuan.cn

J. Zu · G. Liu
Zhengzhou Bioyuan Biotech Co., Ltd., Zhengzhou, Henan, China

H. Song, L. Dai (eds.), *In Vitro Diagnostic Industry in China*,
https://doi.org/10.1007/978-981-99-3110-1_35

ISO18153, which put forward the path and requirements for the traceability of clinical laboratory results. The General Conference of Weights and Measures (CIPM), the International Federation of Clinical Chemistry and Laboratory Medicine (IFCC), and the International Laboratory Accreditation Cooperation (ILAC) jointly established the Joint Committee on Traceability on Laboratory Medicine (JCTLM) to identify and evaluate existing measurement procedures and reference materials, and publish qualified measurement procedures and reference materials, thereby promoting the standardization of test results worldwide.

Reference materials and certified reference materials were first proposed by the ISO in 1977, and then are continuously revised by the Committee on Reference Materials (REMCO) of ISO. In ISO/REMCO Guide 34 (Version 3, 2009) and Guide 35 (Version 2, at the end of 2006), a Reference Material (RM) is defined as a material with one or more specific properties that are sufficiently uniform and stable, and has been determined to conform to the intended use in measurement. Meanwhile, the use of reference material is clearly described, that is, it can be used for calibration of measurement systems, evaluation of measurement procedures, assignment of values to other materials, and quality control (QC). Reference materials with documents issued by the authority to provide one or more property measurement values obtained by testing of effective procedures with the statement of uncertainty and measurement traceability are called certified reference materials.

In the process of clinical laboratory measurement, calibrators or calibrator materials are used to calibrate the measurement procedure. Calibrator or calibrator material is a reference material that has an independent assigned value used in a calibration function. So, calibrators are intrinsically also reference materials. In clinical laboratory, calibration materials can be divided into primary calibrators (reference materials), secondary calibrators, manufacturers' working calibrators, and manufacturers' product calibrators according to traceability hierarchy. Hierarchy of different calibrators in a traceability chain and institutes responsible for implementation are shown in Fig. 35.1.

To better understand the actual traceability of different calibrators in measurement procedures, Fig. 35.2 illustrates the traceability diagram of serum calcium measurement, and the actual traceability process can be understood according to the measurement procedures and calibration substances shown in the diagram.

The importance of traceability of clinical laboratory results is required for the development of clinical laboratory quality assurance. The traceability of clinical laboratory results can reduce not only the inconsistency between different laboratories and different detection methods, but also the cost of health care. The earliest standardization of cholesterol determination in the USA has reduced the uncertainty of cholesterol analysis from 18% in 1969 to 5.5–7.5% in 1994, which can reduce the medical expenditure caused by wrong diagnosis and classification by 100 million US dollars every year. Therefore, the reference system of clinical laboratory is not only to guarantee health care quality, but also it is of great significance for saving social resources.

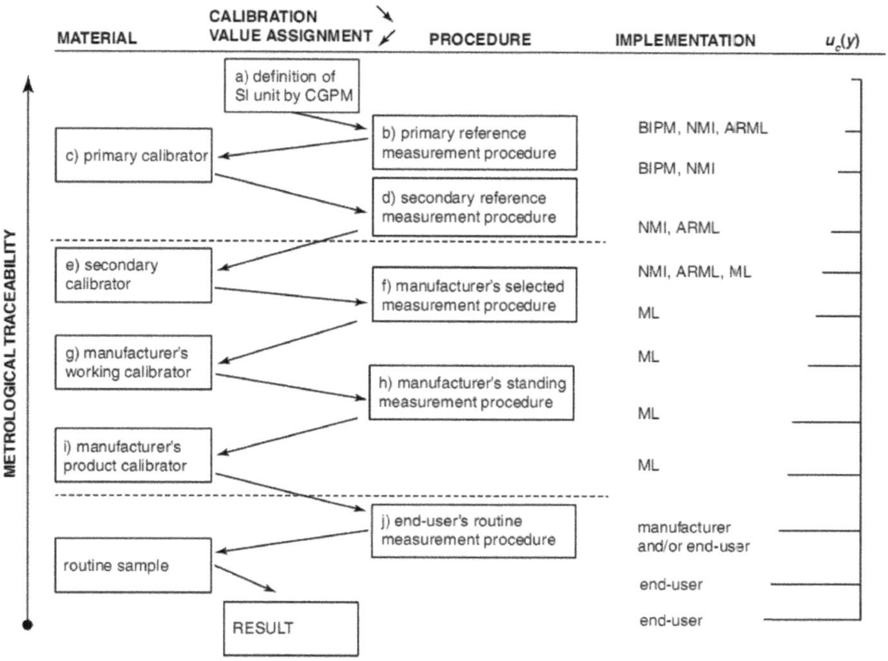

Fig. 35.1 Measurement procedures and measurement value traceability diagram of calibration substances [1]. *CGPM* General Conference on Weights and Measures, *ARML* Accredited Reference Measurement Laboratory, *BIPM* International Bureau of Weights and Measures, *NMI* National Measure Institute, *ML* Manufacturer's Laboratory

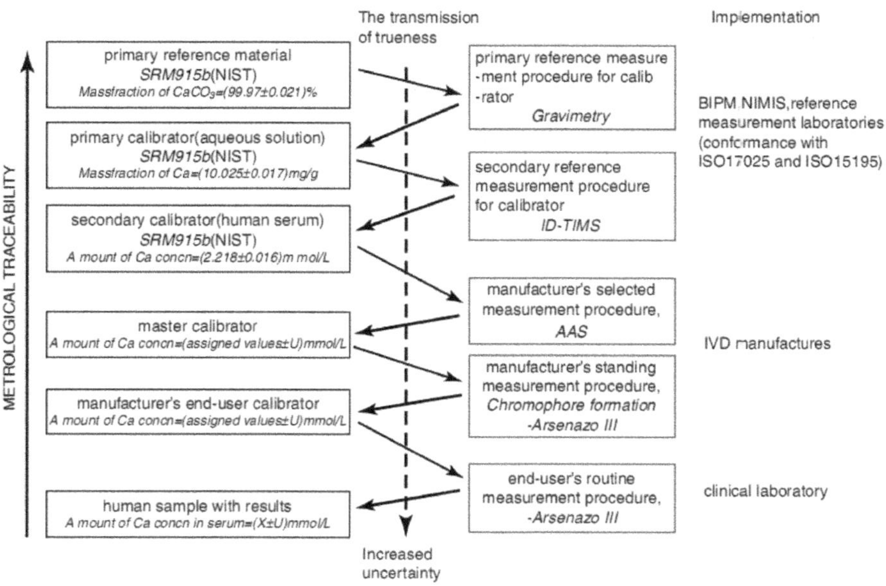

Fig. 35.2 Measurement value traceability diagram of serum calcium measurement. *AAS* Atomic Absorption Spectroscopy, *BIPM* International Bureau of Weights and Measures, *ID-TIMS* Isotope dilution thermoionization mass spectrometry, *NIMIS* National Institute of Metrology In Standrads, *NIST* National Institute of Standards and Technology, *IVD* in vitro diagnosis, *SRM* Standard reference material

35.2 Supervision and Management of Domestic Reference Materials

Reference materials, which are of great significance to the traceability of laboratory results, are under the unified management of countries. In accordance with the provisions of the *Metrology Law of the People's Republic of China*, the *Detailed Rules for the Implementation of the Metrology Law*, and the *Measures for the Administration of Reference Materials*, reference materials are legally managed as measuring instruments in China. According to the *Administrative Licensing Law of the People's Republic of China*, the grading review of reference materials is a national administrative licensing project.

35.2.1 Grading of Reference Materials

The properties of reference materials include homogeneity, stability, and measurement value accuracy meeting intended use. The accuracy of property measurement values of reference materials determines the use scope thereof, and is also an important basis for grading. Reference materials are divided into two categories in China, namely primary (national) reference materials and secondary (departmental) reference materials. Table 35.1 illustrates major similarities and differences of primary reference materials and secondary reference materials.

35.2.2 Classification of Reference Materials

According to different industries and use scopes, reference materials are classified into 13 types in China, as shown in Table 35.2.

By the end of 2021, 3088 kinds of primary reference materials and 12,392 kinds of secondary reference materials have been approved and released by China. These reference materials include 1617 kinds for clinical chemistry and drug composition analysis, mainly including human serum composition, whole blood composition, body fluid composition, gene detection, animal body fluid composition analysis, cosmetic composition analysis, clinical drug composition, and other reference materials.

35.2.3 Management of Reference Materials

The Metrology Department of the State Administration for Market Regulation (SAMR) is responsible for the supervision and administration of certified reference materials. SAMR has made clear provisions on the declaration, technical review,

Table 35.1 Comparison of primary reference materials with secondary reference materials

Comparison	Primary reference material	Secondary reference material
Producers	The national metrological institution or the institution confirmed by the national metrological authority	Industry, enterprise laboratories, research institutes, and other research institutions
Characterization	1. Absolute method of measurement 2. Using two different principles of demonstrable accuracy methods 3. Using the same demonstrable accuracy method in multiple laboratories	1. Methods for comparative measurement with primary reference materials 2. Method of primary reference material
Homogeneity and accuracy	The highest level in China, and the homogeneity is within the accuracy range	The homogeneity and accuracy do not reach the level of primary reference material, but can meet the needs of general measurement
Stability	At least 1 year or reach the advanced level of similar international reference materials	More than half a year, meeting the needs of reagent measurement
Main applications	1. Calibration of measuring instruments 2. Research and evaluation of standard measurement methods 3. Secondary reference material identification 4. Field application of high accuracy measurement	1. Calibration of measuring instruments 2. Research and evaluation of field measurement methods 3. Quality control of daily analysis and measurement (field application)

grading review, approval, and release of reference materials. SAMR entrusts the Chinese Society for Measurement to organize relevant experts to establish the National Certified Reference Material Management Committee, which is responsible for accepting the application for grading reference materials, and organizing the review and assessment. The National Technical Committee for the Measurement of Reference Materials is set up under the National Certified Reference Material Management Committee, and the secretariat is affiliated to the National Institute of Metrology, China, which is responsible for the daily work of the National Technical Committee for the Measurement of Reference Materials.

To effectively implement national laws, regulations, and norm, the National Technical Committee for the Measurement of Reference Materials has also formulated a series of technical norms to regulate and require research, development, and production of reference materials, as shown in Table 35.3.

Table 35.2 List of primary and secondary reference materials approved and issued

Catalog	Primary reference material (GBW)	Secondary reference material (GBW(E))
Ferrous metals	355	598
Non-ferrous metals and gases in metals	209	251
Building materials	42	8
Nuclear and radioactivity	261	24
Polymetric materials	2	9
Chemical products	142	2969
Geology	732	328
Environmental	354	4946
Clinical chemistry, biomedical, and pharmaceuticals	399	1218
Food	244	796
Energy resources	86	134
Technological and engineering	53	198
Physics and physicochemistry	209	913
Total	3088	12,392

Note: The data are from the National Sharing Platform for Reference Materials

Table 35.3 Technical norms for research and production of reference materials

Standard number	File name
JJF 1006–1994	*Technical norm of primary reference material*
JJF 1218–2009	*The rule for drafting in report of reference materials*
JJF 1342–2012	*General requirement for reference material producers*
JJF 1343–2012	*Characterization, homogeneity, and stability assessment of reference materials*
JJF 1344–2012	*General technical requirements for producing gas reference materials*
JJF 1507–2015	*The selection and use of reference materials*
JJF 1005–2016	*General terms and definitions used in connection with reference materials*
JJF 1644–2017	*The production of reference materials for clinical enzymology*
JJF 1646–2017	*The production of reference materials for Geoanalysis*
JJF 1718–2018	*The production of genetically modified plant nucleic acid reference materials*
JJF 1186–2018	*Requirements of reference materials certificates and labels*
JJF 1854–2020	*Metrological technical specification for establishment, evaluation, and expression for metrological traceability of reference materials*
JJF 1855–2020	*Metrological technical specification for purity assessment of certified reference materials—Organic purity certified reference materials*

35.3 Use Demand and Situation of Reference Materials in the Industry of IVD Reagents

With the economic globalization, more and more attention has been paid to analysis quality assurance and management. Standards, guidelines, and directives related to analysis quality assurance and management, such as ISO17025 *General Requirements for the Competence of Testing and Calibration Laboratories*, ISO15189 *Special Requirements for the Quality and Competence of Medical Laboratories*, and EN45001, are widely used in various laboratories engaged in analysis and measurement in certified and accredited forms.

Reference materials, as metering standards, have special functions and effects. Particularly in terms of quality control in laboratories, reference materials are used without limitations of instruments, equipment, or laboratory scale, and can achieve the purpose of quality control only with the testing capability. China has started to develop certified reference materials for clinical tests since the 1980s, which started late and is still in the initial stage, so the relevant national standards are lagging behind. By the end of 2021, there are more than 200 certified reference materials for IVD reagents, as shown in Table 35.4. According to the *Catalog of Clinical Laboratory Items in Medical Institutions (2013)* issued by the National Health Commission of the People's Republic of China, there are 1465 test items that can be carried out by clinical laboratories at present, so the existing reference materials are far from meeting the clinical needs. For the research and development of national certified reference materials for IVD reagents, the National Institutes for Food and

Table 35.4 Test items of certified reference materials for IVD reagents

Classification	Quantity	Test items
Clinical chemistry	74	Inorganic ions, metal ions, proteins, lipids, amino acids
Molecular diagnosis	82	Hepatitis B, hepatitis C, AIDS, Epstein-Barr virus, *Mycobacterium tuberculosis* IS110, epidermal growth factor receptor, COVID19, Newcastle disease virus, lung cancer KRAS and other related gene detection, human genome
Clinical immunology	47	Hepatitis B, hepatitis C, hepatitis E, AIDS, syphilis, Epstein-Barr virus, rubella virus, *Toxoplasma gondii*, cytomegalovirus, tetanus, rabies virus, COVID19, tumor, hormone, myocardial inflammation, and other related antigens and antibodies
Clinical hematological	13	Whole blood metal ions, red blood cells, white blood cells, platelets, etc.
Other	6	Fibrinogen, coagulation factor, *Bacillus subtilis* spore, etc.

Note: The data are from the National Sharing Platform for Reference Materials. *AIDS* acquired immunodeficiency syndrome, *COVID-19* Coronavirus Disease-2019

Drug Control issued a notice in February 2017 to widely collect the demand for new varieties of reference materials for IVD reagents from the society. Later, 759 kinds of reference materials were collected from nearly 100 enterprises, mainly including infectious diseases, tumor markers, hormones, proteins, small molecule metabolites, personalized diagnosis materials, and chemical drugs.

35.4 Major R&D Institutes and Products of Domestic Reference Materials

1. *National Institute of Metrology, China*

   Founded in 1955, under the State Administration for Market Regulation, the National Institute of Metrology (NIM), China, is the highest metrological research center and national legal metrological technology institution. It is responsible for ensuring nationwide consistency and international equivalence of quantity values, maintaining the highest measurement capabilities in China, supporting the improvement in the quality of development of China, and facing the challenges of the new technological revolution. At present, the NIM has developed more than 2000 kinds of reference materials, including 888 national primary reference materials and 1124 secondary reference materials, along with 106 reference materials for clinical testing. The NIM has strong advantages in the fields of high-purity materials, foods, inorganic solutions, organic solutions, biological nanometers, new materials, gases, etc.
2. *National Center for Clinical Laboratories*

   The National Center for Clinical Laboratories (NCCL) was established in the Beijing Hospital of the Ministry of Health in 1982. NCCL carries out relevant scientific research by undertaking the national clinical laboratory quality management and control entrusted by the Ministry of Health, implementing quality evaluation plans of national clinical laboratories, and establishing and applying the clinical laboratory reference system with the main work of control and improvement of clinical laboratory quality. At present, about 40 kinds of reference materials for routine test items have been developed and approved as national primary or secondary reference materials by relevant departments.
3. *Beijing Institute of Medical Device Testing*

   Beijing Institute of Medical Device Testing (BIMT), founded in 1983, is responsible for the standardization of medical devices such as medical biological protection products nationwide. The institute has organized to draft, formulate, and revise 362 national and industrial standards for medical devices, and successfully developed 31 national secondary reference materials.
4. *Beijing Controls & Standards Biotechnology Co., Ltd.*

   Beijing Controls & Standards Biotechnology Co., Ltd., founded in 2009, is a high-tech enterprise focusing on development, production, and marketing of third-party reference materials and serum plates in China. Since its establishment, the company has made remarkable achievements in the development and production of certified reference materials. By the end of 2021, nearly a total of 150 reference materials have obtained the *National Certified Standard Material Classification Certificate*, mainly involving products such as antigen antibody and nucleic acid reference materials related to infectious diseases.

5. *Guangzhou BDS Biological Technology Co., Ltd.*

   Guangzhou BDS Biological Technology Co., Ltd., founded in 2015, is a joint-stock company of Daan Gene Co., Ltd., and is mainly engaged in integral research, development, production, and marketing of national certified reference materials and serum plates. By the end of 2020, nearly a total of 80 reference materials have obtained the *National Certified Standard Material Classification Certificate*, mainly involving research and development of nucleic acid reference materials of hepatitis B, hepatitis C, syphilis, AIDS, etc.

6. *Shanghai Bioyuan Biotech Co., Ltd.*

   Shanghai Bioyuan Biotech Co., Ltd., was founded in 2016, and established its subsidiary Zhengzhou Bioyuan Biotech Co., Ltd., in the same year. It is mainly engaged in research, development, production, and marketing of third-party QC materials and national certified reference materials. A total of 90 reference materials have passed the review of national authoritative institutions, and obtained the *National Certified Standard Material Classification Certificate* issued by the General Administration of Quality Supervision, Inspection, and Quarantine of the People's Republic of China, including products of fields such as hepatitis B, hepatitis C, syphilis, AIDS, tumor-related immune detection, and nucleic acid testing.

Declaration Jian Zhang is an employee of Shanghai Bioyuan Biotech Co., Ltd.
Junli Zu is an employee of Zhengzhou Bioyuan Biotech Co., Ltd.
Gongcheng Liu is an employee of Zhengzhou Bioyuan Biotech Co., Ltd.

Reference

1. ISO 17511:2003, In vitro diagnostic medical devices-measurement of quantities in biological samplesmetrological traceability of values assigned to calibrators and control materials[S].

36 Research and Development, Production, and Application Status of Quality Controls for in Vitro Diagnostic Reagents

Junli Zu, Jian Zhang, and Gongcheng Liu

36.1 General

As per requirements of ISO15189 *Medical Laboratories-Requirements for Quality and Competence (2012)*, clinical laboratories providing medical laboratory services should meet the basic requirements of quality management. The *Measures for the Administration of Clinical Laboratories in Medical Institutions* (Wei Yi Fa [2006] No.73) issued by the National Health Commission of the People's Republic of China also requires that "clinical laboratories in medical institutions should conduct internal quality control over clinical laboratory items carried out and draw quality control charts," and "they should participate in the external quality assessment of clinical tests organized by external quality assessment institutions authenticated by the Ministry of Health." Therefore, internal quality control (IQC) and external quality assessment (EQA) are core works of clinical laboratory quality management required by domestic and internal standards and regulations.

The internal quality control (IQC) of a clinical laboratory is a series of inspection and control methods to monitor and evaluate the quality of work and determine whether the routine test report can be issued, aiming at detecting and controlling the precision of the routine work of the laboratory, testing changes in accuracy, and improving the consistency of inter-batch and inter-day specimen detection in the routine work of the laboratory. According to the requirements of the health industry standard *WS/T 641–2018 Internal Quality Control for Quantitative Measurement in Clinical Laboratory*, the internal quality control methods of clinical laboratories

J. Zu (✉) · G. Liu
Zhengzhou Bioyuan Biotech Co., Ltd., Zhengzhou, Henan, China
e-mail: zujunli@bioyuan.cn

J. Zhang
Shanghai Bioyuan Biotech Co., Ltd., Shanghai, China

H. Song, L. Dai (eds.), *In Vitro Diagnostic Industry in China*,
https://doi.org/10.1007/978-981-99-3110-1_36

include two modes, namely quality control (QC) methods based on testing of QC materials and quality control methods based on the application of patient sample measurement data. At present, the first mode is majorly taken in actual operation in clinical laboratories.

External quality assessment (EQA) of clinical laboratories is to determine the test capability of laboratories by comparison between laboratories. Comparison between laboratories refers to organization, implementation, and assessment for measuring or testing identical or similar items by two or more laboratories according to prespecified conditions. Participating in the external quality assessment is the basic requirement in laboratory management in the *Measures for the Administration of Clinical Laboratories in Medical Institutions*, and is also a key indicator for grading hospitals. According to the *ISO/IEC 17043:2010 Conformity Assessment—General Requirements for Proficiency Testing*, external quality assessment is also called proficiency testing (PT). Proficiency testing (PT) plan includes modes of quantitative plan, qualitative plan, sequential plan, concurrent plan, and other organization modes, but the basic mode is to reflect the testing quality of the laboratory by testing the external quality assessment samples that are generally supplied by QC materials.

Therefore, since the use of QC materials is the main way of internal quality control and external quality assessment, research, development, production, and supply of QC materials also become an important part of in vitro diagnostics (IVDs).

36.2 Classification, Performance Requirements, and Management of QC Materials

36.2.1 Classification of QC Materials

QC materials can be classified according to their properties, divided into liquid QC materials and lyophilizated QC materials. They can also be classified into assayed QC materials and unassayed QC materials according to assigned values. According to the new version of CLSI C-24 A4 *Statistical Quality Control for Quantitative Measurement Procedures: Principles and Definitions* [1], samples that can be used for internal quality control can be classified into four main categories according to their sources, namely: (1) QC materials prepared and produced by manufacturers themselves, mainly for supporting use of their own diagnostic reagents or equipment; (2) QC materials customized by other institutions entrusted by the manufacturer, also mainly for supporting the use of their own diagnostic reagents or equipment; (3) QC materials independently prepared and produced by a third party, independent from the manufacturers of diagnostic reagents and instruments, and used by multiple detection platforms; and (4) QC materials made in laboratories, mainly used in the laboratories.

In addition, under special circumstances, certified reference materials can also be used for internal quality control, but due to their price and quantity, the cost is high, so this rarely happens. National secondary reference materials prepared by primary reference material measurement value transferring can be used as internal quality control samples for internal quality control due to their large quantity and relatively reasonable price. However, no matter the primary or secondary reference materials, attention should be paid to the commutability between these materials and clinical samples, and they can be used for internal quality control only when their matrix effects are acceptable when compared with those of clinical samples.

36.2.2 Performance Requirements for QC Materials

36.2.2.1 Homogeneity

Quality control is to control the repeatability of test results. In the control process, assume that the QC material is a homogeneous sample, since it is difficult to evaluate the stability in the analysis process by using a QC material with poor homogeneity. Therefore, attention should be paid to the homogeneity of samples during production of qualified QC materials, and, especially for lyophilizated QC materials, the precision of sample adding should be strictly controlled during redissolution. In general, the variation coefficient of the added sample shall be controlled within 0.5%. For liquid QC materials, although the error in the sample-adding process is reduced, such QC materials are prone to affect the matrix of the sample due to added anti-corrosion solvents, stabilizers, etc.

36.2.2.2 Stability

Stability is another important indicator of QC materials. The property values of test items included in QC materials change with storage conditions and time. Therefore, the stability can only be controlled within a certain time, that is, the validity period of a material. QC materials of different specialties have different validity periods; generally, biochemical and immune QC materials can be stored for 2–3 years, while most blood QC materials can only be stored for 3–6 months. Clinical laboratories should try to purchase QC materials of the same batch number with a long validity period; then the quality change can be observed and controlled in a longer process. Besides, each QC material shall also have an unpacking validity period, and the QC material should be used for quality control within the unpacking validity period by users.

36.2.2.3 Commutability

QC materials are tested together with clinical samples to predict the test quality of the clinical samples through quality control measurement values. Therefore, the QC materials should be as consistent as possible with the clinical samples in terms of the matrix. At present, human serum is used as the matrix for most commercialized QC materials. However, to ensure the validity period and unpacking validity period of a QC material, preservatives, stabilizers, and other additives should be added to maintain the service life of the QC material during production. These additives have an impact on the matrix of the QC material, which is known as matrix effects.

Therefore, due consideration should be given to the matrix effects when preparing and selecting QC materials.

36.2.2.4 Suitability

The testing of QC materials is used to evaluate the testing quality of clinical samples; therefore, due consideration should be given to the setting of the concentration level of quality control materials, which should be suitable for the analysis and measurement range of the testing method for the test items and should cover the levels of significant medical decision as far as possible. Generally, two levels of quality control materials (normal concentration and pathological concentration) are used for quantitative test items, which is a more economical and applicable method. However, for test items with clinically significant increases and decreases in concentrations, such as thyroid stimulating hormone (TSH), three levels of QC materials should be considered to cover the analysis and measurement range that is clinically significant.

36.2.3 Management of QC Materials

36.2.3.1 Assayed QC Material

Assayed QC materials should provide the target values and ranges of each analyte (test item) contained in the QC material under different testing system in the Instruction for Use, from which users can select the assignment table of the same testing system as their own as a working reference. According to Article 112 of the *Measures for the Administration of Registration and Recordation of* In-Vitro *Diagnostic Reagents* (Order No. 48 of State Administration for Market Regulation (SAMR)), calibrators and QC materials can be applied for registration with the supporting in vitro diagnostic reagents or applied for registration alone. The calibrators and QC materials used in conjunction with the first category of in vitro diagnostic reagents shall be registered as the second category of products; the calibrators and QC materials used in conjunction with the second and third categories of in vitro diagnostic reagents are registered in the same category as the reagents when applied for registration separately; while multiple calibrators and QC materials are registered according to the higher category.

In accordance with the relevant requirements of the newly revised *Regulations on the Supervision and Administration of Medical Devices* (Order No. 739 of the State Council) and *Measures for the Administration of Registration and Recordation of* In-Vitro *Diagnostic Reagents* (Order No. 48 of SAMR), QC materials are subject to classified management according to medical devices, and the supervision and management agencies for their registration and filing, production, and business activities are listed in Table 36.1.

Under the leadership of SAMR, a series of industry standards with respect to the QC materials have been drafted, released, and implemented in recent years to guide the industrial development, as provided in Table 36.2.

Table 36.1 Requirements for classified management of medical devices

Classification		Class I	Class II	Class III
Registration	Domestic	Municipal medical products administration for record	Registration with medical products administration of provinces, autonomous regions, and municipalities	Registration with National Medical Products Administration
	Import	Registration with National Medical Products Administration		
Production		Municipal medical products administration for record	Permission of medical products administration of provinces, autonomous regions, and municipalities	
Business		–	Municipal medical products administration for record	

Table 36.2 List of industry standards relating to QC material

Standard number	File name
GB/T 20468–2006	*Guideline for internal quality control for quantitative measurements in clinical laboratory*
GB/T 21415–2008	In vitro *diagnostic medical devices-measurement of quantities in biological samples-metrological traceability values assigned to calibrators and control materials*
YY/T 0638–2008	In vitro *diagnostic medical devices-measurement of quantities in biological samples-metrological traceability of assigned values for catalytic concentration of enzymes in calibrators and control materials*
YY/T 0702–2008	*Control material for hematology analyzer*
YY/T 0501–2014	*Urine dry chemistry analysis control material*
YY/T 1652–2019	*General technical requirement of quality control materials for* in vitro *diagnostic reagents*
YY/T 1662–2019	*Quality control material for clinical chemistry analyzer*

36.2.3.2 Unassayed QC Material

Unlike the assayed QC material, no assignment table is provided for the unassayed QC material. According to the 2013 *Notice of the General Office of the China Food and Drug Administration on the Classification and Definition of 53 Products Such as Degradable Lacrimal Duct Emboli* ([2013] No. 11 of China Food and Drug Administration (CFDA)), "unassayed QC material is prepared by serum or plasma, and is used for internal quality control of laboratory testing of in vitro diagnostic reagents and for the observation and precision control of the testing process. It is not regulated as a medical device."

36.3 Development Status of Domestic QC Materials

36.3.1 Certification of NMPA QC Materials

According to the statistical data of "Domestic Approved Medical Devices (Registration)" of the National Medical Products Administration (NMPA), as by the end of 2021, the number of QC products approved by NMPA has reached 1384, with about 400 clinical laboratory items, mainly involving biochemical, immunological, hematological, and microbial testing and Point of Care Testing (POCT) platform, etc. Figure 36.1 shows the number of QC materials registered with NMPA from 2014 to 2021. According to the *Catalogue of Clinical Laboratory Items in Medical Institutions (2013)* promulgated by the National Health Commission, there are currently 1462 test items that can be carried out by clinical laboratories, and about 1000 test items have been carried out by Large tertiary general hospital in China. More than 2000 test items have been actually carried out in independent laboratories. Therefore, the number of commercial QC materials available is far from meeting clinical needs.

In terms of the types of markers covered by the registered QC materials, the QC materials currently registered in NMPA are mainly for routine clinical laboratory items. As shown in Fig. 36.2, the immunological test items account for 42.33%, and the clinical biochemical test items account for 36.51%, while the body fluid test items account for 17.46%. The QC materials in the fields of flow cytometry, drug concentration detection, and nucleic acid and sequencing detection develop slowly and lag behind.

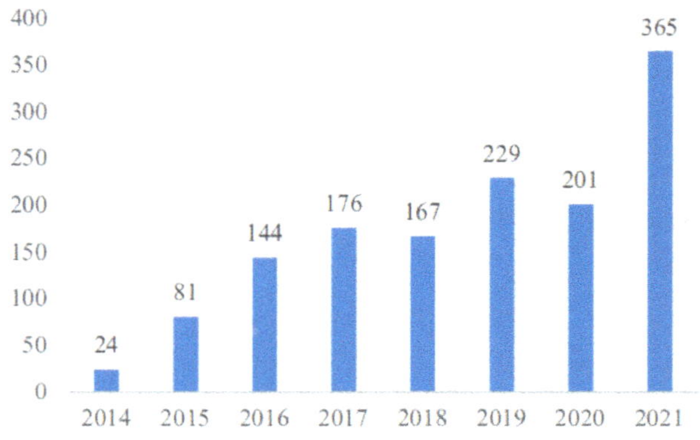

Fig. 36.1 Cumulative number of domestic QC materials approved by NMPA. (Note: Data are derived from the NMPA website)

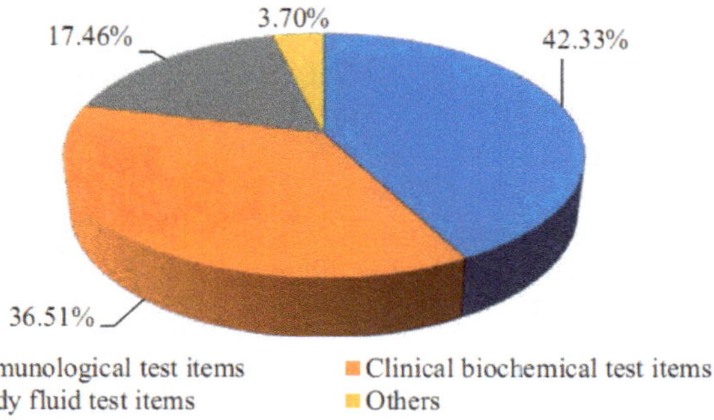

Fig. 36.2 Classification of application fields of NMPA QC material markers. (Note: Data are derived from the NMPA website)

Table 36.3 Some manufacturers' R&D and production of QC materials and the number of produced NMPA QC materials

Region	Registrant	Quantity
Guangdong	Shenzhen Mindray Bio-Medical Electronics Co., Ltd.	81
Jiangsu	Jiangsu MDK Biotech Co., Ltd.	55
Sichuan	Maccura Biotechnology Co., Ltd.	39
Henan	Autobio Diagnostics CO., Ltd.	36
Chongqing	Chongqing Zhongyuan Biotechnology Co., Ltd.	36
Guangdong	Guangzhou Wondfo Biotech Co., Ltd.	30
Nanjing	Lansion Biotechnology Co., Ltd.	27
Beijing	Beijing Kangche Sitan Biotechnology Co., Ltd.	24
Jiangsu	Suzhou Evermed Biomedical Co., Ltd.	24
Guangdong	Guangzhou Yichuan Biological Technology Co., Ltd.	22
Jiangsu	Vazyme Biotech Co., Ltd.	22

Note: The data are derived from the NMPA website

36.3.2 Major Domestic Manufacturers and Their Products

With the continuous development of laboratory medicine and the continuous progress of medical level, the clinical laboratories are carrying out more and more test. The laboratory quality is closely related to the level of clinical diagnosis and treatment, so higher requirements for clinical laboratory are proposed. Carrying out internal quality control and regularly participating in external quality assessment have become a normalized work for the clinical laboratory. By the end of 2021, there are a total of 237 companies that engage in research and development (R&D), registration, and production of NMPA QC materials nationwide, mainly in Guangdong, Beijing, Jiangsu, Shanghai, etc. These companies are mainly manufacturers of in vitro diagnostic reagents to produce supporting QC materials. The number of registered QC materials of some manufacturers is listed in Table 36.3.

36.3.2.1 Shenzhen Mindray Biomedical Electronics Co., Ltd.

Shenzhen Mindray's in vitro diagnostic business services cover eight areas (hematology, chemiluminescence, biochemistry, hemagglutination, urine, flow cytometry, microbiology, and glycation), involving more than 100 product models. By the end of 2020, it has 81 NMPA registration certificates for QC materials (147 test items). The QC materials are mainly used in conjunction with kits, including single QC materials and composite QC materials.

36.3.2.2 Maccura Biotechnology Co., Ltd.

Maccura's in vitro diagnostic products cover the technological platforms of biochemistry, immunity, POCT, coagulation, blood transfusion, blood cells, urine, molecular diagnosis, pathology, etc. It is professional in developing and manufacturing in vitro diagnostic equipment, reagents, calibrators, and QC materials. It owns 56 NMPA registration certificates for QC materials, and the QC materials are mainly used in conjunction with the company's kits.

36.3.2.3 Autobio Diagnostics Co., Ltd.

Autobio focuses on the R&D, manufacturing, integration, and service of in vitro diagnostic reagents and instruments. Its products (instruments + reagents + QC material) cover the testing fields of immunity, microorganisms, biochemistry, molecules, blood coagulation, etc. It has 30 NMPA QC materials that are used in conjunction with supporting kits, and 167 test items. Most of them are composite QC materials, which provide the assignment results of multiple platforms and can be used as third-party QC materials.

36.3.3 Third-Party Manufacturers of QC Materials and Their Products

36.3.3.1 Beijing Controls and Standards Biotechnology Co., Ltd.

Beijing Controls & Standards Biotechnology Co., Ltd., a wholly owned subsidiary of Beijing Wantai Biological Pharmacy Enterprise Co., Ltd., is the first professional QC material manufacturer in China. It mainly engages in the development and production of QC materials and reference materials. Presently, it has 36 NMPA registration certificates for QC materials, and mainly detects immunological test items, including infectious disease series, myocardial series, inflammation series, and tumor series markers. The products can be used as third-party QC materials.

36.3.3.2 Shanghai Bioyuan Biotech Co., Ltd.

Shanghai Bioyuan Biotech Co., Ltd., and its subsidiary Zhengzhou Bioyuan Biotech Co., Ltd., are holding subsidiaries of Autobio Diagnostics Co., Ltd. It specializes in the research and development, production and sales of third-party QC materials, and has been committed to the development and promotion of third-party QC materials. Its products cover the immunological testing of hepatitis B, hepatitis C, syphilis, AIDS, tumor, hormone, myocardial inflammation, clinical biochemical series, clinical testing series, POCT platform, and molecular testing. It owns 90 certificates of reference materials, and its single and multiple composite QC materials include various disciplines such as biochemistry, clinical testing, immunity, microbiology, and molecules covering more than 160 test items. The products can be used as third-party QC materials, and the samples of external quality assessment for more than 90% of the domestic agencies for external quality assessment.

36.3.3.3 Beijing Shuimu Jiheng Biotechnology Co., Ltd.

As a domestic comprehensive service provider of independent research and development of full category of reference standards and QC materials, Beijing Shuimu Jiheng Biotechnology Co., Ltd., is committed to the whole process of in vitro diagnostic product R&D, registration, supervision, and use, focusing on the R&D of in vitro diagnostic reagent standards and QC materials. As a high-tech enterprise with core advantageous resources for related product R&D, production, and service, it has five R&D technology platforms, namely biochemistry, immunity, molecular, mass spectrometry, and clinical testing, and can provide third-party QC materials and contracted R&D and production services of customized references standards, calibrators, and QC materials Contract Development Manufacture Organization (CDMO).

Declaration Jian Zhang is an employee of Shanghai Bioyuan Biotech Co., Ltd.
Junli Zu is an employee of Zhengzhou Bioyuan Biotech Co., Ltd.
Gongcheng Liu is an employee of Zhengzhou Bioyuan Biotech Co., Ltd.

Reference

1. CLSI Statistical Quality Control for Quantitative Measurement Procedures: Principles and Definitions. C24 A4. Clinical and Laboratory Standards Institute, 2016.

Part XII

In Vitro Diagnosis of Listed Enterprises Development and Investment, Financing, Acquisition and Merger Status in China

Performance of Listed Companies in 2021

37

Xunzhi Su, Lei Wang, and Jianmeng Cao

After the initial period in the 1980s, the development period in 1990s, and the high-speed development period since the twenty-first century, the in vitro diagnostic (IVD) industry has grown into a complete range, with numerous production and research and development (R&D) enterprises, circulation enterprises with comprehensive layout, and industrial chain become increasingly perfect, continuously improving its product quality, with the fastest development speed of medical equipment. The sudden Coronavirus Disease-2019 (COVID-19) outbreak in 2020 has greatly improved the IVD industry in China, and the sense of social responsibility and the mission of enterprises have been fully reflected.

37.1 IVD Industry Revenue and Net Profit

According to Wind database, IVD segment 2021 annual report data show that IVD segment revenue reached 86.173 billion yuan, with year-on-year growth of 59.22% (Fig. 37.1). The net profit deducted from non-return income reached 27.098 billion yuan, up 77.38% year on year, as shown in Fig. 37.2. Compared with 2020, IVD segment still maintained rapid growth, operating revenue and non-attributable net profit have increased significantly, but the growth rate is slower than 2020. The main reason is that the scale and market share of IVD enterprises have become stable due to the influence of the normalization of the epidemic, which can cover the demand of in vitro diagnosis at home and abroad.

Table 37.1 reports 52 IVD listed companies' operating revenues. Compared with the same period last year, 44 companies realize positive growth in operating

X. Su
GuoRong Securities Co., Ltd., Beijing, China

L. Wang (✉) · J. Cao
Northeast Securities Co., Ltd., Changchun, Jilin, China

H. Song, L. Dai (eds.), *In Vitro Diagnostic Industry in China*,
https://doi.org/10.1007/978-981-99-3110-1_37

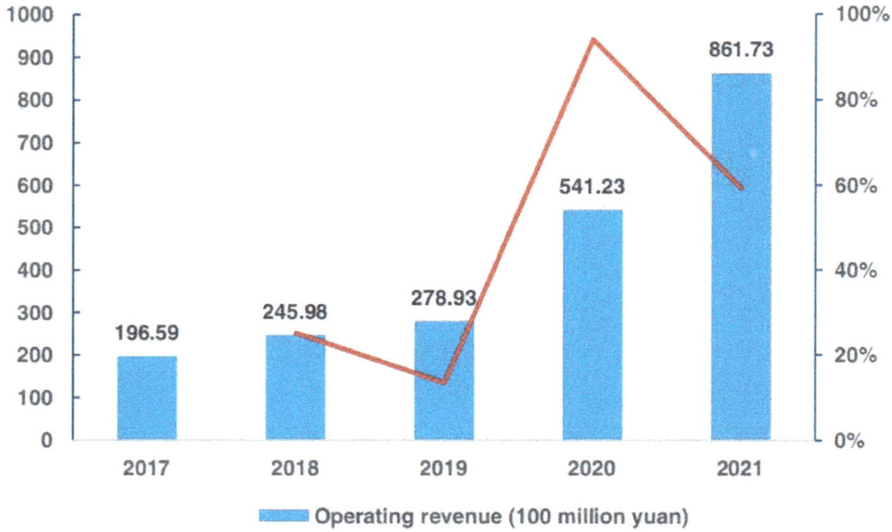

Fig. 37.1 Revenue growth of IVD segment from 2017 to 2021. (From: Wind)

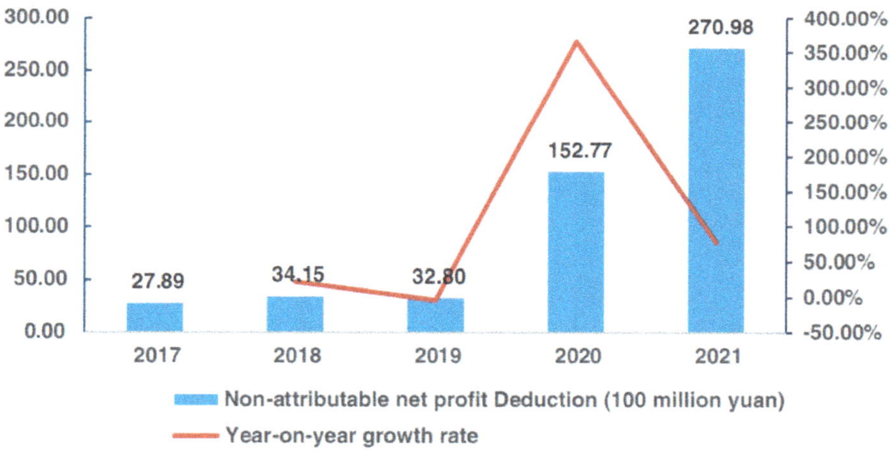

Fig. 37.2 Growth of non-attributable net profit of IVD segment from 2017 to 2021. (From: Wind)

revenue, which shows that most companies in our IVD industry still have room for improvement at present. Among them, Hotgen Biotech and Orient Gene Biotech, relying on their overseas business, seized the opportunity of the spread of COVID-19 overseas and promoted the surge in orders for COVID-19 testing products, with year-on-year revenue growth of 945.54% and 211.43%, respectively. In addition, the total revenue of New Horizon Health, Easy Diagnosis Biomedicine, WANTAI Biological, and BIOTEST BIOTECH in 2021 all increased by more than 100% year on year.

Table 37.1 Operating income of major IVD listed companies in 2021

Stock code	Company	Time to market	Operating income (100 million yuan)	Year-over-year growth rate of operating revenue (%)
300244.SZ	Dian Diagnostics	2011-7-19	130.83	22.85
603882.SH	Kingmed Diagnostics	2017-9-8	119.43	44.88
688298.SH	Orient Gene Biotech	2020-2-5	101.69	211.43
603108.SH	Runda Medical Technology	2015-5-27	88.6	25.33
002030.SZ	Daan Gene	2004-8-9	76.64	43.49
300676.SZ	BGI Genomics	2017-7-14	67.66	−19.42
603392.SH	Wantai Biological	2020-4-29	57.5	144.25
688068.SH	Hotgen Biotech	2019-9-30	53.69	945.54
688289.SH	Sansure Biotech	2020-8-28	45.15	−5.22
002022.SZ	Kehua Bio-Engineering	2004-7-21	42.68	2.71
300463.SZ	Maccura Biotechnology	2015-5-28	39.81	7.47
603658.SH	Autobio Diagnostics	2016-9-1	37.66	26.45
300482.SZ	Wondfo Biotech	2015-6-30	33.61	19.57
688399.SH	Bioperfectus Technologies	2019-12-5	28.39	63.19
002932.SZ	Easy Diagnosis Biomedicine	2018-7-10	28.30	195.05
01931.HK	Huajian Health Chekup	2019-7-12	27.31	12.46
300639.SZ	Hybribio Biotech	2017-4-12	26.73	97.34
603716.SH	Thalys Medical Technology	2016-10-31	26.00	22.30
300832.SZ	New Industries Biomedical Engineering	2020-5-12	25.45	15.97
300298.SZ	Sinocare	2012-3-19	23.61	17.17
300439.SZ	Medicalsystem Biotechnology	2015-4-22	22.52	−2.19
688317.SH	ZJ Bio-Tech	2021-1-18	20.19	−1.62

(continued)

Table 37.1 (continued)

Stock code	Company	Time to market	Operating income (100 million yuan)	Year-over-year growth rate of operating revenue (%)
688606.SH	Alltest Biotech	2021-3-25	18.73	64.98
688105.SH	Vazyme Biotech	2021-11-15	18.69	19.44
688315.SH	Novogene	2021-4-13	18.66	25.26
688767.SH	Biotest Biotech	2021-9-8	18.18	110.09
300406.SZ	Strong Biotechnologies	2014-10-30	15.99	88.58
688075.SH	Assure Tech	2021-11-18	15.89	32.47
000710.SZ	Berry Genomics	1997-4-22	14.22	−7.67
603387.SH	Getein Biotech	2017-7-17	14.02	24.78
605369.SH	Gongdong Medical Technology	2020-9-16	11.94	43.95
688575.SH	YHLO Biotech	2021-5-17	11.78	17.91
09960.HK	Kindstar Global	2021-7-16	9.31	4.41
300685.SZ	Amoy Diagnostics	2017-8-2	9.17	25.90
300396.SZ	Dirui Industrial	2014-9-10	9.06	−3.35
300030.SZ	Improve Medical Instruments	2009-12-25	8.00	−12.99
688389.SH	Lifotronic Technology	2019-11-5	7.78	40.50
300318.SZ	Bohui Innovation Biotechnology	2012-5-23	7.15	−3.24
300642.SZ	Tellgen Corporation	2017-4-21	6.55	33.70
300289.SZ	Leadman Biochemistry	2012-2-16	5.64	19.63
GTH	Bebetron Health	2020-6-19	5.32	25.47
BNR	Burning Rock Dx	2020-6-12	5.08	18.14
688468.SH	Chemclin Diagnostics	2021-4-9	4.71	12.57
688393.SH	LBP Medicine Science & Technology	2020-8-20	4.39	16.93

Table 37.1 (continued)

Stock code	Company	Time to market	Operating income (100 million yuan)	Year-over-year growth rate of operating revenue (%)
08247.HK	Biosino Bio-technology and Science Inc	2006-2-27	3.48	7.06
688656.SH	HOB Biotech	2020-12-15	3.18	43.20
688193.SH	Rendu Biotechnology	2021-2-30	2.92	16.97
688217.SH	Rightongene Biotechnology	2021-5-17	2.91	2.11
688338.SH	Succeeder Technology	2020-8-6	2.40	7.88
06606.HK	New Horizon Health	2021-2-18	2.13	201.50
688067.SH	AVE Science & Technology	2021-6-16	2.11	16.91
08622.HK	Huakang Biomedical Holdings Company Limited	2018-12-13	0.26	18.94

From: Wind

Dian Diagnostics ranked first in 2021 with total revenue of RMB13.083 billion, mainly due to the continued strong demand for large-scale COVID-19 nucleic acid screening and routine testing across the country, and the gradual recovery of routine independent medical laboratory (ICL) business, which promoted the overall performance improvement. Kingmed Diagnostics, also a leading third-party medical laboratory company, followed with total revenue of 11.943 billion yuan due to the contribution of its COVID-19 nucleic acid business.

Table 37.2 reports the net profit of 52 IVD listed companies. Orient Gene Biotech ranked first with net profit, attributable to its parent, of 4.92 billion yuan, and Daan Gene ranked second with net profit, attributable to its parent, of 3.618 billion yuan. From the perspective of the year-on-year growth of net profit, Hotgen Biotech ranked first again, with a year-on-year growth rate of 1850.41% in net profit attributable to its parent. In addition, the net profit of Novogene increased significantly, reaching 515.74%, mainly because of the expansion of the company's revenue and the application of falcon flexible intelligent production line, which made the cost reduction and efficiency increase obvious. The net profits of Strong Biotechnologies and Easy Diagnosis Biomedicine also increased by more than 200% year on year, thanks to the sharp increase in the sales of COVID-19 testing products and the continuous deepening of overseas markets. The year-on-year growth of overseas market revenue of Jiuqiang and Mingde in 2021 was 130.39% and 191.9%, respectively.

Among the 52 IVD listed companies and 23 IVD-related listed companies, in the 2021 annual financial results, more than 80% of the companies achieved good results. With the high density of COVID-19 nuclear testing nationwide and the high demand for foreign testing, many IVD-related companies delivered impressive

Table 37.2 Net profit attributable to parent of major IVD listed companies in 2021

Stock code	Company	Net profit attributable to its parent (100 million yuan)	Year-on-year growth rate (%)
688298.SH	Orient Gene Biotech	49.2	193.33
002030.SZ	Daan Gene	36.18	47.74
603882.SH	Kingmed Diagnostics	22.2	47.03
688068.SH	Hotgen Biotech	21.86	1850.41
603392.SH	Wantai Biological	20.21	198.59
300676.SZ	BGI Genomics	14.62	−30.08
002932.SZ	Easy Diagnosis Biomedicine	14.13	201.37
688399.SH	Bioperfectus Technologies	11.93	45.59
300244.SZ	Dian Diagnostics	11.63	44.83
603658.SH	Autobio Diagnostics	9.74	30.20
300832.SZ	New Industries Biomedical Engineering	9.74	3.68
300463.SZ	Maccura Biotechnology	9.57	20.49
300639.SZ	Hybribio Biotech	8.52	134.97
688767.SH	Biotest Biotech	8.34	91.57
688606.SH	Alltest Biotech	7.66	12.73
688317.SH	ZJ Bio-Tech	7.59	−18.61
688075.SH	Assure Tech	7.39	13.80
002022.SZ	Kehua Bio-Engineering	7.21	6.76
688105.SH	Vazyme Biotech	6.78	−17.46
300482.SZ	Wondfo Biotech	6.34	0.04
300406.SZ	Strong Biotechnologies	4.06	261.29
603387.SH	Getein Biotech	3.99	30.93

Table 37.2 (continued)

Stock code	Company	Net profit attributable to its parent (100 million yuan)	Year-on-year growth rate (%)
603108. SH	Runda Medical Technology	3.8	15.23
605369. SH	Gongdong Medical Technology	3.11	37.68
300685. SZ	Amoy Diagnostics	2.4	32.86
688315. SH	Novogene	2.25	515.74
300396. SZ	Dirui Industrial	2.1	−21.39
688575. SH	YHLO Biotech	2.05	−2.75
688389. SH	Lifotronic Technology	1.9	32.23
01931. HK	Huajian Health Chekup	1.75	9.97
300642. SZ	Tellgen Corporation	1.61	33.62
688468. SH	Chemclin Diagnostics	1.43	21.99
300298. SZ	Sinocare	1.08	−42.44
688338. SH	Succeeder Technology	0.97	40.73
688656. SH	HOB Biotech	0.86	52.24
688393. SH	LBP Medicine Science & Technology	0.8	−5.86
688193. SH	Rendu Biotechnology	0.65	5.28
688217. SH	Rightongene Biotechnology	0.47	22.26
688067. SH	AVE Science & Technology	0.31	3.90
688289. SH	Sansure Biotech	0.2243	−14.29
300289. SZ	Leadman Biochemistry	0.22	143.97
300030. SZ	Improve Medical Instruments	0.19	−88.57
300439. SZ	Medicalsystem Biotechnology	0.0179	−40.07
08247. HK	Biosino Bio-technology and Science Inc	−0.01	−141.94

(continued)

Table 37.2 (continued)

Stock code	Company	Net profit attributable to its parent (100 million yuan)	Year-on-year growth rate (%)
08622. HK	Huakang Biomedical Holdings Company Limited	−0.04	63.71
603716. SH	Thalys Medical Technology	−0.5	−186.00
000710. SZ	Berry Genomics	−1.11	−152.60
300318. SZ	Bohui Innovation Biotechnology	−3.22	−4394.40
GTH	Bebetron Health	−4.96	83.84
BNR	Burning Rock Dx	−7.97	−68.86
09960. HK	Kindstar Global	−14.54	−49.32
06606. HK	New Horizon Health	−30.85	−291.18

From: Wind

performance in 2021, and their performance soared in the first quarter of this year. However, for IVD-related enterprises, how to maintain stable growth in the post-epidemic era is the top priority.

37.2 Proportion of R&D Expenses in IVD Industry

According to the data of IVD sector R&D expenses in Wind, the R&D expenses of IVD industry increased year by year from 2017 to 2021, and the year-on-year growth rate also increased, as shown in Fig. 37.3. In terms of R&D as a percentage of revenue, as shown in Fig. 37.4, R&D accounted for the highest percentage in 2019, while R&D as a percentage of revenue declined in 2020 and 2021 due to the COVID-19 pandemic. In combination with the R&D expenses shown in Fig. 37.3, it can be seen that in the past 2 years, under the influence of COVID-19, IVD enterprises have paid more attention to the investment in product and technology R&D, but at the same time the revenue of IVD industry has increased substantially, and the proportion of R&D expenses in total revenue is bound to decrease. In the field of in vitro diagnosis, homogenization competition is more intense, and the quality of some products needs to be further improved. Therefore, companies should strengthen innovation and technology research and development to improve product quality and better meet people's testing needs, in order to let the IVD industry in the domestic and international markets have a broader stage.

Table 37.3 reports the published research and development expense data; there are 16 companies that spend more than 10% of their revenue on R&D. Among them, Rightongene Biotechnology's research and development investment accounted for the highest proportion of 23.59%. According to the change in ratio of

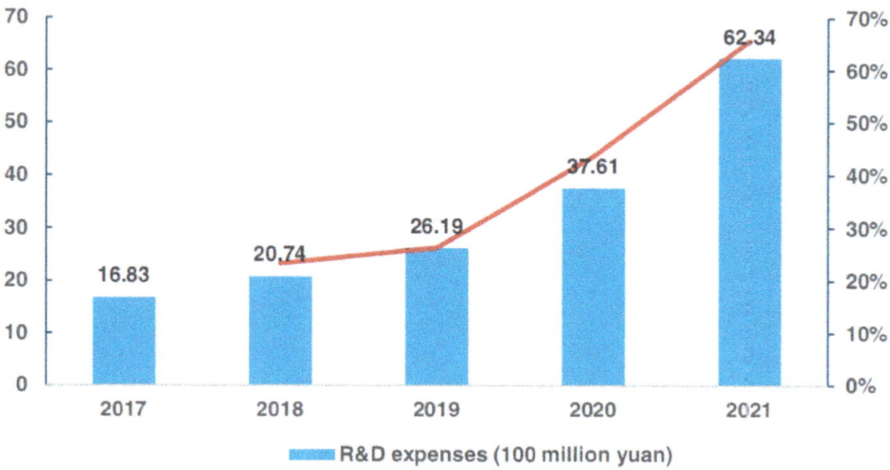

Fig. 37.3 Research and development expenses of IVD segment from 2017 to 2021. (From: Wind)

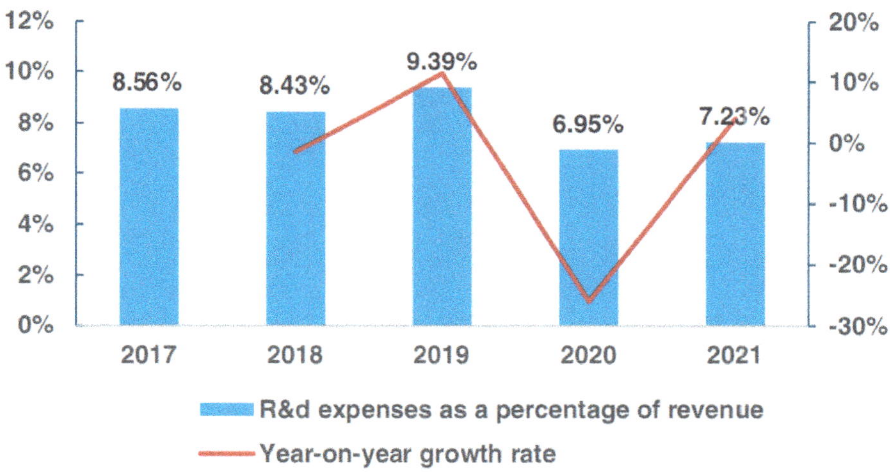

Fig. 37.4 Ratio of R&D expenses in revenue of IVD segment from 2017 to 2021. (From: Wind)

R&D to revenue for the whole year 2021, 29 enterprises achieved positive growth, which indicates that more and more domestic enterprises continue to increase investment in R&D. Although Lifotronic Technology is small in size, it is involved in many fields such as treatment and rehabilitation and in vitro diagnosis, so it has a large investment in research and development. Strong R&D team and high investment in R&D cast the core competitiveness of the enterprise. No matter how the revenue and profit of the enterprise, continuous and stable R&D investment to constantly improve the core competitiveness is the key to maintaining long-term stable growth of the enterprise.

Table 37.3 Research and development expenses of major IVD listed companies in 2021

Stock code	Company	R&D expenses (100 million yuan)	Year-on-year growth rate of R&D expenses (%)	R&D expenses as a percentage of revenue (%)	Growth rate of R&D expenses as a percentage of revenue (%)
06606. HK	New Horizon Health	0.59	1.36	27.69	−8.21
688217. SH	Rightongene Biotechnology	0.69	−7.69	23.59	−2.51
688389. SH	Lifotronic Technology	1.56	50.79	20.03	1.36
300685. SZ	Amoy Diagnostics	1.56	35.63	17.02	1.22
688067. SH	AVE Science & Technology	0.31	37.94	14.79	2.26
688468. SH	Chemclin Diagnostics	0.67	19.33	14.29	0.81
603658. SH	Autobio Diagnostics	4.81	40.30	12.77	1.27
688105. SH	Vazyme Biotech	2.30	83.47	12.32	4.31
603392. SH	Wantai Biological	6.82	116.91	11.86	−1.49
603387. SH	Getein Biotech	1.63	37.23	11.65	1.31
300482. SZ	WONDFO Biotech	3.91	39.96	11.64	2.30
300318. SZ	Bohui Innovation Biotechnology	0.81	69.13	11.40	2.41
300642. SZ	Tellgen Corporation	0.73	18.29	11.10	−1.45
688575. SH	YHLO Biotech	1.31	26.72	11.10	1.12
300396. SZ	Dirui Industrial	0.95	−1.00	10.49	−0.66
688393. SH	LBP Medicine Science & Technology	0.46	65.52	10.46	3.07
688656. SH	HOB Biotech	0.32	31.72	10.00	−0.88
09960. HK	Kindstar Global	0.90	0.20	9.70	1.25
08622. HK	Huakang Biomedical Holdings Company Limited	0.02	0.04	9.33	−0.89
000710. SZ	Berry Genomics	1.28	1.93	9.02	0.97

Table 37.3 (continued)

Stock code	Company	R&D expenses (100 million yuan)	Year-on-year growth rate of R&D expenses (%)	R&D expenses as a percentage of revenue (%)	Growth rate of R&D expenses as a percentage of revenue (%)
688193. SH	Rendu Biotechnology	0.26	11.06	9.01	−0.48
300832. SZ	New Industries Biomedical Engineering	2.15	42.81	8.45	1.59
300406. SZ	Strong Biotechnologies	1.27	60.66	7.94	−1.38
688315. SH	Novogene	1.45	29.36	7.79	0.52
300298. SZ	Sinocare	1.82	−0.03	7.73	−1.33
300676. SZ	BGI Genomics	4.87	−21.38	7.20	0.43
300439. SZ	Medicalsystem Biotechnology	1.51	11.22	6.69	0.80
002030. SZ	Daan Gene	5.09	204.77	6.64	3.80
688338. SH	Succeeder Technology	0.15	13.82	6.34	0.33
300289. SZ	Leadman Biochemistry	0.33	−14.86	5.81	−2.35
688317. SH	ZJ Bio-Tech	1.09	107.51	5.39	2.84
300030. SZ	Improve Medical Instruments	0.42	−9.09	5.29	0.02
300463. SZ	Maccura Biotechnology	2.07	2.57	5.21	0.30
688606. SH	Alltest Biotech	0.95	73.22	5.10	0.25
605369. SH	Gongdong Medical Technology	0.58	57.62	4.88	0.42
002932. SZ	Easy Diagnosis Biomedicine	1.33	89.82	4.69	−2.60
688075. SH	Assure Tech	0.70	20.42	4.43	−0.44
603882. SH	Kingmed Diagnostics	5.18	30.40	4.34	0.48
300639. SZ	Hybribio Biotech	1.15	60.98	4.31	−1.39
688298. SH	Orient Gene Biotech	4.29	357.09	4.21	1.34
688289. SH	Sansure Biotech	1.88	126.53	4.15	2.41

(continued)

Table 37.3 (continued)

Stock code	Company	R&D expenses (100 million yuan)	Year-on-year growth rate of R&D expenses (%)	R&D expenses as a percentage of revenue (%)	Growth rate of R&D expenses as a percentage of revenue (%)
688399.SH	Bioperfectus Technologies	1.07	47.97	3.76	−0.38
688767.SH	Biotest Biotech	0.62	49.85	3.41	−1.37
300244.SZ	Dian Diagnostics	4.25	33.11	3.25	0.25
002022.SZ	Kehua Bio-Engineering	1.07	−27.22	2.51	−0.34
688068.SH	Hotgen Biotech	1.32	177.07	2.46	−6.81
603108.SH	Runda Medical Technology	1.23	40.88	1.38	0.15
603716.SH	Thalys Medical Technology	0.35	81.62	1.36	0.44
08247.HK	Biosino Bio-Technology and Science Inc	0.03	−0.11	0.72	−16.54
01931.HK	Huajian Health Chekup	NaN	NaN	NaN	NaN
GTH	Bebetron Health	NaN	NaN	NaN	NaN
BNR	Burning Rock Dx	NaN	NaN	NaN	NaN

From: Wind
NaN Not a Number

37.3 EBITDA of IVD Listed Enterprises

According to Fig. 37.5 data, the earnings before interest, tax, depreciation, and amortization (EBITDA) of IVD listed companies have increased year by year since 2017. Especially in 2020, the IVD industry's earnings before interest, tax, depreciation, and amortization under the impact of the pandemic reached 21.619 billion yuan. In 2021, as the COVID-19 situation stabilized, the IVD industry EBITDA increased compared with 2020, but the year-on-year growth rate was significantly lower. EBITDA represents the ability of enterprises to generate cash flow through operating activities, which indicates that the operating cash flow of IVD industry has maintained a steady growth trend in the past two years, and the outbreak of the pandemic has brought the in vitro diagnostics market into a period of rapid development.

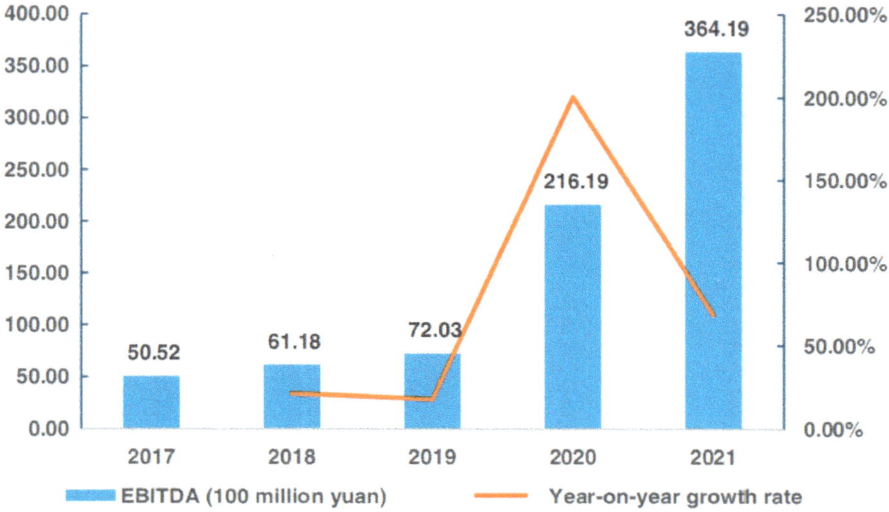

Fig. 37.5 IVD segment EBITDA from 2017 to 2021 (From: Wind)

Table 37.4 reports 16 companies whose earnings before interest, tax, depreciation, and amortization exceeded 1 billion yuan, with Orient Gene Biotech topping the list with 5.872 billion yuan. Due to the impact of the global COVID-19 epidemic, there is a large demand for overseas testing, and Orient Gene Biotech's COVID-19 testing reagents continue to be exported to the European market, achieving significant sales results. According to the year-on-year growth rate data, 35 enterprises achieved positive growth in EBITDA, among which Hotgen Biotech achieved the highest year-on-year growth rate of 1578.50%, which is closely related to the company's active development of overseas markets. At the beginning of 2021, the novel corona virus antigen self-test product developed by Hotgen Biotech was the first to gain market access in Germany, and also obtained self-test registration and filing in the European Union, the UK, France, and other major economies, which greatly increased the sales scale. In the fourth quarter of 2021, when the epidemic situation in foreign countries continued to worsen, Hotgen Biotech foreign trade orders surged, achieving revenue of 368 million yuan in a single quarter, a year-on-year growth of 407%. Due to the impact of COVID-19 overseas, the performance of many IVD enterprises in China has greatly improved. In the long run, COVID-19 products are just a stepping stone to open the international market, and the future growth point needs more comprehensive products to maintain.

Table 37.4 EBITDA of major IVD listed companies in 2021

Stock code	Company	EBITDA (100 million yuan)	Year-on-year growth rate (%)
688298.SH	Orient Gene Biotech	58.7201	189.80
002030.SZ	Daan Gene	41.8142	59.40
603882.SH	Kingmed Diagnostics	33.3785	51.75
300244.SZ	Dian Diagnostics	27.5246	20.37
688068.SH	Hotgen Biotech	26.6143	1578.50
688289.SH	Sansure Biotech	26.0845	−16.31
603392.SH	Wantai Biological	24.3343	183.41
300676.SZ	BGI Genomics	21.2972	−28.30
002932.SZ	Easy Diagnosis Biomedicine	17.1575	197.71
002022.SZ	Kehua Bio-Engineering	15.5862	1.66
300463.SZ	Maccura Biotechnology	15.1494	19.62
603658.SH	Autobio Diagnostics	14.03	21.96
688399.SH	Bioperfectus Technologies	13.9304	45.36
603108.SH	Runda Medical Technology	13.2729	24.41
300832.SZ	New Industries Biomedical Engineering	12.0516	4.14
300639.SZ	Hybribio Biotech	11.5864	123.01
688767.SH	Biotest Biotech	9.7779	82.60
688317.SH	ZJ Bio-Tech	9.2355	−20.22
300482.SZ	Wondfo Biotech	8.9935	−9.82
688075.SH	Assure Tech	8.8944	11.33
688606.SH	Alltest Biotech	8.6855	7.03
688105.SH	Vazyme Biotech	8.2762	−16.06

Table 37.4 (continued)

Stock code	Company	EBITDA (100 million yuan)	Year-on-year growth rate (%)
300406. SZ	Strong Biotechnologies	5.8783	212.74
300439. SZ	Medicalsystem Biotechnology	4.9312	3.89
603387. SH	Getein Biotech	4.8155	28.02
300298. SZ	Sinocare	3.7926	−23.63
688315. SH	Novogene	3.6732	126.61
605369. SH	Gongdong Medical Technology	3.5895	23.17
688575. SH	YHLO Biotech	3.3773	0.23
1931. HK	Huajian Health Chekup	2.9958	12.84
300685. SZ	Amoy Diagnostics	2.9375	23.69
300396. SZ	Dirui Industrial	2.2807	−22.31
688389. SH	Lifotronic Technology	2.1235	40.04
300642. SZ	Tellgen Corporation	2.107	17.72
688468. SH	Chemclin Diagnostics	2.0267	18.15
603716. SH	Thalys Medical Technology	2.0153	−23.32
300289. SZ	Leadman Biochemistry	1.3088	232.35
9960. HK	Kindstar Global	1.1761	−19.93
688656. SH	HOB Biotech	1.1205	64.46
688338. SH	Succeeder Technology	0.8983	10.53
300030. SZ	Improve Medical Instruments	0.8792	−43.69
688393. SH	LBP Medicine Science & Technology	0.8589	−15.29
688193. SH	Rendu Biotechnology	0.7952	8.40
000710. SZ	Berry Genomics	0.7486	−75.78

(continued)

Table 37.4 (continued)

Stock code	Company	EBITDA (100 million yuan)	Year-on-year growth rate (%)
688217.SH	Rightongene Biotechnology	0.7413	−2.19
8247.HK	Biosino Bio-technology and Science Inc	0.3984	235.07
688067.SH	AVE Science & Technology	0.381	−3.10
300318.SZ	Bohui Innovation Biotechnology	0.148	−88.93
8622.HK	Huakang Biomedical Holdings Company Limited	−0.0131	−45.87
6606.HK	New Horizon Health	−2.4836	130.35
BNR.O	Burning Rock Dx	−7.493	97.65
GTH.O	Bebetron Health	NaN	NaN

From: Wind

Declaration Xunzhi Su is an employee of GuoRong Securities Co., Ltd.
Lei Wang and Jianmeng Cao are employees of Northeast Securities Co., Ltd.

38 Investment, Financing, and Merger of Listed Companies in 2021

Xunzhi Su, Lei Wang, and Jianmeng Cao

With the increasing trend of the aging population in China and the growth of per capita medical expenditure and technological progress, the growth rate of in vitro diagnostic (IVD) field in China has remained high in recent years. In recent years, due to the impact of the Coronavirus Disease-2019 (COVID-19) pandemic, competition on IVD tracks has become increasingly fierce. In new enterprises and enterprises with a history of accumulation, how to flexibly adjust the window period for innovation and transformation, and make differentiated value, has become a new challenge faced by the domestic IVD industry. Under the influence of the epidemic, IVD enterprises have rapidly expanded their scale in recent years, taking advantage of the capital market to develop their scale and obtain more financial support. The representative cases of investment, financing, and merger and acquisitions (M&A) among listed IVD companies in 2021 are summarized as follows.

On May 16, 2021, Mindray Medical intends to acquire 100% of the equity interest of Finland's Hytest Invest Oy and its subsidiaries in cash for a total purchase price expected to be approximately €545 million.

On June 21, 2021, Sansure Biotech signed an investment agreement with GeneMind and its shareholders, Shenzhen Zhongke Darui Gene, Shenzhen Shanduo Industrial, and Shenzhen WanRio E-commerce. The company acquired 14.77% of Zhenmai Biology at a total price of 255.2 million yuan through equity transfer and subscription of new registered capital. Sansure Biotech will complete the aforementioned transaction with its own funds, and upon completion of the transaction, Sansure Biotech will become the second largest shareholder of Zhenmai. Through this transaction, Sansure Biotech and GeneMind will reach a strategic cooperation, where the two sides can fully reap the synergistic effects in the intellectual property

X. Su
GuoRong Securities Co., Ltd., Beijing, China

L. Wang (✉) · J. Cao
Northeast Securities Co., Ltd., Changchun, Jilin, China

H. Song, L. Dai (eds.), *In Vitro Diagnostic Industry in China*,
https://doi.org/10.1007/978-981-99-3110-1_38

talent team technology platform and other aspects, along with complementary advantages, so as to carry out more in-depth research and development in the field of gene sequencing polymerase chain reaction (PCR) and other molecular diagnosis, thus fully tapping the potential of sustainable development.

On June 23, 2021, Deng Guanhua, the controlling shareholder and actual controller of Guangzhou Improve Medical Instruments Company, signed the Share Transfer Agreement and the Irrevocable Waiver of Voting Rights Agreement with Zhuhai Gree Financial Investment Management Co., Ltd. Improve Medical Instruments Company authorities said that state-owned capital and private capital will complement each other, promote each other, and integrate the advantages of the resources conducive to the company to carry out financing, asset restructuring, and capital operation, and to further enhance the company's overall ability to resist risks and get rid of the real control through 100% limit of pledge of shares, thus further promoting the orderly and healthy development of the business of the company in line with the company's strategic development planning conducive to the sustainable development of the company.

On July 6, 2021, Berry Gene entered into the "Shareholders' Agreement on Fujian Herui Gene Technology Co., Ltd. (the Third Amendment)" with Fujian Herui Series B investors and related parties. The B-round investors of Fujian Herui subscribed for 11,961,757 yuan of Fujian Herui's newly registered capital with a total of 640 million Yuan, which corresponds to 13.83% of Fujian Herui's equity after the completion of the transaction.

On September 3, 2021, Beijing Strong Biotechnologies was publicly delisted from Fuzhou Maixin Biotechnology Development Co., Ltd., by China Pharmaceutical Investment Co., Ltd., with a delisted price of 947.5 million yuan. Mai Xin Bio is the company's holding subsidiary, mainly engaged in the immunohistochemical diagnostic business. Through the acquisition of 30% equity of Maixin Biological, Strong Biotechnologies improves the company's shareholding ratio of Maixin Biological, and improves the service level and competitive strength of the company's testing business.

On November 9, 2021, Kehua Bio-Engineering based on the long-term market development of this segment, but also in order to promote the company, and Sansure Biotech, in the field of chemiluminescence immune segmentation, agreed to cooperate with each other to achieve complementary advantages, mutual benefit, and win-win results. Kehua Bio-Engineering signed a Letter of Intent for Investment Framework with Sansure Biotech Co., Ltd. Kehua Bio-Engineering and Sansure Biotech jointly invested 50 million yuan to establish a joint venture company "Hunan Sansure Immunotech Co., Ltd." (proposed name). The joint venture company was established in the form of a target company held by Kehua Bio-Engineering. The financial statements of the joint venture company shall be included in the consolidated statements of Kehua Bio-Engineering. The equity ratio of the joint venture company is 50% held by Kehua Bio-Engineering and 50% held by Sansure Biotech.

On December 22, 2021, BGI transferred its equity to Shenzhen Zao Know Technology Co., Ltd., with a registered capital of 353,368 yuan held by Shenzhen Zao Know Investment Co., Ltd., with its own capital of 9.53 million yuan. With its own capital of RMB 8.47 million yuan, the company transferred its equity to Shenzhen Zao Know Science and Technology Co., Ltd., with a registered capital of RMB 311,397 million Yuan held by the Shenzhen uncertain investment enterprise (limited partnership).

As can be seen from the above events, the IVD industry is favored by the capital markets. When an enterprise cannot meet the market demand by relying on its own endogenous development speed, it is undoubtedly the most effective means to complete the product line through merger and reorganization and strengthen its own development potential and power by supplementing the product shortcomings. In 2021, more than 100 IVD enterprises reached strategic cooperation. Two-way empowerment through cooperation between enterprises promotes complementary advantages, deepens resource integration, and achieves mutual benefit and win-win results. The strong alliance also injects new vitality into the IVD industry, cultivates new momentum, jointly writes a new chapter of leapfrog development, and pushes forward the high-quality development of the industry.

Declaration Xunzhi Su is an employee of GuoRong Securities Co., Ltd.

Lei Wang and Jianmeng Cao are employees of Northeast Securities Co., Ltd.

Appendix: List of Selected Chinese IVD Manufacturers

Nanjing Norman Biological
Getein Biotech, Inc.
LandwindBIO
EUROIMMUN Medical Diagnostics (China) Co., Ltd.
Beijing Hotgen Biotech Co., Ltd.
Shanghai Medconn Diagnostics Technology Co., Ltd.
BioSino Bio-Technology and Science Inc.
Biobase Biodustry
HOB Biotech Group
Chongqing Biostec Biological Technology Co., Ltd.
Beijing Applied Biological Technologies Co., Ltd.
Suzhou Lihe Biomedical Engineering Co., Ltd.
Zhejiang Shengyu Medical Technology Co., Ltd.
Rayto Life and Analytical Sciences Co., Ltd.
Hipro Biotechnology Co., Ltd.
Xiamen Biotime Biotechnology Co., Ltd.
Sunostik Medical Technology Co., Ltd.
Sekisui Medical Technology(China) Ltd.
Guangzhou Improve Medical Instruments Co., Ltd.
Beijing BGI-GBI Biotech Co., Ltd.
Anhui Iprocom Biotechnology Co., Ltd.
Hebei Archi Biological Technology Co., Ltd.
Acon Biotech (Hangzhou) Co., Ltd.
Guangzhou LBP Medicine Science & Technology Co., Ltd.
Beijing Sjodax Biotechnology Co. Ltd.
Nanchang Biotech A&C Biotechnical Industry Incorporated Co., Ltd.
Neusoft Whitman
Coyote Bioscience Co., Ltd.
Hangzhou Matridx Biotechnology Co., Ltd.
Hangzhou Proprium Biotech Co. Ltd.
COBIO Smart Healthcare Technology Co., Ltd.
Hangzhou Bioeast Biotech Co., Ltd.

H. Song, L. Dai (eds.), *In Vitro Diagnostic Industry in China*,
https://doi.org/10.1007/978-981-99-3110-1

Jiangsu Kangjian Medical Apparatus Co., Ltd.
Agilent Technologies (China)
Suzhou AstraBio Technology Co. Ltd.
Suzhou Evermed Biomedical Co., Ltd.
Zhuhai Encode Medical Engineering Co., Ltd.
Shanghai Upper Bio-Tech Co., Ltd.
Shenzhen XPENARRAY Biotechnology Co., Ltd.
Jiangsu Mole Bioscience Co., Ltd.
Beijing Beier Bioengineering Co., Ltd.
Beijing Topu Analytical Instruments Co. Ltd.
Beijing Zhongjian Antai Diagnostic Technology Co., Ltd.
Beijing Sainuopu Biological Technology Co., Ltd.
Shenzhen Ultra-Diagnostics Biotec. Co., Ltd.
Ningbo Elejech Biological Technology Co., Ltd.
Anhui Zhongke Duling Commercial Appliance Co., Ltd.
Shandong Lifei Biological Group
Blue Cross Bio-Medical (Beijing) Co., Ltd.
Co-Health (Beijing)
Beijing MagicNurse Surgical Robot Technology Co., Ltd.
Hangzhou Allsheng Instruments Co., Ltd.
Shanxikangjianen
Innovita Biological Technology Co., Ltd.
Hua Sin Science Co., Ltd.
Shenzhen Lightlife Technology Co., Ltd.
Kingsbio
WeiHai NeoproBio. Technologies Co., Ltd.
Liaoning DIHO Biotechnology Co., Ltd.
Beijing Techlink Biomedical Technology Co., Ltd.
Tigsun Diagnostics Co., Ltd.
Beijing Share-Sun Oet
Dewei Medical Equipment
Beijing Unidiag Technology Inc.
Beijing Quantobio Biotechnology Co., Ltd.
Core Technology Co., Ltd.
Beijing JINWOFU Bioengineering Technology Co., Ltd.
Chengdu VACURE Biological Technology Co., Ltd.
HD Standard Diagnostics Co., Ltd.
BRED Life Science Technology Inc.
Xiamen Wiz Biotech Co., Ltd.
Primus Medical (Shanghai) Co. Ltd.
XEMA Co. Ltd.
CanAg Diagnostics (Beijing) Co., Ltd.
ShenZhen ChanSon Precision Mold Co., Ltd.
SHMY Healthdigit Biochips Co., Ltd.
Beijing GeneseeBiotech, Inc.

Beijing Jinghua Biotechnology Co., Ltd.
Hangzhou Sejoy Electronics & Instruments Co., Ltd.
Changde BKMAM Biotechnology Co., Ltd.
Shanghai Heamo-Pharmaceutical&Biological Co., Ltd.
Guangzhou Xueba Special Equipment Co., Ltd.
One Clone Biotech Inc.
Nantong HJT Trading Co., Ltd.
Nantong Manzhen Biotechnology Co., Ltd.
Chengdu One-Chip Biotechnology Co., Ltd.
Hebei Aiolos Biotechnology Co., Ltd.
Haimenfeihong Mechanical Manufacture Company Limited
Suzhou Usane Precision Tooling & Molding Co., Ltd.
Jiangsu Maike Medical Devices Co., Ltd.
Precisionist Diagnostics Co., Ltd.
Guangzhou Embedsky Computer Technology Co., Ltd.
Welltop
Zhang jia kou fuxi Biotechnology Co., Ltd.
Hangzhou Binhe Microorganism Reagent Co., Ltd.
Guangzhou Huantong Bioscience Co., Ltd.
Nanjing Zhongke Tony Technology Co., Ltd.
Guangxi IVD Biotechnology Co., Ltd.
Zhejiang Kangte Bio-Tech Co., Ltd.
Sichuan Mingshi Biotechnology Co. Ltd.
Beijing ebio-top Biotechnology Co., Ltd.
The Binding Site Group Ltd., Birmingham, UK
Hangzhou Yooning Instruments Co., Ltd.
Sysmedical
Hunan JoyRealm Biomed Co., Ltd.
Hubei Jinjian Biological Co., Ltd.
Guangzhou Mecart Sensor Technology Co., Ltd.
NanoMagBio
Nanjing Liming Bio-Products Co., Ltd.
Tsingke Biotechnology Co., Ltd.
Beijing Baibin Medical Instruments Co., Ltd.
BRAND (Shanghai) Trading Co., Ltd.
Jiangsu huaerkang Medical Instrument Co., Ltd.
Biologix Corporation
Shenzhen Stone Intelligent Industrial Design Co., Ltd.
Shanghai Maike Biotech Co., Ltd.
Hangzhou Jianli Biotechnology Co., Ltd.
Jiangxi huitai Biotech Co., Ltd.
Guangzhou BayBio Bio-tech CO., Ltd.
Suzhou Borui Sunga Medical Technology Co., Ltd.
ReLIA Biological Engineering (Shanghai) Co., Ltd.
Suosi (Suzhou) Medical Treatment Technology Co. Ltd.

Guangzhou iGene Biotechnology Co., Ltd.
Nordson EFD
Guangzhou Mac Laser Marking Co., Ltd.
Haimen Rotest Labware Manufacturing Co., Ltd.
Tianjin Geneally Biotechnology Co., Ltd.
Guangzhou Dongsheng Biotech Co., Ltd.
Beijing Springup Scientific Co., Ltd.
The EmerTher Company
Union Medical & Pharmaceutical Technology (Tianjin) Group Co., Ltd. (Union)
New England Biolabs (Beijing), Ltd.
Poyton
Zhejiang Sanch Laboratory Equipment Co., Ltd.
Tianjin Meritmedtech Co., Ltd.
Baoding Sino fluid Technology Co. Ltd.
Suzhou NovoCom Biotechnology Co., Ltd.
Carl Zeiss (Shanghai) Co., Ltd.
Medix Biochemica China
Roche Diagnostics (Shanghai) Ltd.
Hzymes Biotechnology Co., Ltd.
Toyobo (Shanghai) Biotech Co., Ltd.
BioDot Trading (Shanghai) Co., Ltd.
Shanghai DEFT lutelligent Technology Co., Ltd.
Merck Chemicals (Shanghai) Co., Ltd.
MBL Beijing Biotech Co., Ltd.
Zhejiang Gongdong Medical Technology Co., Ltd.
Haier Biomedical
Holmes (Beijing) Diagnostics Co., Ltd.
Vazyme Biotech Co., Ltd.
Cytiva
Yuhuan Kangjia Enterprise Co., Ltd.
Shanghai Reigncom Biotechnology Co., Ltd.
Beijing Deaoping Biotechnology Co., Ltd.
Hangzhou Sonice Biotechnology Co., Ltd.
Rapid Novor Inc.
Hangzhou Special Paper Industry Co., Ltd.
Kang Yuan Biology
Guangzhou Jet Bio-Filtration Co., Ltd.
Beijing KEY-BIO Biotech Co., Ltd.
Suzhou Vdo Biotech Co., Ltd.
Kunshan Wisepac Desiccant Co., Ltd.
R.P.H. (Xiamen) Import & Export Co., Ltd.
BBI Solutions
Suzhou Chanshow Biotechnology Co., Ltd.
Shenzhen Keyto Fluid Control Co., Ltd.
Cangzhou Shengfeng Plastic Product Co., LLtd.

Nanjing Nanoeast Biotech Co., LLtd.
Suzhou Cellpro Biotechnology Co., Ltd.
Fapon Biotech Inc.
Hangzhou NeuroPeptide Biological Science and Technology Incorporation, Ltd. (NUPTEC)
Realbio Group
HyTest Ltd.
LGC Science (Shanghai) Ltd.
Yeasen Biotech Co., Ltd.
Novoprotein Scientific Inc.
Qingdao AUCMA Ultra Low Temperature Freezing Machines Co., Ltd.
Shanghai Jiadao Bio-technology Co., Ltd.
YareWell Biotechnology Ltd.
Changzhou Fulling Motor Co., Ltd.
Genstars Biotech Co., Ltd.
Fujian Hitronics Technologies Inc.
Fantibody
Shanghai Jiening Biotech Co., Ltd.
GenScript Biotech Corporation
Cnpair Biotech Co., Ltd.
Wuhan Huamei Biotech Co., Ltd.
Beijing APIs Bioscience Co., Ltd.
Kactus Biosystems
Wuhan Tacro Technology Co., Ltd.
Nanjing Diannuo Biotechnology Co., LLtd.
Shenzhen Topoct Biomedical Technology Co., Ltd.
Taizhou Huangyan Fangye Technology Development Co., Ltd.
Beijing Biosynthesis Biotechnology Co., Ltd.
Sartorius (Shanghai) Trading Co., Ltd.
Suzhou NanoMicro Technology Co., Ltd.
Hangzhou Cobetter Filtration Equipment Co., Ltd.
Zhejiang huanuo pharmaceutical
Ebiocore Biotechnology Co., Ltd.
Beijing Shouyi Clinical Medicine Scientific Co., Ltd.
MC Healthcare China Co., Ltd.
Nuhigh Biotechnologies Co., Ltd.
Shanghai Janzy Biotechnology Co., Ltd.
Cangzhou Xingyuan Plastic Products Co., Ltd.
Shanghai Nodel Biotech Co., Ltd.
Ningbo Hongding Medical Equipment Technology Co., Ltd.
CIMC Cold Cloud (Beijing) Supply Chain Management Co., Ltd.
Chengdu Hyrux Bioscience Co., Ltd.
Biocare Diagnostics Ltd.
Chongqing Ilinda Bio-Technology Co, Ltd.
Sunshiny Advertisment-MIR Magzine

Guilin Immunetech International, LLC
Beijing Biobridge Biotechnology Co., Ltd.
Chang Zhou THINKER Electrical Mechanical Equipment Co., Ltd.
Shanghai Laya Biotechnology Co., Ltd.
Shenzhen HeavyBio Science and Technology Co., Ltd.
Yesen Biotechnology (Shanghai).Co. Ltd.
Guangzhou Xiang-kang Medical Devices Technology Services Co., Ltd.
Xiamen Tongrenxin Biotech Co. Ltd.
Shanghai BioSun Sci&Tech Co., Ltd.
Scantibodies Laboratory, Inc.
Ningbo Liudeng Medical Technology Co., Ltd.
Shanghai Bio-chem Biological Technology Co., Ltd.
JiangSu DeNeng Medical Technology
BEAVER Biomedical Engineering Co., Ltd.
HuiYou Automation Co., Ltd.
Sumika Electronic Materials (Shanghai) Corporation
ABclonal
ShenZhen AIVD Biotech Inc.
Avantor VWR (Shanghai) Co., Ltd.
DiagnostikNet-BB e.V.
Changsha Xiangzhi Centrifuge Instrument Co., Ltd.
Beijing Jyton and Kannel Medical Tech. Co., Ltd.
Qingdao Kangda Biotechnology Co., Ltd.
ZYSJ Medical Polymer Technologies Co., Ltd.
Pall (China) Co., Ltd.
Shanghai BiOligo Biotech Co., Ltd.
Jiangsu Jingchuang Electronics Co., Ltd.
Sangon Biotech (Shanghai) Co., Ltd.
ShangHai WenQiang Technology Co., Ltd.
Bioantibody Biotechnology Co., Ltd.
Beijing Maris Medical Technology Co., Ltd.
Adhesives Research
Nanjing Chuanbo Biotech Co., Ltd.
Meridian Life Science, Inc.
3M China Limited
Jiangsu Changfeng Medical Industry Co., Ltd.
Changzhou Wheeler Linear Motors Co., Ltd.
Changsha Yingtai Instrument Co., Ltd.
Takara Biomedical Technology (Beijing) Co., Ltd.
Igenesis (Shanghai) Co., Ltd.
Zhejiang Runlab Technology Co., Ltd.
Shanghai Brookline Scientific Co., Ltd.
Shandong Elek Biotechnology Co., Ltd.
Bestflos Precision Dispensing Pump
Ningbo Daxie Development Zone Soken Chemical Co., Ltd.

Tianjin Kede Biotechnology Co., Ltd.
Shanghai yuanye Bio-Technology Co., Ltd.
Zhengzhou Cell to Antibody&antigen Biotech., Ltd.
Biointron Biological Inc.
Shanghai Blueripple BIO Technology Co., Ltd.
Shanghai Jierui Information Technology Co., Ltd.
Hunan-Tech New Medical Systems Co., Ltd.
Shenzhen Bao Run Lin Health Technology Co., Ltd.
Shanghai Arjoin Industry Trading Co., Ltd.
Housmabn
Knowledge & Benefit Sphere Tech. Co., Ltd.
Suzhou Zeman Biological Technology Co., Ltd.
Chengdu VACURE Biological Technology Co., Ltd.
Cobioer Biosciences Co., Ltd.
Haimen Hosentest Labware Manufacturing Co., Ltd.
Shanghai Biohandler Life Sci-Tech Co., Ltd.
Jiangsu DaXin Medical Devices Co, Ltd.
Zhuhai Nikka-Shinkoh Electronics Co., Ltd.
Hunan Yunbang Bio-pharmaceutical Co., Ltd.
Wuhan Yuangu Biotechnology Co., Ltd.
WuHan Dia-An Biotech Co. Ltd.
Changzhou Dedakangcheng Medical Technology Co., Ltd.
Baoding Ditron Electronic Technology Co., Ltd.
Jiangxi Province JinHuan Medical Instrument Co., Ltd.
Altech New Materials (Suzhou) Co., Ltd.
Qingdao Libbot Biotech Co., Ltd.
Xiamen Xinshengxiang Desiccant Co., Ltd.
Wuxi Hebo Automatic Machinery Manufacturing Co., Ltd.
J&K Scientific Ltd.
Unogen Biotechnology Co., Ltd.
Shenzhen XRD LCD Technology Co., Ltd.
Xiamen Hi-Check Medical Technology Co., Ltd.
Nantong Pakion Medical Material Co. Ltd.
Shenzhen Yisheng Technology Co., Ltd.
Ningbo Bio Sciences Co Ltd.
Ningbo SNEpro Biotechnology Co., Ltd.
Letswin Biotechnology Co., Ltd.
Shenzhen GeneSeqtools Bio-science and Technology Co., Ltd.
Beijing Best IVD MD Technology Co. Ltd.
Changzhou Dreure Packaging Material Co., Ltd.
Wuxi Jingpai Machinery Co., Ltd.
GenStar Biosolutions Co., Ltd.
Chengdu BK Biotech Co., Ltd.
Suzhou Haiheng Pharmbiotech Co., Ltd.
Abgree Biotechnology Co., Ltd.

Hangzhou Hongene Biotech Co., Ltd.
Beijing Haojia Biological Engineering Technology Co. Ltd.
Shanghai Be Fluidics Co., Ltd.
Pharmtech Machinery Co., Ltd.
Pulse Electronics (Dongguan) Co., Ltd.
SHIMA Laboratories Co., Ltd.
Ademtech
Ahlstrom-Munksjo Germany GmbH
Shanghai Jiemen Bio-Tech Co., Ltd.
Shanghai Reagent Biotech Co. Ltd.
HS Medical Technology Limited
HuNan Gokvision Intelligent Technology Co., Ltd.
US-China Xinxin Biotechnologies Co., Ltd.
Angus Chemical Company
Bestchrom (Shanghai) Biosciences Co., Ltd.
Ambigen (Shanghai)Biotech Co., Ltd.
Jiangsu Qianchun Biotechnology Co., Ltd.
Anhui Beiming Biotech Inc.
Chongqing Bolanying Biotechnology Co., Ltd.
IFCAN
NeoBioscience
Assurance (Suzhou) Biotechnology LLC
Kairui Biotech
Changsha Bioadvantage Ltd., Inc.
DBS Cooling Technology (Suzhou) Co., Ltd.
HangZhou LangChuan automation equipment Co., Ltd.
Hebei Chaoran Medical Instruments Co., Ltd.
Cangzhou Weikang Food & Pharmaceutical
Suzhou Genemill Biotechnology Co., Ltd.
Seebio Biotech (Shanghai) Co., Ltd.
Wuxi Guosheng Bio-Eng. Co., Ltd.
Shanghai Rong Tai Biochemical Engineering Co., Ltd.
Hunan RunKun Pharmaceutical Co., Ltd.
HuNan RunMei Gene Technology Co., Ltd.
Suzhou Kaho Polymer Technology Co., Ltd.
Taizhou Weierkang Medical Supplies Co., Ltd.
Jiangsu Yuli Medical Instrument Co., Ltd.
General Biosystems, Inc.
City Express
Suzhou ConRem Biomedical Technology Co., Ltd.
Nanjing Robiot Co., Ltd.
Zhejiang Tianhang Biotechnology Co. Ltd.
Beijing Chun-Lei Biotechnology Co., Ltd.
Shanghai Epiprobe Biotechnology Co., Ltd.
Beijing Bioforce Bioscience Co., Ltd.

Shenzhen Chiplink Electronics Co., Ltd.
Beijing ExpertMedical Technology Co., Ltd.
Zhuhai Uni-Technology Co., Ltd.
Shanghai Linc-Bio Science Co., Ltd.
Beijing Dacheng Biotechnology Co., Ltd.
Beijing Poly Microchip Technology Co., Ltd.
Wenzhou Bacet Medical
Suhzhou Huajing Air-Condition Purification Engineering Installation Co., Ltd.
Yikon Genomics
Baoding Forlinx Embedded Technology Co., Ltd.
Beijing Dewei Medical Technological Service Co., Ltd.
Biomex
Nanjing Hanrui Baike Biotechnology Co., Ltd.
Shanghai ZJ Bio-Tech Co., Ltd.
Beijing Bohui Innovation Biotechnology Co., Ltd.
HORIBA Medical
PerkinElmer Healthcare Diagnostics (Shanghai) Co., Ltd.
Beion Medical Instrument (Shanghai) Co., Ltd.
Shanghai Kinbio Tech. Co., Ltd.
Genius Biotech Inc.
Hangzhou RoBothink Technology Co., Ltd.
Shandong Oriental Ocean Sci-Tech Co., Ltd.
Beijing Leadman Biochemistry Co., Ltd.
Hangzhou Genesis Co., Ltd.
Merit Choice Bioengineering (Beijing) Co., Ltd.
DLAB Scientific Co., Ltd.
Beijing Labgic Technology Co., Ltd.
Citotest Labware Manufacturing Co., Ltd.
Beijing BMH Instruments Co., Ltd.
Vastec Medical Ltd.
Shenzhen Living Water POCT Co., Ltd.
Jiangsu ZECEN Biotech Co., Ltd.
InTec Products Inc.
Jiangxi Leandia Biotechnology Co., Ltd.
Shanghai Chemtron Biotech., Ltd.
Cellomics (Shenzhen) Co., Ltd.
Beijing Baiyang Medical Instruments Co., Ltd.
Chongqing South NC Equipment Co., Ltd.
Shenyang BCT Biotechnologies Co., Ltd.
Micropoint Biotechnologies Co., Ltd.
Wuhan Life Origin Biotech Joint Stock Co., Ltd.
Zhejiang Quark Biotechnology Co., Ltd.
Guangzhou Kofa Biotechnology Co., Ltd.
Ustar Biotechnologies (Hangzhou) Ltd.
Zhejiang Hongchuang Aoge Trading Co., Ltd.

Suzhou Topmedlab Medical Science and Technology Co., Ltd.
Joinstar Biomedical Technology Co., Ltd.
Sino-Swed TongKang Bio-Tech Limited
Integrated Technologies Ltd. (ITL Group)
Shanghai Dizi Precision Machinery Co., Ltd.
Shanghai Biodell Biotechnology Co., Ltd.
Suzhou Precise Biotechnology Co., Ltd.
Goldstandard Diagnostics Inc.
Zhejiang PushKang Biotechnology Co., Ltd.
Lansion Biotechnology Co., Ltd.
Reliable Medical Technology CO., Ltd.
Beijing Diagreat Biotechnologies CO., Ltd.
Moons
Genskey
Dongguan Nabai Medical Technology Co., Ltd.
Beijing Microread Genetics Co., Ltd.
Shenzhen xilaiheng Medical Electronics Co., Ltd.
Beijing FenYang Technology Co., Ltd.
Shenzhen HEFA Gear Machinery Co., Ltd.
Shanghai B&C Biological Technology Co., Ltd.
Suzhou Molarray Biological Technology Co., Ltd.
Boson Biotech Co., Ltd.
Shanghai Lu Xiangyi Centrifuge Instrument Co., Ltd.
BGI PathoGenesis Pharmaceutical Technology Co., Ltd.
Render Biotech Co., Ltd.
Ningbo Scientz Biotechnology Co., Ltd.
Shanghai Chuanzhi Biotechnology Co., Ltd.
Guangdong Uniten Biotechnology Co., Ltd.
VivaChek Biotech (Hangzhou) Co., Ltd.
Beijing Huashengyuan Medical Technology Co., Ltd.
GuangZhou HEAS Biotech Co., Ltd.
Sugatsune Shanghai Co., Ltd.
Weihai LiHua packaging Co., Ltd.
Guilin Biotoo Medical Technology Co., Ltd.
Sichuan Shuke Instrument Co., Ltd.
NanJing LaoLa Electronic Co., Ltd.
Beijing ALT Bio
Hochuen Medical Technology Co., Ltd.
QingDao SanKai Science&Tech. Co., Ltd.
R-Biopharm China
Anhui Deepblue Medical Technology Co., Ltd.
Anhui Daqian Bio-Engineering Co., Ltd.
Chengdu Excellent Medical Scientific Co., Ltd.
Zhuhai Foyen Technology Co., Ltd.
Aivde Medical

Wuhan YZY Medical Science and Technology Co., Ltd.
Wuhan UNscience Biotechnology Co., Ltd.
Shanghai Shensuo Unf Medical Diagnostic Articles Co., Ltd.
Shanghai GeneoDx
Tianjin Xinda Technology Co., Ltd.
Sichuan Hapyear Bio-Engineering Co., Ltd.
Shang Hai i-Reader Biotech Co., Ltd.
Shandong Meiyilin Electronic Instrument Co., Ltd.
Eikin China Co., Ltd.
Copan Innovation Shanghai Limited
INTEGRA Biosciences
Changzhou Biowin Biopharm Co., Ltd.
Jiangsu DINGS' Intelligent Control Technology Co., Ltd.
Haydon Linear Motor (Changzhou) Co., Ltd.
Hangzhou Clongene Biotech Co., Ltd.
Vision Bio-Tech(hefei)
TB Healthcare
Shen Zhen Zi Jian Biotechnology Co., Ltd.
Nanjing Youyuan Medical
Hangzhou Miu Instruments Co., Ltd.
Hefei Kejiusheng Biopharmaceuticals Co. Ltd.
Jsuniwell
Jiangsu Kehua Medical Instrument Technology Co., Ltd.
Hunan Qankorey Technology Co., Ltd.
Beijing Tianshi Tianxing Technology Co., Ltd.
HC Scientific (Chengdu) Co. Ltd.
Shenzhen Hycreate Biotech Co., Ltd.
Humanwell Diagnosis
Qingdao Jianma Gene Technology Co., Ltd.
Zhousi Life-Tech (Changzhou) Co., Ltd.
Xi'an GoldMag Nanobiotech Co., Ltd.
SDR Diagnostics Co., Ltd.
Saint-Gobain Performance Plastics (Shanghai) Co., Ltd.
Suzhou Helmen Precision Instrument Co. Ltd.
Shenzhen Mejer Medical Technology Co., Ltd.
Shenzhen Medicom Packaging Technology Co., Ltd.
Hangzhou Alltest Biotech Co. Ltd.
Randox Laboratories
Shanghai Shengqian Industrial Co., Ltd.
Zhejiang Delta
Zhejiang Ikon Biotechnology Co., Ltd.
MyGenostics Inc.
Wenzhou Kont Biology & Technology Co., Ltd.
W.H.P.M Bioresearch and Technology Co., Ltd.
Suzhou Chenxi Biological Technology Co., Ltd.

MyGene Diagnostics Co., Ltd.
Henan FangZheng Medical Electronics Co., Ltd.
Ningbo Ziyuan Medical Device Co., Ltd.
Shanghai Anting Healthcare Industry Development Co., Ltd.
GenMagBio
Shenzhen Jiarui Hand Model Technology Co., Ltd.
DeKangRun Biotechnology (Beijing) Co., Ltd.
Qingdao Ama Co., Ltd.
Senboll Biotechnology
Shanghai Zhikun Automation Equipment Manufacturing Co., Ltd.
Zhengzhou Zhijie Biotechnology Co., Ltd.
Huiyu weiye (Beijing) Fluid Equipment Co., Ltd.
Dalian Dongfang Yonghe Biological Technology Development Co., Ltd.
Jingchuang Technology
Taizhou City Kangwei Medical Instruments Co., Ltd.
Hangzhou KBM Life sciences Co., Ltd.
Changzhou Prostepper Co., Ltd.
Beijing Botai Reagent Co., Ltd.
Ningbo Co-healthy Biotechnology Co., Ltd.
Guangzhou Ewell Bio-Technology Co., Ltd.
Cida (Guangzhou) Biotechnology Co., Ltd.
HangZhou Bio-Gechnology Co., Ltd.
IMADEK
Guangzhou Yilaifa Mechanical and Electrical Equipment Co. Ltd.
Suzhou Gallant Biotech Biotechnology Co. LTD.
Zenith Lab (Jiangsu) Co., Ltd.
Jiangsu Rongye Technology Co., Ltd.
ZheJiang Anji Seinofy Biotech Co., Ltd.
LuoYang Giant-bio Technology Co., Ltd.
Shandong Chengwu Medical Products Factory
Hunan Herexi Instrument & Equipment Co., Ltd.
Chongqing Kangju Quanhong Biological Technology Co., Ltd.
Zhenjiang Dantu Keda Medical Supplies Factory
Guangzhou Hearty Expression Medical Technology Co., Ltd.
Taizhou Zhenzhong Medical Equipment Co., Ltd.
Shenzhen Yizhan Hongtu Industrial Design Co., Ltd.
BioPredia Biotech Co., Ltd.
Wuhan kangyisheng biological technology Co., Ltd.
Ningbo Inarray Biomedical Systems Co., Ltd.
Amyr Fluid Technology (Changzhou), Ltd.
UniTech Bioscience Co., Ltd.
Shenzhen Jia'an Automation Technology Co., Ltd.
Wuhan Ammunition Life-tech Co., Ltd.
Shenzhen GEREKE Machinery Co., Ltd.
Dongguan Juray Electrical Technology Co., Ltd.

PERWIN Packing Machinery Co., Ltd.
Shenzhen Reetoo Biotechnology Co., Ltd.
Beijing 4A Biotech Co., Ltd.
Taicang Port Economic and Technological Development Zone
Shandong Angshi Group
Hebei Xinle Sci&Tech Co., Ltd.
Shanghai PD Machinery Co., Ltd.
Shanghai Stac Biotechnology Co., Ltd.
Tailored Medical
3H Group
Quidel China Ltd.
Bring Biology
Beijing SMJH Biotechnology Co., Ltd.
Yong Yue Medical Technology (Kunshan) Co., Ltd.
Shaman (Kunshan) Medtech Co., Ltd.
JetKeen Biotechnology Co., Ltd.
Shenzhen Colibri Hi-Tech Co., Ltd.
Qingdao Huajing Biotechnology Co., Ltd.
Bioway Bioengineering (Shanghai) Co., Ltd.
Huizhoucity bestam precision machine Co., Ltd.
Shenzhen Wellgrow Blo-tech Ltd.
Quaero
RocGene Technology Co., Ltd.
Jiangsu Medomics Medical Technology Co., Ltd.
Runlian Eco-Tech
BioTeke Corporation(wuxi) Co., Ltd.
Suzhou Wendi Photoelectric Technology Co., Ltd.
Medica Corporation
Jiangsu Lonray Electronic Technology Co., Ltd.
OriGene WuXi Biotechnology, Inc.
Zhengzhou Kodia Biotechnology Co., Ltd.
Blove light plastic Mould (Dong Guan) Co., Ltd.
Madenew
WWHS Biotech, Inc.
Techpool Bio-Pharma Co., Ltd.
Xiamen Haifei Biotech Co., Ltd.
Suzhou Servo Dynamics Co., Ltd.
Sichuan Shuisiyuan Environment Technology Co., Ltd.
Shenzhen LeQin Technology Co., Ltd.
Zhejiang Xuankang Medical Scientific Co., Ltd.
Leide Biosciences Co., Ltd.
Zhenzhun Bio-Tech (Shanghai) Co., Ltd.
Beijing Baicare Biotechnology Co., Ltd.
Atlas Link Technology Co., Ltd.
QH Medical Technology Ltd.

PerGrand bioTech Development Co., Ltd.
Assure Tech (Hangzhou) Co., Ltd.
Artron Bioresearch (Shandong) Inc.
Kamoer Fluid Tech (Shanghai) Co., Ltd.
Baoding Lead Fluid Technology Co., Ltd.
Anhui Leagege Biotechnology Co., Ltd.
Chromai Technologies Co., Ltd.
Chroma Technology Corp.
Shenzhen GeneBioHealth Co., Ltd.
Shenzhen Uni-medica Technology Co., Ltd.
Shandong Aosaite Medical Devices Ltd.
Beijing XMJ Scientific Co., Ltd.
Guangzhou Fenghua Bioengineering Co., Ltd.
Guangzhou Hexin Kangyuan Medical Technology Co., Ltd.
Chongqing Novegent Biotech Co., Ltd.
Beijing Sihuan Qihang Technology Co., Ltd.
Yantai Sandem Medical Laboratories Co., Ltd.
Jiangsu Kangjianhua Medical Apparatus Co., Ltd.
Nanjing Medical Deviceland Co., LTD.
Shenzhen Foreach Technology Co., Ltd.
IWAKI China
Haemonetics
Huizhou Sunshine Biotechnology Co., Ltd.
Chongqing Kejie Medical Technology Co., Ltd.
AMTK, Inc.
NAYO Biotechnology (Shanghai) Co., Ltd.
Pilot Gene Technologies
Nanjing Leading Biotechnology Co., Ltd.
Hangzhou Goodhere Biotechnology Co., Ltd.
Shenzhen EbyTon Technology Ltd.
Foring Technology Development (Beijing) Co., Ltd.
HVHV Design
Genfine Biotech (Beijing) Co., Ltd.
Guangzhou Micro-shot Technology Co., Ltd.
Meling Biology & Medical
Jian Wei Biological
Wishtech Medical Technology Co., Ltd.
Nanjing Santa Scott Biotechnology Co., Ltd.
BioWavelet Co., Ltd.
Guangzhou Forevergen Biosciences Co., Ltd.
Guangdong Yimaikang Biotechnology Co. Ltd.
Shanghai Genstech Technology Co., Ltd.
HiComp Microtech (Suzhou) Co., Ltd.
Xi'an Abborbio Co., Ltd.
Changchun Chenyu Biomedical Technology Co., Ltd.

Jinan Bohang Biotechnology Co. Ltd.
Xiamen Winbio Biotechnology Co., Ltd.
Guangzhou Targene Biotech co. Ltd.
Beijing XinQiaoYiKang Biotechnology Co., Ltd.
Sunresin New Materials Co. Ltd.
Virion Serion Biotechnology (Shenzhen) Co., Ltd.
Wuhan Aoke Botai Biotechnology Co., Ltd.
Guangdong Wesail Biotech Co., Ltd.
Saylloni (Shanghai) Biotechnology Co., Ltd.
REEGEN Bioengineering (Beijing) Co., Ltd.
ShenZhen City RUNWU Medical
Jiangsu Maiyuan Biological Technology Co., Ltd.
Longer Precision Pump Co., Ltd.
Zhejiang CSB Plastic Bearing Technology Co., Ltd.
Shenzhen Anqun Biotech Co., Ltd.
Shenzhen iCubio Biomedical Technology Co., Ltd.
Hunan Demeter instrument Co., Ltd.
Nanjing Synthgene Medical Technology Co., Ltd.
Zhuhai Biori Biotechnology Co., Ltd.
GoldanBio(Shenzhen) Co., Ltd.
Cangzhou Yongkang Medical Devices Co., Ltd.
Haining Werfen automation equipment Co., Ltd.
Hangzhou Ruijian Technology Co., Ltd.
Hangzhou Dahe Thermo-Magnetics Co., Ltd.
Xiamen Talent Biomedical Technology Co., Ltd.
ZSUP Medical Technology Co., Ltd.
ZEMIC
Yadepack Desiccant Co., Ltd.
Taizhou Taiji Packaging Technologies Co., Ltd.
Hangzhou Yizhijie Supply Chain Management Co., Ltd.
Beijing Weihua Electronics Co., Ltd.
Beijing DiagMed Instrument Co., Ltd.
Wenzhou Zhangshi Packaging Equipment Technology Co., Ltd.
Beijing Zhongnuokangjian Technology Co., Ltd.
Shenzhen Kerch Technology Co., Ltd.
Guangzhou Ascend Precision Machinery Co., Ltd.
Beijing Solarbio Science & Technology Co., Ltd.
Suzhou Thunder Weiye Information Technology Co., Ltd.
Core Biotechnology Co., Ltd.
Baizhen Biotechnologies Inc.
AtaGenix Laboratories
Volterpump (GZ) Fluid Equipment Co., Ltd.
Zhejiang Aicor Medical Technology Co. Ltd.
Zhejiang Bioland Biotechnology Co., Ltd.
Changzhou Apollomics Medical Technologies, Inc.

Beijing Vince Technology Co., Ltd.
ShanDong HengChen Biotech Co., Ltd.
BJHK (Beijing) Biotech Co., Ltd.
Tianjin Henghai Electromechanical Equipment Trade Co., Ltd.
Shenzhen Rayming Industrial Design Co., Ltd.
Dongguan Ji Kerr Automation Technology Co., Ltd.
Suzhou GenePharma Co., Ltd.
Wason Biotech Inc.
Beijing Bodian Optical Tech. Co., Ltd.
Porex Corporation
Expeclin Ltd.
Guangzhou Zhipu Pharmaceutical Technology Co., Ltd.
Zhejiang Juli Medical Technology Co., Ltd.
Global Health Qinhuangdao Biological Technology Co., Ltd.
Wuhan Healthgen Biotechnology Corp.
Shanghai Eco Polymer Sci. & Tech. Co., Ltd.
Shanghai Jieyi Biotechnology Co., Ltd.
Sure Biotech(Hangzhou) Co., Ltd.
Zhengzhou Immuno Bio-Tech Co., Ltd.
Nittobo America Inc.
Multi Sciences (Lianke) Biotech, Co., Ltd.
GenSure Biotech Inc.,
Qing Dao Guang Da Sen Plastic Co., Ltd.
Uetbiotec Co., Ltd.
Zoonbio Biotechnology Co., Ltd.
Takasago Fluidic Systems
Shenzhen Cholun Medical Engineering CO., Ltd.
Shanghai Generay Biotech Co., Ltd.
Guan County Chrancy Bio-Technology Co., Ltd.
Shanghai Si-Gene Bio-tech Co., Ltd.
Beijing MDTK Biology Technology
Hangzhou Guidling Technology Co., Ltd.
Shenzhen Haisi'an Biotechnology Co., Ltd.
Inner Mongolia Jin Yuan Kang Biotechnology Co., Ltd.
Shenzhen zhitongcheng Industrial Development Co., Ltd.
Hebei Xiangyuan Medical Devices. Co., Ltd.
Taizhou Qiujing Medical Devices Co., Ltd.
Wenzhou Gaode Medical Instruments Co., Ltd.
Sepure Instruments
Water Purifier
Ease-Medtrend Biotech, Ltd.
Hebei Kangweishi Medical Technology Co., Ltd.
Shenzhen Braveds Biotech Co., Ltd.
Beijing Newshidaibeili Medical Equipment Co. Ltd.
Yugong Biolabs Co., Ltd.

Sinnowa Medical Science & Technology Co., Ltd.
Fubio (Suzhou) Biotechnology Co., Ltd.
Beijing Kangda century Biotechnology Co. Ltd.
Shanghai Eizhi Technology Co., Ltd.
Concare
Wuhu Huaren Science and Technology Co., Ltd.
Yangzhou Chuangxin Medical Device Factory
Shenzhen Wontec Co., Ltd.
Zhuhai Kanglilai Medical
Senlan Medical Science & Trading Co., Ltd.
Senhui Microsphere Technology (Suzhou) Co., Ltd.
Jiangsu Tianli Medical Devices Co., Ltd.
Changzhou Hetai Electric Motors & Appliance Co., Ltd.
Shanghai SOCON Electronic Technology Co. Ltd.
Cang Zhou Fukang Medical Care Co., Ltd.
Hefei Huana Biomedical Technology Co., Ltd.
Baoding Chuangrui Precision Pump Co., Ltd.
ChangZhou Smart-Lifesciences Biotechnology Co., Ltd.
Jiangmen Caring Trading
Beijing Med-Logistics Medical Device Co., Ltd.
Microkn Medical Technology Service (Shanghai) Co., Ltd.
Amoy Diagnostics Co., Ltd.
Wu Xi Bresight Medical Technology Co., Ltd.
Mettler Toledo
Nanjing Superyears Gene Technology Co., Ltd.
Dong Guan Hannotech Co., Ltd.
Easy Biotech Co., Ltd.
Zhengzhou Puwan Medical Technology Co., Ltd.
Xi'an Way-on Industrial Limited Company
Wuhan Huiyan Biotechnology Co., Ltd.
Huirui (Shandong) Environmental Technology Co., Ltd.
TransGen Biotech Co., Ltd.
ShenZhen Youjie Machinery Manufacturing Co., Ltd.
Taizhou Liangpu Medical Technology Co., Ltd.Ltd.
Taizhou City Rongfei Apparatus Factory
Bioda Diagnostics (Wuhan) Co., Ltd.
Jiangsu Winlong Pharmaceutical Machinery Co., Ltd.
Chengdu Hilin Technology Co., Ltd.
Guangzhou Deaou Bio-technology Co., Ltd.
Beijing Metz MS Biotech Co., Ltd.
CoWin Biosciences, Inc.
Beijing Lepu Medical Technology Co., Ltd.
Medcaptain Medical Technology Co., Ltd.
E-LAB Biological Science & Technology Co., Ltd.
Jiangsu Süd-Chemie Performance Packaging Material Co., Ltd.

Beijing Gaugene Bio-technology Co., Ltd.
Guangdong Hybribio Biotech Co., Ltd.
Health Gene Technologies
Xiamen Zeesan Biotech Co., Ltd.
IVD Alliance International Medical Equipments Co. Ltd.
Zhongshan BGH Biochem. Co., Ltd.
Shenzhen Lifotronic Technology Co., Ltd.
Zhejiang Kuaye Biotechnology Co., Ltd.
Anbio (Xiamen) Biotechnology Co., Ltd.
Bioneovan Co., Ltd.
Nantong Diagnos Biotechnology Co., Ltd.
Hunan Xiangyi Laboratory Instrument Development Co., Ltd.
JiangSu LIBO Medicine Biotechnology Co., Ltd.
Alibio Technology Taizhou Co., Ltd.
Hangzhou Cellgene Biotech Co., Ltd.
Zhongshan Chuangyi
Shenzhen Kangmei Biotechnology Co., Ltd.
LongSeeMed
Eppendorf
Suzhou Yiman Biological Technology co., Ltd.
Ningbo Ruiyuan Biotechnology Co., Ltd.
Zhejiang Erkn Biological Technology Co., Ltd.
Sanming Bofeng Biotechnology Co., LTD.
HUMAN Diagnostics Products (Beijing) Co., Ltd.
Changsha Xieda Biotechnology Co., Ltd.
Wuhan Zhongzhi Biotechnologies Inc.
Shanghai BioGerm Medical Technology Co., Ltd.
Zhejiang Orient Gene Biotech Co., Ltd.
Ningbo Geneinn Biotechnology Co., Ltd.
Funotec(Dalian) Co., Ltd.
Shenzhen Diasia Technology Co., Ltd.
Shenzhen Yuanqin Biotechnology Co., Ltd.
Lumigenex (Suzhou) Co., Ltd.
Shenzhen Huisong Technology Development Co., Ltd.
Henan Wayray Biotech Co., Ltd.
Xiamen BaiErJie Biological Technology Co., Ltd.
Qingdao Raisecare Biotechnology Co., Ltd.
Taizhou SunTrine Biotechnology Co., Ltd.
Bio-Medical
Anhui Beichi Biotech Co., Ltd.
Tecom Science
Merlin Biomedical (Xiamen) Co., Ltd.
Beijing OriginGene-Tech Biotechnology Co., Ltd.
Sichuan, C-luminary Biotech Co., Ltd.

Hangzhou Biotest Biotech Co., Ltd.
Beijing CapitalBio Technology Co., Ltd.
Guangzhou Kangrun Biotech Co., Ltd.
Beijing O&D Biotech Co., Ltd. China
Biozon
Beijing Succeeder Technology Inc.
Sophonix Co., Ltd.
Zhuhai Keyu Biological
Shanghai Long Island Biotec. Co., Ltd.
Shenzhen AmTech Bioengineering Ltd., Inc.
Shenzhen NORCO Intelligent Technology Co., Ltd.
Chengdu Rich Science Industry Co., Ltd.
Zhengzhou Fortune Bioscience Co., Ltd.
Shanghai Lepzi Medical Devices Co., Ltd.
Jinan Diman Biotechnology Co., Ltd.
Hefei TianYi Biotech Institute Co., Ltd.
Jilin Province Love Noble Biological Engineering Co., Ltd.
Hunan Uzer Technology Co., Ltd.
Guangzhou Jinde Biotech Co., Ltd.
Tianjin Kang Volcker Biotechnology Co., Ltd.
AnHui HuiBang Biological Engineering Co., Ltd.
Zenmindes Biotech Co., Ltd.
Changzhou Haite Ciren Transmission Technology Co., Ltd.
Bio-Mapper Technology Co., Ltd.
Suzhou IntelUnion Automation Co., Ltd.
Shanghai Turtle Technology Co., Ltd.
Wuxi Techstar Technology Co., Ltd.
ATS Engineering Limited
Syno Bio
DaAn Gene Co., Ltd.
Wuxi Shenrui Bio-Pharmaceuticals Co., Ltd.
Zhuhai Meihua Medical Technology Limited
Apexbio Biotechnology (Suzhou) Co., Ltd.
Zhe Jiang Dongou Diagnostics Co., Ltd.
Lanzhou Yahua Biotechnology Co., Ltd.
Shandong Jining Tiancheng Electronic Technology Co., Ltd.
Shenzhen Highcreation Technology Co., Ltd.
Huachenyang (Shenzhen) Technology Co., Ltd.
Zhengzhou Bangqi Bio Technology Co. Ltd.
Shanghai Fullgene Biotechnology Co., Ltd.
Shenzhen Hongmed-infagen
Zhuhai Lituo Biotechnology Co., Ltd.
Wuhan HealthCare Biotechnology Co., Ltd.
Hangzhou Bailing (Biolynx) Biotechnology Co., Ltd.

KNF China
Hunan Michael Laboratory Instrument Co., Ltd.
Henan Tuoren Medical Technology Co., Ltd.
Hubei NewZongke Viral Disease Control Bio-Tech Ltd.
Hangzhou Dalton BioSciences, Ltd.
Jinhua Xinke Medical Devices Co., Ltd.
Hangzhou Zheda Dixun Biological Gene Engineering Co., Ltd.
Suzhou Yacoo Science Co., Ltd.
Caretium Medical Instruments Co., Ltd.
Jiangsu Mojin Bioengineering & Technology Co., Ltd.
Targeting One
Zhongshan MyVision Medical Technology Co., Ltd.
Jiangsu Nuoge Biotechnology Co., Ltd.
Hangzhou Bigfish Bio-tech Co., Ltd.
Beijing Promed Med-tech Co. Ltd.
Suzhou Rainsure Scientific Co., Ltd.
Jiangsu KeyGEN BioTECH Co., Ltd.
Baiming Biotechnology Co., Ltd.
Sichuan Zhuoyue Water Treatment Equipment Co., Ltd.
Oxford Immunotec (Shanghai) Medical Device Co., Ltd.
GeSiM
Jiangsu Well Biotech Co., Ltd.
Chongqing Jingyin Bio-Science Co., Ltd.
Nanjing Qlife Medical Technology Co., Ltd.
Nantong Biaoyuan Biotechnology Co., Ltd.
Hubei Taikang Medical Equipment Co., Ltd.
GenDx Biotech Co., Ltd.
Zhejiang Zhongshen Biology Technology Co., Ltd.
Wuxi Jiangyuan Industrial
Chongqing IVD Biotechnology Co., Ltd.
Chongqing Swson Automation Technology Co., Ltd.
Guilin Bao Tong Technology Co., Ltd.
Foshan Jiachen MedicalTech Co., Ltd.
Beijing Co-Brilliant Instrument Co., Ltd.
Yantai Protgen Biotechnology Development Co., Ltd.
Icomes Lab Co., Ltd.
Anhui Triumph Medical Science and Technology Co., Ltd.
BoLai Bio-technology Corp., Ltd., Jinan
Chongqing UMot technology Co., Ltd.
Zhongshan Taolue Biological Technology Co., Ltd.
Chongqing Pulse Robot Control System Co., Ltd.
Tsingmu Biotechnology Co., Ltd.
Ameritech Diagnostic Reagent (Jiaxing) Co., Ltd.
Jiangsu Macro&Micro-Test Med-Tech Co., Ltd.

Shandong Baiou Medical Technology Co., Ltd.
Jiangsu Kangjie Medical Devices Co., Ltd.
Xincheng Precision Mould
Jiangsu Assay Specialist
LINK(Shanghai) Fluid Technology Co., Ltd.
Shenzhen Biorain Technology Co., Ltd.
SAIS Co., Ltd.
Wuhan Hygeianey Biological Technology Co., Ltd.
Xiamen My Electronic Technology Co., Ltd.
Suzhou Biogene Technology Co., Limited
Tianjin Reagent Biotech Co., Ltd.
JoysBio (Tianjin) Biotechnology Co., Ltd.
Xi'an Lianer Technology Co., Ltd.
Jiangsu Chaohua Glasswork Co. Ltd.
Hemosmart Medical Technology Co., Ltd.
Sichuan ULUPURE Ultrapure Technology Co., Ltd.
Changchun Brother Biotech Co., Ltd.
Guangdong Huayin Medicine Science Co., Ltd.
Shenzhen Poweray Biotechnology Co., Lt..
Enriching Biotechnology
Shenzhen Precise Technology Co., Ltd.
Jiangsu Xinkang Medical Instrument Co., Ltd.
Suzhou Kgene Diagnostic Co., Ltd.
Shenzhen Huizhong Medical Equipment Co., Ltd.
Tianjin Huayu Bioresearch Co., Ltd.
Lanbiao (Tianjin) Electronic and Technology Co., Ltd.
Byron Diagnostics (Shanghai) Co. Ltd.,
Shandong Tianai Medical Devices Co., Ltd.
Jiangsu Xinjin Medical Devices Co., Ltd.
Shenzhen USK Bioscience Co., Ltd.
Gilson
Shenzhen Maxchemtech Co., Ltd.
DIAGAST
Haimen Shengbang Laboratory Equipment Co., Ltd.
Hunan Xiangxin Instrument and Meter Co., Ltd.
Shanghai Pramers Chemi-tech Co., Ltd.
Shanghai TaoYu International Co., Ltd.
Zhanjiang Bokang Marine Biological Co., Ltd.
Xiamen Wumen Automation Technology Co. Ltd.,
Shenzhen Oriental Yi Chen Industrial Co., Ltd.
Beijing Highgene-tech Automation Ltd.
Qingdao Hope Bio-Technology Co., Ltd.
Wuhan Biotgene Engineering
Foshan Xiongqi Intelligent Technology Co., Ltd.

Beijing H&J NoVoMed Ltd.
Yingsheng Biology
Sansure Biotech Inc.
Ailex Technology Group Co., Ltd.
Sichuan Xincheng Biological Co., Ltd.
Edan Instruments, Inc.
Shanghai Sun Biotech Co., Ltd.
Fosun Diagnostics
Shanghai Fermat Biotech Co., Ltd.
Shandong AccurDx Biotech Co., Ltd.
Beijing ZONCI Technology Development Co., Ltd.
Suzhou Jianyi Biotechnology Co., Ltd.
Avalue Technology (Shanghai) Inc.
MedicalSystem Biotechnology
Shandong Kanghua Biotechnology Co., Ltd.
Beijing Savant Biotechnology Co., Ltd.
Hybiome
ReachGen
Chongqing Tianhai Medical
Zhongxiu Science and Technology Co., Ltd.
Wuhan Thalys Biotechnology Co., Ltd.
Aikang MedTech Co., Ltd.
Jiangsu Sunlant Bioengineering Co., Ltd.
ULS
Scenker Biological Technology Co., Ltd.
Zhuhai Livzon Diagnostics Inc.
Jinan Babio Biotechnology Co., Ltd.
Shanghai Juchuang
Sino Biological Inc.
Beijian·Xinchuangyuan
Tianjin MNCHIP Technologies Co., Ltd.
Shanghai Outdo Biotech Co., Ltd.
Shanghai Trans-Age Medical Technology Co., Ltd.
Jiangsu Bioperfectus technologies Co.
Chengdu IXING Biotechnology Co., Ltd.
Shenzhen YiCube Biotechnology Co., Ltd.
Jiangsu konsung Bio-Medical Science and Technology Co., Ltd.
Weihai Wego Biotech
Guangzhou Biotron Technology Co., Ltd.
Dynamiker Biotechnology (Tianjin) Co., Ltd.
Luoyang constant biological technology Co., Ltd.
Ningbo Purebio Biotechnology Co., Ltd.
Shanghai Rongsheng Biotech Co., Ltd.
ACROBiosystems

Shanghai Advanced Clinical Laboratory Science Co., Ltd. (ACLS)
Shanghai Rendu Biotechnology Co., Ltd.
Nanjing Realmind Biotech Co., Ltd.
Denogen(Beijing)Bio-Sic&Tech Co., Ltd.
Geneway Biotech Co., Ltd.
Tianjin Era Biology Technology Co., Ltd.
NewScen Coast Bio-Pharmaceutical Co.
Hunan Yuan Jing Biotechnology
Diascie Technology
Liuyang SANLI Medical Technology Development Co., Ltd.
Amerom Scientific Co., Ltd.
Cladogram
Biocomma Limited
Luoyang Ascend Biotechnology Co., Ltd.
Shenzhen Tiachen Medical Technology CO., Ltd.
3V Bioengineering Group Co., Ltd.
Asiatiger
Beijing Homa Biological Engineering Co., Ltd.
Ningbo Aucheer Biotechnology Co. Ltd.
Beijing North Institute of Biotechnology Co., Ltd.
Chongqing Micro Identification Technology Co., Ltd.
B&E Bio-technology Co., Ltd.
Shanghai Zhicheng Biological Technology Co., Ltd.
Zhengzhou LabScience Co., Ltd.
Yunnan HaoXu Biological
MD Pacific (Tianjin)Biotechnology, Ltd.
SysCan MedTech (SuZhou) Co., Ltd.
Shenzhen Prokan Electronics Inc
Deheng Medical Technology Co., Ltd.
Hitachi Chemical Diagnostics Systems (Shanghai) Co., Ltd.
Shandong Stars Biological Industry Co., Ltd.
Wuhan New Cangdo Biotechnology Co., Ltd.
Shanghai Ryan Biological Engineering Co., Ltd.
Triplex International Biosciences (China) Co., Ltd.
NepQD Science & Technology Co., Ltd.
Jinan Lanjie Bio-Technology Co., Ltd.
Beijing Macro-Union Pharmaceutical Co., Ltd.
Beijing Biochem Singene S&T Development Co., Ltd.
Hangzhou Watson Biotech, Inc.
Guangzhou Tebsun Bio-tech Development Co., Ltd.
GuangDong Hecin Scientific, Inc.
Nanjing VPS Semiconductor Technology Co., Ltd.
Boyang Experimental Equipment Factory
Onco Biomedical Technology (Suzhou). Co., Ltd.

Xiamen Bioendo Technology Co., Ltd.
Shenzhen Mdern Biotechnology Co., Ltd.
RayKol Group Corp., Ltd.
FS (Beijing) Technology Co., Ltd.
PoraBio
Shanghai Taip-Bio Technology Co., Ltd.
Guangzhou Global Biotech Co., Ltd.
Genetel Pharmaceuticals
Shenzhen GLD Biotechnology Ltd.
Jiaxing Chicheng Automation Equipment Co., Ltd.
Synbio Technologies
Glilin Ucon Technology Co. Ltd.
Shanghai Leqi Fluid Technology Co., Ltd.
Huakang Biomedical
Taizhou Bomaidi Biological Technology Co., Ltd.
Nanjing Dashu Bio-Medical Technology Co., Ltd.
Tianjin Rongtai Mould Manufacturing Co., Ltd.
Nanjing Rebece Biotechnology Co., Ltd.
Everbest Biotechnology Co., Ltd.
ZhuHai Langfeng Biotech Co., Ltd.
Shenzhen Kerunda Co., Ltd.
Yixing Jingke Optical Instruments Co., Ltd.
Scienion AG
Suzhou Danbao Medical Technology Co., Ltd.
Suzhou Fengtai Medical Products Trade Co., Ltd.
Liangzhun(Shanghai) Medical Technology Co., Ltd.
Bono Plastics (Beijing) Co., Ltd.
Jiangsu Audicom Medical Technology Co., Ltd.
Beijing Innochem Science & Technology Co., Ltd.
Guangdong Jinyu
LEONI Fiber Optics
CangZhou HuaAo Plastic Products Co., Ltd.
Shenzhen Huian Bioscitech Co., Ltd.
Shenzhen Medico Technology Co., Ltd.
Haimen Kylin-Bell Lab Instruments Co., Ltd.
Wuxi Tzong-Ejoin Bio-technology Ltd.
Suzhou CretBiotech Ltd.
Inscinstech., Ltd.
Gardner Denver Thomas Pneumatic Systems (Wuxi) Co., Ltd.
N-Lab Technology Center Pte. Ltd.
Shanghai Genesci Medical Technology Co., Ltd.
Shenzhen UImotion Technology Co., Ltd.
Shanghai Guixing Packaging Equipment Co., Ltd.
Sichuan Chunjie Technology Co., Ltd.

Shanghai Gous Optics Co., Ltd.
Alluxa Inc.
Wheisman Medical Technology Co., Ltd.
Beijing Preintell Intellectual Property Agent Co., Ltd.
Qingdao Yangshen Biopharmaceutical Co., Ltd.
Beijing Huirui Industrial Technology Development Co. Ltd.
Chongqing Defang Information Technology Co. Ltd.
TIANJIN PAP-Days InstrumentTech Co., Ltd.
Shanghai Jiaqi Biochemical Technology Center
Hebei Shenghuaer Biomedical Technology Co., Ltd.
Ningbo Kaida Medical Technology Co., Ltd.
Shenzhen Dakewe Bio-engineering Co., Ltd.
Miraclean Technology Co., Ltd.
Huapu (Tianjin) Testing technology Co., Ltd.
Shenzhen, Healthbless Biomedical Technology Co., Ltd.
Yixing City Tianhe Optical Instruments Co., Ltd.
Shanghai Yihua Medical Science & Technology Corporation Limited
Labnovation Technologies, Inc.
Yangzhou Boyang Medical Supplies Co. Ltd.
Science Laboratories Limited
Anhui USTC Zonkia Scientific Instruments Co., Ltd.
Burkert Fluid Control Systems (Shanghai) Co., Ltd.
SwissOptic (Wuhan)
Boopu Biotechnology Co. Ltd.
Beijing KeyGen Gene Technology Co., Ltd.
Beijing LangFeiLin Technology Research and Development Co. Ltd.
Guangdong Hao Jiang Laboratories Co., Ltd.
Hennan TaiyuGaofen Medical Devices Co., Ltd.
Puton Fluid Technology (Shenzhen) Co., Ltd.
Goodwill Precision Machinery (Dongguan) Co., Ltd. (GPM)
Hangzhou Xinrui Technology Co., Ltd.
Shanghai Nagase Trading Co., Ltd.
Beijing Strong Biotechnologies, Inc.
Beckman Coulter Commercial Enterprise (China) Co., Ltd.
Guangzhou Wondfo Biotech Co., Ltd.
Tellgen Corporation
Autobio Diagnostics Co., Ltd.
Shenzhen Mindray
Zybio Inc.
Bioscience
Guangzhou Weimi Bio-Tech Co., Ltd.
SNIBE
About YHLO Shenzhen YHLO Biotech Co., Ltd.
Chongqing Keysmile Biological Technology Co., Ltd.

Wuhan Easy Diagnosis Biomedicine Co., Ltd.
Maccura Biotechnology Co., Ltd.
Shanghai Kehua Bio-Engineering Co., Ltd.
Hitachi High-Tech Diagnostics (Shanghai) Ltd.
Guilin Urit Electronic Group Co., Ltd.
Beijing WANTAI Biological Pharmacy Enterprise Co., Ltd.
Shen Zhen Dymind Biotechnology Co., Ltd.
Chemclin Diagnostic Technology Co., Ltd.
Dirui Industrial Co., Ltd.
Intelligene Biosystems (Qingdao) Co., Ltd.
Sinocare Inc.
Tecan (Shanghai) Trading Co., Ltd.
Stago Diagnosis Technology (Tianjin) Co., Ltd.
Ortho Clinical Diagnostics Trading (China) Co. Ltd.
Nanjing Vazyme Medical Co., Ltd.
Abbott (Shanghai) Diagnostics Sales Co., Ltd.
Guangzhou Labsim Biotech Co., Ltd.
Hangzhou Bioer Technology Co., Ltd.
Chongqing iSIA BIO-Technology Co., Ltd.
Thermo Fisher Scientific
ET Health
AVE Science & Technology Industry Co., Ltd.
Dian Diagnostics Group Co., Ltd.
Boditech(Guangxi) Biotechnology Co., Ltd.
Baso Diagnostic Ltd.
Copyright Shandong Bioway
Henan Jianshilaijie Medical Technology Co., Ltd.
Chengdu Seamaty Technology Co., Ltd.
Zircon Biotech Co., Ltd.
Beijing Pro-med Technology Co., Ltd.
Shanghai Taywell Biotechnology Co., Ltd.
Shenzhen Channel Biotechnology Co., Ltd.
Geno China
Wuhan Milloway Lowtemper Aturelogistics Co. Ltd.
Shanghai Hongene Biotech Corporation
Cognex Vision Inspection System (Shanghai) Ltd.
Jiangsu HanHeng Medical Technology Co., Ltd.
Shenzhen TISENC Medical Devices Co., Ltd.
Shenzhen Microprofit Biotech Co., Ltd.
Shenzhen Watmind Medical Co., Ltd.
ZOPOMED Ltd. Co.
Celula China Med-Technology Co., Ltd.
Jusbio Sciences (Shanghai) Co., Ltd.
Jiangxi Yeli Medical Apparatus Co., Ltd.
Zhejiang A-Gen Biotechnology Co., Ltd.

Hangzhou Laihe Biotech Co.
GuiLin HuaTong Medical Instrument Co., Ltd.
Guangzhou Yichuan Biological Technology Co., Ltd.
Guangzhou Phicon Biotech Co., Ltd.
Shenzhen Cornley Bio-Medical Co., Ltd.
Wuxi BioHermes Bio & Medical Technology Co., Ltd.
Beijing DDM Technology Co., Ltd.

(Note: The above data is from the list of exhibitors of the 18th China International Laboratory Medicine and Blood Transfusion Instrument Reagent Expo in 2021. Listed in no particular order.)

www.ingramcontent.com/pod-product-compliance
Lightning Source LLC
Chambersburg PA
CBHW041301210926
51847CB00010B/97
* 9 7 8 7 5 4 7 8 6 5 8 4 2 *